Operative Endoscopy and Endoscopic Surgery in Infants and Children

Artwork by Azad Najmaldin, assisted by Paul Brown
except in Chapters 1, 2, 3, 5, 8, 24, 30, 32C, 35, 45, 48, 50, 53 and 62A

Operative Endoscopy and Endoscopic Surgery in Infants and Children

Chief Editor

Azad Najmaldin MS FRCS FRCSEd
Consultant Paediatric Surgeon
St James's University Hospital
Leeds
UK

Associate Editors

Steven Rothenberg MD
Chief of Pediatric Surgery
Mother and Child Hospital at PISL
Denver, CO
USA

David C.G. Crabbe MD FRCS
Consultant Paediatric Surgeon
The General Infirmary at Leeds
Leeds
UK

Spencer Beasley MS FRACS
Clinical Professor of Paediatrics and Surgery
Christchurch Hospital
Christchurch
New Zealand

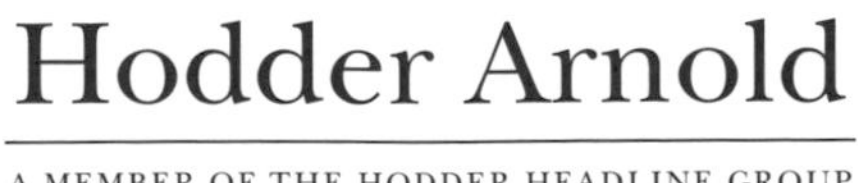

First published in Great Britain in 2005 by
Hodder Education, a member of the Hodder Headline Group,
338 Euston Road, London NW1 3BH

http://www.hoddereducation.com

Distributed in the United States of America by
Oxford University Press Inc.,
198 Madison Avenue, New York, NY10016
Oxford is a registered trademark of Oxford University Press

Whilst the advice and information in this book are believed to be true and accurate at the date of going to press, neither the author[s] nor the publisher can accept any legal responsibility or liability for any errors or omissions that may be made. In particular, (but without limiting the generality of the preceding disclaimer) every effort has been made to check drug dosages; however, it is still possible that errors have been missed. Furthermore, dosage schedules are constantly being revised and new side-effects recognized. For these reasons the reader is strongly urged to consult the drug companies' printed instructions before administering any of the drugs recommended in this book.

British Library Cataloguing in Publication Data
A catalogue record for this book is available from the British Library

Library of Congress Cataloging-in-Publication Data
A catalog record for this book is available from the Library of Congress

ISBN 0 340 80725 3
ISBN-13 978 0 340 80725 5

1 2 3 4 5 6 7 8 9 10

Commissioning Editor: Sarah Burrows
Project Editor: Naomi Wilkinson
Production Controller: Joanna Walker
Cover Design: Georgina Hewitt
Index: Indexing Specialists (UK) Ltd

Typeset in 10/12 Minion by Charon Tec Pvt. Ltd, India
www.charontec.com
Printed and bound in the UK by CPI Bath

To our families, and children everywhere

Contents

Contributors

Satish K. Aggarwal MS MCh
Department of Paediatric Surgery
Leeds Teaching Hospital NHS Trust
Leeds
UK

Niyi Ade-Ajayi FRCS (Paed. Surg)
Department of Paediatric Surgery and Radiology
Great Ormond Street Hospital for children NHS Trust
London
UK

Spencer Beasley MS FRACS
Professor of Paediatrics and Clinical Surgery
Christchurch Hospital
Christchurch
New Zealand

François Becmeur MD
Paediatric Surgeon
Department of Paediatric Surgery
Hôpital Hautepierre
Cedex
France

Peter A. Borzi MBBS FRACS FRCS
Associate Professor of Paediatric Surgery and Urology
University of Queensland
Royal and Mater Children's Hospitals
Brisbane
Australia

Paolo Campisi MSc MD FRCSC
Assistant Professor Otolaryngology – Head and Neck Surgery
The Hospital for Sick Children
Toronto
Canada

John-Paul Capolicchio MD FRCS(c)
Assistant Professor of Surgery (Urology)
Montreal Children's Hospital
McGill University Health Centre
Montreal
Canada

Beverly E. Chaignaud MD
Department of Surgery
Children's Mercy Hospital
Kansas City, MO
USA

John C. Chandler MD
Attending Pediatric Surgeon
The Children's Hospital of the Greenville
Greenville, SC
USA

Zahavi Cohen MD
Department of Pediatric Surgery
Soroko Medical Center
Ben-Gurion University of the Negev
Beer-Sheba
Israel

David C.G. Crabbe MD FRCS
Consultant Paediatric Surgeon
The General Infirmary at Leeds
Leeds
UK

Peter M. Cuckow FRCS(Paed Surg)
Consultant Paediatric Urologist
Great Ormond Street Hospital for Children NHS Trust
London
UK

Antoine de Backer MD
Assistant Professor of Pediatric Surgery
Department of Paediatric Surgery
Academic Hospital Vrije Universiteit Brussel
Brussels
Belgium

Ciro Esposito MD PhD
Associate Professor of Pediatric Surgery
Department of Pediatric Surgery
'Magna Graecia' University
Catanzaro
Italy

Walid A. Farhat MD
Assistant Professor Division of Urology
University of Toronto
Hospital for Sick Children
Toronto
Canada

Thierry A. Folliguet MD
Department of Cardiac Pathology
L'Institut Mutualiste Montsouris
Paris
France

Vito Forte MD FRCS
Associate Professor of Otolaryngology
Department of Otolaryngology
Hospital for Sick Children
Toronto
Canada

Israel Franco MD FACS FAAP
Associate Professor of Urology and Pediatrics
New York Medical College
Valhalla, NY
USA

Uwe Friedrich MD
Professor of Paediatric Surgery
Helios Hospital Erfurt
Germany

Takao Fujimoto MD PhD
Director of Pediatric Surgery
The Imperial Gift Foundation
The Aiiku Maternal and Children's Medical Center
Tokyo
Japan

Michael W.L. Gauderer MD
Chief of Pediatric Surgery
The Children's Hospital of the Greenville Hospital System
Greenville, SC
USA

Munther J. Haddad FRCS FRCPCH
Consultant Paediatric Surgeon
Department of Paediatric Surgery
Chelsea and Westminster Hospital
London
UK

Carroll M. Harmon MD PhD
Associate Professor of Surgery
The Children's Hospital of Alabama
The University of Alabama
Birmingham, AL
USA

Klaus Heller MD
Chief of Paediatric Surgery
Johann Wolfgang Goethe University Hospital
Frankfurt
Germany

George W. Holcomb III MD MBA
Surgeon in Chief
Children's Mercy Hospital
Kansas City, MO
USA

John M. Hutson MD FRACS
Director, Department of General Surgery
Royal Children's Hospital
Victoria
Australia

Thomas H. Inge MD PhD
Assistant Professor of Surgery and Pediatrics
Cincinnati Children's Hospital and Medical Center
Cincinnati, OH
USA

Henry C. Irving FRCR
Consultant Radiologist
St James's University Hospital
Leeds
UK

Natalie K. Jesch MD
Department of Paediatric Surgery
Hannover Medical School
Hannover
Germany

Tamir H. Keshen
Assistant Professor, Surgery
Division of Pediatric Surgery
Assistant Professor, Pediatrics
Washington University in St Louis
St Louis, MO
USA

Antoine Khoury MD FRCS(c)
Head, Division of Urology
Professor, Department of Surgery
University of Toronto
Hospital for Sick Children
Toronto
Canada

Chris Kimber FRACS
Consultant Paediatric Surgeon
Department of General Surgery
Royal Children's Hospital
Victoria
Australia

François Laborde MD
Chief of Cardiac Surgery
Department of Cardiac Pathology
L'Institut Mutualiste Montsouris
Paris
France

Göran Láckgren MD
Associate Professor
Section of Urology
Department of Paediatric Surgery
University Children's Hospital
Uppsala
Sweden

Anthony D. Lander PHD FRCS (Paed Surg)
Senior Lecturer in Paediatric Surgery and Consultant Paediatric Surgeon
Birmingham Children's Hospital
Birmingham
UK

Alex C.H. Lee FRCSEd
Specialist Registrar
Department of Paediatric Surgery
Queen's Medical Centre
Nottingham
UK

Marc A. Levitt MD
Attending, Pediatric Surgery
Assistant Professor of Surgery and Pediatrics
Cincinnati Children's Hospital
University of Cincinnati
Ohio
USA

David A. Lloyd MChir FRCS FCS(SA)
Professor of Paediatric Surgery
Department of Child Health
Alder Hey Children's Hospital
Liverpool
UK

Stuart N. Lloyd FRCS
Pyrah Department of Urology
St James's University Hospital
Leeds
UK

Thom E. Lobe MD
Chairman, Section of Pediatric Surgery
Health Science Center
College of Medicine
University of Tennessee
Memphis, TN
USA

N.J. Magnsoc MD
Department of Surgery
The Chinese University of Hong Kong
Prince of Wales Hospital
Shatin, NT
Hong Kong

Kiki Maoate FRACS
Department of Paediatric Surgery
Christchurch Hospital
Christchurch
New Zealand

Garrett S. Matsunaga MD
Clinical Instructor
Department of Urology
University of California, Irvine
Orange, CA
USA

Ranjiv Mathews MD
Associate Professor
Pediatric Urology
The Johns Hopkins Hospital
Baltimore, MD
USA

Milós Merksz MD
Head of Department
Department of Paediatric Urology
Heim Pál Children's Hospital
Budapest
Hungary

Philippe Montupet MD
Paediatric Surgical Unit
Centre Hospitalier
Universitaire de Bicetre
Paris
France

James T. Moore MD
Assistant Professor of Surgery
Division of Pediatric Surgery
University of Maryland School of Medicine
Baltimore, MD
USA

Azad Najmaldin MS FRCS FRCSEd
Consultant Paediatric Surgeon
St James's University Hospital
Leeds
UK

Rainer Nustede MD
Professor of Paediatric Surgery
Department of Paediatric Surgery
Hannover Medical School
Hannover
Germany

Peter Nyirády MD
Assistant Professor
Urological Clinic
Semmelweis University
Budapest
Hungary

Kalpana K. Patil FRCS(Paed Surg)
Consultant Paediatric Urologist
Guy's Hospital NHS Trust
London
UK

Craig A. Peters MD FACS FAAP
Associate Professor of Surgery
Department of Urology
Children's Hospital
Harvard Medical School
Boston, MA
USA

Stephen Potts FRCS
Consultant Paediatric Surgeon
Royal Hospital for Sick Children
Belfast
Northern Ireland

Prem Puri MS FRCS(Ed) FACS
Consultant Paediatric Surgeon and Director of Research
Our Lady's Hospital for Sick Children
Dublin
Ireland

Yann Revillon MD
Service de Chirurgie Pédiatrique
Hôpital Necker-Enfants Malades
Paris
France

Derek Roebuck FRCR FRANZCR
Consultant Paediatric Radiologist
Department of Paediatric Surgery and Radiology
Great Ormond Street Hospital for Children
London
UK

Steven S. Rothenberg MD
Chief of Pediatric Surgery
Mother and Child Hospital at PISL
Denver, CO
USA

Frédérique Sauvat MD
Department of Pediatric Surgery
Hôpital Necker-Enfants Malades
Paris
France

Klaus Schaarschmidt
Direktor der Kinderchirurgischen Klinik
Chefarzt Kinderchirurgische Klinik
Helios Klinikum
Berlin
Germany

Felix Schier MD
Department of Paediatric Surgery
University Medical Centre Jena
Jena
Germany

Jurgen Schleef MD
Department of Paediatric Surgery
Graz University Medical School
Austria

Allan M. Shanberg MD
Clinical Professor of Urology
Director, Pediatric Urology
University of California Irvine
Irvine, CA
USA

Rang N.S. Shawis MBChB FRCS Ed M.Ed
Consultant Paediatric Surgeon
Sheffield Children's Hospital
Sheffield
UK

Paul Simpson BSc
Marketing Director
Erbe Medical UK Limited
Leeds
UK

Lewis Spitz MBChB PhD MD FRCS FAAP FRCPCH
Nuffield Professor of Paediatric Surgery
Department of Paediatric Surgery
Institute of Child Health
London
UK

Theodore H. Stathos MD
Rocky Mountain Pediatric Gastroenterology
Lone Tree, CO
USA

Henrik A. Steinbrecher BSc MBBS MS FRCS(Paeds)
Consultant Paediatric Surgeon
Wessex Regional Centre for Paediatric Surgery
Southampton General Hospital
Southampton
UK

Arne Stenberg MD
Associate Professor
Section of Urology
Department of Paediatric Surgery
University Children's Hospital
Uppsala
Sweden

Richard J. Stewart FRCS
Consultant Paediatric Surgeon
Department of Paediatric Surgery
Queen's Medical Centre
Nottingham
UK

Mark D. Stringer MS FRCS FRCP FRCPCH
Consultant Paediatric Surgeon
Children's Liver and Gastrointestinal Unit
St James's University Hospital
Leeds
UK

Ian D. Sugarman FRCS(Paed Surg)
Consultant Paediatric Surgeon
Department of Paediatric Surgery
The General Infirmary at Leeds
Leeds
UK

Arash K. Taghizadeh MD
Specialist Registrar
Great Ormond Street Hospital for Children
London
UK

Paul K.H. Tam MD
Professor and Chief
Division of Paediatric Surgery
The University of Hong Kong
Queen Mary Hospital
Hong Kong

Joselito G. Tantoco MD
Chief Pediatric Surgical Registrar
Department of Pediatric Surgery
Women's and Children's Hospital
Adelaide
South Australia

Benno M. Ure MD
Director and Professor of Paediatric Surgery
Department of Paediatric Surgery
Hannover Medical School
Hannover
Germany

François Varlet MD
Centre Hôpitalier Universitaire de Saint Etienne
Service de Chirurgie Pédiatrique
Cedex
France

R. Vetter MD
Consultant Paediatric Surgeon
Helios Hospital Erfurt
Germany

Emmanuel Villa MD
Department of Cardiac Pathology
L'Institut Mutualiste Montsouris
Paris
France

Duncan T. Wilcox MD
Associate Professor of Pediatric Urology
University of Texas
Southwestern Medical Center
Dallas, Texas
USA

Alun R. Williams FRCS(Paed Surg)
Locum Consultant Paediatric Urologist
Nottingham City Hospital
Nottingham
UK

Keneth K.Y. Wong PhD FRCS(Ed)
Assistant Professor
Division of Paediatric Surgery
The University of Hong Kong
Queen Mary Hospital
Hong Kong

Robert E. Wood MD PhD
Professor of Pediatrics
Chief, Division of Pulmonary Medicine
Children's Hospital Medical Center
Cincinnati, OH
USA

Chung K. Yeung MD FRCS FRACS FACS
Department of Surgery
Prince of Wales Hospital
Shatin
Hong Kong

Zacharias Zachariou MD PhD
Professor of Pediatric Surgery
Inselspital, Kinderchirurgische Klinik
Bern
Switzerland

Preface

Over the last few decades, first intraluminal rigid and flexible endoscopy, and more recently laparoscopic and thoracoscopic surgery have become established in pediatric medical and surgical practice. This change has been brought about by the combined efforts of innovative surgeons and physicians as well as scientists and industry the world over. As a consequence, all clinicians who use endoscopes within the tubes lumen, cavities and tissue planes of the body are now united into a multi-disciplinary group of minimal access practitioners who have undoubtedly enriched the culture of our practice and minimised the surgical trauma and morbidity of the patients.

Advances in science and technology have rendered the majority of clinical procedures possible within the scope of endoscopy and endoscopic surgery, and the desire to search for more and new procedures which might be adapted to these techniques will continue. However, the importance of placing safety first, meticulous attention to detail, familiarity with instrumentation and appropriate training cannot be over-emphasized.

Progress in pediatric medicine in general, and surgery in particular, has become so fast and is so broad that it has become difficult for any one clinician to master the breadth of the subject, and consequently a need for multi-author texts covering sub-specialized areas of pediatric practice including endoscopy and endoscopic surgery is now overwhelming.

In this book we have been fortunate to be able to draw upon the vast experience of physicians and surgeons at the forefront of clinical practice in the field of percutaneous procedures, endoscopy and endoscopic surgery. The aim has been to provide a step-by-step guide to the established endoscopic techniques in infants and children. The text also describes some not yet established and experimental but potentially significant procedures, where appropriate. While the authors have forwarded their own (often strong) views as well as some other commonly held but differing views and techniques, the emphasis throughout is on a practical guide to the areas of endoscopy and endoscopic surgery for the relative novice. A significant section of nearly all chapters is devoted to potential pitfalls and problems and their solutions and complications are highlighted throughout. This feature of the book is unique and seen vital particularly to those who are on the steep part of the learning curve.

While this text is aimed primarily at trainee and qualified pediatric surgeons and urologists, it will also prove a useful resource for pediatricians and adult surgeons and physicians undertaking endoscopy and/or endoscopic surgery for thorax, gastrointestinal, urological and other conditions in infants and children.

The vast majority of surgical line diagrams are either re-drawn or created out of the descriptive text by A Najmaldin assisted by P Brown. We are ever grateful to the publishing staff of Hodder Arnold, especially Sarah Burrows and Naomi Wilkinson, for their hard work, patience and support during the production of this volume. The preparation and writing of the text would have been impossible without the great help we have received from the hardworking secretary Parmjit Jajuha.

Azad Najmaldin
Steven Rothenberg
David Crabbe
Spencer Beasley

Section A: Introduction

1

Rigid endoscopes

JURGEN SCHLEEF

INTRODUCTION

Modern endoscopy has revolutionized the practice of medicine. Although the history of endoscopy can be traced back to ancient times, there is no doubt that the current era of minimally invasive surgery was only made possible by the development of fiberoptics and the rod-lens telescope.

HISTORY

Hippocrates (460–377 BC) described the use of a speculum for examination of the rectum. He also described the insufflation of air through the speculum to relieve an intestinal obstruction. Quite advanced specula were recovered from the ruins of Pompeii (AD 79), but inspection of body cavities must have been very limited in the absence of decent illumination.

There is little evidence of significant further development until the beginning of the nineteenth century. In 1806 Philip Bozzini published his observations using an invention he named the *lichtleiter*. Bozzini's instrument consisted of a beeswax candle light source and a silvered mirror to reflect the light down a variety of specula. The endoscopist would peer through a small hole in the center of the mirror. (**See Figure 1.1**)

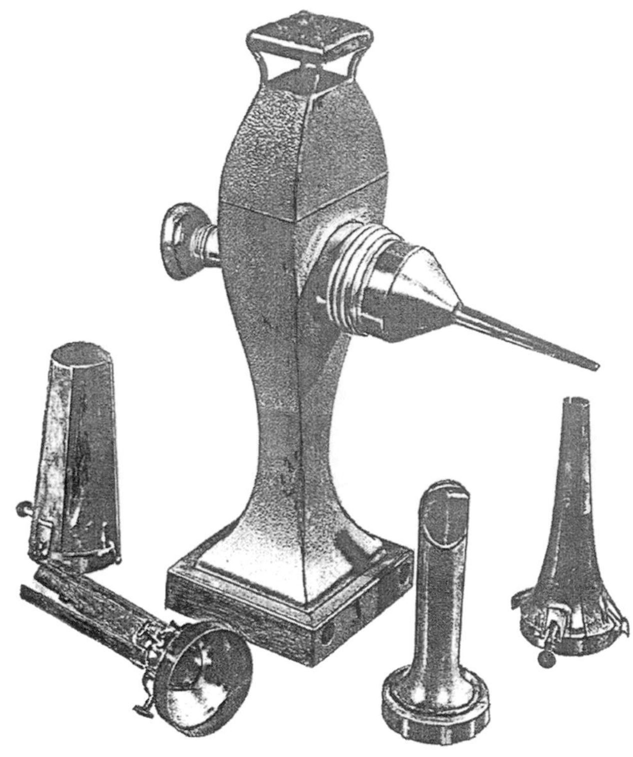

Figure 1.1 *Bozzini's instrument. Kindly supplied by Professor Hans J. Reuter, President of the Max Nitze Museum, Stuttgart, Germany.*

A generation later, Max Nitze developed a cystoscope that embodied the basic principles of all subsequent cystoscopes – namely, an electric light source located close to the field to be examined, a lens system and an instrument channel. The instrument was built by the Viennese instrument maker Josef Leiter in 1877. Illumination was provided by a platinum wire at the tip of the instrument heated by electricity. This was replaced within a few years by an incandescent bulb. Both light sources generated substantial amounts of heat and necessitated a complex system of cooling with iced water to prevent thermal damage to the urethra and bladder. **(See Figure 1.2)**

Rigid endoscopes for esophagoscopy and bronchoscopy appeared during the late nineteenth and early twentieth centuries. However, the practical problem of illumination hampered development until the late 1950s. A light source placed at the end of the endoscope provided reasonable illumination at the risk of thermal injury to the patient. Conduction of light from a source at the proximal end of the instrument was more desirable.

Quartz rods were used for this purpose, but they were fragile, expensive and awkward to use. The problem was really only solved satisfactorily in the early 1960s by the fiberoptic cable. Finally light could be transmitted safely from a bright 'cold' light source outside the body to the distal end of the endoscope.

The next major development was the introduction of the rod-lens system, developed by Hopkins in the early 1960s. Conventional telescope lens systems consisted of thin glass lenses separated by air and this incurred high transmission losses. The Hopkins rod-lens telescope was introduced by Storz in 1966. The revolutionary change was the use of long glass rod lenses separated by thin segments of air. This resulted in a major increase in light transmission and a wider viewing angle. As a consequence, instrument diameter could be reduced without diminishing the image quality.

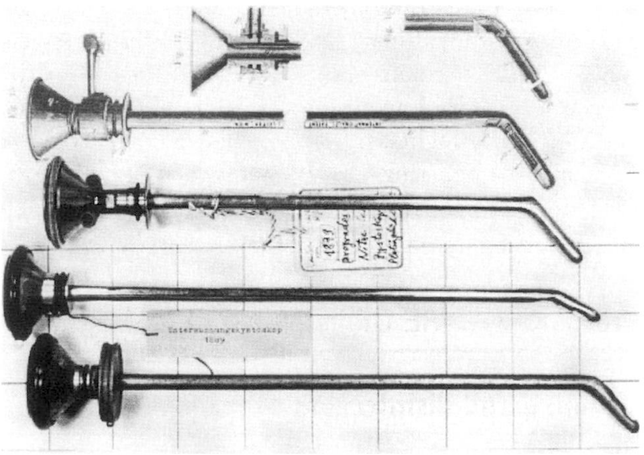

Figure 1.2 *Nitze and Leiter cytoscopes. Kindly supplied by Professor Hans J. Reuter, President of the Max Nitze Museum, Stuttgart, Germany.*

Around the mid-1970s, endoscope manufacturers introduced a range of black and white television cameras. The charge-coupled device (CCD) was invented by Boyle and Smith in 1969, although, curiously, a patent was not applied for. In March 1987, Philippe Mouret in Lyons, France, performed the first human laparoscopic cholecystectomy. Since that time there have been further developments in CCD camera technology, including three-dimensional imaging, and manufacturers are now focusing on the ergonomics of minimally invasive surgery with improved instruments and robotic arms.

ENDOSCOPE OPTICS

Basic principles: optics

Vision down a hollow tube is poor, regardless of lighting. Magnification is needed to improve the view and also increase the field of vision. Typically the optical relay system is composed of a number of identical stages. The objective lens allows acceptance of light from a wide field, typically 60–70°. A prism may be placed before the objective lens for oblique viewing endoscopes. The objective lens forms an inverted image of the subject and a field lens placed near the image redirects the chief ray towards the center of the relay lens system. Another field lens keeps the chief ray confined to the narrow diameter of the lens system. This succession of relay and field lenses is repeated as necessary according to the length of the instrument. The lenses are separated by air. At the eyepiece, light is magnified, inverted and focused by an ocular lens. **(See Figure 1.3)**

The rod-lens telescope

Modern telescopes are constructed with rod lenses of the Hopkins design in place of thin lens field/relay elements. The glass rod lens acts as a very efficient optical wave-guide compared to the thin lens system. The length to diameter ratio of these lenses may be as high as 10. Light is tightly confined to the optical axis by reducing ray divergence in the air gaps between the lenses. Consequently, light

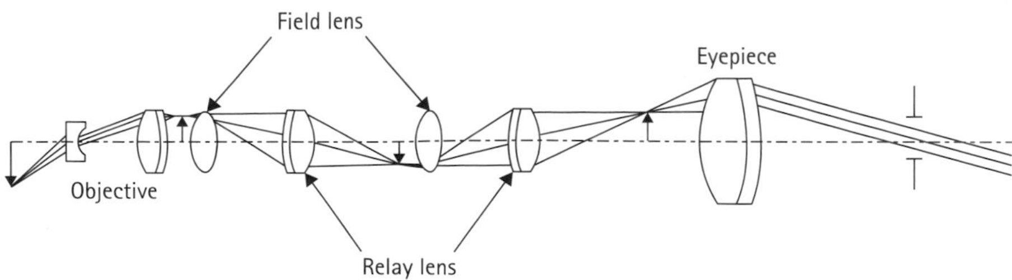

Figure 1.3

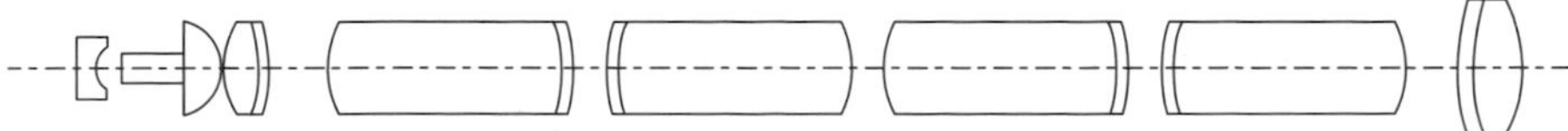

Figure 1.4

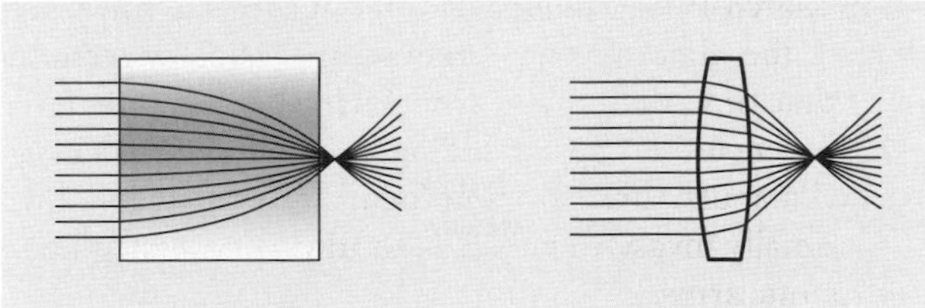

Optics of the Gradient Index (GRIN) lens compared to a conventional thin lens

Figure 1.5

transmission is increased and telescope diameter can be reduced. Vignetting (darkening of the image away from the center due to light fall-off), which is a major problem with thin lens telescopes, is virtually abolished. Construction is simplified because rod lenses are much simpler to align during telescope assembly. **(See Figure 1.4)**

Gradient-index (GRIN) rod lens

A conventional lens refracts light at its surface. At the air–glass interface, rays of light are bent by the abrupt change in refractive index. Focal length is determined by the curvature of the lens. GRIN lenses refract light by virtue of a continuous variation in the refractive index of the lens material rather than curvature of the surface of a conventional lens. The refractive index is highest in the center of the lens and declines with radial distance from the central axis. The rate of this decline determines the lens's optical performance. As a consequence, the trajectory of light rays through a GRIN lens varies progressively from center to periphery. If the light passes through a longer lens, it will follow a sinusoidal path. The length of lens that is required for light to traverse one cycle of the sine wave is termed the pitch of the lens. The key to manufacturing GRIN lenses is controlled variation of the refractive index. At present, the production of high-quality lenses is a complex process involving high-temperature ion processes within molten liquid glass. **(See Figures 1.5 and 1.6)**

Gradient-index lens relay systems are likely to appear in surgical endoscopes over the next few years. The GRIN system works best with a small diameter telescope (0.7–1 mm). The advantages to the pediatric surgeon will be immense – light transmission efficiency will increase dramatically and endoscope diameter will decrease. There will be fewer optical components in the relay system and these endoscopes will be more robust than conventional rod-lens telescopes.

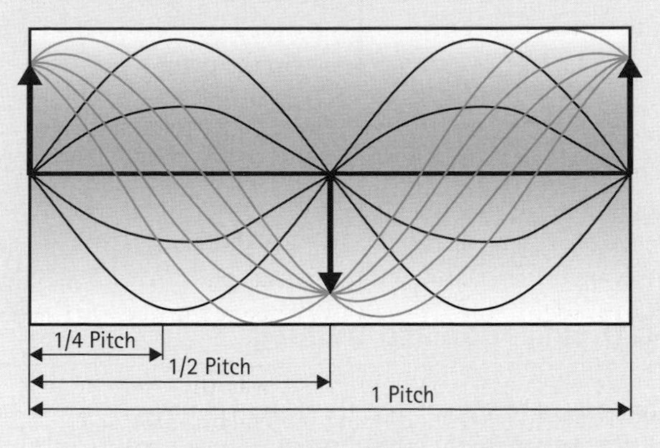

GRIN lens pitch

Figure 1.6

MODERN RIGID TELESCOPE DESIGN

Modern rigid telescopes are manufactured by assembling a rod-lens system within a metal sleeve. The sleeve protects the lenses and maintains optical alignment. The body of the telescope consists of an adapter for a fiberoptic light cable and an eyepiece. Light is transmitted down the telescope via a narrow fiberoptic ring surrounding the rod-lens elements. **(See Figure 1.7)**

PRACTICAL CARE OF PEDIATRIC ENDOSCOPES

Cleaning and disinfection of rigid telescopes

Endoscopes should be disassembled and cleaned after use by manually washing all surfaces using a mild detergent and a soft brush or by soaking in enzymatic cleaning solutions. After washing, endoscopes should be rinsed to remove residues of the cleaning agents. Automatic instrument washing machines may be used for this process. Lens surfaces should be cleaned with 70 percent alcohol. Endoscopes should be inspected for damage and then wrapped and placed in sterilization containers. They can be stored in the sterilization containers until needed.

Protective metal or plastic sleeves are available for most telescopes. The sleeves provide protection to the telescope when not in use and also provide additional stability and safety when the telescope is being transported, sterilized or stored.

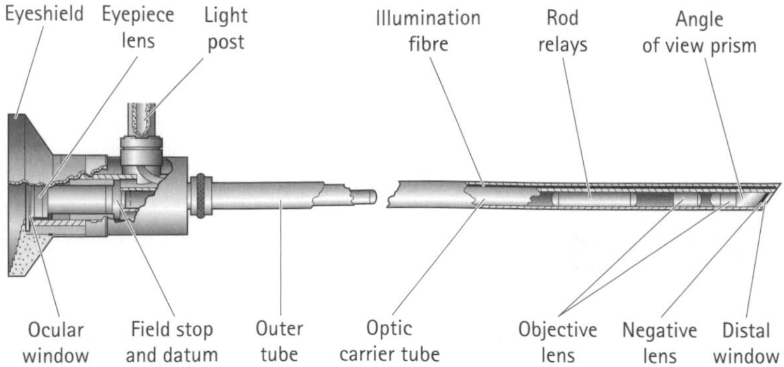

Figure 1.7

Staff education and training

The costs of repair and replacement of damaged endoscopic equipment are high. Education of staff can reduce this bill. Once the complexity and workings of endoscopic equipment are understood, the fragility of the equipment can be appreciated. Educating physicians to handle instruments correctly during endoscopic procedures is a particularly important part of this process but, unfortunately, it is often overlooked.

RIGID ENDOSCOPY IN CHILDREN

Rigid endoscopy is used in newborns, babies and children. Endoscopic techniques have been developed to gain access to body cavities for diagnostic and therapeutic purposes:

- tracheo-bronchoscopy
- rigid endoscopy of the upper and lower gastrointestinal tract
- cystourethroscopy
- laparoscopy
- thoracoscopy
- arthroscopy
- endoscopic neurosurgery.

This broad range of endoscopic surgery requires telescopes of different sizes (diameter, length) and different viewing angles (from 0° to 120°). Telescopes may need to be introduced through trocars, puncture cannulae or the optic channels of combined instruments. The choice of telescope will be influenced by the circumstances, the indication for the examination (diagnostic or therapeutic) and, finally, by the size and age of the patient.

Flexible endoscopes are replacing rigid instruments for many endoluminal applications, e.g. upper gastrointestinal endoscopy. However, image quality and instrument technology for flexible endoscopes remain far behind those of rigid equipment. Furthermore, robotic telescopic assistance and control are built on the concept of rigid endoscope technique.

THE FUTURE

New CCD chip technology and nanotechnology are beginning to change the design of surgical endoscopes. Rigid telescopes with a CCD chip at the tip will provide better image quality and better illumination. Digital transmission of three-dimensional images should abolish the problem of depth perception encountered with conventional two-dimensional imaging. Endoscopic ultrasound and optical coherence tomography, which is a laser-based imaging technology similar to B-mode ultrasound imaging, are being developed to provide real-time tissue imaging. GRIN lens technology will result in progressive reduction in endoscope diameter. Over the next few years the seemingly disparate fields of engineering and surgery will undoubtedly converge further.

FURTHER READING

Boppart SA, Deutsch TF, Rattner DW. Optical imaging technology in minimally invasive surgery – current status and future directions. *Surgical Endoscopy* 1999; **13**:718–22.

Hulka GF, Wilmott RW, Cotton RT. Evaluation of the airway. In: Meyer CM, Cotton RT, Shott SR (eds), *The Pediatric Airway – An Interdisciplinary Approach*. Philadelphia: Lippincott, 1995.

Reuter MA, Reuter HJ. *Geschichte der Endoskopie*, Vols. 1–4. Stuttgart: Krámer, 1998.

2

Flexible endoscopes

ANTHONY D. LANDER

INTRODUCTION

The desire to look inside the hollow viscera of the human body has been driven by curiosity and the potential advantages to be gained from diagnosing and treating disease at an early stage. Progress has been fueled by ingenuity and technological advances borrowed from many diverse fields. Rigid endoscopes came first. The development of a flexible endoscope had to await a solution to the problem of a flexible optical wave-guide. The answer came in the form of the fiberoptic cable. Subsequently, advances in electronics, computing and material science contributed to the array of modern reliable endoscopes available today.

The flexible endoscope in historical context

The earliest serious attempts at alimentary endoscopy are attributed to Adolf Kussmaul (1822–1902), who developed a rigid gastro-esophagoscope with the help of a circus sword swallower in 1868. Illumination was a major obstacle and Kussmaul used an alcohol and turpentine lamp, lens and reflector. The incandescent electric light bulb had yet to be invented. Mikulicz (1850–1905) recognized the need for a flexible endoscope, observing that the axes of the esophagus and stomach were not in the same plane. In 1881 Mikulicz made a 65 cm long endoscope with a slight angle in its distal quarter and he also insufflated air to distend the esophagus and stomach.

In the early 1930s, the Munich physician Rudolf Schindler and the Berlin instrument maker George Wolf devised a semi-flexible endoscope. The lower end of the instrument consisted of a flexible bronze spiral filled with an array of short focus lenses that could be bent to an angle of 34° without distorting the image. Schindler's gastroscope remained in clinical use until the later 1950s and Munich became the Mecca of endoscopy.

John Logie Baird is best known for inventing the television. What is less well known is that he also patented a fiberoptic means of light transmission in 1928, although he did not develop the idea any further. In 1954 Hopkins and Kapany reported transmission of an image through a coherent fiberoptic bundle in the journal *Nature*. Basil Hirschowitz, a South African gastroenterologist working in Michigan, worked with colleagues to develop the first flexible gastroscope using fiberoptics and this appeared in 1957. The instrument had a joystick to control the direction of the tip, although, in comparison with modern instruments, the range of movement was limited. Over the following decade a number of flexible endoscopes were developed and the diameters of these instruments gradually decreased.

Early work was driven by the American firm American Cystoscope Makers Incorporated (ACMI), which produced the first commercial gastroscope in 1960. It soon became apparent that the potential market for flexible endoscopes was large, and the might of industrial research and development was used to bring material science and advanced manufacturing techniques into play. Japanese optical companies entered the marketplace with endoscopes, light sources and cameras developed by Olympus, Fujinon, Pentax and Machida. As the market expanded, it was evident that clinicians wanted instruments with smaller diameters, larger working channels, greater flexibility and better optics. Early instruments were fragile and difficult to sterilize. These problems were solved and progress continued at a pace. The most significant development in recent years has been the charge-coupled device (CCD).

FIBEROPTICS

Transmission of light by total internal reflection

The principle of light transmission down a single fine flexible glass fiber is the cornerstone of modern fiberoptic endoscopy. The optics of fiberoptic light transmission are complicated but, in simple terms, transmission relies on repeated reflections of the light beam down the fiber. This occurs without loss by virtue of the principle of total internal reflection.

When light travels in a transparent material and meets the surface of another transparent material, two things happen. First, light is reflected, and second, some light is transmitted into the second transparent material. The light that is transmitted changes direction or bends. This is refraction. Refraction is a result of the fact that light travels at different speeds in different transparent materials. The two materials are said to have different refractive indices. The refractive index is defined as $n = c/v$ where n is the refractive index, c the speed of light in a vacuum, and v the speed of light in the material.

When light passes from a material of high refractive index n_1 into a material of lower refractive index n_2, θ_2 will always be greater than θ_1 (**See Figure 2.1**). Now consider what happens when θ_1 increases: θ_2 will reach 90° before θ_1 does. θ_1 is said to have reached the critical angle, θ_c, when θ_2 equals 90°. When θ_1 equals θ_c, light might be expected to travel in both mediums simultaneously. For complex physical reasons this is impossible and all the light energy is reflected. So for any θ_1 equal to or greater than θ_c there is what is called total internal reflection. The phenomenon of total internal reflection causes 100 percent reflection to occur. This does not happen in any other reflection, for example at a mirrored surface. The unique principle of total internal reflection explains why fiberoptics can be used to transmit data many miles. The light path down an optical fiber is a zig-zag path of total internal reflection for all rays that strike the fiber within a defined arc, which is termed the acceptance angle. (**See Figure 2.2**)

Even though the fibers are flexible, there is a limit to bending. Fibers do fracture and dots may be seen when looking at the end of a transmitted light source and on the image of poorly handled endoscopes. Bending can also lead to loss of light when total internal reflection is not achieved. However, in practice, light losses are minimal and a collection of fibers can carry sufficient light around a bend or even in a loose knot to illuminate an object. (**See Figure 2.3**)

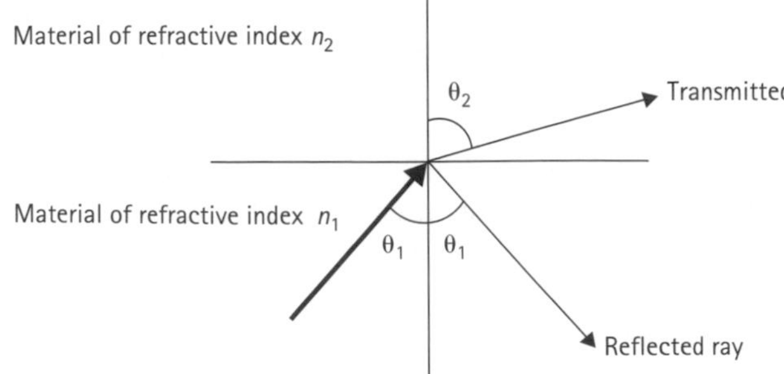

Figure 2.1

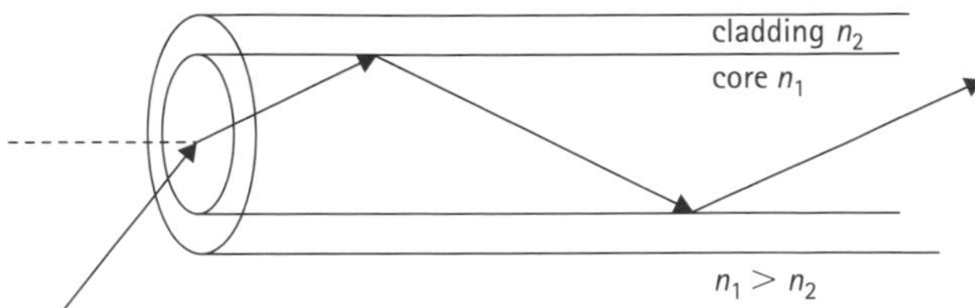

Figure 2.2

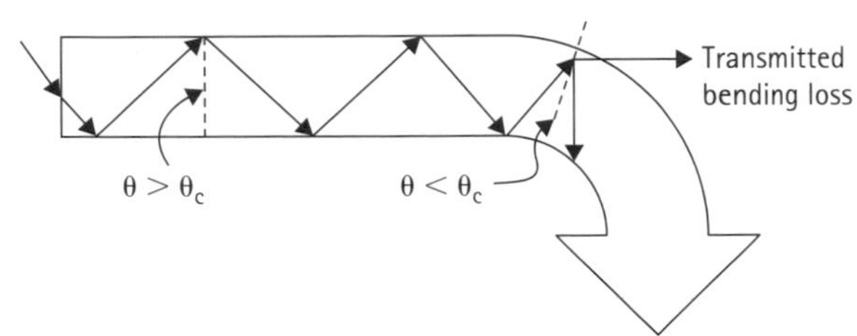

Figure 2.3

Modern fiberoptics

Manufacturing fine, high-quality fibers is technically difficult. By the 1980s, good quality glass fibers had come down from 20 μ to 8 μ in diameter, allowing clearer, brighter and sharper images. A thinner diameter endoscope could be produced for similar optical performance, which allowed greater flexibility. Angulation became possible up to 210°, with angles of view up to 120°. Fibers as thin as 6 microns are now available and performance is improved by optimizing the fiber design. Modern optical fibers are constructed from borosilicate glass, which has a high refractive index to maximize the total internal reflection, and each fiber is surrounded by an outer sheath of optical grade epoxy resin with a lower refractive index, which helps to reduce dispersion on bends.

Image production

Fiberoptic bundles may be coherent or non-coherent. A coherent array maintains the spatial organization of the individual fibers and this is necessary for accurate image transmission. Coherent bundles used to contain around 20 000–40 000 fibers, but as smaller fibers have been possible, bundles now contain as many as 66 000–120 000 fibers.

Each fiber in the bundle effectively conveys one pixel of information about the image. The fibers only need to be fixed to each other at the ends of the endoscope to maintain coherence. Most of the length of the endoscope can thus be made flexible to allow passage down a viscus.

A non-coherent bundle lacks the spatial organization of a coherent bundle and is therefore unsuitable for image transmission. However, this type of array is less costly to manufacture and can be used to transmit light to the endoscope tip. A typical light bundle will contain around 80 000 fibers.

Packing fraction

The outer sheath of each fine glass fiber and the space between the circular cross-sections of sheathed fibers do not transmit any of the image. They appear as dark areas on the image. These dark areas are known as the packing fraction and account for the 'mesh' effect evident on the image as seen on the monitor. This explains why the image quality of a fiberoptic endoscope can never be as good as one produced from a rigid Hopkins rod-lens telescope. However, a rigid telescope cannot be bent around a corner or tied in a knot.

Depth of field

Depth of field is important in a useful endoscope. Depth of field is the difference in the distance from the lens between near and far objects that are both in reasonable focus. The pinhole camera has an infinite depth of focus – the smaller the aperture, the better the depth of focus available. Unfortunately, a small aperture reduces the amount of light that is transmitted. The aperture at the distal lens of an endoscope is not adjustable. Modern endoscopes use lenses with a pinhole aperture and have depths of field of 3–150 mm. This is quite sufficient for all clinical applications. At the top end of the scope, an adjustable lens system produces a focused image for the observer's eye or a camera.

CURRENT ENDOSCOPE DESIGN

There are a number of manufacturers producing endoscopes of many different designs. Unfortunately, light sources and even adapters from different companies are not always interchangeable. Nonetheless, there are common features to most systems.

Light source

There is a light source, typically a 300–500 watt xenon arc lamp, although some halogen tungsten filament systems are still in use. The light source lies at the focus of a parabolic mirror to produce a near-parallel beam of light. The intensity of the light entering the endoscope is controlled by filters or a diaphragm. Light is transmitted to the endoscope and then down to the tip by a non-coherent fiberoptic bundle contained within the umbilical cord. The umbilical cord also transmits one or more specialized channels.

Control head

There is a control head and a flexible shaft with a maneuverable tip. Buttons on the control head allow water and suction to be controlled. If there is a coherent fiber bundle bringing light back to an operator, the control head has a lens system for the operator to look into or for the attachment of a camera. If a CCD is used at the tip of the scope, wires take data from the scope along the umbilical cord and the control head may have buttons to control focus, magnification, gain or other image functions such as to take a picture or control recordings.

Direction control

Control wires attached just beneath the outer protective shaft are connected to the tip direction controls on the side of the control head. The angling wheels for left/right and up/down usually incorporate friction brakes to allow the tip to be temporarily locked in any desired position. Some small endoscopes such as narrow flexible bronchoscopes may only have one angling wire and rely on torsion being applied through the instrument to control one direction of movement. In some instruments there is a deflector to adjust the instrument's tip; a thumb lever usually controls this elevator. Torque applied to the shaft is transmitted to the tip if the shaft is relatively straight. It is important to know about the use of specific scopes because it is easy to damage fine pediatric scopes if torque is applied to the wrong part of the structure. It may be safe to twist the control head or the body just below the control head, but the fine shaft of the scope itself may be damaged if the torque is applied directly to the protective sheath.

Operating channels

These are usually between 2 and 4 mm in diameter and a channel may be dedicated for a particular use or for more than one function. A channel may be used to direct water over the lens to clean it, to insufflate air both to distend organs and to clear debris, to allow suction to remove air or fluid, and to pass instruments to allow procedures to take place such as diathermy, injecting, snaring, biopsying and brushing. In single-channel endoscopes, suction is markedly limited when an instrument occupies the channel.

Video-endoscopes

In the late 1980s, the first video-endoscopes appeared with CCDs. These are computer chips that act as cameras at the very tip of the endoscope. This avoids the need for a coherent fiber bundle transmitting the image from the endoscope tip to the eyepiece, which reduces endoscope diameter. The first CCDs were monochrome devices that needed high levels of illumination. These early CCDs had around 33 000 pixels or picture elements, but devices of up to 480 000 pixels are now available. These silicone chips are only 1.8 × 2 mm in surface area and are connected directly to further local etched devices that process data for transmission up a fine cable to the umbilical cord, computer and monitor.

High-quality color vision is important to visualize pathology satisfactorily. Color images can be obtained in two ways: by the use of either a color-sensitive or monochrome chip with sequential pick-up of red, green and blue images provided by sequential illumination using red, green and blue light. At the end of the umbilical cord away from the scope, a rotating disc containing filters lies in front of a bright white light, thus providing the sequential color illumination. A color chip is larger than a monochrome chip and consists of a CCD capable of detecting only light and dark but lying under a mosaic color filter and so generating color information.

Overall design

There are variations in size, flexibility, stiffness, sophistication, channels, optics and distal lens orientation. For gastrointestinal work, 90–130° wide angle lenses are used. For CCDs, the images are square rather than round and the angle is measured across the diagonal of the square images. There are lateral viewing scopes for endoscopic retrograde pancreatography, but other oblique and moveable systems were never popular. It is important to stress again that the strength of tubes, wires and fiber bundles is greater when they are bigger, and so narrow pediatric instruments are more fragile. A colonoscope could be 15 mm in diameter to allow resilience and torque stability to get round the colon, but this is not appropriate for neonatal upper gastrointestinal work, for which 8–11 mm is better. Making scopes smaller also compromises durability, image quality and, of course, channel size and number.

PRACTICAL CARE OF PEDIATRIC ENDOSCOPES

Immersible endoscopes

Cleaning of early endoscopes was difficult because the control head could not be immersed or autoclaved. Cross-infection was a real risk and clinicians were understandably reluctant to pass instruments that were only 'socially clean' into, for example, the trachea and bronchi. In the 1980s, the first practical fully immersible endoscope became available.

Cleaning and disinfection of flexible endoscopes

The cleaning and decontamination of fiberoptic endoscopes is a complex task. Endoscopes cannot be sterilized by autoclaving. In North America, guidelines for the decontamination of fiberoptic endoscopes have been published by the Society of Gastroenterology Nurses and Associates (SGNA), endorsed by the American Society for Gastrointestinal Endoscopy. In Europe, the European Society for Gastrointestinal Endoscopy has published similar guidelines.

Endoscope decontamination and maintenance should be left in the hands of a dedicated endoscopy team trained in the appropriate procedures. Endoscopes should be decontaminated at the beginning and end of each endoscopy session and between patients. The endoscope should be wiped clean of body fluids and the instrument channels should be sucked through or irrigated with clean water. The importance of this step cannot be overestimated: it is impossible to disinfect an instrument that has not been adequately cleaned.

After manual pre-cleaning, the endoscope must be chemically disinfected. Automated endoscope reprocessing machines are now available and should be regarded as mandatory. These machines expose all internal and external components of the endoscope to disinfection followed by rinsing with bacteria-free water. Of equal importance is the fact that these machines prevent atmospheric pollution with disinfectant and avoid exposure of personnel to potentially hazardous chemicals. If automatic washer–disinfection equipment is not available, manual disinfection must be undertaken. The instrument has to be fully immersed and all channels flushed with disinfectant. Commonly available products include alkaline 2 percent glutaraldehyde, 0.55 percent orthophthalaldehyde and a variety of peracetic acids. All these chemicals are hazardous and must be used in accordance with the manufacturers' instructions. After sterilization, instruments must be rinsed thoroughly with water, internally and externally, and then dried. Drying of the instrument channels can be facilitated by irrigation with 70 percent isopropyl alcohol.

Prior to each disinfection, the endoscope must be tested for leaks. This involves filling the free space inside the endoscope sheath with air under a measured pressure. A fall in pressure as the tip of the instrument is moved suggests a leak in the flexible outer sheath. Provided this damage is detected early, the endoscope can usually be repaired. Good relationships and communication with manufacturers for backup, repair and staff training are essential.

ENDOSCOPY TEACHING AND IMAGE DOCUMENTATION

Cameras and teaching

Until the 1990s, endoscopes required the operator to look directly into a lens system at one end of a coherent fiber bundle. At the other end was another lens gathering light reflected from the inside of the organ. The operator would stand with the scope to his or her eye for many minutes, twisting and turning it whilst steering the tip. Assistants watched but could not see what the operator was visualizing. Trainees got occasional glimpses when the trainer had something to show. When teaching side-arms involving a semi-silvered mirror became available, continuous observation by the trainee was became possible, but the light level was reduced so that neither operator nor trainee could see much. The advent of video cameras had a major impact on teaching. Initially, the cameras were mounted on the optics of the scope above the eyepiece and pictures were viewed on black and white and later color cathode ray monitors. This system enabled all in the theater or endoscopy suite to see what was happening, and training improved significantly.

New developments are often poorly received at first. It is only with further developments and sometimes changes in practice that the full benefits are brought to the fore. Cameras, now almost universally accepted, were poorly received by many in the early days. Early cameras were modified industrial devices designed for quite different functions. They were so large and cumbersome that many required a gantry to support them. No wonder many endoscopists preferred to peer down scopes on their own.

The influence of the use of computers is obvious in the image processing, recording and editing now available on most systems. Computer data-handling facilitates record keeping, the delivery of peer-reviewed clinical care, and education and training. However, the advances in computer power must not be underestimated in the role they have played in lens design, control head design and manufacturing processes.

THE FUTURE

What does the future hold? Endoscopes will undoubtedly become smaller and video-endoscopes universal. As CCD cameras become smaller and more sensitive, two adjacent images might be brought to the two eyes of the operator, giving a three-dimensional image. Another exciting possibility might be to look at pathology under illumination by other parts of the electromagnetic spectrum; infrared and ultraviolet light could be used, but with visualization in transposed colors on familiar monitors. Combining visual endoscopy with ultrasound images generated from crystals at the tip of the scope might prove useful so that the nature of neighboring tissue echodensity could guide biopsy selection, for example.

The following chapters outline the details of instruments and endoscopic procedures widely performed today. Interventional endoluminal endoscopy is still in its infancy. Further advances in endoscope technology will undoubtedly accelerate progress in this field.

FURTHER READING

European Society for Gastrointestinal Endoscopy. Guidelines on cleaning and disinfection in GI endoscopy. *Endoscopy* 2000; 31:77–83.

ASTM International. *Standard Practice for Cleaning and Disinfection of Flexible Fiberoptic and Video Endoscopes Used in the Examination of the Hollow Viscera.* F1518-00. West Conshohocken, PA: American Society for Testing and Materials.

Guidelines for the Use of High-level Disinfectants and Sterilants for Reprocessing of Flexible Gastrointestinal Endoscopes. Chicago: Society of Gastroenterology Nurses and Associates, Inc., revised 2003 (www.sgna.org).

3

Imaging equipment

ZACHARIAS ZACHARIOU

INTRODUCTION

The era of modern endoscopy began in the 1950s with the development of fiberoptics by Hopkins and Kapany. The first prototype fiberoptic gastroscope was demonstrated in 1957 by Hirschowitz. Charge-coupled device (CDD) cameras became available in the 1980s and the first televised laparoscopic cholecystectomy was performed in 1987. Laparoscopy went from being a gloomy solo procedure to a Technicolor spectator sport. Developments in imaging technology have transformed the practice of endoscopy and paved the way to the gamut of current minimally invasive surgery.

TECHNOLOGY

Light sources

The quality of the endoscopic image depends to a large degree on the light source. A typical light source consists of a lamp, a focusing lens or mirror, a heat filter and some form of intensity control.

Three types of lamp are in regular use today: quartz halogen, xenon short arc and metal halide vapor. Xenon arc lamps are the preferred choice. Halogen bulbs are cheap and efficient. The light emitted is crisp white with excellent color rendering. The color temperature is 5000–5600 °K. Halogen lamps use tungsten electrodes because this is the only metal capable of withstanding the high temperature and pressure. Halogen bulbs operate at a low voltage and have an average life of 2000 hours. Xenon arc lamps consist of a spherical or ellipsoidal envelope of fused silica quartz glass, which is usually doped to absorb ultraviolet radiation. The color temperature of a xenon lamp is 6000–6400 °K, which ensures good color rendition. The arc is generated between a small thorium-coated cathode and a larger anode. The optimum working temperature of the cathode is 2000 °C. To maintain a constant operating temperature, the tip of the cathode is pointed and often grooved to act as a heat choke. The anode is usually cylindrical to dissipate heat.

Metal halide lamps consist of an internal arc tube made of quartz enclosed in an outer glass envelope. The quartz tube is filled with argon gas to which a small amount of liquid mercury is added. Sodium iodide and scandium iodide are often also added to increase the luminous efficiency and produce an output that approximates to 'white' light as perceived by the human eye.

The running time of any lamp used in an endoscopic light source should be monitored and the lamp replaced before the end of the indicated service life.

The bulb is placed at the focus of a parabolic mirror to produce a near-parallel beam of light. All light sources are inefficient and produce substantial amounts of heat, mainly in the form of infrared radiation. An infrared heat filter has, therefore, to be included in the light path to prevent unacceptable heating of the fiberoptic cable and endoscope. The heat:light ratio is reduced by filtering, but care must still be taken to protect the patient from inadvertent thermal injury from the light source. Finally, some form of manual or automatic intensity control is included in the light source. This usually takes the form of an adjustable iris diaphragm.

Light is transmitted from the light source to the laparoscope through one of two types of cable – fiberoptic or fluid. Fluid cables are capable of transmitting more light but they are rigid and inherently fragile. Furthermore, they cannot be sterilized by autoclaving. Fiberoptic cables are flexible but do not transmit a precise light spectrum. Whilst they are more robust than fluid cables, they are still prone to damage in the course of normal use. Broken fibers reduce the efficiency of light transmission. A cable should be replaced when more than 15 percent of the fibers have broken.

Charge-coupled device cameras

Charge-coupled devices consist of a collection of charge storage cells with the ability to pass charge from one to the next, in a line, like a bucket brigade (i.e. like a group of fire fighters passing buckets from one to the next). The CCD was originally developed in the 1960s as an analogue delay line for processing RADAR images. Subsequently, light-sensitive storage cells were developed. Advances in large-scale integration technology enabled the production of miniature light-sensitive CCD arrays and thus was born the replacement for the cumbersome TV camera tube. Each light receptor in the CCD array contributes one unit (pixel) to the total image. The resolution or clarity of the final image thus depends upon the number of pixels on the chip: standard laparoscopic cameras contain 250 000–380 000 pixels.

Single-chip cameras use a single CCD array with a color stripe filter to separate red, green and blue light. More sophisticated cameras split the light into red, green and blue optically, and use three CCD arrays. The resulting images are of extremely high resolution and outstanding color fidelity and this makes them ideal for pediatric endosurgical work. CCD camera systems for clinical work often incorporate facilities for digital signal processing, including adjustable gain, contrast enhancement and anti-moiré filters for fiberoptic endoscopes.

Although endoscopic surgery is performed in most centers using two-dimensional imaging, three-dimensional imaging offers a number of potential advantages. Despite the fact that the current three-dimensional camera systems do not provide perfect depth perception, endoscopic maneuvers such as suturing, cutting and knot tying may be performed with increased speed and accuracy. To generate a true stereoscopic three-dimensional picture, the imaging system has to match the resolution, color and contrast equivalents of the best two-dimensional equipment. This involves converting a field sequential stereoscopic video signal (left eye image in one field and right eye image in the other) into a high-resolution three-dimensional image. Proprietary digital processing techniques interpolate both luminance and chroma to provide smooth, step-free edges. These images can then be viewed through comfortable passive-shutter glasses on a time-sequential stereoscopic monitor with a polarized screen. This technology is still expensive, but the increased use of robotics will undoubtedly result in more widespread application.

Another promising development in the field of digital video technology is automatic image righting. Automatic image righting ensures the correct orientation of endoscopic images regardless of the position of the laparoscope. Manual rotation of the camera on the laparoscope becomes redundant. At present this facility is only available with 10 mm laparoscopes, which are rarely used for pediatric surgery.

Monitors

Surgical monitors are no different from the domestic television set: the image is produced by a horizontal beam of electrons scanning the face of the cathode ray tube. The inside of the tube is coated with a fluorescent phosphor, which emits visible light when struck by the beam of electrons. The beam is swept rapidly across the tube in a series of horizontal lines – a technique called horizontal linear scanning. Each picture frame consists of several hundred lines, depending on the type of system used.

The number of scanning lines represents the number of lines of information that are displayed on the monitor. The standard NTSC (National Television Systems Committee) format used in North America and Japan consists of 525 lines scanning at a rate of 30 frames per second. The PAL (Phase Alternating Line) and SECAM (Sèquentiel Couleur et Mèmoire) systems used in other parts of the world use 625 lines at 25 frames per second. High-definition television systems under development will probably have more than 1000 scanning lines. The human eye, in comparison, can distinguish the equivalent of 1600 scanning lines, and the resolution of 35 mm photographic film is equivalent to about 2300 scanning lines.

The quality of the final image displayed on the monitor depends upon a number of factors, including the number of pixels in the CCD chip, the number of scanning lines used by the monitor and the dot pitch. More scanning lines provide greater resolution. The more pixels in the camera, the better the detail. The final limiting factor for detail on the monitor is the dot pitch size, which represents the phosphor element size.

Flat panel liquid crystal displays (LCDs) are replacing conventional cathode ray tube monitors. These devices use a multi-layer sandwich of liquid crystal segments that transmit varying amounts of light, depending on the applied voltage. This light is then filtered with red, green and blue filters and the whole display is backlit with cold cathode fluorescent tubes. Thin film transistor (TFT) arrays provide the enormous number of crystals required for a high-resolution display. LCDs are lighter and less bulky than cathode ray tubes. Of more practical importance to the surgeon, LCDs are non-reflective and almost completely flicker-free, which reduces viewing fatigue.

Recording equipment

Documentation of minimally invasive procedures is optional – conventional open surgical procedures are rarely recorded. However, imaging technology is an integral part of minimally invasive surgery and this makes documentation of operative findings far simpler than with conventional surgery. A number of options exist, but most commonly videotape recorders or still video printers are used, depending on whether a continuous recording or a still picture is required.

The best quality still images are photographs taken with a 35 mm camera attached directly to the eyepiece of the laparoscope, but this method is too inconvenient for routine use. In practice, still images are usually obtained from video printers. Endoscopic images can also be stored in digital format on floppy disks or compact discs for later retrieval and this preserves image quality.

The way in which the recording equipment is connected to the imaging system has a major effect on the quality of the final recording. Super-VHS (S-Video) systems split the signal into luminance (Y) and chroma (C), whereas RGB systems split the image into the three primary colors. If the camera system has outlets for component signals, both the recorder and the primary monitor can be connected to the camera directly.

In a serial hook-up, the camera, recorder and monitor are connected in a line. If the signal goes to the recorder first and to the monitor second, the image on the monitor will be degraded. If the signal goes to the monitor first, the quality of the recorded image will not be as high. If the camera system has dual Y/C outlets or Y/C and RGB outlets, the monitor and recorder can be connected in parallel without degradation of the image. For example, one Y/C port can be connected to the recorder and the second Y/C outlet or the RGB port can be connected to the monitor.

ERGONOMICS

Loss of binocular vision with endoscopic surgery is a major disadvantage. A three-dimensional image has to be interpolated by the surgeon from the two-dimensional image displayed on the monitor. The counter-intuitive movements of the surgeon's hands and the instruments compound the problem. Furthermore, the restricted field of view means that instruments are effectively uncontrolled when they are beyond this area. Processing this complex information requires intense concentration by the surgeon throughout the operation.

Under these circumstances it becomes imperative to establish the best possible endoscopic view of the operative field at the outset. This requires the creation of a constant working space (e.g. a pneumoperitoneum), followed by insertion of trocars for the endoscope and instruments. No matter how sophisticated the imaging equipment is, a good view of the operative site will only be obtained if the optical and instrument ports are correctly placed. As a general rule, working ports should be sited in front of the telescope port at an angle of 60–120° to each other. **(See Figure 3.1)**

Use of a telescope with a 30°, 45° or 70° viewing angle separates the physical (A) and optical (B) axes. This enables the laparoscope to be positioned above the operative field and prevents competition for space between the telescope and instruments. **(See Figure 3.2)**

Image quality and light intensity both increase dramatically with larger diameter telescopes. Although high-definition CCD camera systems will compensate to some degree for these variations, the largest diameter telescope compatible with the optical port should always be selected. Laparoscopes are available in two lengths, 25 cm and 36 cm. Normally, about two-thirds of the telescope lies outside the body. The longer instrument physically separates the camera from the space used by the surgeon to hold the instruments. Unfortunately, this additional length increases visual artifacts caused by movement of the assistant holding the camera. The shorter laparoscope provides a more compact field and is generally preferred for infants and small children. In our hands, a 25 cm long, 4 mm diameter, 30° oblique viewing laparoscope offers the best overall performance for pediatric work.

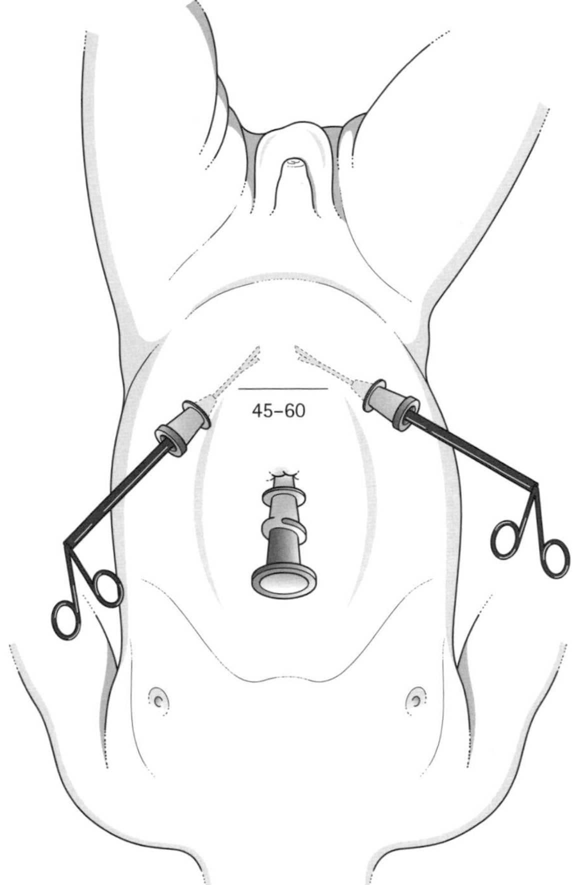

Figure 3.1

The ergonomic layout of the imaging equipment is of great importance. The viewing monitor should be placed a short distance in front of the surgeon so that his or her visual axis includes the laparoscope, the hands controlling the instruments and the monitor in one straight line. The optimal position for the monitor is therefore at manipulation level, usually the abdominal wall, permitting so-called gaze-down viewing. **(See Figure 3.3)**

Gaze-down viewing allows the surgeon to bring both sensory (visual) and motor (instrument manipulation) signals close together. This arrangement ensures the best performance from the surgeon attempting to compensate for the two-dimensional view. Body posture is improved and fatigue is reduced.

If for any reason it is not possible to position the monitor at manipulation level, the second best position is at the surgeon's eye level. However, the surgeon's efficiency

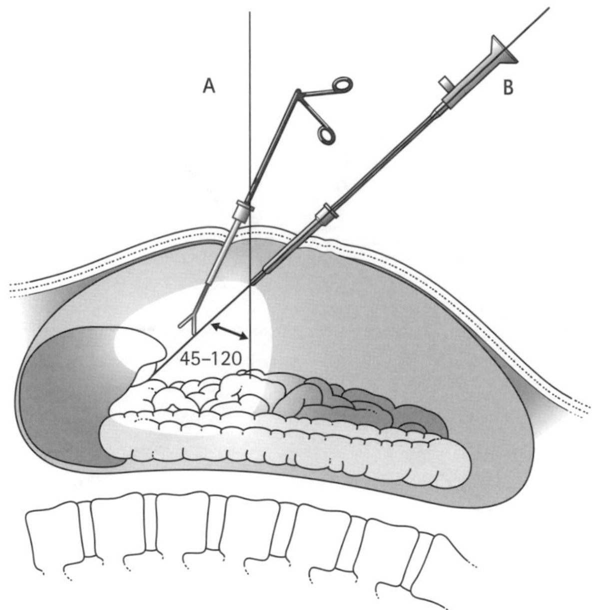

Figure 3.2

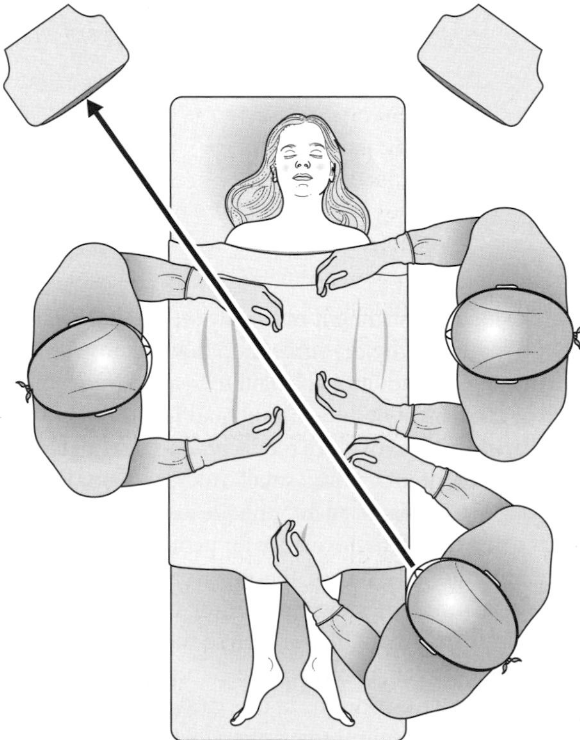

Figure 3.3

declines if he or she has to shift gaze continually from monitor to instruments. This problem is exacerbated if the monitor is positioned some distance away from the operating table because this induces spatial disorientation. Safe and efficient minimally invasive surgery requires the use of ergonomically efficient systems for image display and instrument control.

TROUBLESHOOTING

As the complexity of equipment used for minimally invasive surgery increases, technical problems with the image display become more likely. These can be critical and invariably end in frustration for the whole team.

- Poor projection on the monitor or even complete blackout is usually due to a faulty connection. All connections should be checked before each operation.
- Interference from other equipment, such as the diathermy generator, can be minimized by physical separation of the diathermy and camera systems.
- Dark images can be due to a number of causes. Low levels of illumination may be the result of either a low output from the light source or the reaction of the automatic exposure control on the camera to high light reflection from polished instruments or trocars. Blood on the end of the endoscope absorbs a considerable amount of light and invariably degrades the image quality.
- A blurred image is usually the result of an out-of-focus camera or contamination of the laparoscope tip with blood or other body fluids. The focus should be corrected and the tip of the laparoscope cleaned inside or outside the abdomen.
- Fogging is due to condensation on a cold laparoscope tip. The laparoscope should be immersed in hot water before use to minimize fogging. Cold CO_2 insufflated through the optical trocar may cause the same problem, and this can be avoided by connecting the gas supply to one of the instrument ports.
- Intraperitoneal tissue coagulation produces smoke that disturbs the image. An intermittent short desufflation or controlled discharge of CO_2 from a partly open valve on the trocar will clear the working space.

MAINTENANCE

Modern imaging equipment has become very sophisticated and requires special care – ideally by a dedicated technician. This would reduce frustration on the part of the surgeon and theatre staff, to the undoubted benefit of the patient. Considerable expense can be saved in the long term by preventive maintenance.

FURTHER READING

Scott-Conner CEH (ed.). *The SAGES Manual: Fundamentals of Laparoscopy and GI Endoscopy.* New York: Springer, 1999.

4

Energy used in endoscopic surgery

HENRIK A. STEINBRECHER AND PAUL SIMPSON

INTRODUCTION

The recent advances in endoscopic surgery are due, in no small part, to the development of new energy generators and instruments to perform tasks previously requiring suturing, ligation or conventional diathermy. It is vital that the endoscopic surgeon has a working knowledge of this technology to maintain safe and efficient practice. This field is developing rapidly and new technology is likely to alter the practice of minimally invasive surgery substantially over the next few years.

Ultimately, all energy sources used in clinical surgery produce thermal effects in tissues, some desirable and some undesirable. The effect of increasing temperature at a tissue level is shown in **Table 4.1**.

Table 4.1 *Effects of temperature on living tissues*

Temperature (°C)	Effect
40	Reversible tissue damage, depending on exposure time
49	Irreversible tissue damage
65–70	Coagulation. Collagen is converted into glucose, collagenous tissue shrinks, hemostasis
100	Dehydration/desiccation. Intracellular and extracellular liquid vaporizes. As a result of dehydration, glucose has a sticking effect. The coagulated area shrinks
200	Carbonization. The tissue carbonizes similarly to a fourth-degree burn; this can lead to a delay in the postoperative course of healing

Endoscopic surgery brings a number of unique problems which must be considered if energy is to be used safely.

- The working space is limited and instruments outside the immediate field of vision have the potential to damage surrounding tissues.
- Even small amounts of blood or smoke prejudice vision. As a consequence, hemostasis must be quick, efficient and reliable.
- Tactile feedback and depth perception are absent or substantially diminished.

ENERGY SOURCES

Electrosurgery

Electrical energy is the oldest and most widely used external energy source. The passage of an alternating current through living tissues produces three effects, depending on its intensity and frequency. **(See Table 4.2)** In clinical practice, useful effects are only seen with high-frequency alternating current (>300 kHz), which produces predictable effects as the tissue temperature rises:

- coagulation (60 °C)
- vaporization/desiccation (100 °C)
- carbonization (>200 °C).

The electrical energy can be delivered through monopolar or bipolar electrodes. In monopolar electrosurgery, current is delivered through an active point electrode to the target tissue, where intense heating occurs. The current then passes through the patient's body to a dispersive pad, which is the ground electrode, and back to the generator. The ground

Table 4.2 *Effects of passage of electrical current through living tissues*

	Frequency	Effect	Use in surgery
Electrolytic	Direct current or low frequency Alternating	Causes ions in tissue to travel and may cause electrolytic heating damage.	Undesirable
Faradic	Alternating <20 000 Hz	Direct stimulation of nerve and muscle cells, leading to muscle contraction	Undesirable
Thermal	High frequency Alternating >300 000 Hz	Causes cell death and destruction	Desirable

electrode must cover a large area of the patient's body relative to the size of the active electrode to prevent significant heat build-up and thermal injury at the pad site. In bipolar electrosurgery, current flows between two adjacent electrodes, typically forceps. A dispersive pad is not required and the risk of collateral tissue damage is greatly reduced.

Monopolar electrosurgery is widely used for endoscopic surgery because of its versatility and effectiveness. A constant low voltage produces a cutting effect, whereas a higher voltage produces a coagulative effect. In pure cut mode, a constant low voltage rapidly produces heat, which turns the intracellular fluid to steam, exploding the cells, with tissue separation. In pure coagulation mode, a brief high-voltage burst of energy is followed by a long tissue-cooling period. This interrupted waveform produces less heat, and tissues are desiccated rather than vaporized. The collapsed cells form a coagulum, which is hemostatic. If the voltage is increased further (>4000 V), the electrode can be held over the tissue, rather than in direct contact, spraying the electrical energy over a larger area and thereby creating a larger coagulum. This effect is enhanced further with argon plasma beam coagulation (APC). Current is delivered through a beam of ionized argon gas, which distributes the electrons more evenly than spray coagulation alone.

Electrosurgery burns occur when a stray conductor, usually with a small area, comes in contact with the active electrode, creating an alternative circuit for current to flow to the return electrode. The risk is increased if the return electrode pad is badly applied. A pad of adequate size for the weight of the child should be selected and applied to a flat muscular area of the body, to minimize contact resistance. Bony prominences, scar tissue, tattoos, excessively hairy surfaces, pressure points and areas of skin over implanted metal prostheses are unsuitable sites for the return pad.

The use of monopolar electrosurgery in an endoscopic environment brings additional risks. Arcing to metallic instruments in the abdomen (ports, other instruments) is perhaps the most serious complication of laparoscopic electrosurgery. This is often termed 'coupling'. Direct coupling occurs when an active electrode makes unrecognized contact with another metal instrument. This may cause burns and damage which pass unnoticed because they are outside the field of vision. Poor instrument insulation and using the diathermy when not all the instrument tips are within the visual field are risk factors. Capacitative coupling arises when a non-conductor separates two conductors to set up an electrostatic field. This field may discharge at any time, causing tissue damage at the point of discharge. The risk of electrosurgical injury is substantially lessened with bipolar equipment. However, if monopolar diathermy has to be used, the risk of inadvertent tissue damage can be minimized by taking a number of precautions. **(See Box 4.1)**

Box 4.1 Minimizing risk with endoscopic diathermy equipment

- Examine instrument insulation regularly.
- Use lowest possible power settings.
- Use low-voltage (cutting) waveforms for cutting tissues; reserve high-voltage (coagulating) waveforms strictly for coagulation.
- Use brief intermittent electrosurgery activation instead of prolonged activation.
- Do not activate electrosurgery in close proximity to other instruments.
- Metal cannulae are safer than plastic cannulae, and hybrid (metal/plastic) cannulae systems should be avoided.

Modern electrosurgery generators contain sophisticated regulatory circuitry to optimize power delivery and maximize safety. The power output of a conventional electrosurgery machine varies according to the tissues through which current is conducted. Cutting muscle requires a lower power than cutting fat. Autoregulation of the power output enables a consistent effect to be achieved regardless of tissue characteristics. Return electrode monitoring systems minimize the risk of skin damage at the return pad/patient interface by detecting changes in contact resistance. They also ensure that the generator operates within the preset safe parameters. Active electrode monitoring systems are available to monitor the level of stray current between endoscopic electrosurgery instruments and the patient. This minimizes the risk of capacitative coupling.

Bipolar electrosurgery is inherently safer for endoscopic surgery because the risk of coupling is eliminated. It provides precise and very effective coagulation of tissues for hemostasis, but is poor at cutting tissues unless very high voltages are used. Therefore, to overcome this problem, hybrid instruments have been developed, e.g. ultrasonic dissectors with bipolar coagulators, bipolar scissors.

Ultrasound

Ultrasound refers to frequencies between 20 000 and 50 000 Hz, which are inaudible to the human ear. Ultrasonic dissectors, or 'harmonic scalpels', divide tissues with heat generated by friction from a rapidly oscillating instrument tip. All these instruments utilize the piezoelectric effect. Ultrasound waves are generated by applying an electrical potential across the face of a piezoelectric crystal. This causes deformation of the structure of the crystal, which then oscillates at its resonant frequency with an amplitude proportional to the applied potential.

The dissector consists of an electrical generator that regulates the amount of energy delivered, a transducer which converts the electrical energy into ultrasonic waves, and a hand-piece which delivers the energy to the tissues. The basic element of the transducer is a pair of piezoelectric discs coupled together to produce a sinusoidal waveform at the harmonic frequency of the crystal. In practice, the transducer contains a number of crystal pairs sandwiched between two metal cylinders inside the hand-piece. A metal rod is then attached, which forms the operating tip of the instrument. This vibrates at 55 kHz, with an adjustable amplitude of 50–100 μm.

Three phenomena occur at the interface between an ultrasonic dissector and living tissues.

- Cavitation: this occurs as a result of the rapid vibration of the operating tip. Intracellular water is vaporized, with cell death. The cavitation effect is dependent on the water content of the tissues and the frequency and amplitude of the harmonic wave.
- Tissue division: cutting is achieved by a combination of the effect of cavitation and direct tissue trauma from the vibrating tip of the dissector. Temperatures of up to 100 °C are generated at the tip of the dissector, which also contribute to this effect.
- Tissue coaption and hemostasis: this effect is achieved by denaturation of protein to form a coagulum to occlude blood vessels. To achieve this, the walls of a vessel must be coapted because flow through the blood vessel disperses the ultrasound wave. Coagulation occurs best at low energy settings and at a temperature of 37–63 °C.

Optimal tissue division depends on power settings, the shape of the blade tip, pressure exerted on the dissector and tension applied to the tissues. High power settings produce faster cutting but less hemostasis.

Ultrasonic tissue dissection has advantages and disadvantages compared to conventional techniques. Damage to adjacent tissues is limited to 1–2 mm. Blood vessels can be divided in a single stage, avoiding the need for coagulation with Bovie and then division with scissors. Ultrasonic dissection does not generate smoke and the instrument tip does not char. Ultrasonic dissectors work efficiently in fluid-filled compartments.

However, ultrasonic instruments are still large and heavy. The range of instruments is limited and 3 mm equipment is not available. Although the risk of electrical burns is eliminated, there is still a risk of tissue injury from inadvertent contact with the vibrating instrument tip. Ultrasound dissectors are still expensive.

LASER

Laser – light amplification by stimulated emission of radiation – harnesses the ability of atoms to store and emit light. Electrons in the atoms of the lasing medium are first energized, or pumped, to an excited state by an external energy source (e.g. the xenon flash tube in a Ruby LASER) and then 'stimulated' by external photons to emit the stored energy in the form of additional photons, a process known as stimulated emission. The emitted photons are of the same wavelength, travel in the same direction and are in phase with the stimulating photons. These photons in turn collide with other excited atoms to release more photons. Light amplification is achieved as the photons move back and forth between two parallel mirrors, triggering further stimulated emissions. At the same time the intense, directional and monochromatic laser light 'leaks' through one of the mirrors, which is only partially silvered. The beam is then focused and aimed at a target. Definition of beam path and target aiming are usually achieved with a coaxial helium neon laser which produces low-intensity visible red light.

Laser energy has a number of effects on living tissues. Low-level laser energy produces biostimulation. Atomic and molecular excitation occurs without significant thermal effects. Beneficial effects on wound healing and pain relief after sports injuries have been observed. As the energy level is raised, thermal effects predominate. Above 60 °C, coagulation begins as protein denaturation causes tissue contraction. Above 100 °C, intracellular water boils. Above 400 °C, residual debris is burnt. There is little lateral spread of the injury as there is poor thermal contact between destroyed and normal tissue. Laser energy can be pulsed rather than applied continuously. This produces a non-thermal photomechanical effect in the form of a shock wave, which can be used to fragment calculi.

The thermal effects seen in living tissues subjected to laser energy depend partly on structure, water content, pigmentation and perfusion and partly on the properties of the laser beam. The thermal power of a laser beam depends on the following characteristics.

- Beam power: high power causes more tissue destruction.
- Power density: any laser will have a greater effect if delivered to a small area. Power density is calculated by dividing the power by the area of the laser imprint and is measured in watts/cm^2.

Table 4.3 *Laser types and their clinical characteristics*

Type	CO_2	Argon	ND:YAG	KTP
Medium	Gas	Gas	Crystal	Crystal
Wavelength (μm)	10.6 infrared	1.002 red	1.06 infrared	0.532 green
Preferential absorption	Water	Hemoglobin/melanin	Tissue protein	Hemoglobin/melanin
Cutting ability	High	Low	Fair	Low
Hemostatic ability	Low	Fair	High	Fair
Tissue penetration (mm)	<1	2–3	5–7	2–3

- Total energy delivered: the total energy delivered to a tissue area is the output power/second multiplied by the exposure time. Pulsed dye lasers for lithotripsy produce photomechanical effects as a result of an intense discharge of very short duration.
- Wavelength: the CO_2 laser produces infrared light which is absorbed by water. This results in a very superficial thermal injury, with more than 90 percent of the energy absorbed within a distance of 30 μm. Carbon dioxide laser cannot be delivered through fiberoptics and requires a cumbersome system of lenses and mirrors. These constraints limit the use of CO_2 to epithelial surgery, e.g. laryngeal surgery. The Nd:YAG laser also produces infrared light, but at a wavelength of 1064 nm, which is poorly absorbed by water and tissue pigments. As a consequence, the thermal injury in tissues extends to a depth of 5–7 mm with good hemostasis. Argon and KTP lasers both produce visible light (red and green, respectively), which is preferentially absorbed by hemoglobin and melanin. The ensuing thermal injury extends to a distance of 2–3 mm. These lasers can be delivered through fiberoptic cables, which facilitates endoscopic use. **(See Table 4.3)**

Water jet dissection

Water jet dissection uses the force of pulsatile irrigation with crystalloid solutions to separate tissue planes. Hemostasis is poor and early equipment provided unpredictable depth control and excessive mist, which obscured the view of the operative site. Recent technological developments that address these problems include the use of a fine rotating helical jet, which selectively cleaves tissues, and coaxial suction to remove excess spray. Clinical experience remains limited.

LITHOTRIPSY

Mechanical breakdown on the surface of a solid occurs when the tensile force is greater than the strength of the solid. Shock waves from a variety of sources will produce this effect. Some are suitable for endoscopic use and others for extracorporeal lithotripsy.

Endoscopic lithotripsy

ELECTROHYDRAULIC LITHOTRIPTER

Energy is generated from an electrical sparkplug discharge system. The machine was first developed in St Petersburg in the 1930s. An electrical spark lasting 2–5 microseconds is created within a fluid (water) medium. The surrounding water vaporizes, causing a 'cavitation bubble' that expands and then implodes to create a shock wave which fragments the calculus.

Advantages

- Energy is delivered through a thin probe that is suitable for use with rigid and flexible endoscopes.
- Lithotripsy is performed under direct vision.
- Stones may be fragmented sufficiently to retrieve by basket or may pass spontaneously.
- The instrument is compact and relatively inexpensive compared to lasers.

Disadvantages

- The probe will damage any tissue within 2 mm of the active tip.
- It must be used under direct vision.
- There is a risk of luminal perforation if it is used to fragment an impacted ureteric calculus.
- There is no pigment selectivity.

ULTRASONIC LITHOTRIPTER

Energy is generated in a hollow probe that vibrates in four directions. Occasionally, ultrasonic lithotripsy does not cause fragmentation but carves a way through the stone. This is due to a point contact effect rather than a focused shock wave. Stones have to be held rigidly using a Dormia basket for efficient fragmentation.

Disadvantages

- Vibration may cause surrounding tissue damage.
- The instrument is rigid.
- Heat production by the transducer requires continuous cooling of the probe to prevent mucosal injury. This is achieved by irrigation through the endoscope.
- Energy has to be applied in short bursts (10–15 seconds).

PNEUMATIC LITHOTRIPTER

Gas is delivered to the tip of the instrument probe at 5–10 Hz, causing stone fragmentation.

LASER LITHOTRIPTER

Pulsed lasers can be used as an energy source for lithotripsy. Pulsed dye laser (504 nm) acts for 1 ms through a 320 nm core diameter silica-coated quartz fiber to deliver 140 mJ of energy with each pulse. Light is absorbed by the stone and a gaseous plasma is formed on the stone surface. The plasma absorbs subsequent light and expands between the fiber tip and the stone to produce an acoustic shock wave, which causes fragmentation. A brief rise in temperature occurs, but only at the stone surface, thereby not damaging mucosa. Holmium:YAG laser (2100 nm) operates in a 350 ms pulsed mode at 5–30 Hz and energy setting of 0.2–2 J. Cavitation due to vaporization at the stone–fluid interface occurs. This method can damage tissue and the instrument must not come into contact with urothelium.

Extracorporeal lithotripsy

Extracoporeal shock wave lithotripsy (ESWL) was first developed in Munich in the 1970s. A shock wave is produced by a generator outside the body and focused on the stone. Originally, ESWL necessitated acoustic coupling of the shock wave and calculus by partially immersing the patient in a water bath. Most modern machines use a water cushion or an abbreviated bath to achieve the same effect. A number of different shock wave generators are in current use.

SPARK GAP

The shock wave is generated by a spark gap electrical discharge system submerged in a water bath. The spark gap is contained within a Faraday cage to prevent electrical shock. Shock waves in this machine need to be coordinated with the patient's electrocardiograph to prevent arrhythmias.

PIEZOELECTRIC

A high-frequency electrical pulse is used to excite an array of ceramic piezoelectric elements sitting in a concave focusing dish. A wide-aperture focusing dish allows shock waves to enter the body over a large area before the maximum intensity focal point is reached, which reduces discomfort.

ELECTROMAGNETIC

Electrical currents move a metallic membrane within a shock tube to produce waves that are focused by an acoustic lens onto a point of impact. A water cushion is used to transmit the waves into the body.

MICROEXPLOSIVE

Shock waves are produced by lead azide pellet discharges.

MAINTENANCE

Strict national and international standards govern the manufacture of energy generators for clinical use. Regular maintenance is necessary to guarantee continued safety. Despite this, it is imperative that all equipment be checked carefully prior to use.

CONCLUSION

From the range of energy sources available to the endoscopic surgeon, it is obvious that none has proven ideal for all circumstances. All the equipment discussed in this chapter has significant potential to cause unwanted tissue damage with potentially fatal consequences. The choice of equipment depends on suitability and availability and, even more importantly, on personal experience. As the equipment becomes more complicated, the importance of staff training and education increases if problems are to be avoided.

FURTHER READING

Morris PJ, Wood WC (eds). *The Oxford Textbook of Surgery.* Oxford: Oxford University Press, 2000.

Park AE, Mastrangelo MJ Jr, Gandsas A, Chu U, Quick NE. Laparoscopic dissecting instruments. *Seminars in Laparoscopic Surgery* 2001; 8(1):42–52.

5

Instruments used in rigid and flexible endoscopy

PAUL K.H. TAM AND K.K.Y. WONG

INTRODUCTION

In the past 30 years, endoscopy has established itself as an indispensable procedure in both the diagnosis and treatment of many pediatric conditions. In this respect, many accessory instruments have been designed to be used specifically in conjunction with the endoscope. These instruments can broadly be divided into those used for diagnostic procedures and those used for therapeutic purposes. The initial problems with the designs of many accessory instruments for the pediatric population have mainly been technical, namely, the production of miniature instruments small enough to fit inside the working channels of the pediatric endoscopes. These problems have now largely been overcome. Nonetheless, the maximum diameter of the instrument used in the pediatric upper gastrointestinal endoscope is only 2 mm, while the pediatric colonoscope can accommodate instruments of up to 2.8 mm. The relatively small size of these instruments limits their use to biopsy and small treatment areas.

Although the use of flexible endoscopes has superseded that of the rigid ones, rigid endoscopes still remain valuable in performing therapeutic procedures in the airways. The basic use and mechanics of both the rigid and the flexible endoscopes have already been described in detail in previous chapters. This chapter therefore focuses only on the accessory instruments used. Although the majority of the instruments described below are for use in the flexible endoscope, a number of similar instruments can also be used in rigid endoscopes. This chapter divides the instruments into two main sections: those used in diagnosis and those used in treatment.

INSTRUMENTS FOR DIAGNOSTIC USE

Lavage/aspiration cytology

A simple tube can be fit inside the working channel of the endoscope (rigid or flexible). The end of the tube can be connected to suction via a collecting jar. Fluids or secretions can be kept and sent for cytology. **(See Figure 5.1)**

Biopsy forceps

The jaws of these forceps are opened and closed via a single wire pulley mechanism. Many different shapes have been developed, including simple non-toothed forceps and those with alligator-type jaws. The size of the specimen obtained

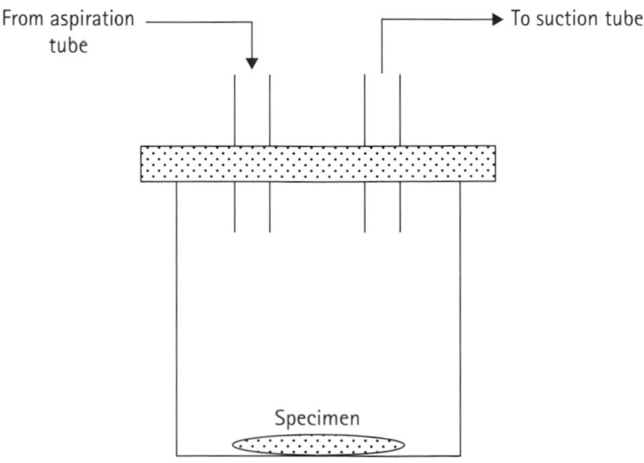

Figure 5.1

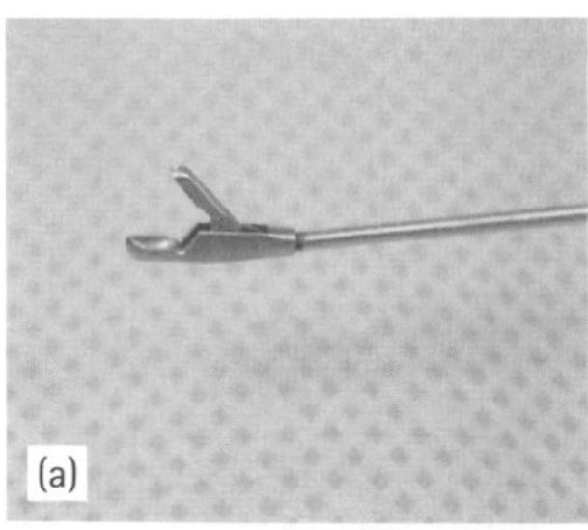

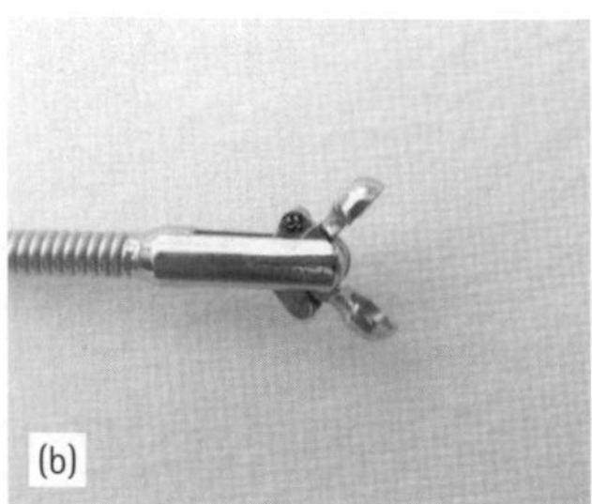

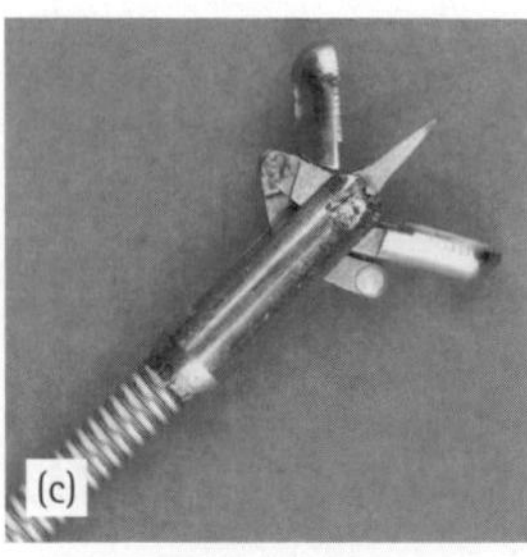

Figure 5.2 *Biopsy forceps. (a) single action jaws; (b) double action jaws; (c) double action with a needle.*

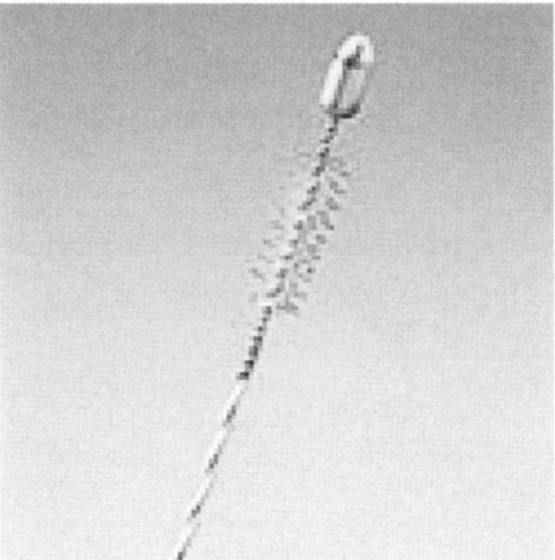

Figure 5.3

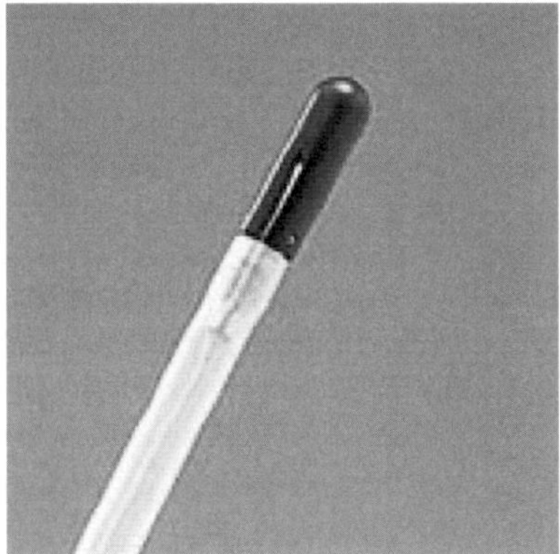

Figure 5.4

is dependent upon both the depth and the length of the cup. In some biopsy forceps, a needle can be present in the center of the cup to minimize slippage on the mucosa and to help secure the specimen. Bipolar diathermy instruments can also be attached to specially designed biopsy forceps ('hot biopsy forceps') for the removal of small polyps. (**See Figure 5.2**)

Brush biopsy

These are designed to collect tissue samples under direct observation and comprise a cytology brush with a bullet-shaped distal tip. Cells for cytology are collected by a combination of rotation and withdrawal. Cytology brushes are also equipped with a radio-opaque sheath and an injection port for contrast media. Brush biopsy can be useful in obtaining specimens from the biliary system during endoscopic retrograde cholangiopancreoatgram (ERCP) or in bronchoscopy. (**See Figure 5.3**)

Ultrasound probe

The use of endoluminal ultrasound has improved the accuracy of detecting abnormal lesions due to the decrease in distance between the scanning probe and the organ to be scanned. Although special endoscopes with the capability of ultrasound have been developed, the purchase of an extra set of hardware can be a financial burden. Instead, an ultrasonic probe can be used which allows the endoscopist to perform ultrasound examination using any endoscope with a channel diameter of 2.8 mm or more. With this probe, the procedure can be performed like a biopsy during a routine endoscopy. It is particularly useful in the examination and diagnosis of lesions where an ultrasonic endoscope cannot pass, such as in luminal stricture. However, the limitation is that as the working channel of the endoscope is occupied by the ultrasound probe, real-time biopsy of any lesion found is not possible. (**See Figure 5.4**)

INSTRUMENTS FOR THERAPEUTIC USE

This section is subdivided according to different therapeutic procedures.

Foreign body retrieval

Foreign body ingestion is one of the most common reasons for emergency pediatric admissions. Although a rigid endoscope has traditionally been used for the retrieval of foreign bodies, flexible endoscopes are now the preferred choice. Foreign body aspiration is less common, but potentially life threatening. The removal of a foreign body from the airways is best achieved with ventilating rigid bronchoscopy. Different types of instruments can be used for this purpose.

GRASPING FORCEPS

The underlying working mechanism of grasping forceps is similar to that of biopsy forceps except that they provide

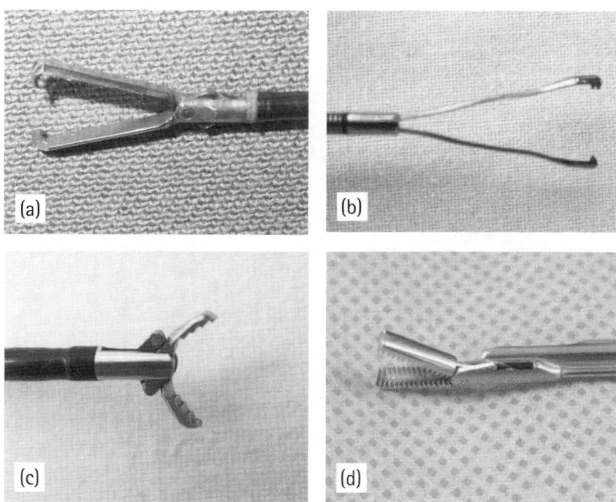

Figure 5.5 *Grasping forceps. (a) rat teeth; (b) prongs; (c) less traumatic; (d) alligator.*

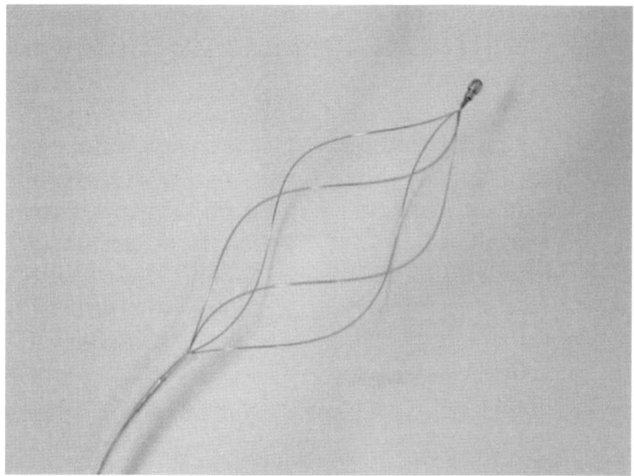

Figure 5.6

better grip and grasping force. Different grasping forceps have been designed, including W-shaped forceps with more pronounced rat teeth, which provide exceptional grasping force, and tripod and pentapod type prongs, which can collect polyps with minimal tissue damage. (**See Figure 5.5**)

RETRIEVAL BASKET

Retrieval baskets can be an alternative to grasping forceps. They are particularly useful for collecting round and slippery objects. The basket at the distal end is opened and closed by a push and pull action using the control at the proximal end. (**See Figure 5.6**)

FOGARTY CATHETER

Vegetable material such as peanuts may sometimes be firmly impacted in the bronchus and difficult to retrieve without

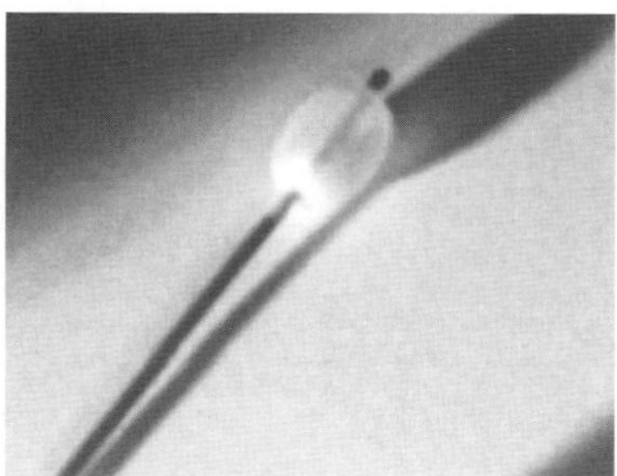

Figure 5.7

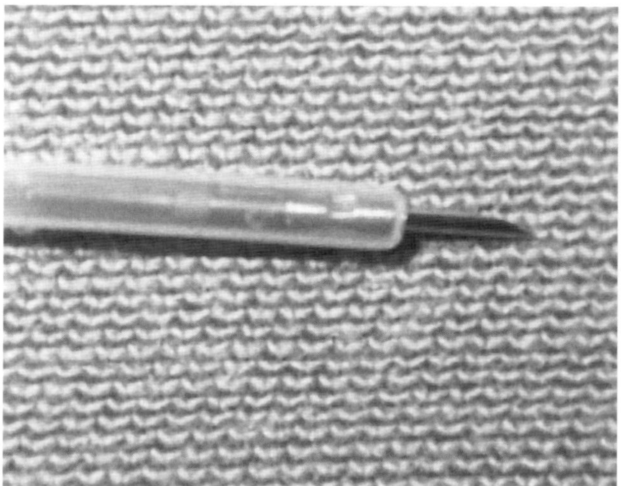

Figure 5.8

fragmentation using forceps. A Fogarty catheter can be used as an alternative and the foreign body can be retrieved upon withdrawal of the bronchoscope and catheter together. (**See Figure 5.7**)

Esophageal varices

Esophageal varices can lead to significant blood loss in pediatric patients with portal hypertension. Varices can be treated by the injection of ethanolamine, a sclerosing agent, clips or band ligation.

INJECTION NEEDLES

Injection needles are particularly useful for sclerotherapy in the treatment of esophageal varices. The needle at the distal end is covered by either a stainless steel or Teflon® sheath. The sheath can be closed or retracted by finger control at the proximal end for easy, safe needle insertion. (**See Figure 5.8**)

BAND/CLIP APPLICATOR

Reliable hemostasis can also be achieved by mechanical means, in the form of either band ligation or clips. Band

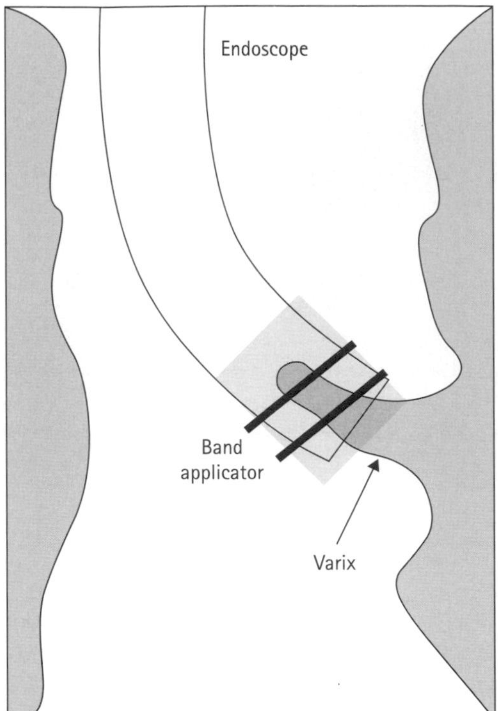

Figure 5.9

ligation is sometimes used for the treatment of esophageal varices. The procedure can be performed when the band applicator is used in conjunction with a distal attachment (straight with rim type). **(See Figure 5.9)**

Clips are also available for a wide range of situations. In some cases, hemostatic clipping may provide almost instant control of gastrointestinal bleeding, which is achieved more rapidly than with electrosurgical and other hemostatic techniques. **(See Figure 5.10)**

Bleeding peptic ulcer

HEATER PROBE

The heater probe controls gastrointestinal bleeding by thermal coagulation. There is a Teflon® coating on the probe tip to minimize tissue adhesion, and a hollow aluminum cylinder with an inner heating coil inside the probe. A thermocoupling device at the tip of the probe maintains a constant temperature. Irrigation ports on the probe tip permit water jets to wash the coagulation site. The amount of heat energy delivered can be adjusted by energy control at the generator or the length of time the probe is in contact with tissue. **(See Figure 5.11)**

INJECTION NEEDLES

The use of injection needles for the treatment of bleeding peptic ulcers is similar to that for esophageal varices (described above). In this case, epinephrine is injected.

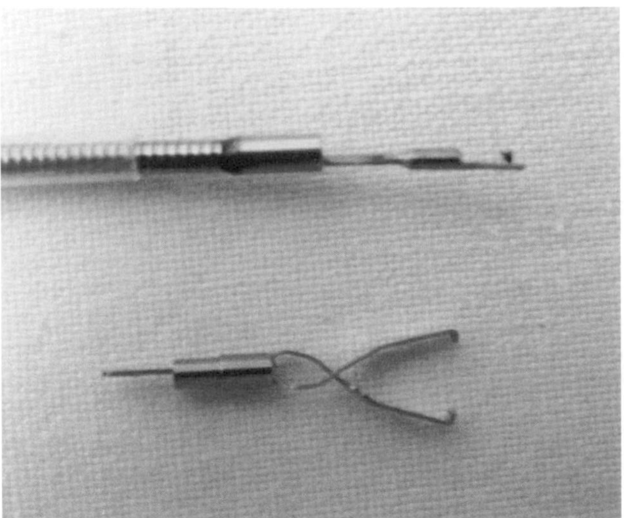

Figure 5.10

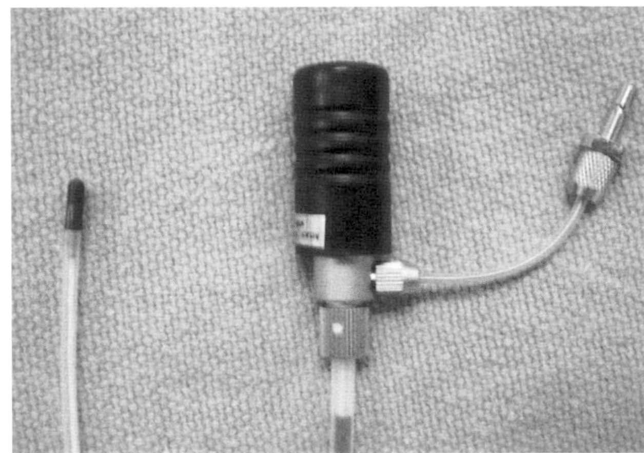

Figure 5.11

CLIP APPLICATOR

The use of clips for hemostasis in the treatment of esophageal varices has been described. Clips can also be applied in a similar way for the treatment of bleeding peptic ulcers.

Endoscopic retrograde cholangio-pancreatogram

Since gall-stone diseases are seen rarely in children, ERCP is performed only infrequently. The main indications for ERCP in the pediatric population are biliary anomalies such as choledochal cyst, anomalous pancreatico-biliary junction and, in some institutions, biliary atresia. The advent of magnetic resonance cholangiopancreatography (MRCP) and other imaging modalities, e.g. ultrasound, computed tomography (CT) etc., has further limited the need of ERCP for the diagnosis of biliary diseases in children. The issue of performing sphincterotomy for common bile

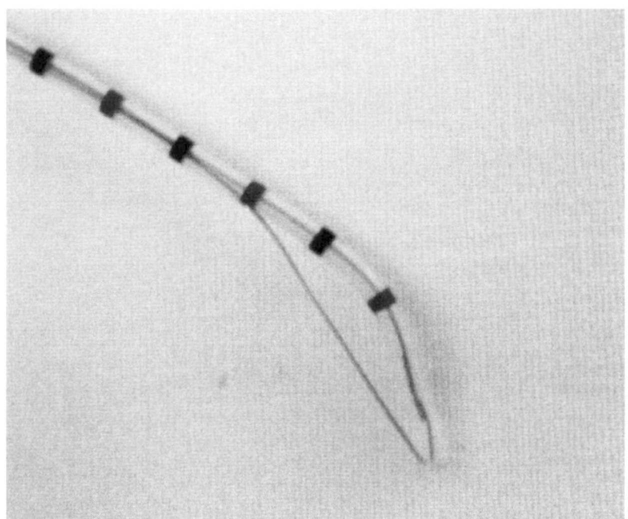

Figure 5.12

duct stones remains controversial in the pediatric population due to possible long-term sequelae.

SPHINCTEROTOMY

The sphincterotomy knife has stiffening wires incorporated into the lumens of the catheter at the distal part. Cannulation of the common bile duct can therefore be performed with significant stability. Markings on the sheath in the distal end indicate the center and the actual cutting portion of the knife. Clear fluoroscopic visualization can be achieved due to the radio-opaque tip. (**See Figure 5.12**)

POLYPECTOMY

SNARES

Juvenile polyps are a relatively common cause of per rectum bleeding in children and can be removed with snares during colonoscopy. Snares of various shapes are available, and there are also different loop sizes with different wire opening widths. The proximal end of the snare is attached to an electrocautery circuit during snaring so that polypectomy can be performed safely and efficiently with hemostasis. (**See Figure 5.13**)

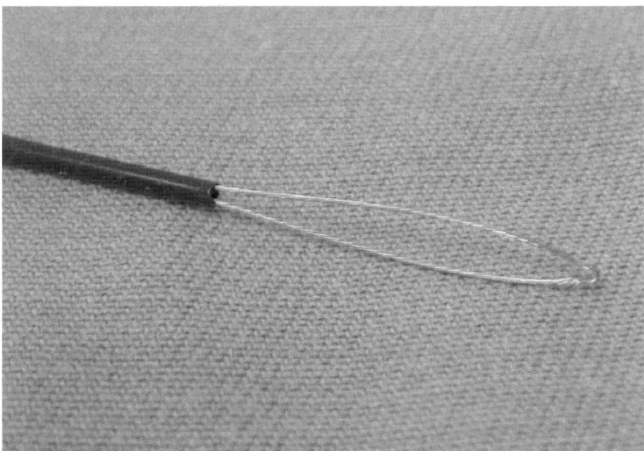

Figure 5.13

Treatment of strictures/stenosis

In the pediatric population, benign strictures are seen more often than malignant strictures. Strictures can be either congenital or acquired; examples of acquired gastrointestinal strictures include esophageal stricture following repair of esophageal atresia or after caustic injury, pyloric stenosis complicating peptic ulcer, and colonic strictures complicating neonatal enterocolitis. Achalasia and hypertrophic pyloric stenosis are more effectively treated surgically than endoscopically. Severe tracheo-laryngomalacia, extrinsic compression (for example from cystic hygroma), and congenital tracheal stenosis will result in narrowing of the airway lumen. Strictures or stenosis can be treated by balloon dilatation, stent insertion or laser ablation.

BALLOON DILATATION

Balloon dilatation has become established as a method for the treatment of esophageal strictures. Traditionally, a radio-opaque guide-wire is first passed through the stricture under endoscopic guidance. Then, with the aid of fluoroscopy, the endoscope is removed and the balloon catheter is slid past the stricture over the guide-wire. With better-designed scopes, both the balloon and guide-wire can be inserted through the working channel at the same time. Various types of guide-wires are available. The authors' preference is to use a straight Teflon®-coated stainless steel guide-wire with a soft tip at one end. The wire is first released from the locked position and advanced distally from the central lumen of the balloon catheter. The floppy tip is then positioned across the stricture using combined endoscopic and fluoroscopic visualization. Once satisfied with positioning, the balloon catheter is advanced over the guide-wire to be at the center of the stricture. With modern catheters, different dilatation sizes can be achieved using different inflation pressures. (**See Figure 5.14**)

For esophageal dilatation, the 'rule of thumb' – the size of the balloon catheter should not exceed that of the patient's thumb – is a useful guide to minimize the risk of iatrogenic perforation.

STENTS

Stents can also be used in the treatment of benign luminal strictures. They are usually made from inert metals that elicit little foreign body reaction and provide a constant radial force to resist any possible collapse of the lumen. There are two main types of stents: self-expandable

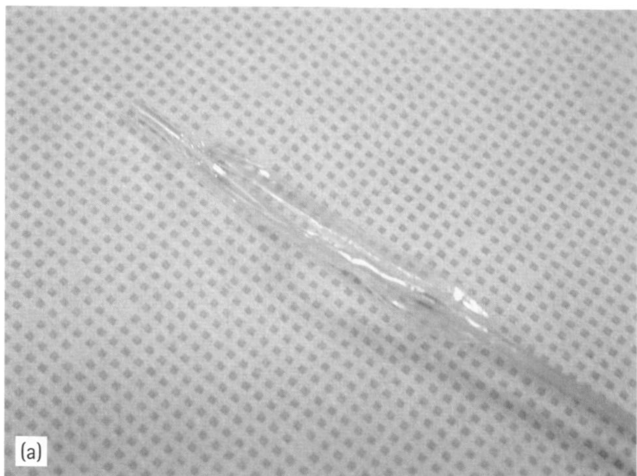

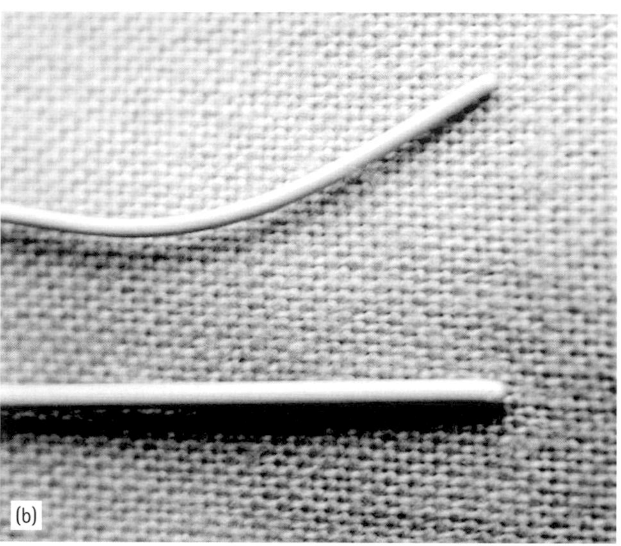

Figure 5.14 *(a) Balloon; (b) teflon-coated guide-wire.*

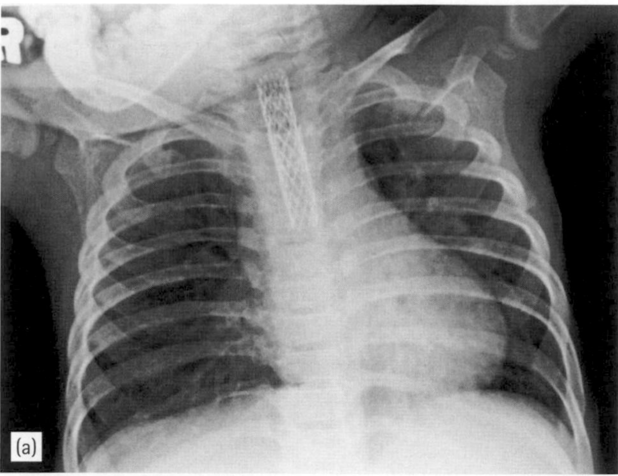

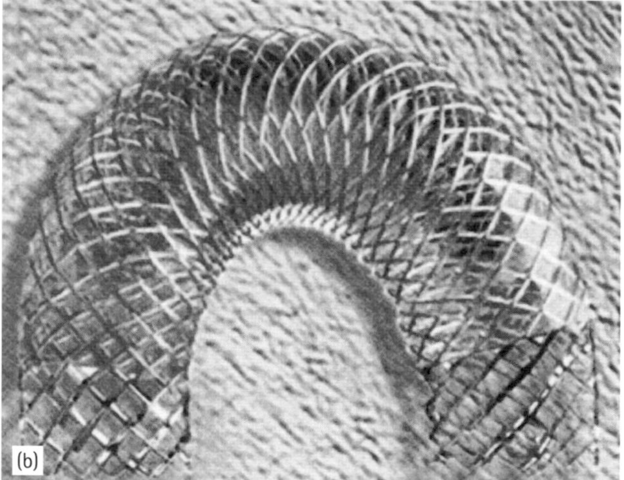

Figure 5.15 *(a) Stent in position; (b) inert mental stent.*

and balloon-expandable. Self-expandable stents are pre-mounted and covered by sheaths. The pre-mounted stent is inserted in a similar fashion to the balloon catheter under endoscopic and fluoroscopic guidance. Once the correct position is attained, the sheath is retracted and the stent is released in situ. Balloon-expandable stents are mounted manually onto the distal tip of balloon catheters before the procedure. These stents have one advantage over the self-expandable stents in that the lumen diameter can be further increased if required. Stent insertion can provide a safe and effective method for the treatment of tracheal stenosis. (**See Figure 5.15**)

LASER

Laser technology represents a practical demonstration of the power of radiant energy and the properties of light amplification. CO_2 and Nd:YAG lasers are most commonly used in endoscopic therapy. Because of its long wavelength, the CO_2 laser currently requires an articulating arm and series of mirrors to apply this therapy and is thus most commonly used in otolaryngology for the management of lesions in the area around the glottic opening. The Nd:YAG laser is more commonly used in the pulmonary area by virtue of the fact that it can be delivered by a flexible cable.

MAINTENANCE AND CLEANING OF ACCESSORY INSTRUMENTS

To avoid unnecessary breakage, the accessory instruments should not be handled with force. Most of the instruments used in endoscopic procedures can be re-used and therefore have to be maintained and cleaned properly, in much the same way as endoscopes. The instrument is immersed in detergent solution immediately after use and left to soak. If the instrument has a channel, it is essential to wash the channel by flushing it with detergent solution. The instrument can also be cleaned ultrasonically for 30 minutes. Following cleaning, the detergent is rinsed off the instrument by running it under clean water. The inside channel is also flushed with water. The instrument is then lubricated on both the outside and inside. The exterior is wiped and the instrument is left to air dry. If sterilization is required, the instrument can be coiled in a sterile pack and autoclaved at 132 °C for 5 minutes.

Proper maintenance of accessory instruments can prolong their lifetime and thus help to reduce the need for frequent re-purchase.

CONCLUSION

From the early days of performing rigid endoscopy for diagnostic purposes only, to the complex therapeutic procedures performed through flexible endoscopes today, endoscopy has come a long way over a relatively short period of time. However, these complex procedures can only be done with the aid of accessory instruments. As technical excellence advances, more sophisticated instruments will become available for use in the pediatric population.

6

Instruments used in urinary tract endoscopy

PETER M. CUCKOW AND KALPANA K. PATIL

INTRODUCTION

The innovations of a rod-lens optical system by Harold H. Hopkins in 1959 and fiberoptic light transmission by Karl Storz in 1960 brought about a revolution in urological endoscopy. In the last four decades the number of possible endo-urological interventions has increased and this has dramatically reduced the need for open surgery. Advances in the management of children have lagged behind those in adult practice, principally due to the size of the pediatric urethra. In an infant boy the caliber of the urethral meatus is approximately 8 Fr, the proximal urethra and bladder neck are often difficult to negotiate and, unless care is taken, trauma is a likely consequence of rigid instrumentation. In girls there are fewer restrictions, as the urethra is shorter, more compliant and straight. Technological progress has brought ever-smaller endoscopes with better illumination and camera technology that can produce clear images from within the smallest infant and even fetal urinary tracts. Optimization of instrument channel size, miniaturization of instruments to use down it and the development of new modalities of power application (laser, electrohydraulic lithotripsy and ultrasound) as well as diathermy allow therapeutic interventions to be carried out.

ENDOSCOPES FOR THE LOWER URINARY TRACT

Endoscopy of the lower tract in children is usually performed per urethra under general anesthetic with a rigid endoscope. Local anesthetic flexible endoscopy has limited application and its use is probably restricted to compliant adolescent patients. Flexible endoscopes do have an application in the reconstructed patient, however (see below).

Rigid endoscopes

There are four basic components to a rigid endoscope: the telescope, the light source, the sheath and the instrument/ irrigation channel(s). The telescope conveys the image back to the eyepiece and, usually nowadays through a camera system, to a video monitor.

Most lower tract telescopes employ a Hopkins rod lens, which produces clear, high-resolution images at the eyepiece. In some makes of telescope, and in particular the smaller ones, fiberoptics are used instead for image transmission. In this case the resolution of the image is limited by the number of fibers in the telescope and may have a 'pixelated' appearance, similar to that seen in flexible telescopes.

The angle of view from the end of the telescope varies from 0° to 70°. Zero-degree telescopes look straight ahead and are most useful for urethroscopy. Orientation with the camera is easiest, and many interventions such as the 'sting', ureteric cannulation and ureterocele puncture are performed in line with the end of the telescope. Whilst 70° telescopes provide the best visual access to the bladder mucosa, they are the most difficult to orientate and are rarely needed in pediatric practice. Thirty-degree telescopes represent a good compromise for diagnostic endoscopy of both the urethra and bladder, but a 0° telescope should also be available for interventions.

Illumination is provided from a remote 'cold' light source via a fiberoptic cable that is attached to a light port on the top or the side of the instrument. Light from here is transmitted to the end of the instrument by optic fibers that run its length and end adjacent to the lens. These are incorporated into the telescope in two-piece instruments. The degree of illumination is directly proportional to the number of fibers.

The instrument and irrigation channels are often combined in a single channel in pediatric endoscopes. This enables the instruments to be of optimal size, but the flow rate of the irrigation (and thus the ability to obtain a satisfactory view) is compromised when an instrument fills the channel. The connections for irrigation and the instrument channel are usually separate, however. The irrigation tube is attached via a Luer-Lok™ port, which is usually on the side of the instrument, and there is an integral tap to control the flow of irrigation. Instrument ports are more in line with the lumen of the instrument and allow rigid and semi-rigid instruments/catheters to be passed. They also have a tap that is closed when they are not in use to prevent loss of irrigation pressure, which is minimized when the port is open by means of a removable plastic nipple that provides a close seal around the instrument.

The outer sheath contains all of the above and its external diameter determines the size of the endoscope – usually expressed by its external circumference in millimeters (the so-called 'French' scale).

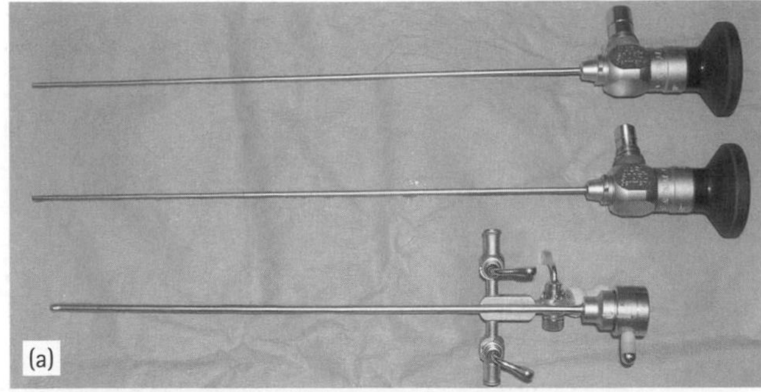

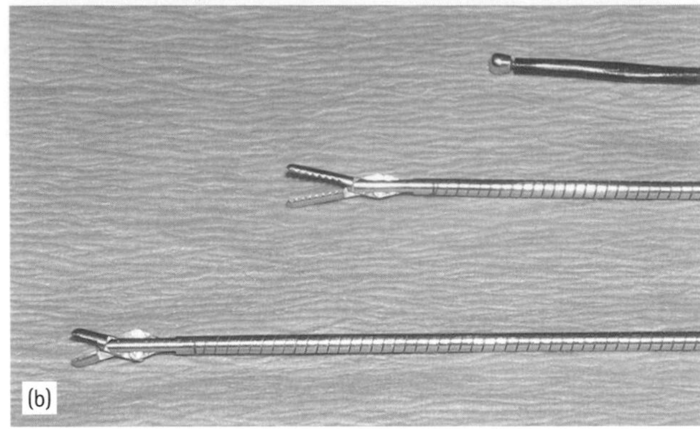

Figure 6.1 *(a) 0° and 30° telescopes and a sheath with irrigation and one working channel; (b) Bugabee electrode, grasping forceps and biopsy forceps.*

Conventional two-piece endoscopes

These are miniaturized versions of the classical adult-type endoscope. Endoscopes with a 0° and 30° telescope are good all-rounders for diagnostic cystoscopy and minor interventions in children. Their channel size permits the passage of insulated diathermy ('Bugabee') electrodes, injection needles (for the 'sting' or bulking injections for continence), guidewires, ureteric catheters and ureteric stents. Specially designed flexible graspers (for stent manipulation and removal) and small biopsy forceps are available, although the latter are only able to take small and often quite superficial biopsies. Baskets, graspers, laser fibers and other instruments for the treatment of bladder and lower ureteric stones are also available. The telescopes may be shared with pediatric resectoscopes, which add further to their versatility. **(See Figure 6.1, Table 6.1)**

An internal blunt-ended trocar locks into the sheath and facilitates its 'blind' passage, although most pediatric instrumentation is performed under direct vision. The telescope connects into the sheath with a watertight locking mechanism at its proximal end.

Unfortunately, optimization of channel size within their small diameter has led to increased malleability of the sheaths of these endoscopes. Heavy-handed use in a large patient or a tight channel (e.g. a scarred Mitrofanoff channel) leads to bending, which soon renders them in need of repair. Flexing of the endoscope against a fixed fulcrum will produce a crescenteric defect in the field of view (e.g. when levering against the pubic symphysis to see the dome of the bladder). This should be taken as a warning that too much force is being used and that the endoscope could be irreversibly damaged.

Table 6.1 *Pediatric two-piece endoscopes*

	Size (Fr)	Angle of vision (°)	Working channel (Fr)	Working length (mm)
Wolf	10.5	0 and 25	5	160
Storz	9.5, 11, 13, 14.5	0 and 30	4, 5, 4, 5	140
Olympus	11–15	0 and 30	5	160

These instruments are most useful in the younger patient, although they are too large for neonatal male urethras. The pubertal male urethra is too long and the bladder too large to be effectively illuminated by their relatively few light fibers. Urologists with older patients and an adolescent practice, in particular, will benefit from having the larger models or small adult endoscopes.

Resectoscopes

In these instruments there is an additional 'working bridge' between the telescope and a correspondingly shorter sheath. Instruments are fixed to the bridge, which can be moved by the operator's forefinger to extend them beyond the end of the sheath and perform simple procedures under direct

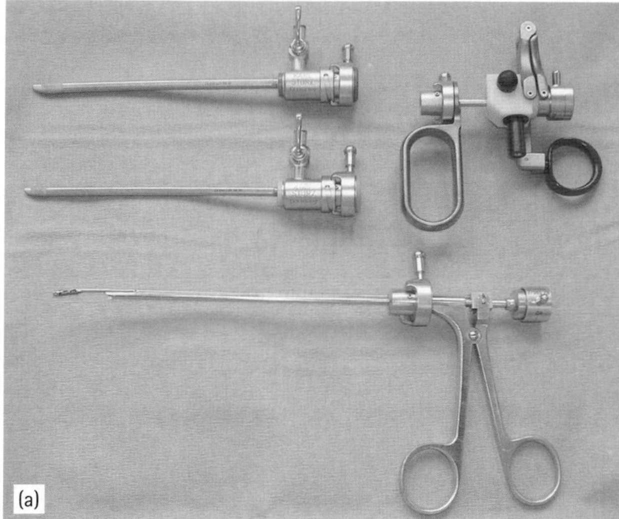

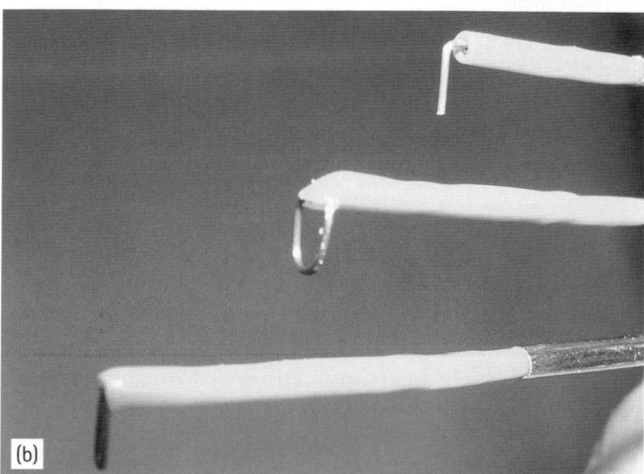

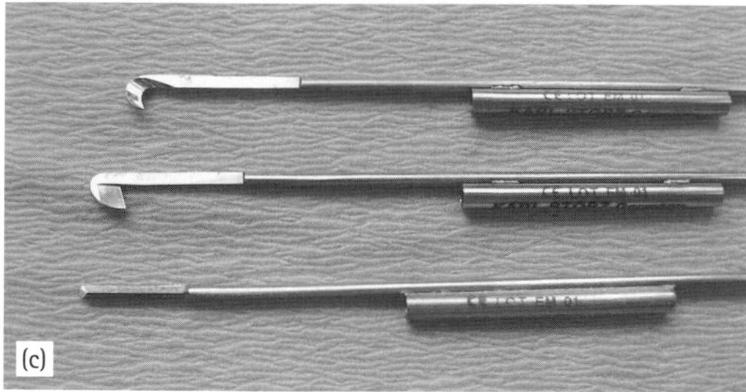

Figure 6.2 *(a) Resectoscope and an integrated biopsy forceps; (b) diathermy electrodes; (c) cold knives.*

vision, usually through a 0° telescope. Insulated sheaths allow diathermy to be applied safely, and loops or hook electrodes permit fulguration or transurethral resection of tissue. Alternatively, there is a selection of cold knives that cut either back towards the telescope or parallel with the line of the instrument. These instruments are useful in the management of posterior and anterior urethral valves, urethral stricture disease (usually iatrogenic in children) and other urethral pathology. **(See Figure 6.2)**

Table 6.2 *Resectoscopes*

	Sheath size (Fr)	Angle of vision (°)	Telescope (mm)
Wolf	8.5, 9, 11.5	0	1.9
			1.9
			2.7
Storz	11, 13	0 and 30	1.9
Olympus	10	0 and 30	1.9

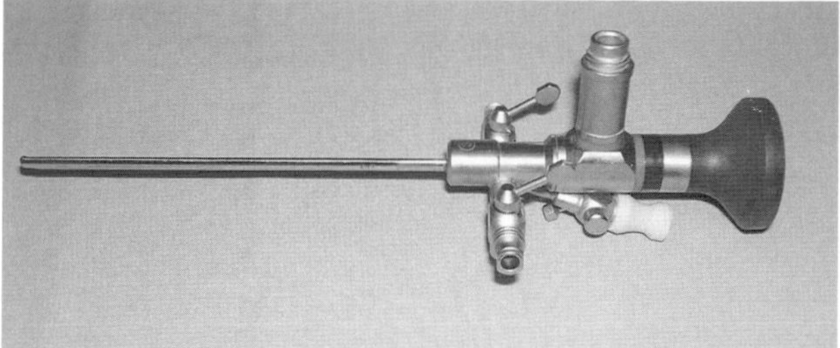

Figure 6.3

There are limited applications for endoscopic bladder resection in children, but biopsies are often needed for diagnostic purposes. An alternative working bridge is available with integral cup biopsy forceps. Although the view is limited with this type of instrument, it allows deep biopsies to be taken which are of greater diagnostic value than those taken with the smaller instruments discussed above. Some surgeons also prefer these for stent removal. If used without their working instruments, an alternative bridge with a large instrument channel may be used for passing larger stents. An Ehrlich's evacuator can be attached to the sheath to wash out blood and clots or stone fragments from the bladder. **(See Table 6.2)**

All-in-one cystoscopes

The need to miniaturize whilst retaining optical quality and a useable instrument and irrigation channel led to the development of small endoscopes in which all the basic elements are combined in a one-piece instrument. These are particularly useful in neonatal male urethras and small channels, where a larger instrument may be traumatic. They are significantly smaller, and their instrument channel may only admit a guide-wire or small ureteric catheter. The authors use these telescopes particularly for the initial fulguration of posterior urethral valves, puncture of ureteroceles and the assessment of neonates with intersex anomalies. **(See Figure 6.3, Table 6.3)**

Apart from their small size, a practical disadvantage of these instruments is the inability to empty the bladder compared to two-piece cystoscopes, with which this can be achieved quite rapidly via the empty sheath on removal of the telescope. Passing a separate catheter or infant feeding tube may be required instead. In addition, their fixed angle

Table 6.3 *'All-in-one' compact cystoscopes*

	Size (Fr)	Angle of vision (°)	Working channel (Fr)	Working length (mm)
Wolf	4.5/6	0	2.4	110
	6/7.5	0	4	140
	10.5	25	5	160
Storz	7.5, 10	0	3.5	110
Olympus	7.9	0 and 30	5	160

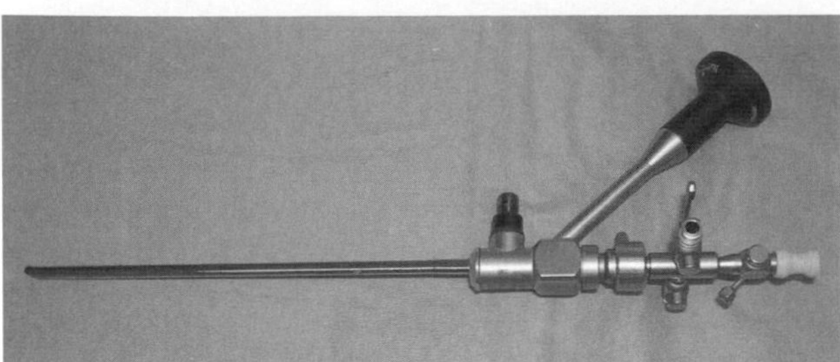

Figure 6.4

of view makes them less versatile and interventions are very limited with the smaller channel.

In some all-in-one cystoscopes, the eyepiece is angled away from the line of the instrument, which is achieved by a deflecting lens. The irrigation/instrument channel runs unimpeded through the middle, which may be particularly useful in larger versions (10 Fr and above) developed for injection therapy or the STING. The straight channel prevents the needle from bending and allows it to be manipulated in line. This also facilitates stent insertion and other interventions. **(See Figure 6.4)**

Flexible endoscopes

Developed for day-case local anesthetic cystoscopy in adult practice, these instruments are too large for most pediatric endoscopy, which is also invariably performed under general anesthesia. Access to the bladder in pediatric patients is generally very good with the range of rigid endoscopes available. The image obtained by a flexible endoscope is inferior to that from a rigid endoscope due to its fiberoptic image transmission. The instrument itself is also much more expensive.

The tip of the instrument flexes in one dimension by a control wire system attached to a lever in the handle, usually activated by the operator's right thumb. By combining this flexion with advancing and rotating the instrument, the tip can be steered into otherwise inaccessible places. Orientation is more difficult than with rigid instruments, but can be achieved with reference to fixed points such as the bladder neck and ureteric orifices. There are a few situations in the authors' practice in which flexible cystoscopes are useful, and they are available to borrow from adult urological colleagues. For example, screening endoscopy of reconstructed bladders may be difficult due to a narrow reconstructed bladder neck. Using the Mitrofanoff channel for access provides a limited view with a rigid instrument, whereas the whole bladder can be seen with a flexible cystoscope. Simple instrumentations – for example stent removal or bladder biopsy via a Mitrofanoff – are possible.

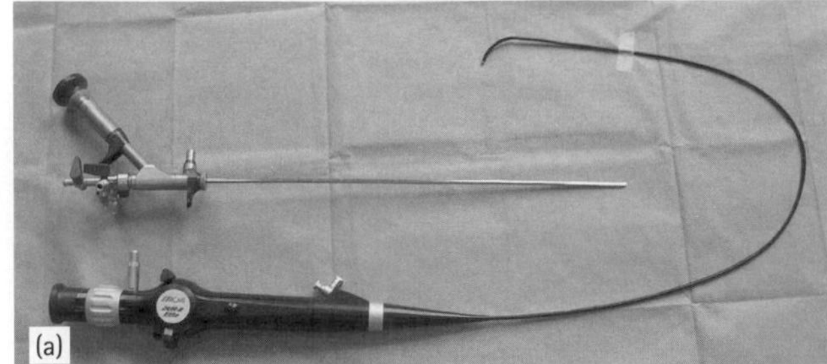

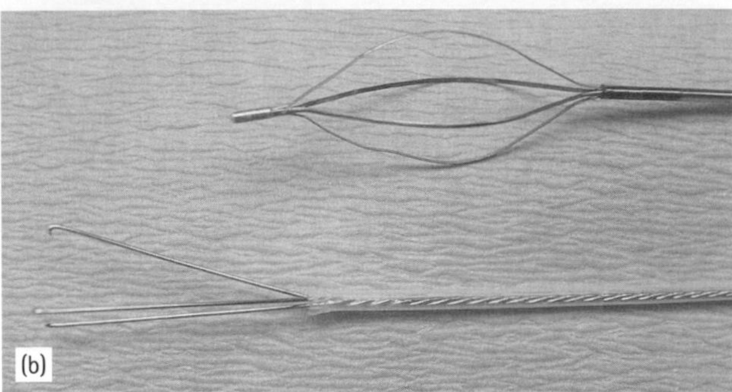

Figure 6.5 *(a) Rigid and flexible ureteroscopes; (b) basket and tripod graspers.*

INSTRUMENTS FOR THE UPPER URINARY TRACT

The upper urinary tract (ureter, renal pelvis and calices) can be instrumented from below via the urethra, from above percutaneously, or directly by laparoscopy (see later chapters). Access from below is with rigid or flexible ureteroscopes.

Rigid ureteroscopes

The availability of rigid or semi-rigid pediatric ureteroscopes has added a new dimension to per-urethral diagnostic endoscopy. These instruments allow visualization of the ureter at least to the level of the pelvi-ureteric junction. Occasionally, the renal pelvis is reached and 'in line' calices are seen. The use of fiberoptics for visualization as well as illumination allows these endoscopes to flex a little without loss of image, reducing the risk of trauma to the ureter, which is nonetheless a significant risk. The image quality is correspondingly inferior to the rod-lens telescopes. **(See Figure 6.5, Table 6.4)**

The diameter of the distal portion of these telescopes is tapered to provide better access to the ureteric orifice (hence

Table 6.4 *Semi-rigid pediatric ureteroscopes*

	Size (Fr)	Direction of view (°)	Irrigation and instrument channel (Fr)	Working length (mm)
Wolf	4.5/6	0	3	310
Storz	7.5/11	5	5.5	340
Olympus	6.5	7	4.2	430
	6.4–7.8	7	4.2	330

the two sizes quoted for some). By pressurizing the irrigation fluid with an external pressure bag, the orifice and ureter are dilated hydrostatically to enable cannulation. The eyepiece is offset to provide a straight, unimpeded channel. For interventions, small graspers, stone baskets and laser fibers are available to fit the 3 Fr instrument channel, as well as small biopsy forceps. The management of ureteric stones is the most common application for these instruments in children, although the authors have also removed retained stents and biopsied ureteric tumors.

Flexible ureteroscopes

Flexible ureteroscopy, combined with a holmium-YAG laser, gives access to the calices from the urethra, and has growing applications in the management of pediatric stone disease. Two-dimensional flexibility of the tip is similar to the flexible cystoscope and enables negotiation of the pelviureteric junction. Acquiring this expensive and fragile instrument will be hard to justify, however, for most pediatric urologists, but it may be loaned from adult colleagues or even hired for a given case. The 5 Fr instrument is very delicate and has a limited lifespan, which may be considerably shortened by inexpert use.

Nephroscopes

The development of percutaneous nephrolithotomy was delayed in pediatric practice until the arrival of smaller endoscopes and a corresponding reduction in the size of track required. Following puncture of the chosen calyx with a guide-wire, a track is formed through the parenchyma using dilators. An Amplatz sheath is placed in this track to tamponade the bleeding and provide access for the telescope. Careful selection of the initial entry point will determine the access available and the success of the procedure. Occasionally, more than one puncture is required. Certainly the assistance of a skilled uro-radiologist is invaluable. **(See Table 6.5)**

Eyepieces are offset and the instrument channels are the largest of any pediatric endoscopes. High-volume irrigation down the endoscope and back out through the sheath prevents bleeding from obscuring the view. All types of power application can be used, but the principal types are the ultrasound probe and the electrohydraulic lithotripter.

Table 6.5 *Pediatric nephroscopes*

	Size (Fr)	Angle of vision (°)	Working channel (Fr)	Working length (mm)
Wolf	15.9	7	7.5	220
Storz	11–15	7	7.5	220
Olympus	11/15.9	7	7.5	220

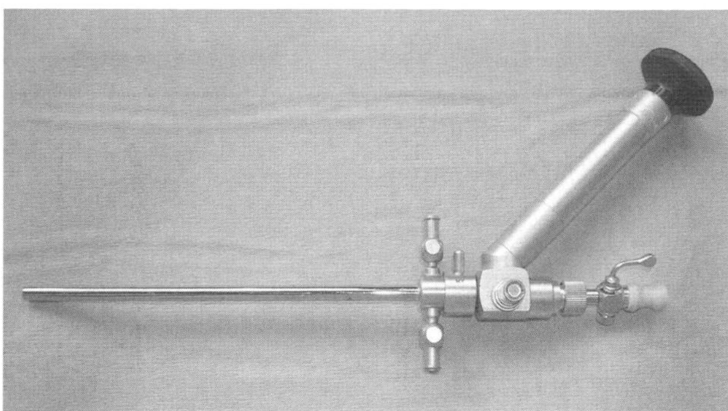

Figure 6.6

Stone fragments are either washed out or removed with graspers. **(See Figure 6.6)**

FETOSCOPY

Endoscopy of the amniotic cavity during pregnancy is a well established, if infrequently used, modality for clarification of fetal anomalies and occasional interventions. Smaller 1.3 mm diameter rigid endoscopes are used and provide access to the bladder by direct puncture through the fetal abdominal wall. This procedure has been performed with a laser fiber for antegrade ablation of posterior urethral valves in the fetus. The technique remains unproven and is limited to a few centers.

FURTHER READING

Aubert D, Rigaud P, Zoupanos G. Double pigtail ureteral stent in pediatric urology. *European Journal of Pediatric Surgery* 1993; 3(5):281–3.

Choong S, Whitfield H, Duffy P et al. The management of paediatric urolithiasis. *British Journal of Urology International* 2000; **86**(7):857–60.

Cockett WS, Cockett AT. The Hopkins rod lens system and the Storz cold light illumination. *Urology* 1998; **51**(5A Suppl.):1–2.

Cuckow PM. Posterior urethral valves. In: Stringer MD, Oldham KT, Mouriquand PDE, Howard ER (eds). *Paediatric Surgery and Urology: Long Term Outcomes.* London: WB Saunders, 1998, 487–500.

Linder TE, Simmen D, Stool SE. Revolutionary inventions in the 20th century.

The history of endoscopy. *Archives of Otolaryngology- Head and Neck Surgery* 1998; **124**(9):1042.

7

Instruments for laparoscopy and thoracoscopy

MARC A. LEVITT AND JOSELITO G. TANTOCO

INTRODUCTION

From the Latin *instrumentum*, an instrument is an implement or tool used for precision work whereby something is achieved, performed or furthered. To achieve the benefits of endoscopic surgery such as less postoperative pain, shorter hospital stays, quicker return to normal activities, and superior cosmetic results, the endoscopic surgeon needs the appropriate tools. The need for elegant and precise instrument is particularly important in pediatric operations.

The introduction of endoscopic surgery presented the surgeon with challenges different from those of traditional open surgery. The surgeon is separated from direct contact with tissues and organs. Tissues are handled and dissected using long instruments, and images are viewed on video monitors positioned across the patient.

Unlike open surgery, in endoscopic surgery the flexibility of the surgeon to approach the surgical field from various directions is limited, visualization is impaired and tactile feedback is significantly dampened. Reversal of movement secondary to the fulcrum effect at the point of instrument entry further compounds the problem. Basic surgical maneuvers such as exposure, tissue dissection, vascular control, suturing and knot tying, and tissue extraction become technical challenges. The problems are not limited to the surgeon performing the procedure, as the surgical assistant needs to hold the telescope and assisting instruments while the surgeon operates.

There are many inherent problems encountered with conventional endoscopic surgery. A common 'language' must be developed so that the individual holding the telescope understands what the surgeon desires. The assistant must understand what the surgeon wants to see and, if wrong, may increase the operating time and the potential for complications. The slightest tremor of the individual holding the telescope is magnified in the operating field. These problems can be minimized as the surgeon and the staff progress along the learning curve and utilize appropriate instrumentation.

Over the past 30 years, particularly during the last decade, endoscopic technology and instrumentation have advanced at a rapid pace to address these challenges. Significant progress has been achieved since Gans introduced the prototypic pediatric endoscopic instruments in the USA in 1969.

Due to the extent of this topic, it would be impossible to describe every instrument available for use. Hence, this chapter focuses on more commonly used, well-established instruments for pediatric endoscopic surgery, and includes instruments used for access, visualization, dissection, vascular control, reconstruction and tissue extraction.

SETTING UP FOR PEDIATRIC ENDOSCOPIC SURGERY

Vital to the success of every endoscopic procedure is proper planning and appropriate set-up of cases. Depending on the pediatric surgical condition, patient position, port placement and the endoscopic approach can be planned. Although the set-up may vary from one surgical condition to another, the 'SCOPe' set-up must, whenever possible, be observed. This places the surgeon, the camera, the organ and the picture in a straight line. Almost always, following this set-up assures smooth conduct of the endoscopic procedure. (**See Figure 7.1**)

Due to the flux of equipment required for the performance of an endoscopic procedure, setting up of cases can be a problem. One may not be able to position the video monitor along the surgeon's line of vision or may have difficulty navigating the operating room because of tangled cables on the floor. Modern endoscopic suites have been developed to address these issues and are designed to improve ergonomics, efficiency and integration of the surgical environment. (**See Figure 7.2**)

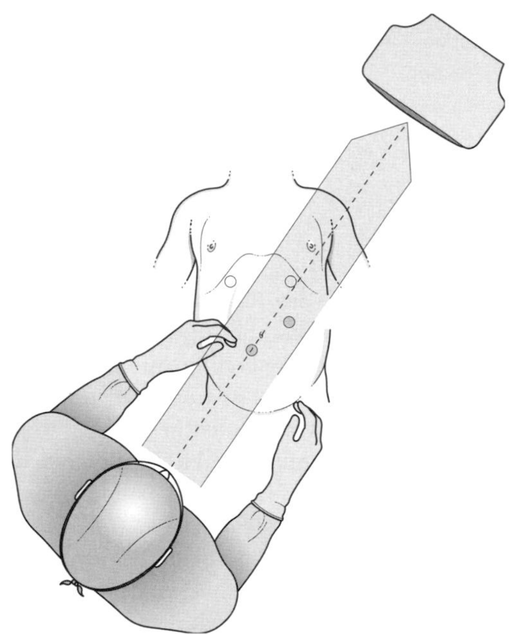

Figure 7.1

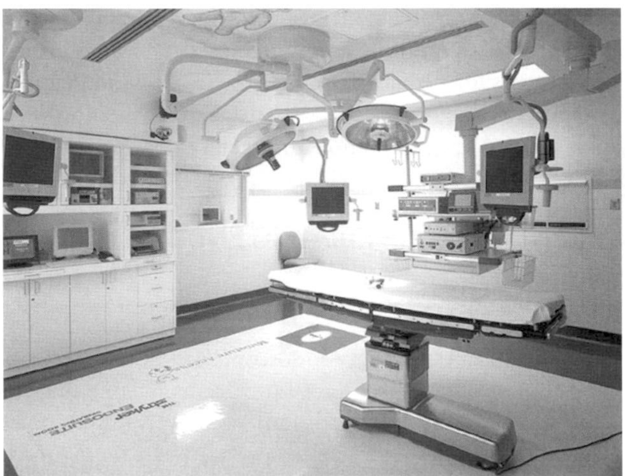

Figure 7.2

Within the room are ceiling-mounted, high-resolution, flat-panel video monitors, which can be easily positioned along the surgeon's visual axis during a procedure and moved out of the way at the end of the operation. Endoscopic devices (which include the triple chip camera, light source, insufflator and energy source) are supported by heavy-duty ceiling-mounted columns. In addition to the endoscopic camera there are two other cameras, the room camera, which provides a bird's eye view of the room, and the in-light camera, which is housed in the operating room light and provides an external view of the patient. These are used mainly for training and teaching purposes. On one side of the wall is the nurses' control station, which houses the central computer and a touch screen control panel that nurses can use to control manually control equipment vital to documentation and communication. Also housed in this control panel are a digital image capture device, voice recognition software and a computer printer. Unlike the traditional endoscopic room, where heavy-wheeled carts and tangled cables and tubes clutter the floor space, the only things on the floor are the operating table and anesthesia machine. The room can be equipped with voice recognition software that allows the surgeon to operate the system using voice control. To adjust the height or angle of the table, move the telescope, zoom the camera in and out, adjust the light intensity and change insufflation pressure and rate, capture and print digital still images, capture and produce digital video, make phone calls and participate in teleconferences.

ACCESS

The process of endoscopic surgery starts with access to the abdomen or chest followed by insufflation to create a space and to move underlying organs away from the wall in preparation for the insertion of the instrument ports. Umbilical access can be achieved either percutaneously using the Veress needle, which was originally introduced by Janos Veress in 1938, or via the open technique introduced by Hasson.

The Veress needle is a sharp needle placed around a blunt inner cannula. The needle is 14 G and its length can be either 12 cm or 15 cm. The inner cannula is spring-loaded and retracts within the sharp needle during passage through the abdominal or chest wall and then springs forward when the needle is inside the cavity to prevent injury to underlying organs. Once in position, insufflation can be started and when the desired insufflation pressure is reached, the instrument port can be inserted. (**See Figure 7.3**)

Opinions vary amongst endoscopic surgeons as to which is the preferred approach.

The expandable trocar system (Step™) comes in a set with a Veress needle, an expandable trocar sheath and a dilator trocar, the last two being available in 3, 5, 10 and 12 mm sizes. The Veress needle together with the expandable trocar sheath is inserted as a set. Once in place, and after insufflation, the Veress needle is removed and the expandable sheath dilated.

Use of the system facilitates umbilical access and trocar placement without complications. **(See Figure 7.4)**

The instrument port (also called a cannula, trocar sheath or sleeve) comes in different sizes (diameter 3, 5, 10, 12 mm and length 75 or 100 mm), colors and configurations (handled or non-handled). For most pediatric endoscopic procedures, 5 mm ports are adequate, but in smaller children, particularly neonates, 3 mm (or even smaller) ports are useful. Occasionally, 10 mm or 12 mm ports are used when either tissue extraction or stapling is anticipated. Hence, the appropriate choice depends on the size of the patient and the contemplated endoscopic procedure. **(See Figure 7.5)**

In addition, trocar sleeves may be valved or non-valved. For most endoscopic procedures, valved trocars are recommended to prevent gas leakage and maintain exposure. The sleeves may also be equipped with an anti-slip device to enhance their fixation in the patient. To prevent displacement of the sleeves, some ports are equipped with special anchors such as balloons, expandable tips or grooves. Finally, trocar sleeves may be disposable or non-disposable. Similar to other endoscopic instruments, disposable devices have the advantage of always being in good condition, but, of course, increase operative equipment expense.

The trocar is the pointed obturator placed inside the trocar sheath or sleeve to facilitate introduction. Trocar tips come in different configurations: bladeless, bladed-dilating, pyramidal and blunt. Bladeless obturators come with a clear optical tip and accommodate an appropriately sized

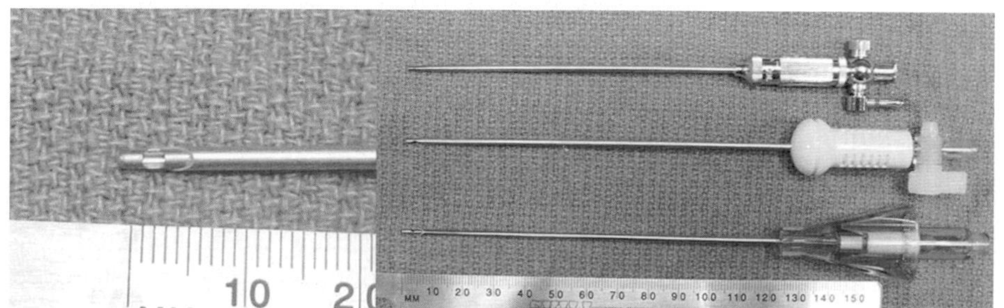

Figure 7.3

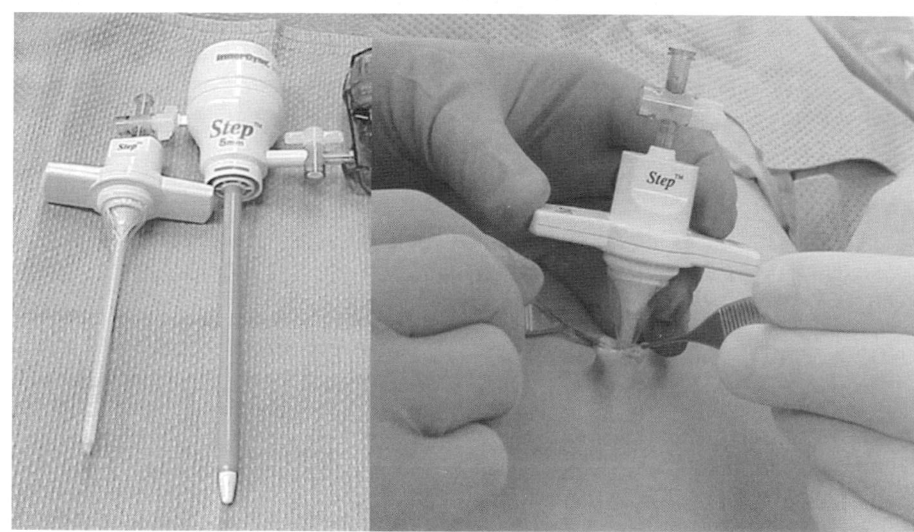

Figure 7.4

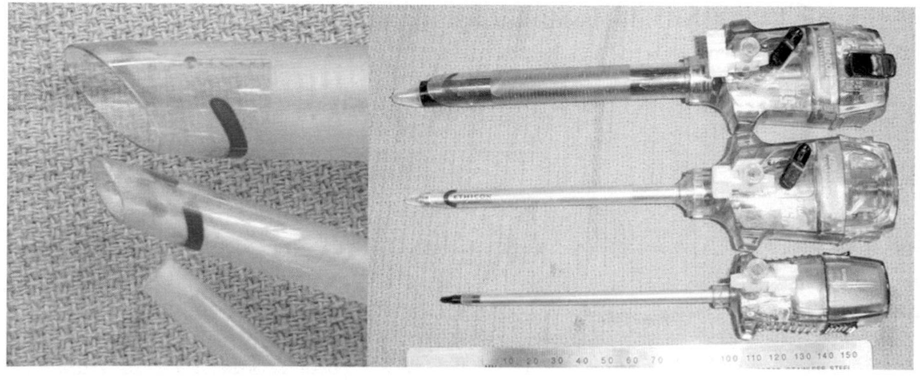

Figure 7.5

0° endoscope. The clear, tapered optical tip, when used with an endoscope, provides visibility of individual tissue layers during insertion. Bladed and pyramidal trocars are equipped with a spring-loaded blade shield designed to cover the sharp tip to protect internal structures from puncture or laceration once the abdominal or thoracic cavity has been entered. Blunt trocars gently move aside any internal viscera that may be adjacent to the abdominal or thoracic wall. Regardless of the type of trocar used, endoscopic visualization at the port entry site is a time-tested technique to avoid complications. **(See Figure 7.6)**

VISUALIZATION

Insufflators are used to create and maintain pneumoperitoneun or pneumothorax to achieve adequate exposure and room for the introduction of endoscopic instruments. Modern versions are designed for longer operating times and flow requirements with multiple trocars and instrument exchanges. **(See Figure 7.7)**

Current insufflators are equipped with a video display and allow the setting of pressure limits and rate of flow. Visual or audible alarms are activated when these limits are reached, alerting the surgical team. Most are also equipped with automatic venting systems and with leakage and occlusion detection capabilities. These features are particularly important in pediatrics, as patient sizes, as well as the effects of carbon dioxide insufflation, are variable. Insufflators can deliver up 40 L/min of gas, but this is rarely needed in pediatric endoscopic surgery. Also, insufflators can heat and humidify laparoscopic gas to physiologic conditions, which provides significant benefits in pediatric patients, as their temperature lowers easily with cold and dry laparoscopic gas. To customize insufflators further for use in children and to address the different physiology and property of the abdominal wall, pediatric insufflator prototypes that allow low-flow and low-pressure insufflation are now being utilized.

Adequate exposure of the operative site often requires some form of retraction. Gravity is the most useful and the cheapest option available. With proper patient positioning and operating table angle, a certain degree of organ exposure can be accomplished. Often, the exposure afforded may be enough to complete the procedure. Occasionally, difficult-to-handle organs such as the liver or bowel may require some form of retraction to facilitate exposure and manipulation, and retraction systems have therefore been developed for a variety of specific uses. Many of these systems involve mechanisms that enter the abdomen in a closed form and are opened at the target site, which means that the instruments are larger but cause less trauma. Due to the delicate nature of the tissues and organs in children, retraction must be applied with caution. Innovations in retraction have been described such as elevating the stomach, falciform ligament or mesentery by attaching it to the abdominal wall with external sutures. **(See Figure 7.8)**

During the procedure, oozing blood and fluid may impair visualization. Irrigation and aspiration systems are available to address this problem. In most instances, aspiration should dominate and irrigation should be limited, because irrigation spreads the blood in the field, making it darker. Currently available systems allow irrigation and aspiration of fluid using the same 5 mm probe.

DISSECTION

Tissue dissections are performed using basic endoscopic graspers and dissectors. The Maryland (a type of atraumatic

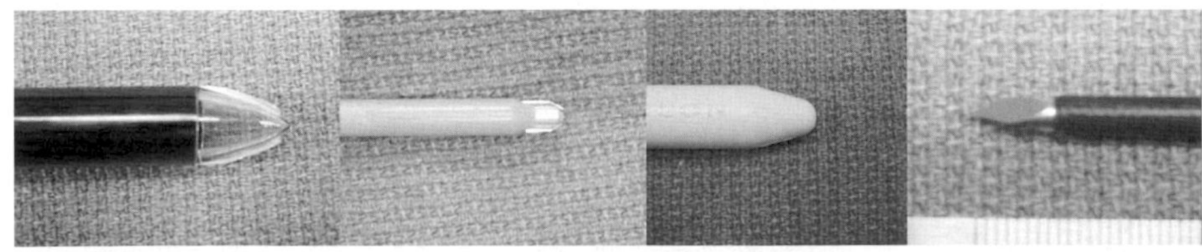

Figure 7.6

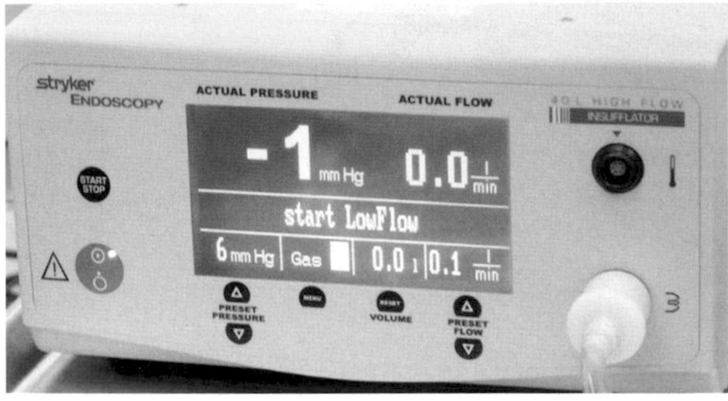

Figure 7.7

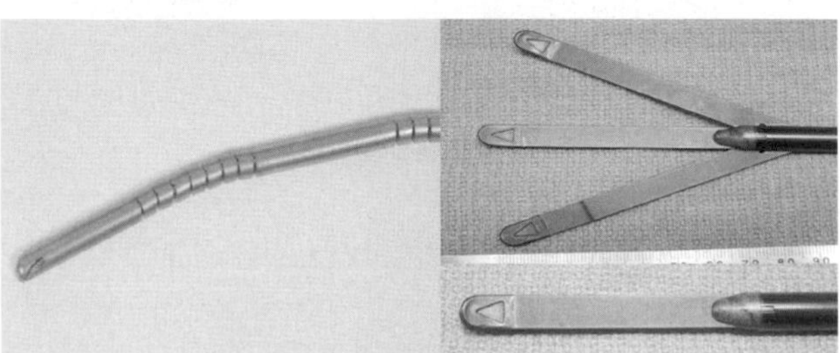

Figure 7.8 *Snake and blade retractors.*

grasper), mixter, Babcock, De Bakey grasping forceps, peanut dissectors and scissors are the instruments preferred by most endoscopic surgeons. Originally only available in 10 mm diameter and 45 cm or longer shafts, these instruments now come in smaller diameters (2, 3 and 5 mm) and shorter lengths (22 and 33 cm). The use of these newer instruments in children has the advantages of enabling the surgeon to work closer to the operative field and to perform more precise tissue manipulation and dissection. **(See Figure 7.9)**

The instrument shafts may be insulated (allowing them to be used with electrosurgery) and rotatable (allowing the surgeon to approach tissue planes at better angles). Instrument handles come in pistol or scissor grip and may be ratcheted or non-ratcheted. In addition, the handles and instrument shafts may be interchangeable, allowing endoscopic surgeons to choose their own preferred combination. **(See Figure 7.10)**

As the organs are smaller and the tissues more delicate in children, the appropriate choice of graspers and dissectors is essential. Blunt dissectors have narrower and flatter tip cross-sections compared to the round configuration of the regular grasping instruments. In addition to the configuration of the tips and the serrations on the jaws, the movement of the jaws must be considered. Double-action jaws are ideal for tissue dissection because they allow balanced spreading of tissues, whereas single-action jaws are preferred for more precise grasping of tissues. The fixed portion of the jaw can be placed in the desired position in relation to a tissue, with just the other jaw moving to grasp the tissue. **(See Figure 7.11)**

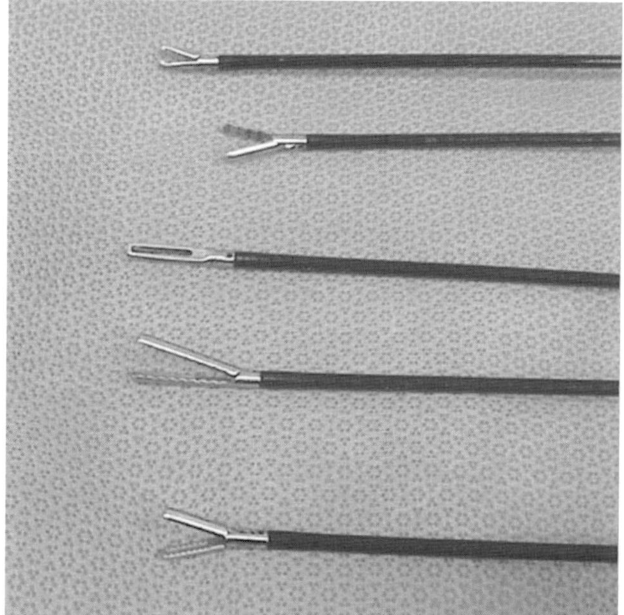

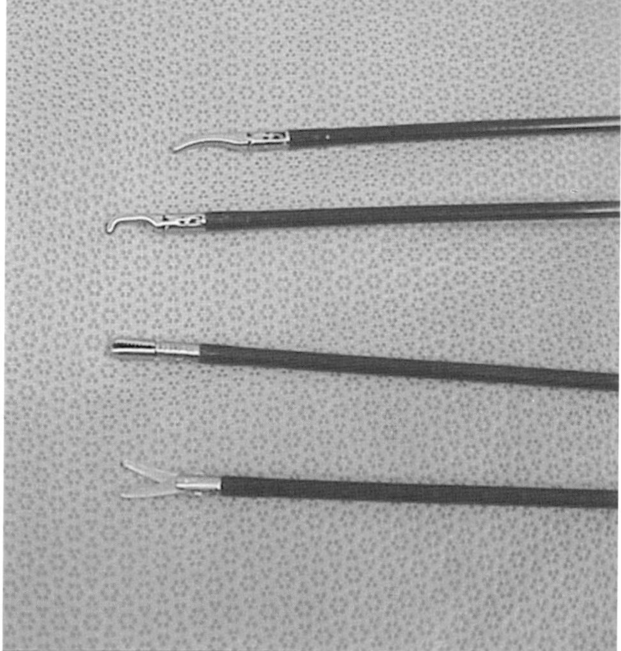

Figure 7.9

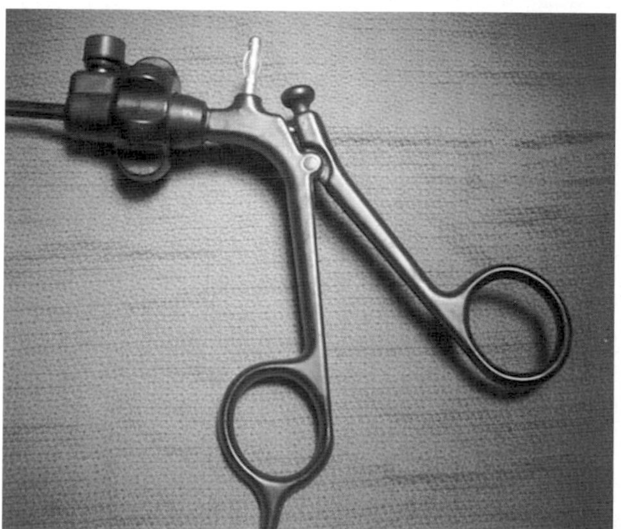

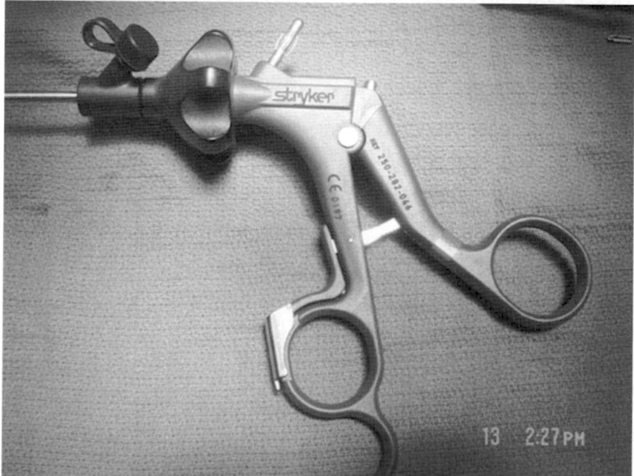

Figure 7.10

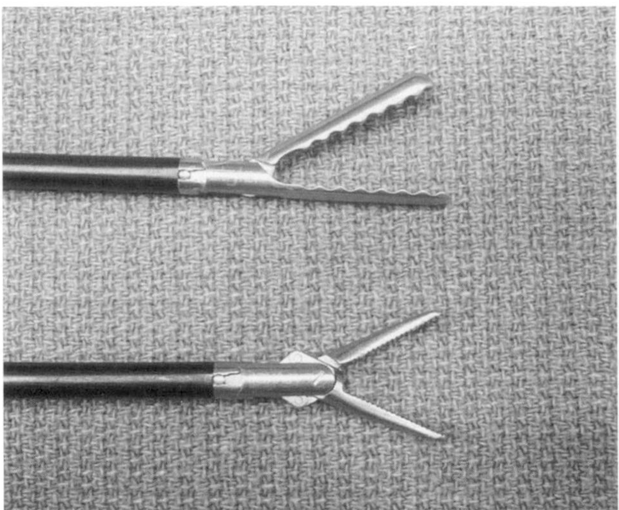

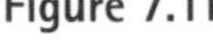

Figure 7.11

Figure 7.12

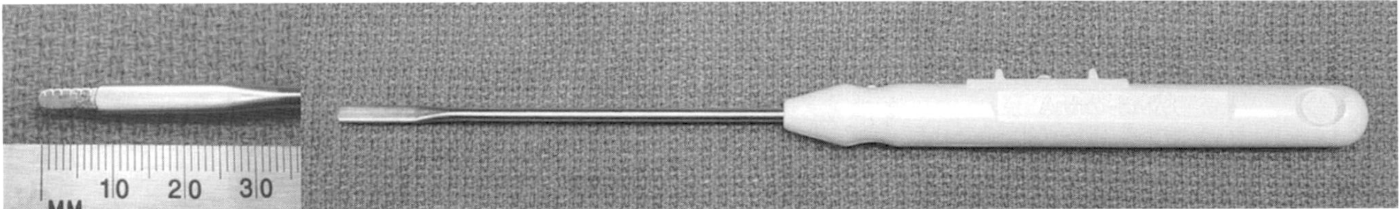

Figure 7.13

Another useful aide to tissue dissection is the monopolar dissector (hook, L-dissector, and spatula). This is the endoscopic counterpart of the popular 'pen' electrosurgery used in open surgery and has various applications in endoscopic surgical procedures, allowing both dissection and hemostasis. **(See Figure 7.12)**

Sharp dissection and cutting can be performed using endoscopic scissors. Scissors come in different blade configurations and can be curved or straight, hooked or saw tooth. Like the endoscopic dissectors and graspers, they are now also available in smaller diameters and shorter lengths. With the advent of versatile or multi-function instruments, which can dissect, cut and coagulate, there is less need for scissors for sharp dissection, and their role in endoscopic surgery is now limited to transecting clipped vessels or ducts, the cutting of sutures and for the lysis of adhesions.

A sheathed, retractable endoscopic blade (Arthro-knife), originally designed for arthroscopic procedures, has been adopted by pediatric surgeons and is useful for making the pyloromyotomy incision. The knife blade is extended and used to perform the myotomy incision and, when retracted, for starting to spread the myotomy. The blade is fully retractable to provide safe, quick and trocar-less introduction and removal from the body cavity. **(See Figure 7.13)**

VASCULAR CONTROL

Hemostasis is a key issue in endoscopic surgery, as adequate visualization can only be achieved in a bloodless field. The prevention of bleeding requires making the appropriate choice and use of the sutures, pre-tied loops, clips, staplers and various energy sources that are available for this purpose. Use of the appropriate modality is also vital, as it is always more difficult to achieve hemostasis at a second attempt, especially in children, because of limited workspace and visualization.

Sutures, clips and staples

As in open surgery, vessels and ducts can be controlled using sutures, clips and staplers. Vessels can be suture ligated using standard suture materials, which can be tied either extracorporeally or intracorporeally. Pre-tied loops are available that can easily be deployed and applied to stumps of transected vessels and ducts. To minimize cost, the loops can be tied preoperatively using regular suture materials. **(See Figure 7.14)**

Endoscopic clips are used primarily to facilitate ligating small- to medium-sized vessels and ducts (2–5 mm). Commonly used disposable multi-clip appliers with either

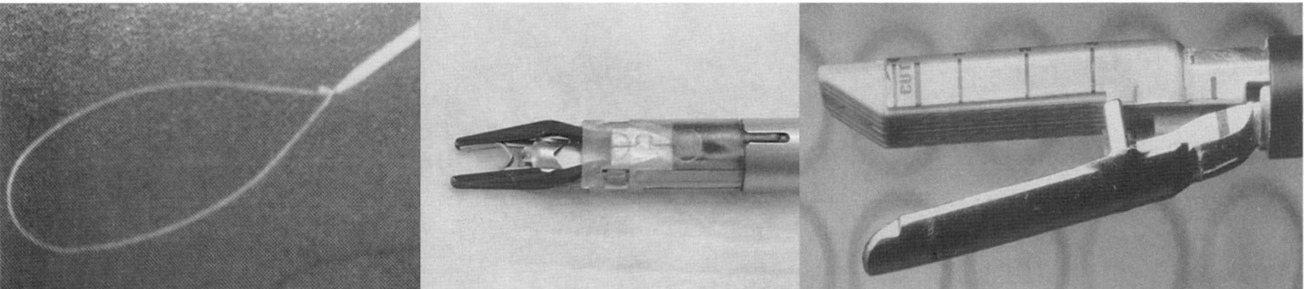

Figure 7.14 *Pre-tried loop, clip applicator and stapler.*

20 or 30 metallic clip loads come in 5 mm and 10 mm shafts. Unlike the older versions, which require a 12 mm port and instrument exchange to reload the clip, the currently available 5 mm multiple clip appliers allow the surgeon to apply all the required clips in one instrument exchange. These are expensive and use must be limited to procedures that require multiple clips to justify the cost. Similar to the application of endoscopic staplers, both sides must be adequately visualized to avoid inadvertent clipping of non-target tissues and ensure proper placement of the clip.

Endoscopic staplers were developed primarily to facilitate tissue approximation, but they can also be useful for hemostatic division of vascular tissue bundles. Staplers deploy parallel rows of staples and come in different staple heights (2.5 mm vascular or 3.5 mm tissue approximation). They also come in different staple line lengths (30–60 mm). Some have a reticulating staple base, which allows stapler application in difficult-to-reach areas such as the pelvis. Some are equipped with a blade that creates a linear incision after a parallel row of staples has been inserted on either side of the incision line, allowing vascular control and tissue division in one motion. However, the smallest endoscopic stapler still has a shaft diameter of 10 mm and requires a suitably sized instrument port. Therefore, in addition to the cost, the size of the instrument is another drawback in its use in pediatric endoscopic surgery. In the near future, the development of miniature stapling devices, with absorbable staples, will enhance many pediatric operations.

Due to the expanding application of ultrasonic scalpel and vessel-sealing systems, the use of sutures, clips and staples for vascular control is decreasing. Vessels less than 3 mm in diameter can be controlled using ultrasonic devices, and those as large as 7 mm can be adequately sealed by vessel-sealing devices. Despite this, sutures, clips and staples will continue to be used in endoscopic surgery due to surgeon preference and when ultrasonic and vessel-sealing systems are not available.

Ultrasonic scalpel

With the ultrasonic scalpel (Harmonic Scalpel®), cutting and hemostasis can be achieved with minimal lateral thermal damage to soft tissue, making it a popular piece of equipment in pediatric endoscopic surgery. The ultrasonic scalpel blade vibrates longitudinally, transferring mechanical energy to tissue. An electrical signal causes piezoelectric ceramics inside the handpiece to expand and contract, converting electrical energy to mechanical motion, which is in turn transferred to the blade extender. As the ultrasonic wave leaves the blade extender, its motion is amplified as it travels to the blade tip, where maximum blade motion occurs. The coagulation effect occurs through the transfer of mechanical energy to the tissue. Internal cellular friction breaks hydrogen bonds, resulting in protein denaturization. As the proteins are denatured, a sticky coagulum forms and seals the small vessels at a temperature under 100 °C, minimizing smoke.

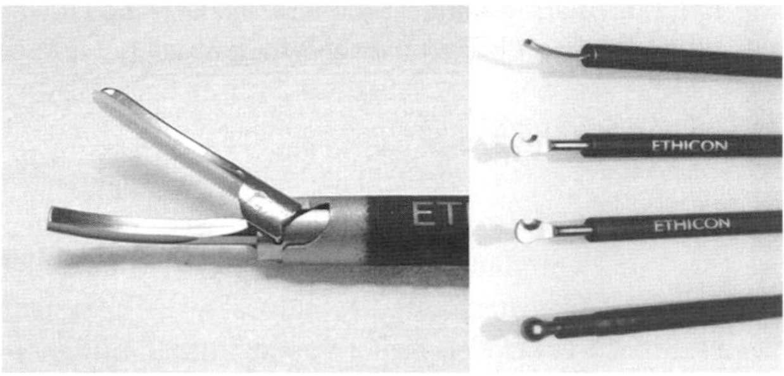

Figure 7.15

Tissue tension, blade sharpness, time, power level and grip force affect ultrasonic cutting and coagulation. Increased tissue tension, a sharper blade, shorter time, higher power level and stronger grip provide faster cutting and less hemostasis. Less tissue tension, a blunt surface, more time, lower power and light grip provide slower cutting and more hemostasis.

The ultrasonic shear, a multifunctional ultrasonic instrument, facilitates the application of ultrasonic energy to unsupported tissues. The shear comes in curve and straight configuration with a choice of pistol or scissor grip. The shaft is 5 mm in diameter and comes in 23 cm or 36 cm length. Using this instrument, the surgeon can grasp, dissect bluntly, cut sharply and coagulate tissues. This multifunction capability not only minimizes instrument exchanges, but also has the potential to minimize cost (fewer clips and sutures, less operative time). **(See Figure 7.15)**

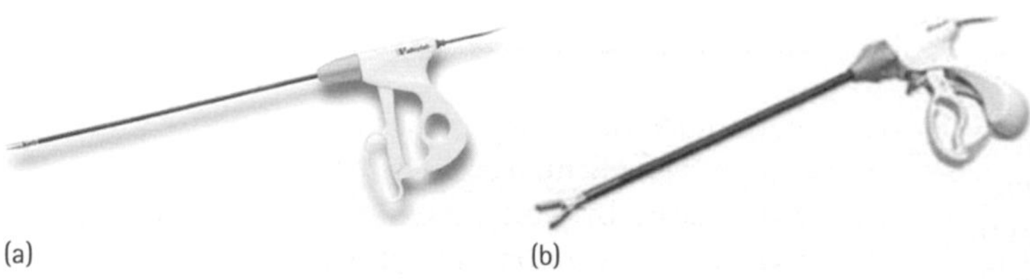

Figure 7.16 *Sealing devices. (a) non-cutting 5 mm; (b) cutting 5 mm and 10 mm device.*

Ultrasonic scalpel blades attached to a 5 mm shaft are also available. The blades come in different configurations: curved, dissecting hook, sharp hook, ball, and sharp curve. Common to each blade is a sharp and blunt surface for cutting and coagulating tissues. The appropriate choice will depend on the specific purpose for which it will be used.

Vessel-sealing system

The vessel-sealing system (LigaSure™) uses optimized pressure and computer-controlled energy to fuse the patient's own collagen and create a natural seal. The system has a feedback-controlled response system that automatically discontinues energy delivery when the seal cycle is complete. The seal appears as a distinctive, possibly translucent area of reformed collagen and maintains plastic resistance to deformation. The vessel-sealing system provides permanent fusion of tissue bundles and vessels up to 7 mm in diameter and can withstand three times the normal systolic pressure. There is minimal sticking and tissue charring and reduced thermal spread compared to standard bipolar electrosurgery. No foreign bodies are left behind and there is the potential for reduced blood loss and time saving compared to suture.

Instruments are available with 5 mm and 10 mm diameter shafts. The 5 mm instrument, which is preferred for most pediatric endoscopic procedures, is 32 cm long, the jaw angle is 15° (non-cutting) or straight (cutting device like the 10 mm instrument) and the seal width is 2–4 mm. The vessel-sealing system has become the option preferred by a number of endoscopic surgeons for procedures such as thoracoscopic lobectomies, excision of a pulmonary sequestration, Nissen fundoplication, and bowel resection. **(See Figure 7.16)**

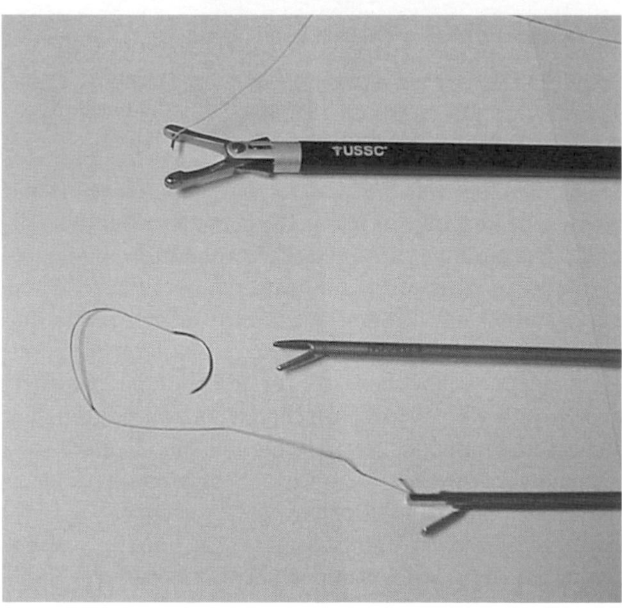

Figure 7.17

RECONSTRUCTION

Endoscopic surgery in children, particularly infants, presents the problem of a small workspace. Structures are not only smaller but also more sensitive to trauma, requiring gentler handling. Therefore suturing and knot tying become technically challenging and take time to accomplish. Often, particularly for the novice, operative time is significantly increased. To address this issue, suture assistants, automatic suture devices, suture applicators and staplers have been developed to aid the surgeon and facilitate the task of reconstruction. Most of these devices deploy a ready-made knot once the needle is passed, thus eliminating the difficult and time-consuming task of knot tying. Despite the availability of these devices, the ability of the endoscopic surgeon to pass sutures and tie knots must not be compromised since, in certain situations, an intracorporeal tie is needed. The appropriate choice of instrument will need to balance the need for properly placed and securely tied knots and the need to minimize operative time. Adequate mastery and knowledge of these devices is essential for their efficient use. **(See Figure 7.17)**

TISSUE EXTRACTION

Pediatric endoscopic procedures that require extraction of tissues, such as appendectomy, cholecystectomy, splenectomy and lung resection, present a unique challenge to pediatric endoscopic surgeons. Often, these organs are larger than the instrument ports used to dissect the tissues and, apart from the variation in size, specimens may differ in their physical characteristics and may be infected or malignant. The best method for removal depends on the nature of the specimen and on whether an intact specimen is required for pathologic examination. Tissue forceps, graspers, retrieval bags and morcelators have been developed to address these problems. To retrieve a specimen, the umbilicus is the ideal portal to the abdomen, as it can be enlarged to accept a 10 mm or 12 mm or larger port without compromising cosmesis. To prevent contamination and specimen loss, specimens are placed inside specially designed retrieval bags and extracted piecemeal. This is particularly important when specimens may be malignant, infected or friable. There are commercially available bags, but sterile gloves, glove fingers and condoms are adequate for most purposes. Important factors to consider when choosing a specimen bag are its size, strength and maneuverability.

CONCLUSIONS

Pediatric endoscopic surgery is instrument intensive and technology dependent. Endoscopic surgeons continue to shape the future by working closely with industry, giving feedback and suggestions about what can be done to improve the currently available tools further. The success of an endoscopic procedure often depends on a number of factors, such as adequate preparation, proper case set-up, the surgical team and the available instrumentation. Familiarity with the instruments available and comfort in their use favorably influence the outcome of endoscopic surgery.

8

Robotic laparoscopic surgery

KLAUS HELLER

INTRODUCTION

The field of surgery is entering a time of great change. The advantages of minimally invasive approaches to conventional surgical operations have become well established. Advances in computer technology have meant that robots, previously regarded as too clumsy and dangerous for use in the operating theatre, are now commercially available to provide intelligent assistance with routine tasks. More significantly, robots are able to manipulate surgical instruments with greater precision than the surgeon's own hand, with unlimited repetition and without fatigue.

Definitions and history

The word robot comes from a play by Karel Capek called *Rossum's Universal Robots*, first performed in 1921. Robot is derived from the Czech word *robota*, meaning forced work or labor. The Robot Institute of America (1979) defined a robot as a 're-programmable, multifunctional manipulator designed to move materials, parts, tools, or specialized devices through various programmed motions for the performance of a variety of tasks'.

The first working industrial robots appeared in the 1960s. Over the following decades, robot technology burgeoned, largely as a result of the automotive and aerospace industries. In 1986 the Organization for Economic Co-operation and Development (OECD) commissioned a feasibility study into the application of robotics to medicine and received over 400 proposals. The first practical application of robotics to surgery appeared in the late 1980s with the development of neurosurgical navigation systems.

CONTEMPORARY ROBOTIC SYSTEMS

Current applications of robotics to surgery can be divided into two groups: image-guided robots and telemanipulators. Image-guidance systems have developed in parallel with advances in medical imaging. They enable the surgeon to decide in advance on the path to the chosen target, based on the medical images obtained during the preoperative planning stage, and for the robot to be preprogrammed. A critical aspect of this type of surgery is the need for accurate registration of the robot, patient and image, so that all three are brought into the same frame of reference. Because image-guided surgery depends on fixed reference points, current applications are restricted to orthopedics (e.g. the Robodoc™ system for hip joint replacement), neurosurgery (e.g. the NeuroMatetrade™ stereotactic navigation system) and maxillofacial/otorhinolaryngology surgery (e.g. the Evolution 1™ system for cochlear implant surgery).

Most surgical robotic systems in current use are not strictly robots but telemanipulators. A telemanipulator is a master/slave device with sensors (force sensors, cameras etc.) and actuators (grasping tools and handles) that is under the direct control of a human operator. The movements of the surgeon's hands are transformed into digital information, which is modified and then translated back into remote mechanical control of the surgical instruments. At present there are two telemanipulators in widespread use: the *Da Vinci*® and the *Zeus*® surgical systems.

The *Da Vinci*® system consists of a master console with an integrated computer interface, a slave patient-side cart, instruments and image-processing equipment. **(See Figure 8.1)**

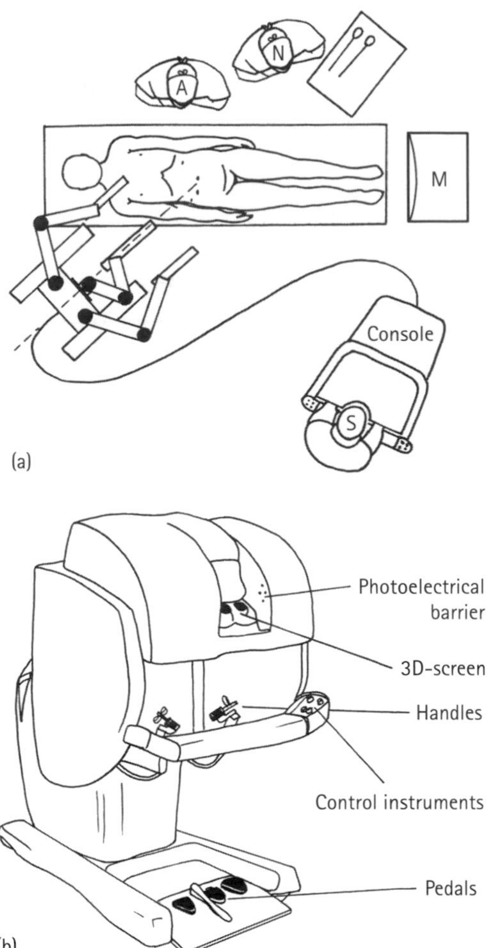

Figure 8.1 *(a) Cart and console; (b) Console.*

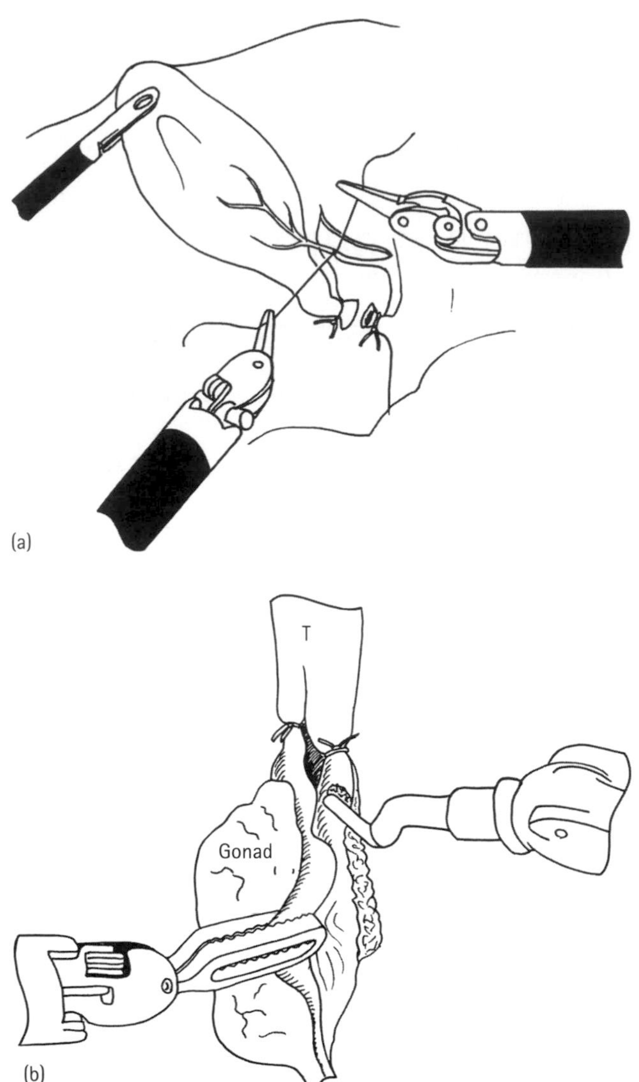

Figure 8.2 *(a) Cholecystectomy; (b) gonadectomy.*

The surgeon operates while seated comfortably at a distance from the patient viewing a three-dimensional image of the surgical field. The surgeon's fingers grasp the master controls below the display. The surgeon's hand, wrist and finger movements are translated into precise, real-time movements of the surgical instruments inside the patient. Three foot pedals control camera position, electrocautery and instrument disengagement to allow repositioning of the control handles in a more comfortable position without altering the position of the instruments inside the patient.

The slave unit (patient-side cart) comprises three or four robotic arms and is placed beside the operating table. One arm controls the camera and two or three arms are available for instruments. Ports for the camera and instruments are inserted in a conventional manner. The camera and intracorporeal instruments are connected to the arms of the robot. A comprehensive range of instruments, *EndoWrist*®, has been designed with 7° of motion to exceed the range of movements of the human hand and wrist. As a result, the direction of suturing is not restricted to 90° relative to the axis of the needle driver. Intracorporeal knot tying is also simplified. (**See Figure 8.2**)

The *Zeus*® system, which is now out of production, is similar in principle. The surgeon is seated at a distance from the patient in front of a video console. The slave unit is attached to the side rail of the operating table so that it does not move in relation to the patient if the table is moved.

Three robotic arms control surgical instruments and the camera. The camera arm incorporates the AESOP® voice-activated control, which provides the surgeon with a steady magnified view of the operative field. Spoken commands by the surgeon guide the movement of the camera with precision. The surgeon controls the right and left instrument arms in the master console and these movements are translated into real-time articulation of the surgical instruments. Electrocautery is activated by a button inside the hand control. The instrument slave arms, with 7° of freedom, mimic the human arm in form and function but without fatigue. The AESOP® system can be used in isolation to replace the surgical assistant as a camera holder for conventional laparoscopy.

CLINICAL APPLICATIONS

As a general rule, any procedure that can be performed with conventional minimally invasive equipment can be performed using a telemanipulation system. However, open conversion may be required on occasions for exactly the same reasons as in conventional minimally invasive surgery. Patient selection is of paramount importance in minimizing this risk.

Once the trocars are in place, any retractors positioned and the robotic arms loaded with instruments, the surgeon can retire to the console. The scrub nurse assumes responsibility for changing instruments and loading sutures. An assistant only becomes necessary for operations such as cholecystectomy or fundoplication in the event that the liver retractor becomes displaced.

ADVANTAGES AND DISADVANTAGES OF ROBOTIC SURGERY

Robotic surgery has all the advantages of minimally invasive surgery compared to open surgery plus a number of additional advantages over conventional laparoscopic surgery.

Advantages

- The surgeon is able to operate from the comfort of the robotic console in a position that ensures optimum manual dexterity.
- Three-dimensional visualization permits rapid and accurate intracorporeal orientation of instruments.
- Voice-operated or foot-operated camera control systems ensure a consistent visual image, eliminating artifact caused by the assistant moving.
- In-built electronic and mechanical safety systems prevent tissue damage.
- Precise control of the instruments, including a tremor filter and variable downscaling of the hand movements, facilitates dissection and manipulation of tissues. Intracorporeal knot tying is considerably easier than with conventional laparoscopic instruments.

Disadvantages

- Robotic systems are expensive to purchase and maintain.
- The absence of tactile feedback is a significant problem. All movements, including knot tying, rely solely on visual control.
- Current robotic equipment is large and cumbersome. Consequently, a large dedicated robotic operating room is required.
- Further miniaturization of instruments and trocars is necessary for pediatric surgical practice.

Initial experience with robotic surgery in children is promising. Robotic telemanipulation systems are reliable and safe. Technological improvements (tactile force feedback, smaller instruments) can all be expected in the near future. Cost remains a major obstacle to widespread use. There is, however, no doubt that robotic surgery represents a revolution in minimally invasive surgery.

FURTHER READING

Ballantyne GH. Robotic surgery, telerobotic surgery, telepresence and telementoring. *Surgical Endoscopy* 2002; **16**:1389–402.

Goh PMY, Lomanto D, So JBY. Robotic-assisted laparoscopic cholecystectomy. *Surgical Endoscopy* 2001; **16**:216–20.

Heller K, Gutt CN, Schaeff B, Beyer PA, Markus B. Use of the robot system Da Vinci for laparoscopic repair of gastro-oesophageal reflux in children. *European Journal of Pediatric Surgery* 2002; **12**:239–42.

Section B: Airway and thoracic

9

Rigid endoscopy of the airway – basic technique

PAULO CAMPISI AND VITO FORTE

INTRODUCTION

Rigid endoscopy of the airway is an invaluable diagnostic and therapeutic tool employed in the practice of pediatric otolaryngology. The applications of rigid endoscopy are numerous and encompass a plethora of clinical scenarios. However, the variety and complexity of endoscopic instruments and the inherent risks associated with manipulation of the pediatric airway underscore the importance of the surgeon's thorough familiarity with equipment and technique.

This chapter provides an overview of the role of rigid endoscopy in infants and children and a description of a standard technique for laryngo-bronchoscopy that emphasizes the importance of ongoing communication between surgeon and anesthesiologist.

Indications

DIAGNOSTIC

- Persistent or progressive aerodigestive symptoms including stridor, dysphonia, dysphagia, odynophagia, hemoptysis and cough.
- Recurrent aspiration pneumonia.
- Cyanotic or apneic spells.
- Suspected foreign body aspiration.
- Assessment of subglottic stenosis.
- Assessment of injury following trauma or burns.
- Evaluation of prolonged intubation trauma.
- Tumor staging and biopsy.
- Bronchoalveolar lavage.
- Radiologic evidence of a mediastinal mass with tracheo-bronchial compression.

THERAPEUTIC

- Emergent airway management.
- Removal of laryngeal and bronchial foreign bodies or tumors.
- Endolaryngeal microsurgery (with or without laser).
- Dilatation of glottic, subglottic and tracheal stenosis.

Contraindications

ABSOLUTE

- Lack of proper equipment and experienced personnel.
- Precarious airway.
- Severe chemical burn (transmural).
- Cervical spine instability (e.g. rheumatoid arthritis, Down's syndrome).

RELATIVE

- Pulmonary insufficiency.
- Cardiac instability.
- Coagulopathy.

A safe and uneventful endoscopic examination of the pediatric airway mandates the presence of an experienced endoscopist and a wide range of pediatric instrumentation. The absence of either component represents a significant risk to the welfare of the patient and is therefore an absolute contraindication to rigid endoscopy.

Even under ideal technical circumstances, rigid endoscopy of the airway should be avoided when there is a risk of further injury to the airway that will inevitably lead to further airway compromise. In the presence of significant glottic, subglottic or tracheal stenosis, rigid endoscopy may induce mucosal edema that results in complete airway obstruction. In these situations, the airway may need to be secured with a tracheostomy prior to performing a diagnostic endoscopy.

Rigid endoscopy of the airway should also be avoided when there is confirmed or suspected transmural injury of the upper aerodigestive lumens following the ingestion of caustic substances. Rigid endoscopy may result in rupture of the trachea or esophagus, predisposing the patient to devastating complications such as mediastinitis and pneumomediastinum. If a transmural injury is noted only on endoscopy, the endoscope should be withdrawn and examination of the airway beyond the injury avoided.

Elective endoscopic procedures should never be undertaken in the setting of an unstable cervical spine to avoid catastrophic neurologic complications. This risk is not isolated to the trauma patient. It is also inherent in patients with rheumatoid arthritis and Down's syndrome. Elective diagnostic procedures may require a delay in patients with pulmonary or cardiac insufficiency and coagulopathy until they are medically optimized.

Advantages

- An effective and rapid means of establishing an airway, which is maintained under direct vision.
- Superior visualization of the airway compared to flexible endoscopy.
- Permits a therapeutic intervention at the time of diagnosis.

Disadvantages

- Requires a general anesthetic.
- Requires experience and proper equipment.
- More traumatic than flexible endoscopy.
- Distortion of normal anatomy and function.

EQUIPMENT/INSTRUMENTS

Laryngoscopy

ESSENTIAL

- Four variably sized open-sided pediatric laryngoscopes.
- Three variably sized operating and intubating pediatric laryngoscopes.
- Anterior commissure pediatric laryngoscope.
- Cupped laryngeal forceps (straight and up-cupped).
- Laryngeal alligator grasping forceps.
- Through-cutting forceps.
- Laryngeal probe.
- Suction catheters (atraumatic and open end).
- Suction tubing.

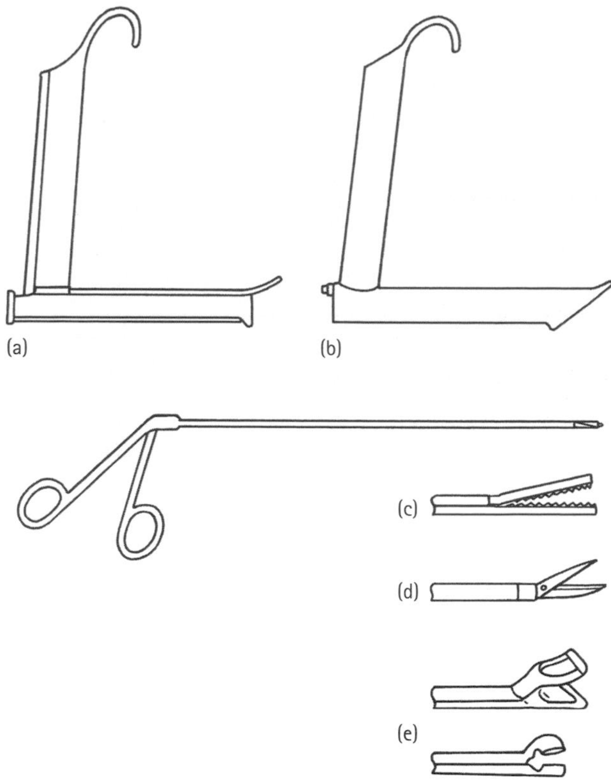

Figure 9.1 *(a) Open-sided laryngoscope; (b) operating laryngoscope; (c) alligator forceps; (d) scissors; (e) cupped forceps.*

- Light source and fiberoptic cables.
- Fiberoptic light clip.
- Rigid telescopes (0°, 30° and 70°).
- Camera, monitor.
- Video-recording or image-printing equipment.
- Suspension apparatus.
- Tracheostomy set.

(**See Figure 9.1**)

DESIRABLE

- Two variably sized laryngoscopes – separate metal cannula for anesthetic gases.
- Three variably sized slotted, small diameter laryngoscopes – difficult intubations.
- Two variably sized operating laryngoscopes – a wide proximal end for microlaryngoscopy and laser surgery.
- Two variably sized subglottiscopes – diagnostics, microsurgery and laser surgery in subglottis and upper trachea in infants and newborns.
- Microlaryngeal instruments:
  - knife, sickle shaped
  - fine scissors
  - fine cupped forceps
  - fine up-cupped forceps (1, 3 and 5 mm)
  - suction tubes, atraumatic (2 and 3 mm diameter).

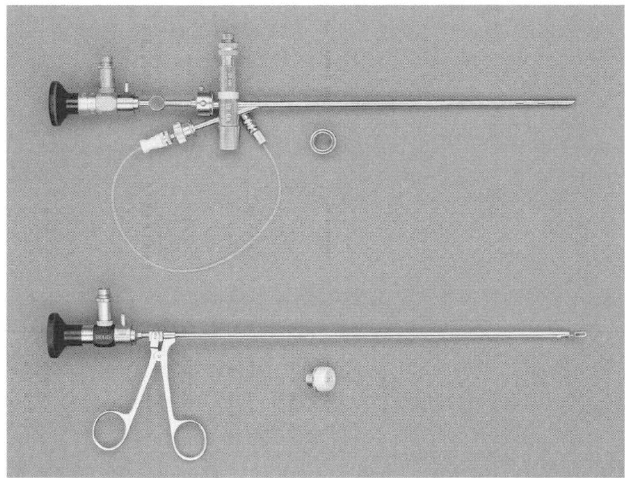

Figure 9.2

- Carbon dioxide laser.
- Carbon dioxide laser coupler.
- Operating microscope.

Bronchoscopy

ESSENTIAL

- Variably sized ventilating open and rod-lens bronchoscopes.
- Anesthesia laryngoscope with straight Miller blade.
- Rigid biopsy, grasping and cupped forceps.
- Flexible grasping and cupped forceps (for side channel port).
- Flexible and rigid suction.
- Suction tubing.
- Light source and fiberoptic cables.
- Rigid telescopes (0°, 30° and 70°).
- Camera, monitor.
- Video recording or image-printing equipment.
- Tracheostomy set.

(See Figure 9.2, Table 9.1)

DESIRABLE

- Optical grasping forceps.
- Aspiration traps for cytology and culture.
- Carbon dioxide laser.
- Carbon dioxide laser coupler.
- Operating microscope.

PREOPERATIVE PREPARATION

For the stable patient, the preoperative preparation begins with a thorough patient history. Symptoms suggestive of aerodigestive tract pathology should be elicited from the caregivers and patient if possible. Specific and detailed information concerning previous endotracheal intubations and the status of the cardiac and pulmonary systems should be documented. A complete head and neck examination that includes a flexible endoscopic nasolaryngoscopy is necessary to obtain as much information as possible about the location and severity of the airway problem. The presence and position of any loose teeth should be noted. Neck and chest plain radiographs, computed tomography and magnetic resonance imaging studies may be required to complete the preoperative database. All radiographic studies should be reviewed with a radiologist prior to performing the endoscopy.

Table 9.1 *Selection of rigid bronchoscopes (Storz) according to age*

Age	Size	Length (cm)
Preterm (1–2.5 kg)	2.5	20
Term–3 months	2.5/3.0	20
3–6 months	3.0/3.5	20
6–12 months	3.5	30
1–4 years	3.5	30
4–7 years	4.0	30
7–12 years	5.0	30

Anesthetic considerations

There are several anesthetic techniques that may be employed during rigid laryngoscopy and bronchoscopy. Decisions concerning the method of anesthesia induction, the use of paralyzing medications or spontaneous respiration, and the need for endotracheal intubation are made on a case-by-case basis. Factors such as the age of the patient, location and degree of airway obstruction and physician preference guide the choice of anesthetic technique. Special circumstances, including craniofacial abnormalities and cervical spine instability, may also need to be addressed. These factors should be considered prior to entering the operating room to define the respective roles of the surgeon and anesthetist and to avoid airway complications.

In infants and young children, it is preferable to induce anesthesia with an inhalational, volatile anesthetic. After induction, intravenous access is established and an anticholinergic medication is administered to minimize airway secretions and to prevent bradycardia caused by vagal stimulation. Local anesthetic is also applied to the glottic and supraglottic areas. For laryngoscopy, we prefer an insufflation technique, with the patient breathing spontaneously and gases delivered via a 15 mm port on the suspension laryngoscope. Alternatively, a small caliber endotracheal tube may be used to secure the airway. For bronchoscopy, the bronchoscope is used as a conduit for ventilation. Jet ventilation is not recommended in children and may be associated with a higher risk of airway injury and pneumothorax.

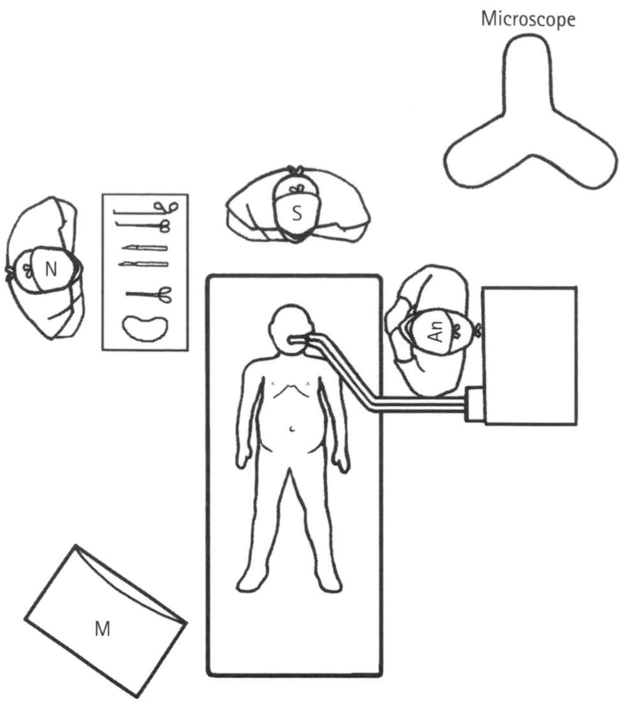

Figure 9.3

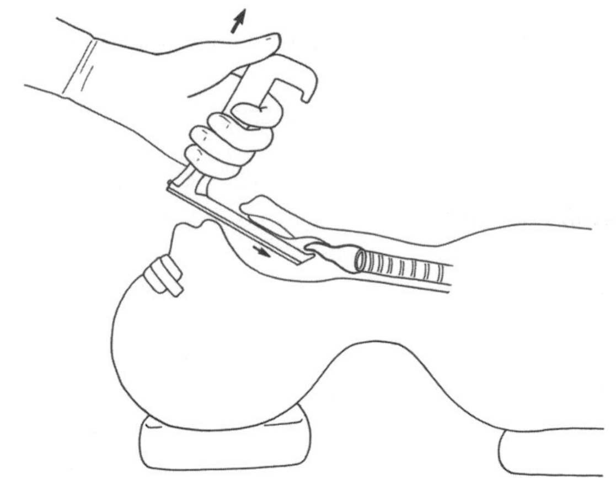

Figure 9.4

At the end of the procedure, the inhalational anesthetic may be discontinued while the surgeon examines the glottic and supraglottic regions to rule out movement abnormalities such as laryngomalacia and vocal fold paralysis.

Once the endoscope has been removed, the surgeon should examine the patient for loose dentition and mobilize the jaw to ensure that the mandible is mobile and not dislocated. Prior to leaving the operating room, the child should have regained a strong respiratory effort to protect the airway from aspiration and laryngospasm.

TECHNIQUE

For both laryngoscopy and bronchoscopy, the equipment must be organized in a logical fashion. The surgeon must be seated in a comfortable position, have easy access to the instrumentation and have an unobstructed view of the video monitor. To achieve these goals, the anesthetist and anesthesia equipment are usually positioned to the left of the patient, and the instrumentation, scrub nurse and video equipment are positioned to the right of the patient. (**See Figure 9.3**)

Laryngoscopy

Following induction of anesthesia, the patient is placed supine on the operating table. The head and neck are extended, placed in a 'sniffing' position and supported with a shoulder roll and ring pillow. The table should be elevated to a height that allows the surgeon to view the larynx while maintaining an upright back posture. Tilting of the table is usually not necessary. The eyes are protected with ointment and gauze pads and the head is draped in sterile fashion. A dental guard or moist gauze is used to protect the teeth and lips. An appropriately sized laryngoscope is then chosen and lubricated with warm saline.

By convention, the laryngoscope is held in the surgeon's left hand and is passed along the right side of the mouth and tongue while taking care to protect the lips and teeth. As the laryngoscope is introduced into the oral cavity, the blade is rotated 90° to facilitate entry. Once the laryngoscope approaches the base of tongue, it is straightened. The laryngoscope is gently lifted forward, taking great care to avoid damaging the teeth, to expose the epiglottis. A systematic examination of the upper airway should be performed in every case and includes an assessment of the base of the tongue, posterior pharyngeal wall, vallecula, piriform sinuses, both surfaces of the epiglottis, aryepiglottic folds, false cords, ventricles, vocal folds and subglottic space. (**See Figure 9.4**)

Depending on which laryngoscope is used, it is placed either anterior or posterior to the epiglottis when further surgery on the larynx is required. For general-purpose diagnosis, an appropriately sized open-sided laryngoscope is most commonly used. A wide variety of closed laryngoscopes are commercially available for use when intubation or further surgical intervention is required. For example, small-diameter slotted laryngoscopes are available for difficult intubations, and operating laryngoscopes with wide proximal ends are ideal for microlaryngoscopy and laser surgery. Regardless of the type of laryngoscope used, care is taken not to fold the epiglottis during suspension, as this can lead to unwanted edema and pain postoperatively. When properly positioned, the laryngoscope is suspended over the patient using a suspension apparatus. Again, various suspension systems are commercially available and the positioning depends on the type of system used. For some patients, anterior pressure on the laryngeal prominence may be necessary to visualize the anterior commissure and anterior end of the vocal folds.

With the laryngoscope suspended over the patient, the surgeon has bimanual access to the larynx. Secretions are suctioned, and rigid, straight and angled telescopes are used to visualize less accessible areas of the larynx such as the ventricles and subglottis. Attaching the telescopes to a camera and video monitor permits an efficient means of communicating the characteristics of the airway lesion to the anesthetist and nursing personnel and documenting the findings for later review or comparison. The telescope is also used to visualize the trachea to rule out a second, distal airway lesion. The microscope may also be used to provide an unparalleled, magnified view of the vocal folds for delicate, microsurgical procedures.

Care must be taken when removing the laryngoscope not to injure the aerodigestive mucosa and teeth. When removed, the jaw should be mobilized to ensure that it has not been dislocated.

Bronchoscopy

The safety precautions employed during laryngoscopy are similarly applied during bronchoscopy. Following the induction of anesthesia, preferably with spontaneous ventilation if obstructive disorders such as by a foreign body, the patient's larynx is exposed using the anesthetist's laryngoscope attached to a straight Miller blade. The laryngoscope is held with the left hand and a rigid 0° telescope is inserted with the right hand to visualize the glottis and subglottis prior to insertion of the bronchoscope. Once assured of the ability to pass a bronchoscope safely, an open or rod-lens bronchoscope is inserted alongside the straight blade of the laryngoscope. An open bronchoscope consists of a metal tube with a glass window at the proximal end. Visualization is with the naked eye, without the use of a telescope or video monitor. A superior view and depth perception can be obtained with a rod-lens bronchoscope, especially when the telescope is coupled to a video camera and monitor. **(See Figure 9.5)**

As the bronchoscope approaches the glottic opening, it is rotated 90° to align its leading beveled edge to the plane of the vocal folds. It is then introduced through the glottis into the trachea. The laryngoscope is then removed and the bronchoscope supported by the fingers and thumb of the left hand. Support provided by the left hand prevents injury to the lips and upper teeth and facilitates advancement of the bronchoscope. The anesthetic fresh gas supply is attached to the ventilating channel of the bronchoscope. Secretions in the trachea and bronchi may be aspirated. Vigorous and prolonged suctioning should be avoided, as it may cause oxygen desaturation in the young patient. **(See Figure 9.6)**

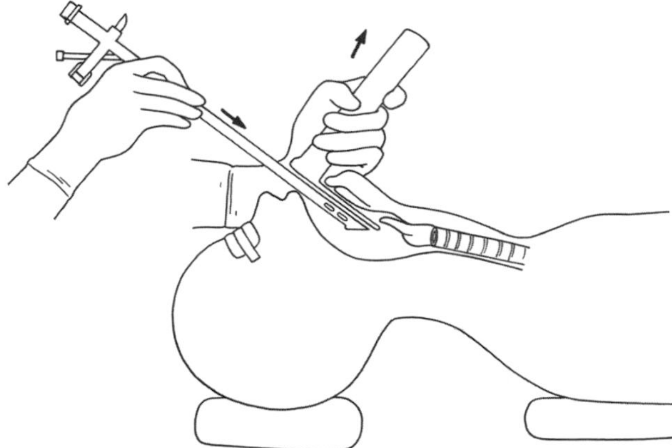

Figure 9.5

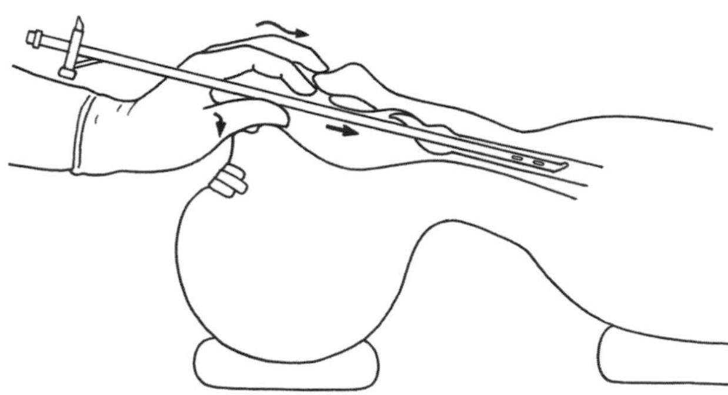

Figure 9.6

With the airway secured, the bronchoscope is advanced and the carina identified. To visualize the right mainstem bronchus, the tip of the bronchoscope is rotated to the right and the head of the patient to the left. To visualize the left mainstem bronchus, the opposite maneuver is performed. In general, the position of the operating table does not require adjustment during these maneuvers. It should be noted that with small caliber rod-lens bronchoscopes (less than 4 mm), the telescope must be removed intermittently to decrease ventilatory resistance. When rod-lens bronchoscopes less than 3 mm are used, ventilation may be impossible without the aid of an ultra-slim infant telescope. In these instances, pre-oxygenation with 100 percent oxygen is mandatory.

With the bronchoscope in position, manipulations of the lower airway such as removal of foreign bodies, biopsies, laser excisions, tracheal dilatations and stent placements can be performed. At the end of the procedure, the bronchoscope is gently withdrawn, avoiding trauma to the aerodigestive mucosa and dentition. The airway is then secured either with an endotracheal tube, inserted by the anesthetist, or by bag-mask ventilation until the patient has fully emerged from anesthesia.

POSTOPERATIVE CARE

Postoperative care begins in the operating theatre. Prior to transferring the patient to the post-anesthetic care unit, it is necessary to ensure that he or she has regained protective airway reflexes to minimize the risk of aspiration. The post-anesthetic care unit should be fully equipped to deal with airway obstruction and laryngeal spasm and be staffed by experienced personnel who can recognize and initiate the treatment of airway complications. Oxygen saturation monitoring may be necessary for several hours if significant postoperative airway edema is anticipated. In these instances, it is recommended that humidified oxygen and intravenous steroids be administered to the patient. Postoperative chest radiographs, especially after traumatic endoscopy, should be considered to rule out pneumothorax.

The timing for discharge from hospital is made on a case-by-case basis. In general, uncomplicated endoscopies should be followed by at least 4–6 hours of observation in a monitored setting. Discharge from hospital will then depend on several factors, such as the age of the patient, the distance of the patient's home from the hospital, the time of day the procedure was performed, the degree of airway compromise and the surgeon's sense of appropriateness. Any concerns should be addressed by an overnight admission to hospital. Complicated cases require the minimum of an overnight admission in a monitored setting.

PROBLEMS, PITFALLS AND SOLUTIONS

The majority of problems that arise during rigid endoscopy of the airway may be avoided by having a complete working knowledge of the endoscopic equipment and technique. The surgeon must possess a sound understanding of the applications, limitations and sizes of the available instrumentation. Moreover, there must be a preconceived technical approach that is clear in the mind of the surgeon and anesthetist.

Endoscopy of the airway, in a child or adult, must never be compromised with the use of inappropriately sized or functioning instrumentation. The mismatching of telescopes, light sources and connectors will invariably lead to frustration, a failed diagnostic assessment and a potentially catastrophic outcome. All instruments should be inspected by the surgeon prior to endoscopy. It is imperative to ensure that the chosen instruments are of an appropriate size and that all of the components, from laryngoscope to suction apparatus, are in proper working order. The instruments must be conveniently placed to the right of the surgeon, and an unobstructed view of the video monitor established. All telescopes should be warmed prior to use to prevent fogging. Warm saline and commercially available anti-fog solutions should also be available.

The endoscopic procedure should not be initiated until an adequate anesthetic state has been achieved. Forcing a laryngoscope or bronchoscope in a 'light' patient may result in injury to the lips, dentition and mandible. A patient that coughs or displays vocal fold movement is inadequately anesthetized. Any endoscopic instrument that is present in the upper airway should be immediately withdrawn in these instances to prevent significant injury to the vocal fold mucosa and the onset of laryngospasm. Topical application of lidocaine to the larynx is useful in preventing laryngospasm and vagally induced bradycardia.

The pediatric airway is susceptible to edema and subsequent airway compromise following manipulation. Therefore endoscopy should be performed with the smallest possible size of instrument that allows for adequate ventilation and visualization. Various sizes of laryngoscopes, bronchoscopes and a tracheostomy set should be readily available for use when examining the precarious airway.

Box 9.1 Complications associated with rigid endoscopy of the airway

Intra-operative

Non-traumatic

- Loss of airway control
- Airway fire
- Laryngospasm
- Anesthetic-induced respiratory depression
- Bradycardia
- Gastric distension
- Contamination of room air by anesthetic gases

Traumatic

- Mucosal tears and/or barotrauma causing:
  - pneumothorax
  - pneumomediastinum
  - subcutaneous emphysema
  - mediastinitis
- Dental trauma
- Mandibular dislocation
- Eye injury
- Burn or laceration injury to lip and gums
- Mucosal bleeding
- Rupture of viscus (trachea, bronchus, esophagus)
- Cervical spine injury

Postoperative

- Airway edema and obstruction
- Laryngospasm
- Post-obstructive pulmonary edema
- Persistent bleeding
- Pneumonia (late)

Difficulty in ventilating a patient even when access to the airway has been clearly established may suggest the presence of an iatrogenic pneumothorax. If this complication is suspected, an intra-operative chest radiograph should be immediately requested. The risk of developing a pneumothorax is significantly decreased when instruments are introduced and advanced gently and when the patient is breathing spontaneously. For this reason, jet ventilation is not recommended in children.

COMPLICATIONS

There are many potential complications associated with rigid endoscopy of the airway. They may occur intra-operatively or postoperatively. The majority can be avoided by maintaining a meticulous and consistent endoscopic approach, as outlined in this chapter. **(See Box 9.1)**

FURTHER READING

Benjamin B. *Endolaryngeal Surgery.* London: Martin Dunitz Ltd, 1998.

Bluestone CD, Rosenfeld RM (eds). *Surgical Atlas of Pediatric Otolaryngology*, 2nd edn. Hamilton, Ontario: BC Decker Inc., 2002.

10

Fiberoptic bronchoscopy – basic techniques

DAVID C.G. CRABBE

INTRODUCTION

The fiberoptic bronchoscope is an indispensable tool for endoscopic examination of the pediatric airway. Reliable endoscopes are now commercially available for fiberoptic bronchoscopy in children of all ages, from premature infants to adolescents.

In many instances, examination of the airway can be accomplished equally well with rigid or fiberoptic bronchoscopes. Fiberoptic bronchoscopy is simpler and probably less traumatic than rigid bronchoscopy for routine diagnostic use. Access to distal bronchi is good, particularly upper lobe bronchi, and bronchoalveolar lavage is simple to perform. At the present time, the main disadvantages of fiberoptic over rigid bronchoscopy are reduced image quality and the limited range of accessory instruments available. Fiberoptic endoscopes are still relatively expensive and fragile instruments. Equipment for rigid bronchoscopy must be available if a foreign body is suspected, even if a preliminary examination is undertaken with a fiberoptic bronchoscope.

Indications

DIAGNOSTIC BRONCHOSCOPY

- Persistent respiratory symptoms, e.g. hemoptysis, wheeze, stridor, persistent cough.
- Persistent atelectasis.
- Suspected chemical or thermal injury.
- Selective sampling of endobronchial secretions.
- Endobronchial lung biopsy.
- Selective bronchography.

THERAPEUTIC BRONCHOSCOPY

- Bronchoalveolar lavage.
- Placement of endotracheal tubes, confirmation of endotracheal tube position and patency.

Contraindications

- Uncorrected hypoxia.
- Uncorrected bleeding diatheses.
- Suspected foreign body.

The range of instruments available for use down a pediatric fiberoptic bronchoscope is too limited for reliable retrieval of foreign bodies. Furthermore, removal of foreign bodies from the airway always carries the potential risks of bleeding and airway obstruction. If a foreign body is suspected, the use of a rigid bronchoscope is advised. A wide range of grasping forceps is available and the bronchoscope will function as a rigid endotracheal tube.

EQUIPMENT/INSTRUMENTS

Essential

- Fiberoptic bronchoscope(s):
  - premature infant– term infant: 2.2 mm ultra-thin bronchoscope, term infant–adolescent: 3.6 mm bronchoscope.

The ultra-thin 2.2 mm bronchoscope lacks a suction channel. The larger 3.6 mm bronchoscope has a 1.2 mm working channel for suction and instrumentation. Both

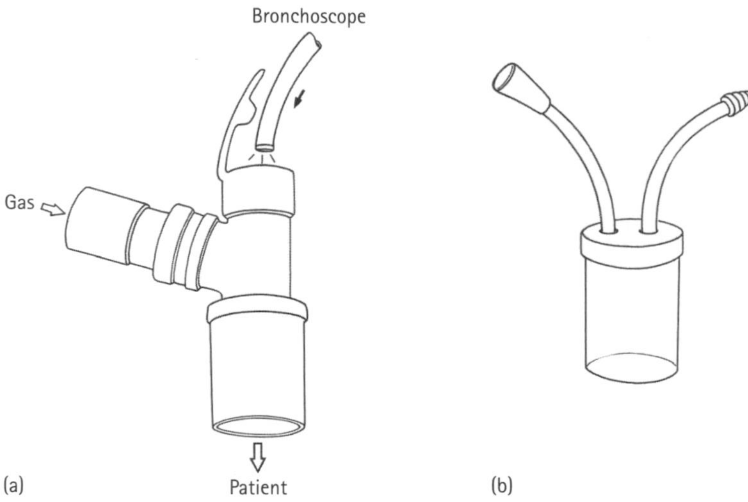

Figure 10.1 *(a) Bronchoscope adapter; (b) trap.*

instruments have a single control to angle the tip. Three-dimensional 'steering' of the bronchoscope involves angulation of the tip and rotation of the shaft.

- Light source (high-intensity xenon or halogen).
- Bronchoscopy swivel adapter for anesthetic circuits.
- Sputum trap.
- Suction apparatus and connecting tubing.
- 0.9 percent sodium chloride for bronchoalveolar lavage, in 10–20 mL aliquots, plus syringes.
- Pulse oximetry, electrocardiography monitoring, oxygen.
- Equipment and skills for endotracheal intubation and mechanical ventilation of the lungs if necessary. **(See Figure 10.1)**

Desirable

- Imaging equipment, including camera, television screen and video recorder/printer.
- Biopsy forceps, guide-wires, brushes etc.
- If interventional work such as bronchography is contemplated, an image intensifier is required and assistance from an experienced radiologist is desirable.

TECHNIQUE

Bronchoscopy inevitably produces some degree of airway obstruction, and constant monitoring for signs of hypoxia is essential throughout the procedure and during the recovery period. For this reason, continuous electrocardiogram (ECG) and oxygen saturation monitoring is essential. The child should be fasted prior to bronchoscopy, whether the procedure is performed under local anesthesia with sedation or under general anesthesia.

General anesthesia offers several advantages for fiberoptic bronchoscopy. The anesthetist will assume responsibility for the sedation of the patient and joint responsibility with the surgeon for oxygenation. Bronchoscopy can be performed via an endotracheal tube in a ventilated patient. This precludes examination of the larynx and upper trachea, and the size of endotracheal tube dictates the bronchoscope that can be accommodated:

- 2.2 mm bronchoscope: size 3.0 endotracheal tube or greater
- 3.6 mm bronchoscope: size 5.5 endotracheal tube or greater.

If the bronchoscope is inserted through an endotracheal tube and examination of the larynx and upper trachea is considered important, direct laryngoscopy will be necessary as a separate procedure, which may be performed under the same anesthetic.

Under most circumstances, routine diagnostic bronchoscopy is performed most easily under light general anesthesia delivered through a laryngeal mask, with the patient breathing spontaneously. This permits complete inspection of the larynx and upper trachea and, using this technique, fiberoptic bronchoscopy can be performed safely in children of all ages. **(See Figure 10.2)**

Bronchoscopy can be performed under sedation with local anesthesia. The child is sedated with intravenous midazolam 0.05–0.1 mg/kg. Mucosal anesthesia is achieved with lidocaine up to a total dose of 3 mg/kg (0.3 mL/kg 1 percent solution). Direct instillation of 1 percent solution into the nose is effective. If bronchoscopy is performed under sedation, it is essential to have equipment available and the expertise to intubate the airway and ventilate the child in the event of excessive sedation and hypoxia.

Topical anesthesia of the vocal cords, larynx and trachea can be achieved by injecting 1 percent lidocaine solution down the suction channel of the bronchoscope once these structures are visualized. This maneuver is also valuable if bronchoscopy is performed via a laryngeal mask airway under general anesthesia.

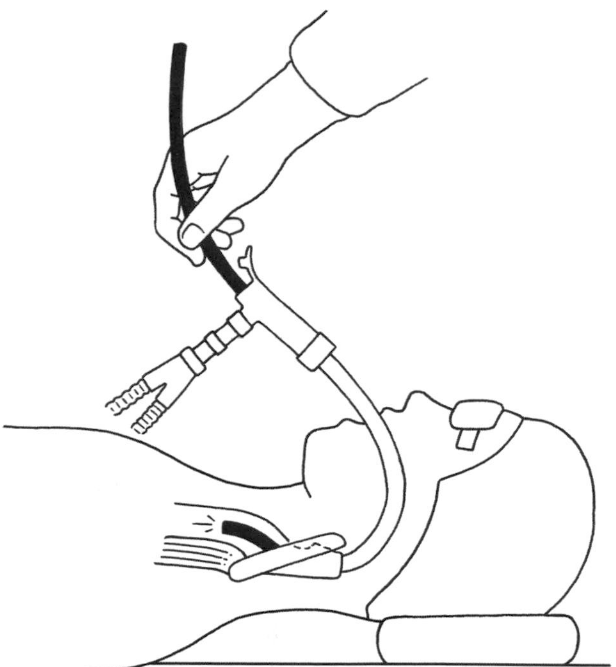

Figure 10.2 *Fiberoptic bronchoscope through a laryngeal mask.*

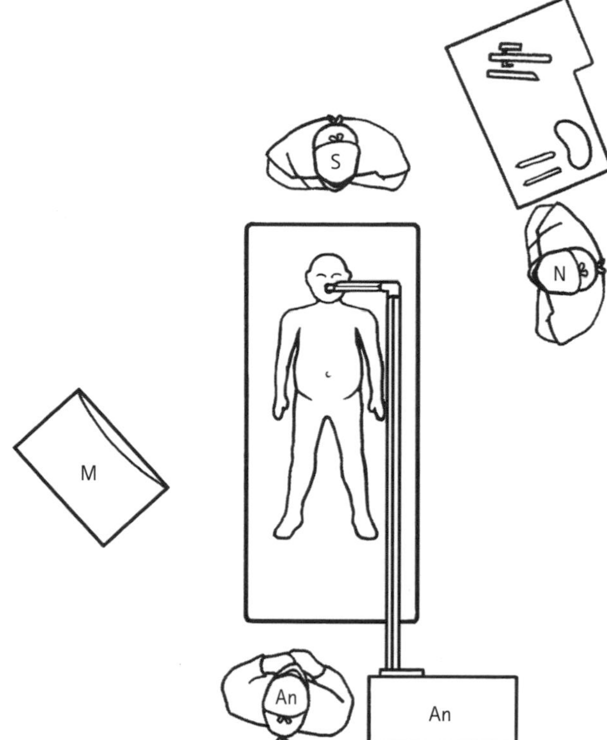

Figure 10.3

After the induction of anesthesia or sedation, the child is positioned supine on the operating table, with his or her head at the foot end. The neck is held in a neutral position using a head ring or sand bags on either side. The child's eyes should be held closed with adhesive paper tape to prevent corneal abrasion. The surgeon stands at the foot of the table with the scrub nurse to his or her left. **(See Figure 10.3)**

The bronchoscope is held in the surgeon's left hand, using the thumb to operate the control wheel and the index finger to operate the suction as necessary. Rotation of the control wheel will angulate the tip of the bronchoscope upwards or downwards. The right hand guides, advances and rotates the shaft of the bronchoscope. Whether sedation or general anesthesia is employed, bronchoscopy involves gentle passage of the instrument down the airway. The instrument is 'steered' down the center of the airway by angulation of the tip and application of torque to the shaft with the right hand, which also advances the bronchoscope. **(See Figure 10.4)**

The supraglottis is inspected and vocal cord movement and the configuration of the trachea and in its caliber with respiration are noted. The airway mucosa is normally pale pink in color and has a smooth texture. The tracheal/bronchial cartilages should be clearly visible. The presence or absence and the consistency of secretions within the airway are noted. Acute and chronic lower respiratory tract infection is invariably associated with copious amounts of purulent secretions. These should be gently aspirated and sent for culture. In children with established bronchiectasis, the secretions are frequently so viscous that the suction channel of the bronchoscope blocks. In this event, the instrument should be withdrawn and the suction channel cleaned by the injection of saline down it.

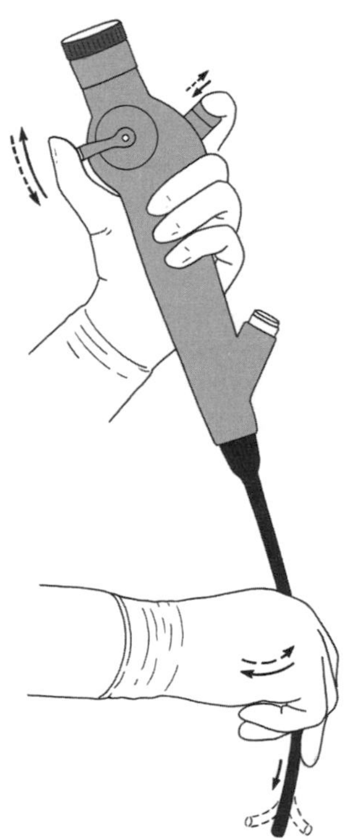

Figure 10.4

As the bronchoscope is advanced down the trachea, the carina comes into view. At this point the bronchoscope

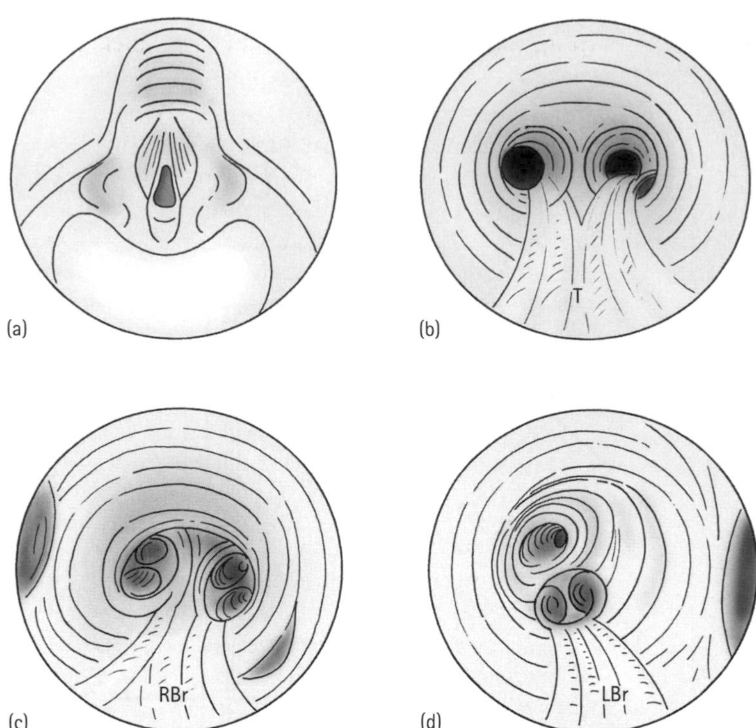

Figure 10.5 *(a) Larynx; (b) carina; (c) right main bronchus; (d) left main bronchus.*

must be rotated 90° clockwise to examine the right main bronchus, which is then entered by upward angulation of its tip. Sequential examination of the lobar and segmental bronchi is then performed. The bronchoscope is then withdrawn, rotated anti-clockwise and the left main bronchus, lobar and segmental bronchi examined in a similar fashion. **(See Figure 10.5)**

Bronchoalveolar lavage is performed using 10–20 mL aliquots of warm saline. The bronchoscope is positioned at the entrance to the lobar bronchus of interest and saline is injected down the suction channel using a syringe controlled by the surgeon's right hand. Gentle suction is applied and the fluid aspirated at the mouth of the bronchus. The yield is very variable and further aliquots of saline often have to be instilled to obtain sufficient aspirate.

An isolated tracheo-esophageal fistula (TEF) is usually seen at thoracic inlet level. This point is easily determined by transillumination of the trachea – the light from the bronchoscope is visible through the neck. Occasionally the TEF will be large enough to be spotted immediately, but most are not so obvious and may only be visible as a small collection of air bubbles on the posterior wall of the trachea. The posterior wall of the trachea may be gently probed with the flexible end of a 0.035 radiologic guidewire passed down the suction channel of the bronchoscope, but great care must be taken to avoid iatrogenic injury to the airway. Distal TEFs, associated with esophageal atresia, are usually located around the carina. These fistulae are invariably large and easily visible.

Tracheomalacia is easy to appreciate with a fiberoptic bronchoscope. The child is able to breathe spontaneously around the bronchoscope with minimal obstruction, particularly if it is inserted through a laryngeal mask. This simplifies anesthetic management considerably and allows the severity of tracheomalacia to be assessed during spontaneous respiration. Tracheomalacia is most frequently encountered in children following repair of esophageal atresia, and in this situation the malacia predominantly affects the middle third of the trachea. The anterior wall of the

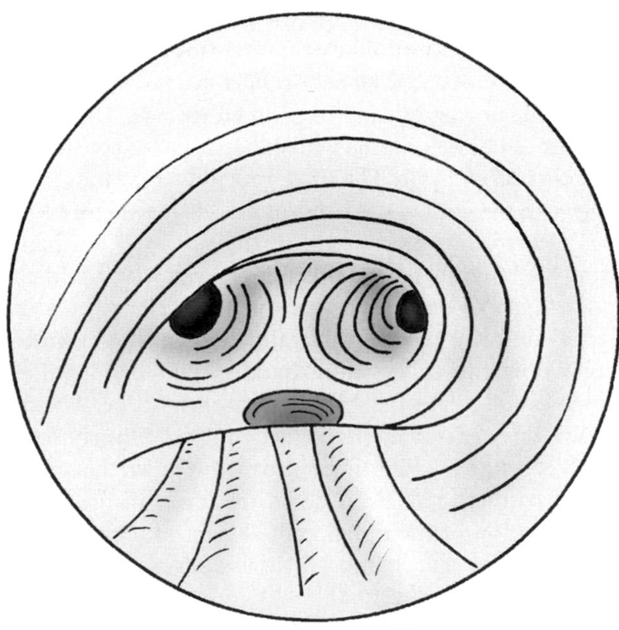

Figure 10.6 *Tracheomalacia. Note the collapsed anterior wall with a repaired fistula just below it.*

trachea collapses and transmits the pulsation of the aortic arch. The magnitude of the collapse can be estimated in terms of the percentage of the cross-sectional area of the trachea occluded and also the length of the malacic segment determined. In addition it is useful to document whether malacia extends down to the carina and whether the main bronchi are involved. **(See Figure 10.6)**

Congenital tracheal stenosis is usually associated with the presence of complete circular tracheal cartilages. If a tracheal stenosis is suspected, no attempt should be made to force the bronchoscope through the stenosis because this will invariably result in mucosal edema and worsening of the airway obstruction. The stenosis should be documented and the bronchoscopy then terminated. Appropriate referral should be made to an expert in pediatric airway reconstruction.

POSTOPERATIVE CARE

Postoperative recovery following fiberoptic bronchoscopy is usually smooth and uncomplicated. If topical anesthesia of the larynx is employed, it is important to keep the child fasted for 2 hours postoperatively to prevent aspiration. Oxygen saturation should be monitored in the early postoperative period by pulse oximetry. Provided there is no concern about airway obstruction/edema, fiberoptic bronchoscopy can be performed safely as a day-case procedure.

PROBLEMS, PITFALLS AND SOLUTIONS

- Hypoxia is a constant and avoidable complication of bronchoscopy. Supplemental oxygen should be administered to the child. Frequently, temporary withdrawal of the bronchoscope is necessary.
- Laryngeal spasm is occasionally encountered whilst attempting to insert the bronchoscope through the larynx. This is preventable to a large degree by anesthetizing the vocal cords with lidocaine, but if this is not successful, the bronchoscope should be temporarily withdrawn and further intravenous sedation given or the anesthetic deepened. Supplemental oxygen should be administered and close cooperation with the anesthetist is essential.
- Loss of anatomical bearings: the precise location of the tip of the bronchoscope can be difficult to discern on occasions in the midst of serial divisions of the airway. If the position is unclear, the bronchoscope should be withdrawn and the landmarks followed distally again, from the trachea if necessary.
- Blurred vision: this is usually due to thick secretions or blood fogging the end of the bronchoscope. Withdrawal and cleaning of the tip of the instrument may be necessary. If the problem keeps recurring, passage of a suction catheter down the airway to clear secretions prior to re-insertion of the endoscope may be helpful.

COMPLICATIONS

- Bronchoscopy-induced hemorrhage is rare in pediatric practice, but alarming and potentially serious. Management consists of attention to the airway, oxygenation and circulation, if necessary. Minor bleeding will usually cease spontaneously. Irrigation with ice-cold saline may be effective. Dilute epinephrine (1:200 000) can be added to the saline. After the hemorrhage has ceased, the child should remain on bed rest with close monitoring for 24 hours. Anti-tussives may be of benefit. In more dramatic cases, endotracheal intubation should be performed to secure the airway. If the bleeding is arising from one particular bronchus, this can be isolated from the airway by occlusion with a Fogarty embolectomy catheter. Should these maneuvers prove necessary, the child should be admitted to the pediatric intensive care facility and should remain sedated and ventilated for 24 hours prior to removal of the catheter and subsequent extubation.
- Occasionally, stridor develops post-bronchoscopy. In mild cases this can be managed with humidified air/oxygen and will settle after 24–48 hours. In more severe cases, nebulized epinephrine (up to 5 mL 1:10 000 solution) may be necessary. Under these circumstances, early involvement of the pediatric intensive care team is wise.

FURTHER READING

Prakash UBS. *Bronchoscopy.* New York: Raven Press, 1994.

11

Foreign bodies in the airway

DAVID C.G. CRABBE

INTRODUCTION

Tracheo-bronchial foreign bodies are not rare in children. Each year approximately 250 children asphyxiate from an inhaled foreign body in the UK. The symptoms can be dramatic or very minor and a low threshold for submitting a child to bronchoscopy is necessary. The classical triad of symptoms – sudden-onset coughing, wheezing and reduced air entry – occurs in less than one-third of children. Removal of inhaled foreign bodies, particularly when a major degree of airway obstruction is present, can be a real challenge for both anesthetist and surgeon.

Indications

- Actual or suspected foreign body inhalation.
- Persistent lobar collapse.
- Persistent wheeze, unresponsive to medical therapy.

Contraindications

- Inadequate equipment.
- Lack of proper equipment and experienced personnel (surgeon, anesthetist and operating room staff).

EQUIPMENT/INSTRUMENTS

Essential

- Full range of Storz ventilating bronchoscopes.
- Optical grasping forceps: optical grasping forceps for the Storz bronchoscopes are available in two sizes. The smaller size can be accommodated within a bronchoscope of at least 3.5 mm. The larger size can be accommodated within a bronchoscope of 4.0 mm or larger. Optical forceps are longer than the bronchoscopes to allow manipulation and grasping of foreign bodies. Consequently, a longer rod-lens telescope is required. The choice of forceps depends on the foreign body to be removed. Peanuts are most easily removed with double-action peanut-grasping forceps, whereas a sharp object is more easily removed with alligator forceps.
- Rigid telescopes (0°) to suit the bronchoscopes and the optical grasping forceps.
- Glass eyepiece for the bronchoscope.
- Rubber gland for the bronchoscope, to ensure an airtight seal around the optical forceps.
- Intubating anesthetic laryngoscope.
- McGill's forceps (anesthesia).
- Flexible and rigid suction.
- Suction tubing.
- Light source and fiberoptic cables.
- Camera, monitor.
- Video recording or image printing equipment.
- Ice-cold saline for irrigation, with syringes.

Desirable

- Fogarty embolectomy catheters.
- Fiberoptic bronchoscope.

PREOPERATIVE PREPARATION

Preoperative preparation depends to some extent on the nature and severity of the child's symptoms. It is inappropriate to delay bronchoscopy in a child with significant airway obstruction for any longer than the time necessary to set up the operating room. On the other hand, bronchoscopy to exclude a foreign body in a child with chronic respiratory symptoms should be performed in an elective setting in a suitably fasted patient. A chest radiograph should be obtained for all children with a suspected inhaled foreign body, although the majority are not radio-opaque. Inspiratory and expiratory films to demonstrate air trapping from a foreign body may be useful in an older child who will cooperate with requests to suspend respiration, but this is rarely possible in the group of children most at risk, i.e. toddlers. In the cervical region it may be difficult to decide whether a foreign body is in the airway or esophagus. In this situation a lateral radiograph of the neck may be helpful. Normal radiographs do not exclude a foreign body.

The procedure should be explained to the child, as appropriate, and to the parents. The parents need to understand the potential risks of the procedure, including airway obstruction and failed extraction.

The importance of checking that all the necessary equipment is present and compatible cannot be over-estimated. The scrub nurse must be familiar with the equipment and the likely sequence of events. Telescopes and bronchoscopes must be kept warm to minimize condensation, which will fog the endoscopic view. The surgeon and anesthetist should discuss strategy and their relative responsibilities prior to the arrival of the child. Failed retrieval of an inhaled foreign body has the potential to produce complete airway obstruction, with predictable consequences.

TECHNIQUE

The presence and position of any loose teeth should be noted. Continuous electrocardiogram and oxygen saturation monitoring is essential. Anesthesia should be induced with volatile agents and spontaneous respiration maintained during the procedure. Mechanical ventilation of the lungs may force a foreign body distally into the airway and may result in a 'ball-valve' obstruction, with worsening hypoxia and/or pneumothorax. The anesthetist maintains the child's airway using a facemask and a T-piece anesthetic circuit until the surgeon is ready to commence the bronchoscopy. If there is significant airway obstruction, the inspired oxygen concentration should be kept at 100 percent for the duration of the procedure.

The technique of rigid bronchoscopy has been covered in detail in Chapter 9. A preliminary examination of the pharynx and larynx should be made with the anesthetic intubating laryngoscope because occasionally foreign bodies can be retrieved from this region using McGill's forceps. The next objective is to assess the airway to confirm or exclude the presence of a foreign body. This is performed using an appropriately sized rigid bronchoscope, as described in Chapter 9. Great care must be taken to ensure the lumen of the airway remains in view at all times to avoid pushing a foreign body further down the tracheobronchial tree. Once the foreign body is located, the bronchoscope is positioned approximately 2 cm above the obstruction and supported by the surgeon.

The scrub nurse then removes the telescope and occludes the open bronchoscope with a glass eyepiece.

The optical biopsy forceps is then assembled with the correct telescope and rubber gland.

This apparatus is then introduced into the bronchoscope. **(See Figure 11.1)**

The jaws of the forceps are opened once they emerge from the end of the bronchoscope and the foreign body is grasped under direct vision. In the case of spherical or globular foreign bodies, it is important to ensure that the blades of the forceps pass beyond the equator of the object to minimize the risk of fragmentation during retrieval. This is a particular problem with peanuts, which must be grasped with great delicacy. **(See Figure 11.2)**

The anesthetist should temporarily suspend ventilation at this point. If the foreign body is small and unlikely to fragment, it may be retrieved through the bronchoscope. This is not usually possible, and foreign body and bronchoscope must be withdrawn together. It is easy to lose the foreign body in the upper trachea or larynx at this stage. After the bronchoscope has been removed, the anesthetist should take over control of the airway with a facemask whilst the retrieved object is inspected.

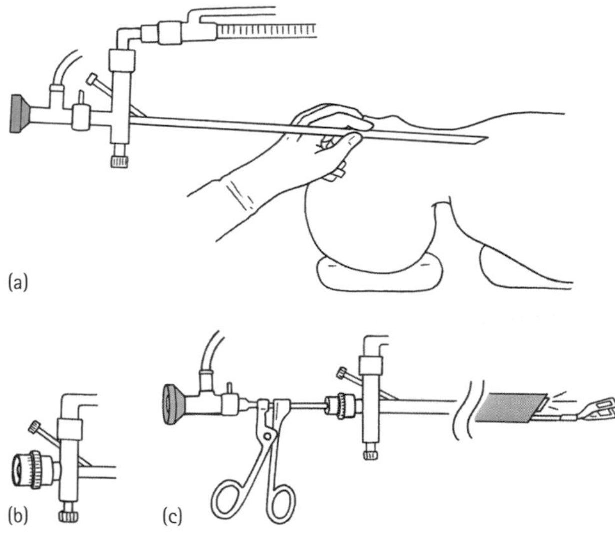

Figure 11.1 *(a) Bronchoscope in position; (b) telescope removed, fenestrated rubber gland in place; (c) optical biopsy forceps in place.*

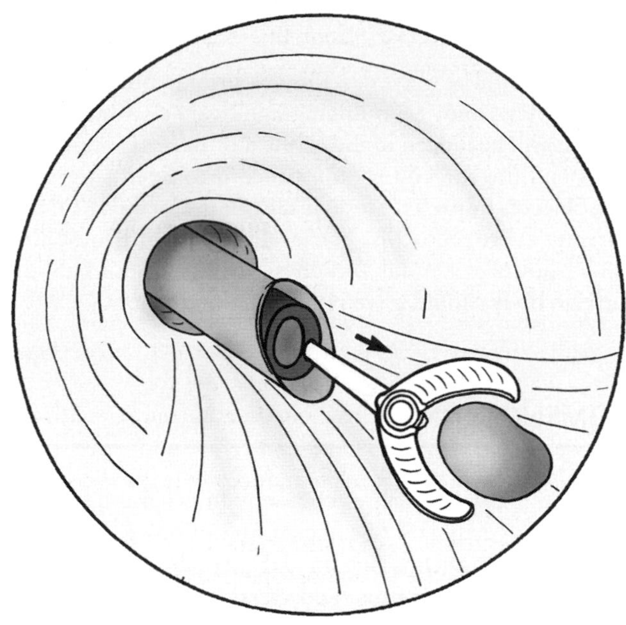

Figure 11.2

It is mandatory to examine the distal airway after removal of a foreign body to exclude additional foreign bodies and to aspirate secretions. This may be performed either with the rigid bronchoscope used for the preliminary examination or with a fiberoptic bronchoscope. Residual foreign body fragments may need to be removed, in which case the procedure described above should be repeated.

POSTOPERATIVE CARE

General postoperative care following bronchoscopy has been covered in Chapter 9. If there is significant lobar collapse distal to a foreign body, chest physiotherapy and antibiotics may need to be continued for a few days postoperatively. Steroids are not generally required. In all cases children should remain in hospital under observation overnight.

PROBLEMS, PITFALLS AND SOLUTIONS

Airway obstruction

Most foreign bodies will produce some degree of airway obstruction. However, foreign bodies in the larynx and upper trachea have the propensity to produce severe obstruction and these cases comprise the majority of the recorded fatalities. In the immediate setting the Heimlich maneuver should be attempted. In hospital these children should be taken immediately to the operating room for bronchoscopy. The foreign body is likely to be relatively large (e.g. a coin) and, as a consequence, attempts to force the object down one

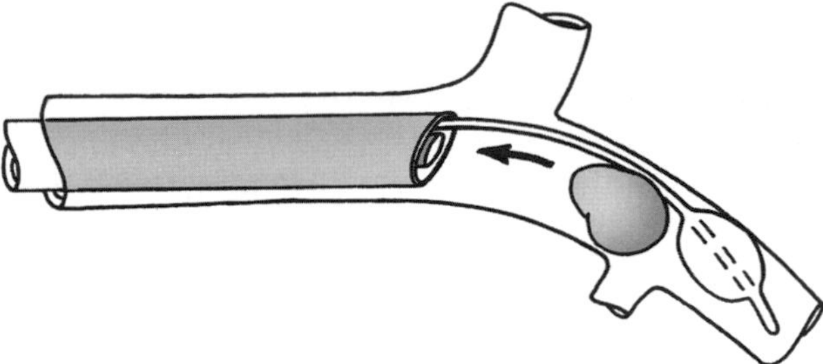

Figure 11.3

or other main bronchus are likely to result in total airway obstruction as the object is impacted in the distal trachea. If the object cannot be grasped through the bronchoscope, retrieval with a Fogarty embolectomy catheter may be successful. The Fogarty catheter is passed either down the bronchoscope or, alternatively, through the larynx alongside the bronchoscope. The catheter is advanced beyond the foreign body and the balloon inflated. Traction is exerted on the catheter to withdraw the foreign body. The bronchoscope should be removed at this stage and the anesthetic laryngoscope inserted. As the object appears in the laryngeal inlet it should be grasped with McGill's forceps and retrieved. **(See Figure 11.3)**

Bleeding

Peanuts provoke a florid inflammatory reaction in the airway and rapidly become surrounded by granulation tissue. The process is less rapid with more inert objects, but nonetheless any longstanding foreign body is likely to be encased in granulation tissue. Granulation tissue obscures the view of the foreign body down the bronchoscope but, more importantly, bleeds as soon as an attempt is made to grasp the object. Ice-cold saline injected down the suction catheter may stop the bleeding. Provided the foreign body can be grasped securely, it should be retrieved. If the view is totally obscured by bleeding, the safest course of action is to abandon the bronchoscopy and make a further attempt after 48–72 hours. Bleeding from granulation tissue invariably ceases spontaneously after the foreign body has been removed, and the granulations will resolve.

Sharp objects

Sharp objects should be retrieved either blunt end first or by drawing the pointed end into the shaft of the bronchoscope. Bronchoscope and foreign body are then removed together.

Distally impacted or upper lobe foreign bodies

Both of these are rare and best located by fiberoptic bronchoscopy. Depending on the nature of the foreign body, it may be amenable to retrieval with a Dormia basket. Prior to attempting this procedure, it should be established that the basket can pass down the suction channel of the bronchoscope. Occasionally it is possible to move the foreign body to a more accessible location by applying suction through the bronchoscope. It may also be possible to retrieve an inaccessible foreign body using a Fogarty catheter. If all these measures fail, bronchotomy or lobectomy may be necessary.

Fragmentation

Organic material (especially peanuts) becomes soggy and friable in the airway. Great care is necessary during extraction to avoid fragmentation. Peanut forceps are recommended and the surgeon should ensure that the jaws of the forceps pass beyond the equator of the object to be retrieved. The jaws should be closed gently and the foreign body, bronchoscope and optical forceps removed together. The object must be inspected to confirm integrity and the bronchoscope re-inserted to exclude residual debris in the tracheobronchial tree.

Lost foreign body

If the foreign body is lost during retrieval, the airway should be secured immediately and then the bronchoscope re-inserted. If the foreign body lies in the trachea and cannot be grasped immediately, it should be pushed back down the bronchus in which it had originally lodged. A second, more controlled attempt should be made to retrieve the object. If the foreign body is not seen, the bronchoscope should be withdrawn and the larynx and hypopharynx carefully inspected. The airway should then be intubated with an endotracheal tube and the mouth, nose and esophagus examined digitally and with an endoscope to ensure that the foreign body is retrieved or at least not in a location from which it can be aspirated again during emergence from anesthesia.

Failed foreign body retrieval

Parents should be warned of this risk prior to bronchoscopy. If the foreign body is producing significant airway obstruction, it will be lodged in the cervical or upper thoracic trachea and the surgeon should proceed to open surgery. If the object is impacted more distally in the airway, a further attempt at bronchoscopic retrieval may be performed after 48–72 hours of steroids and physiotherapy. If this fails, the foreign body should be retrieved at thoracotomy.

COMPLICATIONS

The complications of bronchoscopy in general have been covered in Chapter 9. Specific complications encountered as a result of bronchoscopy for foreign bodies include failed retrieval, airway trauma and persistent lobar collapse. Complications are more likely to occur if the foreign body is longstanding. In most reported series, open surgery to retrieve a foreign body is necessary in less than 1 percent of cases. Airway edema after a difficult bronchoscopy will usually settle after 2–3 days and should be managed expectantly with humidified air/oxygen and intravenous dexamethasone 1–2 mg/kg daily. Persistent lobar collapse may indicate a residual foreign body, bronchial stenosis or, in longstanding cases, bronchiectasis. Repeat bronchoscopy after several weeks of intensive medical treatment may be necessary. In the case of severe symptomatic bronchiectasis, lobectomy may be required.

FURTHER READING

Darrow DH, Holinger LD. Foreign bodies of the larynx, trachea and bronchi. In: Bluestone CD, Stool SE, Kenna MA (eds), *Pediatric Otolaryngology*, 3rd edn. Philadelphia: WB Saunders, 1996.

12

Interventional bronchoscopy

ROBERT E. WOOD

INTRODUCTION

Interventional bronchoscopy in children is a relatively recent development. The discussions that follow are predicated on an understanding that the reader is familiar with the techniques and instrumentation for both rigid and flexible bronchoscopy in pediatric patients. This chapter introduces a number of techniques with the caveat that experience in pediatrics is limited, particularly regarding long-term outcomes.

The commonest reason to perform a therapeutic bronchoscopy in pediatric patients is to remove an aspirated foreign body, which is discussed in detail in Chapter 11. This chapter focuses on advanced endoscopic techniques, including stent placement, laser applications and airway dilatation.

AIRWAY STENTS

Stents were initially developed for intravascular use. More recently, they have been used in the tracheo-bronchial tree to maintain the shape and dimensions of the lumen. In pediatric patients, stents may be considered to treat tracheomalacia, bronchomalacia and tracheal or bronchial stenosis. Despite theoretical attractions, stents should be used with great caution in the pediatric airway because of the potential for complications and uncertainty about the long-term results.

Experience with expandable metallic stents in the pediatric airway is largely confined to the Palmaz stent. These devices are marketed for use as vascular or biliary stents in adults. Expandable metallic stents have a thin wall and a lattice structure that allows the lumen of the airway to epithelialize, promoting the clearance of secretions.

The Palmaz stent is constructed from a stainless-steel cylinder in which longitudinal slits have been cut by laser. Its pre-expansion diameter is approximately 2 mm, and the wall thickness is 0.15 mm. The stent is loaded over an angioplasty balloon catheter and positioned in the airway either under direct visualization with a bronchoscope or by fluoroscopy. The balloon is inflated to expand the stent. **(See Figure 12.1)**

In pediatric patients, it may be desirable to expand the stent initially to a diameter less than maximum because this allows for further dilatation in the future to accommodate growth. Metallic stents are virtually impossible to reposition once expanded into place.

The position of the stent should be verified visually (with a small flexible bronchoscope) and fluoroscopically prior to its expansion. Radiographic contrast medium in the airway will enhance visualization of anatomic landmarks and aid positioning.

Indications for airway stents in children

- Tracheomalacia.
- Bronchomalacia.
- Airway stenoses.

In theory, stents could be used in children with either dynamic or fixed airway obstructions. When the alternative

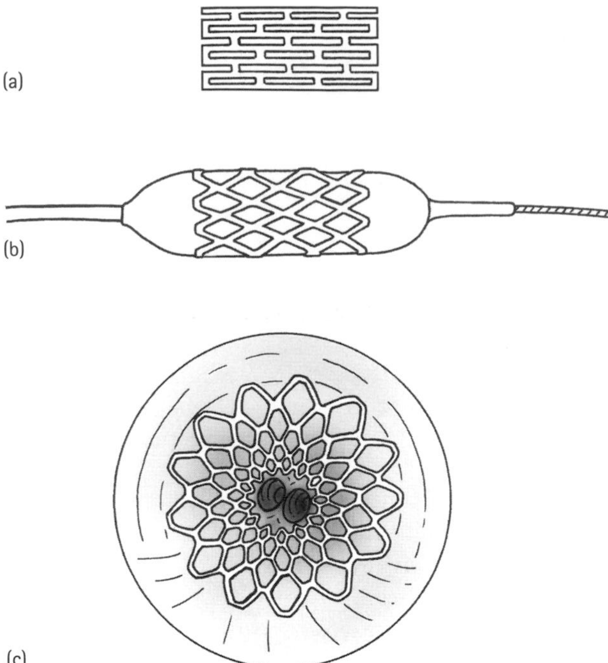

Figure 12.1 *(a) Stent; (b) stent over a balloon; (c) stent positioned in the airway.*

is prolonged intubation and tracheostomy, a stent seems intuitively attractive. However, one should be confident that the underlying pathology will resolve and allow the subsequent removal of the stent. Metallic stents have been used to manage anastomotic stenosis and tracheal resection. It must be stressed that experience in children is limited and data on the long-term safety of airway stents are not yet available.

In practice, stents are most readily employed in the trachea and the left main bronchus. These sections of the airway are sufficiently long that a stent can be positioned with some margin for error. The anatomy of the right main bronchus is not conducive to stent placement, as a very short stent is required in order to avoid obstruction of the right upper lobe bronchus.

Complications of stents

Stents are foreign bodies and some tissue reaction is inevitable. Granulation tissue and scar formation are common complications. Granulation tissue may obstruct the lumen of the airway. There are a number of options for treatment, including piecemeal removal with biopsy forceps, coagulation with laser and balloon dilatation. Balloon dilatation involves negotiating a balloon catheter through the stent and inflating the balloon to compress the granulation tissue. Bleeding, mucus plugging, and migration of the stent are potential complications. Mucus plugging may require urgent bronchoscopy and, if the stent is in the trachea, this complication may be life-threatening.

The natural history of airway obstruction in children is such that if stents are used they may need to remain in place for a prolonged period. Restricted growth of the airway in the years after stent placement may result in an acquired functional stenosis as the patient outgrows the stent. Therefore, the stent may have to be removed at some stage and, unless the condition for which the stent was placed has resolved, a larger one placed. Metal stents can erode through the wall of the airway and there are reports of stent erosion into adjacent blood vessels with fatal consequences. Limited data exist on the lifespan of stent materials and there are no data on the long-term consequences of airway stenting in the growing child.

Stent removal

At some point most stents will require removal, whether because of complications or disintegration of the stent itself, or because the problem for which the stent was initially placed has resolved. The latter can be challenging to define, since one can only determine whether the airway will be adequate by actually removing the stent.

Metal stents may be removed with endoscopic forceps and traction, preceded by rotation to free the stent from the wall of the airway. By necessity, this deforms the lattice of the stent into a sharp, crumpled ball of wire. This is usually associated with brisk bleeding from the airway mucosa. The remains of the stent must then be retrieved either through the larynx, with the attendant risk of damage to the vocal cords, or, more safely, through a short incision in the cervical trachea. If the stent has been in place for a significant period of time, the lattice may fragment during extraction, in which case piecemeal removal is necessary. In any case, bleeding will surely result, and the airway should be evaluated several days to weeks after stent removal to ensure healing.

LASER TECHNIQUES

Lasers are used in the airways to destroy abnormal or excess tissue while producing relatively little damage to surrounding normal tissues. At low energy levels, lasers can also be used to achieve hemostasis. Laser energy has varying effects on tissues, ranging from coagulation to desiccation and vaporization, depending on the intensity and duration of application.

Instrumentation

Several lasers are available for airway use, including the CO_2 laser, argon or KTP laser and Nd:YAG laser. These lasers have different wavelengths and, as a result, different characteristics, which are discussed in Chapter 4. The CO_2 laser must be used in a direct line-of-sight mode, usually with an operating microscope, which limits its use to the larynx. Nd:YAG and KTP lasers can be delivered through a fiberoptic cable, which makes them ideally suited for use with rigid and fiberoptic bronchoscopes in children.

How lasers are used in the airways

The laser beam should be directed parallel to the airway wall, to avoid inadvertent damage to surrounding normal tissue. The lowest effective power should be used in short bursts. KTP or argon lasers can be effective with delivered energy in the range of 2–3 watts and pulse durations of 0.1–1 second.

Removal of obstructing tissue can be accomplished by coagulating or 'cooking' the mass and then removing fragments piecemeal with forceps. This may be accomplished effectively with an open-tube bronchoscope. Alternatively, the target tissue may be vaporized and totally ablated by the laser. This process entails two significant risks: first, steam released from vaporization of the target can produce thermal damage to surrounding normal airway, and second, the laser beam may pass beyond the target lesion and damage deeper or more peripheral structures.

By applying laser energy at a level below that required for charring, the target tissue can be desiccated and then left to involute naturally. This method of ablation is generally best performed in stages, separated by 2–4 weeks, to minimize residual scarring. It is also safer to leave some residual abnormal tissue than to attempt to achieve full resolution in one stage. This is particularly important for annular lesions because if the entire circumference of the airway is coagulated, contracture of the airway may occur during the subsequent healing phase.

The KTP and argon lasers may be used by positioning the tip of the laser fiber close to or in contact with the target tissue. While it is feasible to direct the laser fiber through an open-tube bronchoscope, precise application of the laser energy to the target tissue can be achieved more conveniently with a flexible bronchoscope. The tip of the laser fiber is advanced 3–5 mm beyond the tip of the instrument and the laser is then fired under direct visual control. In small children, a 300 μ laser fiber is generally the best choice. Accurate positioning of the laser fiber is essential to avoid damage to adjacent structures. Surgical lasers are equipped with a low-intensity aiming beam of visible light, which should be used to confirm alignment with the target. Great caution must be taken to ensure that the laser is not operated while the fiber tip is inside the fiberoptic bronchoscope, as severe damage to the instrument will result. *The fiber and the aiming beam* must be seen to exit the bronchoscope before the laser can be fired. Because of the risk of ignition, the inspired oxygen concentration delivered to the patient should not exceed 40 percent during the laser procedure. The laser should not be used where the beam (direct or reflected) may impact on an inflammable object such as an endotracheal or tracheostomy tube. Syringes of saline should be immediately available as a precaution to extinguish an airway fire.

Clinical applications of lasers in the pediatric airways

Subglottic lesions such as granulation tissue or hemangiomas are logical targets of laser therapy. Many patients with such lesions will also have a tracheostomy and care must be taken to minimize the risk of ignition of the tracheostomy tube by stray laser energy. The CO_2 laser is conventionally used in this region, but there is some evidence to suggest that the long-term outcome may be better with the KTP laser. If the patient does not have a tracheostomy, the mass must be debulked sufficiently to ensure a safe airway during the recovery period.

Tracheal lesions such as granulation tissue above a tracheostome are also amenable to treatment by laser. Care must be taken to avoid destruction of cartilage rings proximal to the stoma because these are often displaced into the tracheal lumen by the tracheostomy tube. The tracheostomy tube should be removed momentarily while the laser is operated to avoid the risk of fire. Tracheal tumors are rare in children. Resection is usually the treatment of choice, but occasionally recanalization of the lumen with laser may be appropriate. Whatever method of treatment is employed, a histological diagnosis is essential.

Bronchial lesions amenable to laser therapy in children include granulation tissue and stenoses. Granulation tissue associated with acute bronchial injury (such as with an aspirated foreign body) will usually resolve after the inciting cause is removed. In the case of more mature granulation tissue, or a mass that obstructs a large bronchus, laser therapy may be effective. In the author's experience, the most common indication for laser therapy in the bronchi of children is granulation tissue and stenosis resulting from deep endobronchial suctioning in children with tracheostomies or those who have been intubated for prolonged periods. In this situation the airway obstruction is usually limited to the right lower or right middle and lower lobes. Judicious treatment with low-intensity laser in several sessions generally gives good long-term results. Stenotic lesions may be treated effectively with a combination of laser and subsequent dilatation using an angioplasty balloon catheter.

DILATATION

Stenoses in the subglottis, trachea and mainstem bronchi are amenable to dilatation. Dilatation of airway stenoses invariably provides temporary benefit only, and is usually performed in preparation for definitive surgery.

Dilatation can be achieved by several techniques, including using the endoscope itself, using a dilator which is pushed through the stenosis, and using a calibrated balloon catheter. A rigid or flexible bronchoscope can be used, but it is difficult to gauge the most appropriate diameter of endoscope required from the limited range of sizes available. Flexible bronchoscopes are relatively fragile and easily damaged if force is applied in an effort to dilate a stenosis. It is possible to force a rigid bronchoscope through a soft airway stenosis, but this should be reserved as a technique for intubation of the airway in an emergency situation.

Calibrated angioplasty balloon catheters are very effective for dilating airway stenoses, but are expensive, single-use devices. The catheter may be passed through or alongside a bronchoscope so that the position can be confirmed endoscopically. When the catheter is in the correct location, the balloon is inflated with saline to a pressure of 10–15 atmospheres. The balloon is held inflated for 1–2 minutes, or less if the patient begins to desaturate, and then rapidly deflated so that ventilation can be resumed. If desired, the balloon can be re-inflated for a second dilatation. Positioning of the catheter and progress of the dilatation can be monitored by fluoroscopy. The balloon is inflated with water-soluble contrast medium diluted 50:50 with water (approximately 150 mg/mL iodine concentration). A waist appears at the site of the stricture as the balloon is inflated, and disappears on successful dilatation.

Airway rupture is a potential complication of balloon dilatation, and tight stenoses should be dilated in stages. A theoretical advantage of the balloon technique is that the force applied to the stenosis is radial rather than longitudinal and this may result in less tissue damage.

BIOPSY TECHNIQUES

Biopsy specimens can be obtained for histologic and microbiologic studies from virtually any site in the airway using rigid or flexible instrumentation. Rigid instruments are required for larger specimens and make the biopsy of tracheal lesions easier, whereas flexible instruments are more useful for peripheral lesions. The size of forceps that can be used with a fiberoptic bronchoscope is limited. The instrumentation/suction channel of a pediatric bronchoscope is typically 1.2 mm diameter, whereas the channel of an adult bronchoscope is typically 2–2.7 mm.

Endobronchial biopsy is performed under direct visualization. Suitable forceps are advanced to the desired site (lesion), opened, moved onto the site, and closed while maintaining pressure against the mucosa. After the biopsy has been removed, the site should be examined to assess bleeding. In most cases, bleeding is minor and ceases spontaneously, but it can be brisk and require intervention. Topical application of vasoactive drugs such as phenylephrine is usually effective. Biopsies of the tracheal mucosa can be obtained from the carina, but it is technically difficult to biopsy other areas of the trachea with anything other than rigid up-biting forceps.

Transbronchial lung biopsy is rarely performed in pediatric patients, except in post-lung transplant management. The specimens obtained using this technique are small. Transbronchial biopsy is technically relatively easy, but, especially in small patients, is fraught with risks, including pneumothorax, massive hemorrhage, post-procedure atelectasis, and perforation of other organs. It is best performed under fluoroscopic guidance. The flexible forceps are passed into the selected bronchial segment until the desired depth is reached (usually some resistance will be felt, but it is possible to perforate the pleura relatively easily, especially in children). The forceps are then withdrawn slightly, opened, advanced, closed and then withdrawn to recover the specimen. Some bleeding will always occur and it may be necessary to tamponade the bronchus with the tip of the bronchoscope. For this reason, many operators wedge the bronchoscope in the bronchus before taking the biopsy and then leave the instrument in place until the bleeding stops. Because of the small size of the biopsy specimens obtained and the inherent sampling error, multiple specimens should be taken. This enhances the diagnostic yield but also increases the risk of complications. Sampling should be limited to one lung only because of the high incidence of pneumothorax. It is difficult to assess the adequacy of an individual specimen with the naked eye. In transbronchial biopsy, when the primary goal is to obtain alveolar tissue, a specimen that floats in saline is more likely to contain alveoli than one that immediately sinks.

BRONCHOPLEURAL FISTULA

Bronchopleural fistulas are uncommon in children, but can present many challenges. The first challenge is localization of the bronchus leading to the air leak.

Localization of the leak can be accomplished only if there is a steady flow of air through the fistula during the endoscopic examination. A Fogarty catheter can be passed through the bronchoscope (rigid or flexible) positioned in the bronchial orifice and inflated. If the air leak stops, the bronchus leading to the leak is thus identified. Alternatively, small volumes of saline can be instilled into the bronchial orifice. If the saline is consistently pulled into a bronchus, it is reasonable to assume that there is a one-way flow of air into that bronchus.

Endoscopic treatment of a bronchopleural fistula involves plugging the bronchus leading to the fistula long enough for the fistula to close naturally. A variety of techniques have been used in adults and these may be adapted for children. A Fogarty catheter can be left inflated in the bronchus, but the catheter must be positioned precisely, and endotracheal intubation with sedation or paralysis will be necessary. To minimize the potential for movement of the catheter, it should be passed through a nostril and taped to the endotracheal tube.

A fistula can be occluded with fibrin glue instilled into the bronchus through a catheter passed down the bronchoscope. Fibrin glue does not adhere well to normal bronchial epithelium and, consequently, it is necessary to fill a number of branches in order to achieve an effective plug. This technique may be effective if the fistula heals and seals within approximately 24 hours. In cases where a larger bronchus has been transected, the application of methylmethacrylate or other synthetic glue may be effective.

Finally, a bronchus can be temporarily occluded by packing it with Gelfoam®, Surgicell® or other material which will slowly dissolve or can later be retrieved. This is most readily done with rigid instrumentation.

PULMONARY HEMORRHAGE

Pulmonary hemorrhage presents several potential challenges to the endoscopist. Unless there is active bleeding during the procedure, localization of the bleeding site is difficult. Conversely, if the rate of bleeding is substantial, it may be difficult, if not impossible, to localize the bleeding site because of contamination of the airway. In children, continued airway bleeding often arises from a bronchial artery. Identification of the affected lobe or segment is desirable because selective embolization of the feeding bronchial artery may stop the bleeding.

It is often difficult to clear clots from the bronchi. Fresh blood in a bronchus tends to create an arborizing clot with 'roots' that ramify into the smaller bronchi. Suction is not generally helpful. A rigid bronchoscope and foreign body-type forceps can be used to grasp and extract as much of the clot as possible. Extraction of a fresh clot may stimulate further bleeding.

Endoscopic management of continuing major hemorrhage is difficult. Lavage with iced saline is rarely of substantial value. Instillation of vasoactive drugs such as epinephrine or phenylephrine can also be tried, but this fails more often than it succeeds. The most effective technique is tamponade of the bleeding bronchus. Bronchial tamponade can be achieved in a number of ways. Selective intubation of the contralateral main bronchus allows ventilation of the non-bleeding lung while protecting it from the accumulating blood. The bleeding lung is then allowed to self-tamponade with clot. Intubation with a double-lumen endotracheal tube is the most successful strategy if the patient is of sufficient size. Most children are too small to accept a double-lumen tube, in which case endobronchial intubation with a cuffed tube is preferable.

Balloon-tip catheters, such as a Fogarty, can be directed into the bronchus leading to the bleeding site to achieve tamponade. Care must then be taken to avoid dislodging the catheter once the balloon is inflated. In patients large enough for an adult-size flexible bronchoscope to be used, specially designed balloon catheters may be passed through the suction channel and inflated. The bronchoscope is then withdrawn over the catheter, leaving the balloon in place to tamponade the bronchus. These catheters can be left in place for several days. An endotracheal tube should be passed alongside the catheter for mechanical ventilation.

FIBEROPTIC INTUBATION

The flexible bronchoscope is a useful aid for the management of the difficult airway. Even the smallest infant in whom conventional techniques have failed can usually be intubated with a flexible bronchoscope.

For bronchoscopic intubation, the flexible bronchoscope is lubricated and passed through the appropriate endotracheal tube. The tube is positioned proximally on the shaft of the bronchoscope, which is then passed into the trachea (usually through the nose) in the same fashion as for a diagnostic bronchoscopy (including placement of topical anesthetic solution on the glottis). The tip of the bronchoscope is held just above the carina and the shaft is kept straight to reduce friction. Lubricating jelly is applied to the nostril and the endotracheal tube is slowly advanced over the bronchoscope into the trachea. **(See Figure 12.2)**

The tube should be rotated as it is advanced, to reduce friction and the risk of damage to the turbinates and vocal cords. The position of the tip of the tube is verified visually before the bronchoscope is removed. With practice, it should be possible to perform this procedure in 30–45 seconds.

There are several important technical points related to bronchoscopic intubation. First of all, there is the risk of damaging the bronchoscope itself. A flexible bronchoscope used for intubation should be close to the size of the endotracheal tube's inner diameter. A small bronchoscope can be damaged easily by using it to intubate with a large, relatively stiff endotracheal tube. **(See Table 12.1)**

The operator must ensure that there is adequate lubrication of the flexible bronchoscope and the endotracheal tube lumen. The bronchoscope must slide through the endotracheal tube easily or it will be impossible to remove the instrument once the endotracheal tube is in the trachea.

Bronchoscopic intubation is often performed under adverse conditions, when conventional intubation has failed or is thought likely to fail. Glossoptosis or the presence of abundant adenoidal lymphoid tissue may make it difficult to visualize the glottis as the bronchoscope is inserted. Insufflation of oxygen through the suction port – at a flow rate not exceeding 2–3 L/min – can help distend the airway and improve visualization. Mandibular lift, or even the use of a rigid laryngoscope, may improve visualization of the larynx. Topical application of 1 percent lidocaine to the

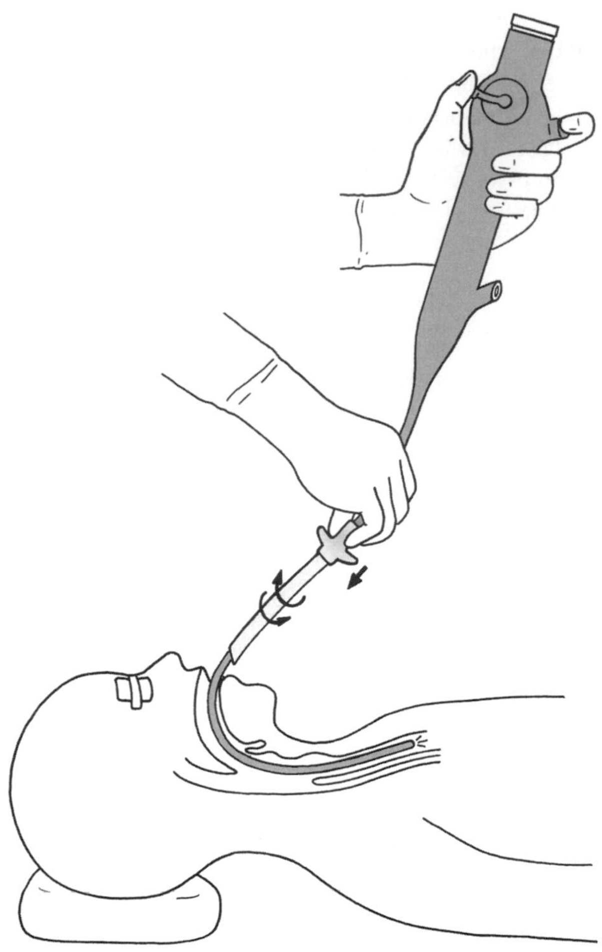

Figure 12.2

Table 12.1

Flexible bronchoscope (mm)	Endotracheal tube (mm)
2.2	2.5–3.5
2.8	3.0–4.5
3.5	4.5–6.0
4.9	6.0–8.5

larynx reduces the likelihood of laryngeal spasm. To save time in emergency situations, 1–2 mL of 1 percent lidocaine can be instilled into the posterior pharynx by an assistant while the operator is advancing the flexible bronchoscope through the nostril.

BRONCHOALVEOLAR LAVAGE

Bronchoalveolar lavage can be performed for diagnostic and therapeutic purposes. This discussion focuses on the latter.

Bronchoscopy for 'bronchial toilet'

Clearing the central airways of thick, purulent secretions can be accomplished with a rigid or flexible bronchoscope, although it is easier in most instances with the latter. Furthermore, many patients who benefit are already intubated and a flexible bronchoscope can be passed through an endotracheal or tracheostomy tube without interrupting ventilation. With currently available flexible bronchoscopes, effective visualization and suctioning can be carried out in patients intubated with endotracheal tubes with an internal diameter as small as 3.5 mm. One limitation of flexible instrumentation, however, is that the suction channel is only 1.2 mm in diameter.

Clearing the bronchi of accumulated secretions may be facilitated by lavage with sterile saline, followed by suctioning. It is important to use small volumes of saline to avoid respiratory embarrassment. In general, no more than 5–10 mL should be instilled at any one time. Sufficient negative pressure must be used for suctioning, but care must be taken to avoid exhausting the patient's functional residual capacity or producing mucosal trauma.

Inspissated mucus may not yield to simple suctioning. Repeated small-volume saline lavage may help clear a mucus plug, but more often prolonged suctioning of the plug is needed. The tip of the flexible bronchoscope or suction catheter is positioned against the mucus plug, suction is maintained for several seconds and then the bronchoscope or catheter is slowly withdrawn, maintaining suction to help extract the mucus plug. Since mucus plugs are often anchored by arborization into distal bronchi, repeated efforts may be required. Occasionally, mucus plugs require forceps extraction. The instillation of 5–10 mL 1 percent N-acetylcysteine into the bronchi distal to the mucus plug may also be helpful.

Bronchopulmonary lavage

Bronchopulmonary lavage (BPL) with very large volumes is used in the treatment of alveolar filling disorders such as alveolar proteinosis. In adults and adolescents, this is most readily accomplished via a double-lumen endotracheal tube, isolating one lung from the other. In smaller children, a single-lumen cuffed tube can be positioned under endoscopic control to isolate one lung whilst the other lung is ventilated via a laryngeal mask airway or a nasopharyngeal tube. The author has successfully lavaged infants as small as 3.5 kg with this technique.

The object of BPL is to clear the alveoli of foreign material while causing as little damage to the airways and alveoli as possible. After positioning the tube through which the lavage will be performed, the lung is ventilated with 100 percent oxygen for several minutes. Then saline at 37 °C is slowly instilled, allowing the lung to fill over several minutes. This allows the alveolar gas to be absorbed before the lung is emptied, preserving surfactant, which is depleted if there are bubbles. The lung is filled with saline to a pressure of 30–50 cmH_2O and then emptied by gravity. The cycle is repeated until the effluent is clear. Mechanical chest percussion during the lavage cycles enhances the efficiency of this procedure.

After the last aliquot of fluid is drained, as much residual saline as possible should be aspirated using a flexible bronchoscope. The lung is re-inflated and the endobronchial tube is removed. Depending on the degree of underlying lung disease, the patient may or may not be able to be extubated immediately. There will be a considerable amount of saline left in the alveolar spaces, which will be absorbed over the subsequent 12–24 hours. Maximum benefit appears to be reached in approximately 3 days.

Because one lung is filled with saline during the lavage procedure, hypoxemia is to be expected. Saturation nadirs during the cycle as low as 50–70 percent are not uncommon. Since the desaturation is transient, no intervention is necessary, and typically the nadirs become less severe as the lavage proceeds and hypoxic vasoconstriction becomes established.

When both lungs require lavage, it is prudent to perform two separate procedures, at least 4 days apart, to allow recovery of the first lung. If both lungs are washed sequentially in the same procedure, ventilation and gas exchange will be markedly impaired while the second lung is washed, and the patient will probably require mechanical ventilation following the procedure.

FURTHER READING

Prakash UBS. *Bronchoscopy.* Baltimore, MD: Lippincott Williams and Wilkins, 1993.

Wood RE. Pediatric bronchoscopy. *Chest Surgery Clinics North America* 1996; **6**:237–51.

Wood RE, Lacey SR, Azizkhan RG. Endoscopic management of large, postresection bronchopleural fistulae with methacrylate adhesive (Super Glue). *Journal of Pediatric Surgery* 1992; **27**:201–2.

13

Thoracoscopy – basic techniques

STEVEN S. ROTHENBERG

INTRODUCTION

Rapid development of technology associated with laparoscopic surgery in the late 1980s and 1990s allowed for much more advanced diagnostic and therapeutic procedures to be performed. These developments, including high-resolution and digital cameras, smaller instruments and better optics, have enabled pediatric surgeons in the twenty-first century to apply minimally invasive techniques to the majority of procedures in neonates, infants and children. One area in which major advances have been made is in the use of thoracoscopy to perform even the most complex intrathoracic procedures. Far from the limited diagnostic evaluations and small biopsies performed by Rodgers and others in the late 1970s and early 1980s, even the most complex thoracic procedure, the correction of a tracheo-esophageal fistula (TEF), can now be safely and efficiently performed using thoracoscopic techniques.

Indications

The indications for thoracoscopy have expanded greatly over the last decade and are somewhat dependent on the experience of the surgeon and the equipment available. A pediatric surgeon with reasonable endoscopic experience and relatively standard equipment can perform the majority of the procedures listed below safely.

- Lung or pleural biopsy: interstitial lung disease, infection, malignancy.
- Lobectomy: sequestration, congenital adenomatoid malformation, bronchiectasis, malignancy.
- Decortication.
- Pleurectomy.
- Bleb resection.
- Pleurodesis.
- Biopsy/resection of mediastinal masses.
- Resection of foregut duplications and bronchogenic cysts.
- Heller's myotomy.
- Thymectomy.
- Sympathectomy.
- Diaphragmatic plication.
- Diaphragmatic hernia repair.
- Ligation of thoracic duct: for congenital or acquired chylothorax.
- Anterior spinal fusion.
- Aortopexy.
- Patent ductus arteriosus ligation.
- Tracheo-esophageal fistula repair.

Contraindications

With the improvement in instrumentation and technique, there are very few contraindications to a thoracoscopic approach. Each surgeon must consider his or her own experience and the particular child and condition to determine if it is reasonable to use thoracoscopy. Size, previous thoracic surgery, and being ventilator dependent are no longer absolute contraindications.

ABSOLUTE

- Severe respiratory distress requiring alternative forms of ventilation, i.e. high frequency or oscillating ventilator.

- Respiratory compromise secondary to a giant anterior mediastinal mass.
- Severe hemodynamic instability requiring multiple pressors.

RELATIVE

- Previous thoracic surgery.
- Extensive infection resulting in dense adhesions (i.e. previous empyema, pneumonia or infected duplication cyst).
- Coagulopathy.
- Extensive tumor or numerous pulmonary metastasis.

EQUIPMENT/INSTRUMENTS

The instrumentation used for thoracoscopy is basically the same as that for laparoscopy. In general, 3 mm and 5 mm instruments are of adequate size and therefore 5 mm or smaller trocars can be used in most cases. In most cases it is helpful to use valved trocars, especially in smaller children, in whom it is difficult to obtain complete one lung ventilation. This allows the insertion of a low flow pressure of CO_2 to help collapse the lung. It is also appropriate to use trocars of a shorter length (50–70 mm), as the chest wall in children is relatively thin and there is limited intrathoracic space. Also, ports with a flat rather than a beveled tip are better, as there will be less risk of lung or tissue injury. Because of the narrow interspaces, there is a risk of cutting the intercostal neurovascular bundle if a sharp-bladed trocar is used; therefore a radially expandable or blunt-tipped trocar is best. Also, because there is relatively little thickness to the chest wall, the trocars are more likely to slip during instrument manipulation. For this reason it is helpful to fix the trocars to the chest wall during prolonged procedures. This can be accomplished by placing a small segment (approximately 5 mm) of Silastic® catheter over the trocar sleeve to act as a stop. A simple stitch can then be used to tie the cuff to the skin and prevent slippage. **(See Figure 13.1)**

Standard equipment should include 5 mm 0° and 30° telescopes. For smaller children and infants it is helpful to have shorter (16–20 cm) 3 mm and 4 mm 30° wide-angle scopes and specifically designed shorter instruments. These tools will allow the surgeon to perform much finer movements and perform more complex procedures, even in neonates. A high-resolution microchip or digital camera and good light source are essential to allow for adequate visualization, especially when using smaller scopes that transmit less light.

Essential

(5 mm and 3 mm): in general, these instruments should be insulated and rotating.

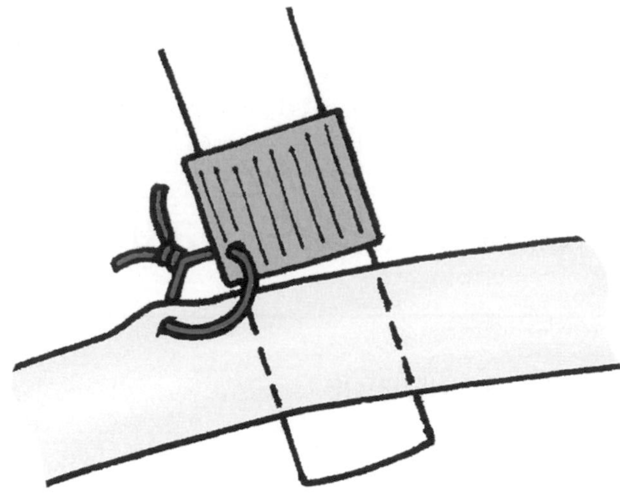

Figure 13.1

- Curved scissors.
- Curved dissector.
- Atraumatic clamps (i.e. bowel or Babcock clamp), racheted.
- Suction/irrigator.
- Fan or snake retractor.
- Needle driver.

Disposable instruments

- Hemostatic clips (5 mm and 10 mm): generally clips 8–10 mm in length.
- Endoloops® (pre-tied ligatures).
- Endoscopic linear stapler. The stapler is an excellent device for performing wedge resections but, because of its current size (12 mm diameter), is of limited use in children weighing less than 10 kg. Both vascular and tissue loads.

Optional instruments/energy sources

- Monopolar and bipolar cautery.
- Ultrasonic dissector.
- LigaSure™: a variation on bipolar technology/ eliminates the need for sutures, clips and staples in most pediatric lung resections (excellent for sealing larger vessels and lung tissue).

PREOPERATIVE PREPARATION

Extensive preoperative preparation is generally not necessary. The appropriate preoperative imaging studies need to be obtained, but extensive physiologic testing to determine if a patient will tolerate a thoracoscopic approach is rarely necessary or warranted. Even ventilator-dependent patients and those with significant cardiac defects can tolerate the limited periods of partial lung collapse necessary to perform most thoracoscopic procedures.

The only procedure that needs to be coordinated closely with radiology is that involving pulmonary nodules that are small (<5 mm) and deep to the pleural surface. These patients are sent to radiology 1–2 hours prior to their procedure so that CT-guided localization can be performed.

TECHNIQUE

Anesthesia

While single lung ventilation is achieved relatively easily in adult patients using a double-lumen endotracheal tube, the process is more difficult in the infant or small child. The smallest available double-lumen tube is a 28 Fr, which can generally not be used in a patient weighing less than 30 kg. Another option is a bronchial blocker. This device contains an occluding balloon attached to a stylet on the side of the endotracheal tube. After intubation, this stylet is advanced in the bronchus to be occluded and the balloon is inflated. Unfortunately, size is again a limiting factor, as the smallest blocker currently available is a 6 mm diameter tube. For the majority of cases in infants and small children, a selective mainstem intubation of the contralateral bronchus with a standard uncuffed endotracheal tube is effective. This can usually be done blindly without the aid of a bronchoscope simply by manipulating the head and neck. It is also important to use an endotracheal tube one-half to one size smaller than the anesthesiologist would pick for a standard intubation or the tube may not pass into the mainstem bronchus, especially on the left.

At times, this technique will not lead to total collapse of the lung, as there may be some overflow ventilation because the endotracheal tube is not totally occlusive. If adequate visualization cannot be obtained, a low-flow (1 L/min), low-pressure (4 mmHg) CO_2 infusion can be used during the procedure to help keep the lung compressed. This requires the use of a valved trocar rather then a non-valved port (Thoracoport). In fact in neonates, such as those with TEF, insufflation alone is enough to cause collapse of the lung, and mainstem intubation is not necessary. In general, hemodynamic and ventilation problems have not arisen as a result of this small amount of positive intrathoracic pressure. This is an important fact, as excessive time should not be wasted trying to get one lung isolation in a baby with TEF or mediastinal mass. If necessary, the pressure can be temporarily increased to even 8 or 10 mmHg without untoward hemodynamic effects. Once the lung has successfully been collapsed, it will stay collapsed at lower pressures.

This technique can also be used in patients who cannot tolerate single lung ventilation. By using small tidal volumes, lower peak pressures and a higher respiratory rate, enough collapse of the lung can be achieved to allow for adequate exploration and biopsy. Whatever method is chosen, it is imperative that the anesthesiologist and surgeon have a clear plan and good communication to prevent problems with hypoxia and excessive hypercapnia, and to ensure the best chance of a successful procedure.

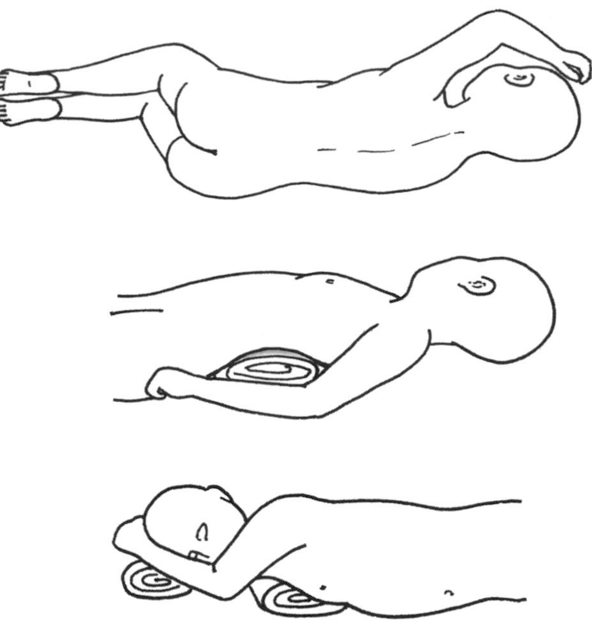

Figure 13.2

Positioning

Positioning depends on the site of the lesion and the type of procedure. Most open thoracotomies are performed with the patient in a lateral decubitus position. Thoracoscopic procedures should be performed with the patient in a position that allows for the greatest access to the areas of interest and uses gravity to aid in keeping the uninvolved lung or other tissue out of the field of view.

For routine lung biopsies or resections, the patient is placed in a standard lateral decubitus position. This position provides for excellent visualization and access to all surfaces of the lung. For anterior mediastinal masses the patient should be placed supine with the affected side elevated 20–30°. This allows for excellent visualization of the entire anterior mediastinum while keeping the lung posterior without the need for extra retractors. The surgical ports may then be placed in the anterior and mid-axillary lines with clear access to the anterior mediastinum. For posterior mediastinal masses, esophageal lesions and work on the esophageal hiatus, the patient should be placed in a modified prone position with the effected side elevated slightly. This maneuver again allows for excellent exposure without the need for extra retractors. The patient can then be placed in Trendelenburg or reverse Trendelenburg, as needed, to help keep the lung out of the field of view. The patient should be placed on a beanbag or secured with rolls and tape to prevent shifting and allow for the table to be rotated as necessary to provide the greatest exposure. **(See Figure 13.2)**

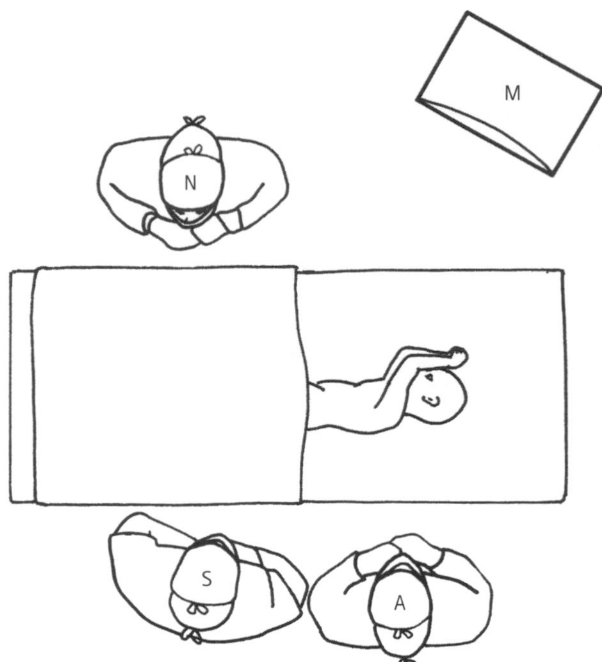

Figure 13.3

Once the patient is appropriately positioned and draped, the monitors can be placed in position. For most thoracoscopic procedures it is advantageous to have two monitors, one on either side of the table. The monitors should be placed near the head of the table, at or near the level of the patient's shoulder. For procedures primarily in the lower third of the thoracic cavity the monitors should be placed near the foot of the table or at the level of the patient's hips. The majority of operations can be performed by the surgeon with one assistant. The surgeon should stand on the side of the table opposite the area to be addressed so that he or she can work in line with the camera during the procedure. In most lung cases it is preferable to have the assistant on the same side of the table as the surgeon so that he or she is not working in a paradox (against the camera) while operating the camera and providing retraction as necessary. This concept is even more important when the field of dissection is primarily on one side. Cases such as a mediastinal mass, isolated lung lesion or more complicated resections require greater surgical skill and it is imperative that both the surgeon and the assistant are working in line with the field of view to prevent clumsy or awkward movements. The scrub nurse is usually on the other side of the patient below the monitor. **(See Figure 13.3)**

Access

ANATOMY

To be successful in thoracoscopy it is imperative that the surgeon has a clear understanding of intrathoracic anatomy and a three-dimensional mental image of the structures of the chest. This is especially true for more complex procedures such as lobectomy, aortopexy and TEF repair. Often structures can be visualized from only one orientation, so it is important to understand the relative relationship between various structures. For instance, when performing a lower lobectomy the surgeon must understand the relative position of the pulmonary artery and lower lobe bronchus, within the major fissure, as these structures cannot be palpated. A clear understanding of the anatomy is also important to aid in appropriate port placement.

PLACEMENT OF PORTS

Port placement is highly dependent on the procedure being performed and is addressed in the various chapters of this book. However, some basic principles can be stated. In general, most procedures can be performed with three ports, although a fourth port is occasionally required to provide retraction if positioning and gravity are not sufficient. The camera port should be slightly superior to and in between the operating ports, in a triangle fashion. This allows the surgeon to look down on the field of dissection, much as in open surgery, and prevents paradoxical movements on the monitor. If possible, the two operating ports should be at approximately 90° to each other with relation to the area of primary dissection or suturing. If using an endoscopic stapler, which requires a 12 mm trocar, this site should be planned carefully. The larger ports are difficult to insert between the ribs of smaller children, and the smaller thoracic cavity can make manipulation of the head of the stapler difficult. Generally the larger port should be placed as low in the thoracic cavity as possible, as the intercostal spaces are larger. Also, if performing a lobectomy in a larger child, this port should be placed so that it is in line with the interlobar fissure.

INSUFFLATION

As already mentioned, insufflation can be extremely helpful in collapsing the ipsilateral lung and providing better exposure. Even in cases where perfect single lung ventilation is obtained, insufflation can be helpful in aiding the initial collapse of the lung. This helps protect against inadvertent lung injury during trocar insertion. There is rarely a disadvantage to using CO_2 during a thoracoscopic procedure. In general, a low flow (1 L/min), low pressure (4 mmHg) is adequate, although a higher pressure is occasionally necessary to facilitate initial collapse. **(See Figure 13.4)**

RETRACTION AND EXPOSURE

As mentioned above, gravity is the best retractor and therefore position plays a key role in the success of any procedure. Further advantage can be gained by rolling the table left or right and increasing the prone or supine position as needed. The patient can also be placed in the head-up or head-down position to facilitate exposure. If the lung needs to be retracted further, there are various 3 mm and 5 mm

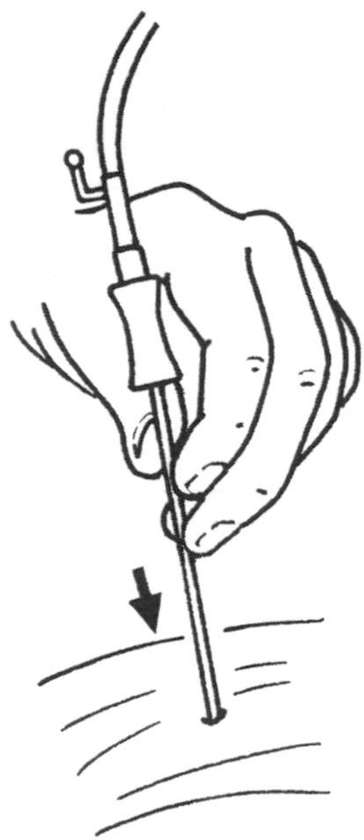

Figure 13.4 *Veress needle in position with an insufflation tube attached.*

fan and snake retractors that work well. Also an atraumatic clamp can be used to grasp the lung without causing injury. When working around the esophagus, it is helpful to have a nasogastric tube, bougie or flexible endoscope in to prevent inadvertent injury to this structure.

SPECIMEN REMOVAL

Because of the improvement in instruments and techniques, all of the procedures listed can be performed via port access alone and a mini-thoracotomy is no longer necessary. Many smaller specimens can be removed via the port or a slightly widened port site. In the case of larger specimens or possible malignancies, these should be placed in an endoscopic specimen bag to prevent contamination of the port site. Most specimens can be brought out morselated, thereby limiting the incision size. If removing a possible malignancy, the surgeon should discuss with the pathologists and oncologist beforehand whether or not surgical margins are important. If they are, morcelation may not be an option and the specimen may need to be brought out intact through an enlarged trocar site.

GENERAL TIPS

The key to any successful thoracoscopic procedure is meticulous attention to detail and hemostasis. Operating around the great vessels is intimidating, and if vascular control is lost, the consequences can be devastating. Therefore, before dividing any vascular structure, the surgeon must be sure he or she has proximal and distal control. Sealing devices such as the LigaSure™ make this technically much easier. Also the surgeon must be sure of the course of any vessel or bronchus that he or she divides; the limited view afforded by the thoracoscope makes it easy to become disoriented. It is imperative that the surgeon preserves the vascular structures to the unaffected parenchyma. The greatest risk is that of uncontrolled bleeding. During major procedures the surgeon should have an open tray of thoracotomy instruments available so that the chest can be opened at a moment's notice.

Exit

After completion of the procedure, the trocars are removed and the incisions are closed in two layers with absorbable sutures. The anesthesiologist should re-inflate the lung and the surgeon should confirm re-expansion. Generally a chest tube is placed through one of the trocar sites to aid this process. In most cases (lung biopsy, resection of smaller mediastinal masses or foregut duplications, sympathectomy, etc.), once the lung is re-expanded and no air leak is seen, the chest tube is removed prior to extubating the patient in the operating room and a standard occlusive dressing is applied. This eliminates much of the patient's postoperative pain. If there is concern about a possible air leak or significant fluid drainage, the tube can be left in for 24–48 hours.

POSTOPERATIVE CARE

Postoperative care in the majority of patients is straightforward. Most patients following biopsy or limited resection can be admitted directly to the surgical ward with limited monitoring (i.e. a pulse oxymeter for 6–12 hours). These patients are generally 23-hour observation candidates and a number are actually ready for discharge the same evening. If a chest tube is left in, it can usually be removed on the first postoperative day. Pain management has not been a significant problem. Local anesthetic is injected at each trocar site prior to insertion of the trocar and then one or two doses of intravenous narcotic are given in the immediate postoperative period. By that evening or the following morning, most patients are comfortable on oral codeine or acetametaphine. The elimination of a chest tube significantly reduces postoperative pain. Because of the limited incisions, intercostal or epidural blocks are rarely needed.

It is very important, especially in patients with compromised lung function, to start early and aggressive pulmonary toilet. The significant decrease in postoperative pain associated with a thoracoscopic approach results in much less splinting and allows for more effective deep breathing. This has resulted in a decrease in postoperative pneumonias and other pulmonary complications.

PROBLEMS, PITFALLS AND SOLUTIONS

- Inability to obtain single lung ventilation. Use CO_2 insufflation; pressures up to 10 or 12 mmHg can be used to cause the initial collapse. Ask the anesthesiologist to hand ventilate. He or she can use lower tidal volumes and pressures that will aid in collapsing the lung. Exposure is the key to success.
- Patient desaturates after mainstem intubation and positioning. This is not uncommon. Single lung ventilation causes a significant initial shunt and a-A gradient. Once the lung is collapsed for a few (3–5) minutes, the shunt diminishes and most patients rebound. Patients often become slightly hypercarbic (pCO_2 in the mid-40 s mg/h), but this is generally tolerated without any untoward effects. If the pCO_2 rises into the 60 s and an increased respiratory rate does not correct the problem, single lung ventilation may have to be abandoned.
- The lung expands every time you use suction. This is very common and another reason to use insufflation.
- Cannot visualize suspected metastatic nodule. Unfortunately, there is little that can be done at this point other than convert to open surgery. The key to this is anticipating the problem and using CT localization. Eventually ultrasound probes may help.
- Cases take too long. This may be an early problem, but with experience, times will quickly improve. The average lung biopsy can be performed in less than 20 minutes, patent ductus arteriosus ligation in 30 minutes, and decortication in less than an hour. The benefits will far outweigh the disadvantages of slightly longer surgical times.
- Inability to gain adequate exposure or awkward dissection. Because of the fixed rib cage there is limited freedom for instrument movement once the trocars are placed. Therefore meticulous planning is imperative. If the desired area cannot be adequately accessed, consider whether another trocar or a change in position is necessary. It is better to add another port than to struggle for added minutes or hours.
- Difficult visualization secondary to bloodstaining and/or adhesions. The key to thoracoscopic surgery, as all endoscopic surgery, is adequate visualization. Therefore meticulous dissection in order to identify and preserve important structures (e.g. phrenic nerve) and avoid bleeding is imperative. A suction/irrigation device should always be set up and ready for major resections and, if necessary, an additional port placed so the device can be used without removing the main dissecting instruments. The best cure is prevention!

COMPLICATIONS

- Need to convert to an open thoracotomy. This should not be considered a complication. Having to abandon a thoracoscopic approach is only a problem if there has been a significant technical mishap. Each case, completed or not, adds experience that will benefit future patients.
- Postoperative air leak. This is a common but usually self-limiting problem. Most raw lung surfaces will seal with chest tube suction/drainage alone. This problem can be lessened by using devices such as the LigaSure™ to seal open lung surfaces and by placing fibrin glue over raw areas. If the leak persists, a bronchopleural fistula should be considered, especially after a lobectomy. Re-exploration may be necessary and can usually be accomplished thoracoscopically.

FURTHER READING

Kogut KA, Bufo AJ, Rothenberg SS, Lobe TE. Thoracoscopic thymectomy for myasthenia gravis in children. *Pediatric Endosurgery Innovative Techniques* 2001; **5**:113–16.

Partrick DA, Rothenberg SS. Thoracoscopic resection of mediastinal masses in infants and children: an evolution of technique and results. *Journal of Pediatric Surgery* 2001; **36**:1165–7.

Rodgers BM, Moazam F, Talbert JL. Thoracoscopy in children. *Annals of Surgery* 1979; **189**:176–80.

Rothenberg SS. Thoracoscopic lung resection in children. *Journal of Pediatric Surgery* 2000; **35**:271–5.

Rothenberg SS. Experience with thoracoscopic lobectomy in infants and children. *Journal of Pediatric Surgery* 2003; **38**:102–4.

14

Principles of lung resection

FRÉDÉRIQUE SAUVAT AND Y. REVILLON

INTRODUCTION

Since the mid-1970s, thoracoscopy has been used primarily for lung and mediastinal biopsy and the management of empyema. With the advances in technology (better optics, miniaturization of instruments, endoscopic stapler and LigaSure™ sealing devices) and the increased experience in minimally invasive surgery and its anesthesia (single lung ventilation), the ability to perform much more complicated procedures, such as lobectomy, has blossomed over the last few years.

Indications

- Pulmonary malformations.
- Pulmonary sequestration.
- Cystic adenomatoid malformations and congenital lobar emphysema. The technique can be challenging and the causes are:
  - limited available space in pediatric hemithorax,
  - reduced working space in the presence of space-occupying lesions and/or hyperinflated lung,
  - previous infection and scarring,
  - lack of tissue plane,
  - the proximity of major vessels and nerves, trunks and heart.
- Whereas thoracoscopic resection of extrapulmonary sequestration is a relatively simple procedure, the resection of intra-lobar sequestration can be very difficult.
- Primary or secondary oncological lesions (localized and/or peripheral lesions): the lack of tactile sensation is a disadvantage. Therefore, only peripheral visible lesions and accurately localized intrapulmonary lesions that can be accurately localized preoperatively by means of imaging and staining are indications for thoracoscopy.
- Recurrent spontaneous pneumothorax: thoracoscopy allows for resecting the sub-pleural blebs and performing a pleurodesis. In cystic fibrosis, repeat surgical pleurodesis may create difficulties for subsequent lung transplantation.
- Bronchiectasis: the resection of the middle lobe is the main indication, while the lower and upper lobes can be extremely difficult because of the large lymph nodes and inflammatory tissues in the hilum.
- Resection of hydatid cysts.

Contraindications

There are few absolute contraindications for thoracoscopic lung resection; however, in some cases, the procedure may prove technically challenging. The relative contraindications include the following.

- Size of the patient. In infants and small children, the application of therapeutic thoracoscopy is limited by the size of the available instruments and lack of tolerance or facility for single lung ventilation if and when required.
- Inability to create a working space:
  - pleural adhesions from previous surgery and inflammation,
  - problems with ventilation,
  - large space-occupying lesions and hyperinflated lung, e.g. giant lobar emphysema.

- Type of pulmonary disease. The boundaries of a cystic adenomatoid malformation can be difficult to define if a limited resection rather than total lobectomy is desired.
- Inability to resect due to severe inflammatory process, e.g. bronchiectasis.

EQUIPMENT/INSTRUMENTS

Essential

- 3 mm, 5 mm or 10–12 mm instruments depending on the size of the patient and nature of the instruments to be used.
- 0° rigid endoscope, usually 5 mm in infants and small children and 10 mm in older children.
  - Three or five cannulae without valves. In thoracoscopy without insufflation (which is the author's choice) instruments may be used through the thoracic wall without cannulae. The EndoGIA® requires a 12 mm cannula.
  - Thoracoscopy with insufflation requires cannulae with valves (see Chapter 13).
  - Atraumatic graspers.
  - Scissors.
  - Hook diathermy.
  - Needle holder.
  - Suction irrigation.
  - Endoscopic linear stapler (EndoGIA®) for lung parenchyma and major vessels. This instrument requires a large space and should therefore be placed low in the chest. It may prove difficult to accommodate in children under the age of 4 years.
  - Alternatively, a LigaSure™ bipolar sealing device is used to secure blood vessels in infants and small children, and intermediate and small-sized vessels in older children.
  - Lung retractor.
  - Pre-tied suture loop or suture ligature for lung biopsy or securing blood vessels or even bronchus.
  - Suture with appropriate sized needle for closure of bronchus and suspected air leak.

Optional

- Ultrasonic dissector for adhesions, lung parenchyma and small vessels.
- Specimen bag.
- Tissue glue.

In all cases, a major open thoracotomy set of instruments must be available for emergency use or conversion to an open technique.

PREOPERATIVE PREPARATION

The preoperative imaging required depends on the underlying lung pathology. In general, however, a plane X-ray and computerized tomography (CT) scan are adequate. In cases of sequestration, an angiogram to look for the systemic feeding vessels is rarely necessary. In patients who have preoperative respiratory insufficiency, functional respiratory tests might be helpful.

TECHNIQUE

General principles

Pulmonary resection is performed under general anesthesia. The use of selective single lung ventilation is essential for lobectomies. The smallest available tube is 4 mm in diameter. Selective left or right main tracheal intubation with a non-cuffed tube requires flexible bronchoscopy guidance. The use of peroperative and postoperative anesthetic agents and epidural or morphine infusion depends on the type of procedure to be executed and the anesthetist's preference.

Appropriate positioning is essential. The patient is usually placed in a lateral decubitus position and appropriately padded and strapped to the operating table. A towel roll or break in the operating table just under the opposite axilla with or without an anterior or posterior lateral tilt may facilitate exposure.

The relative positions of the surgeon and assistant depend on the size of the patient, site of the lesion and the procedure to be performed. In general, the surgeon stands on the side opposite to the lesion with the monitor placed in front of him or her in line with the telescope. In upper thoracic surgery, the monitor is placed near the top end of the operating table, and vice versa for the lower compartment. The assistant and nurse stand on either side of the table.

In the majority of patients, pulmonary resection is performed through three cannulae, the positions of which depend on the size of the patient, the size of instruments to be used, the site of the lesion and the type of procedure to be performed. The primary (telescope) cannula is usually placed in the mid-axillary or posterior axillary line between the fifth and eighth ribs using either open or closed technique thoracoscopy. The working cannulae are placed under thoracoscopic vision using the concept of triangulation.

Lobectomy

Complete lung collapse is essential and achieved by selective pulmonary ventilation and possibly the use of CO_2 insufflation. This, coupled with the lateral positioning of the patient and gravity, usually obviates the need for a lung retractor. Thorascopic lobectomy should follow the same principles as those for open surgery: completion of the fissure, control of vascular structures and division of the bronchus.

Placement of the cannulae depends on the lobe being resected. For middle and lower lobes, most of the difficult dissection takes place in the fissure, and the cannulae are positioned to facilitate this. Usually, the telescope is placed in the fifth or sixth intercostal space in the mid-axillary line so that structures in the fissure can be clearly seen. After an initial survey, the working cannulae are placed in the anterior axillary line one or two intercostal spaces above and below the telescope. If an endoscopic stapler is to be used, care must be taken to ensure that the position of the 12 mm cannula is in line with the fissure.

The dissection should proceed along the fissure going from anterior to posterior. If the fissure is incomplete, monopolar hook diathermy, ultrasound shears, LigaSure™ or a stapler is used to complete it. The artery as it crosses the fissure is then isolated and ligated carefully using suture ligature, clips, stapler or LigaSure™. The pulmonary vein is then isolated and ligated. The bronchus can then be safely divided using a linear EndoGIA® stapler (older children) or intracorporeally tied with multiple absorbable suture ligatures.

For the upper lobe, the approach is also anterior to posterior. In this case the branches of the pulmonary vein are isolated and ligated first to expose the pulmonary artery. The lung can then be dissected off the main pulmonary artery trunk, going from superior to inferior. Segmental branches are identified, isolated and ligated in a sequential fashion. This technique ensures that the blood flow to the lower lobe is preserved. The fissure is then completed and the bronchus is divided.

The lobe is removed, usually piecemeal, through an extended cannula site. A specimen bag is used in cases of malignancy or active infection. Saline is then infused and the bronchial stump is checked for an air leak under thorascopic vision. One or two 15 Fr or 18 Fr chest tubes are then placed through the cannula sites and left in place for 2–3 days.

Segmental resection

The technical approach to segmentectomy is nearly the same as the technique for lobectomy. The relative positions of the three or four cannulae depend on the location of the lesion. The affected part of the lung is pulled with an atraumatic grasper to open the fissure. The dissection is then carried out through the fissure to expose the vessels and bronchus using a diathermy hook or scissors, ultrasound shears or LigaSure™. The vessels of interest and the bronchus are secured and divided as described above. The lung parenchyma is divided using ultrasound shears or endoscopic linear stapler, which minimizes the risks of postoperative hemorrhage and pneumothorax.

Wedge resection or biopsy

The positions of the cannulae are dependent on the location of the lesion to be removed. Usually three cannulae are used: one in the mid-axillary line in the seventh or eighth intercostal space, the second anteriorly in the fourth space, and the third in the posterior axillary line, fourth or fifth space.

Atraumatic grasping forceps are used to expose and pull the lung tissue/lesion while a pre-tied suture ligature or LigaSure™ is used to provide hemostasis and seal the lung tissue. The parenchyma is then divided using scissors. When the patient's size allows the placement of a 12 mm cannula, a single or multiple wedge resection may be carried out using an endoscopic linear stapler.

Pulmonary sequestration

Surgery for pulmonary sequestration depends on the type of sequestration: extra-lobar or intra-lobar. The initial goal of the procedure is the ligation of the systemic vessels. The cannulae are placed according to the site of the sequestration, usually in the inferior and posterior parts of the lung. The lung is then gently retracted with an atraumatic grasper to expose the systemic vessels in the lower posterior mediastinum. The vessels are secured and divided in the usual way. The sequestrated lung is grasped and dissected off the normal lung using a diathermy hook or scissors, ultrasound shears or LigaSure™ devices. The lesion is then removed through a cannula site and a chest drain is placed under direct vision through a cannula site and left in place for 1–3 days.

In cases of intra-lobar sequestration, several approaches have been described.

- Ligation of the systemic artery only, leaving the affected parenchyma in situ – a technique that mimics radiological embolization.
- A complete lobectomy, as described previously.
- Isolated removal of the sequestrated lung and preservation of the surrounding normal lung parenchyma – 'segmental resection'. This technique is difficult and relatively unsafe because of the lack of any clear demarcation between the normal and abnormal lung tissues.

POSTOPERATIVE CARE

Intercostal nerve block and oral analgesia provide adequate postoperative pain relief. Epidural analgesia or intravenous morphine infusion may be used for 12–24 hours postoperatively if required. The chest drains are usually removed 1–3 days postoperatively and the patient is ready to leave the hospital soon afterwards.

PROBLEMS, PITFALLS AND SOLUTIONS

Bleeding

In complicated lung resection, bleeding is the commonest cause of conversion to an open thoracotomy, usually as a result of failure to gain adequate mobilization and control of the vessels, or failure of the chosen sealing device. An anatomic dissection and adequate mobilization of the vessels are mandatory. In infants and small children, the use of a sealing device such as LigaSure™ works well. However, care must be taken to create two proximal seals a few millimeters apart. In older children, an endoscopic linear stapler offers the best way to secure the main pulmonary vessels safely. As a rule, all major vessels are partially divided first, and if the seal is incomplete, the surgeon has the opportunity to achieve hemostasis before finishing the division of the vessel (otherwise the vessel retracts and becomes impossible to control safely).

Persistent air leak

- The risk of parenchymal leak is minimized by careful dissection using sealing devices such as LigaSure™ (in infants and small children) or linear stapler (older children). A simple suture ligature or pre-tied suture is usually adequate for small wedge resection and lung biopsy. Cystic adenomatoid malformation and intralobar sequestration are extremely difficult to shell out. In these situations, most surgeons advocate a total lobectomy. Alternatively, a thoracoscopic-assisted approach using a 5–8 cm muscle-sparing incision in the fifth intercostal space may be considered.
- A single strong transfixation suture, interrupted absorbable sutures or an appropriate sized endoscopic linear stapler is used to prevent bronchial air leak.

Inability to identify pathology

In some cases – often related to the surgeon's experience – visual cues are not adequate to identify the anatomy or suspected pathology, and conversion to an open technique may need to be considered.

The patient does not tolerate single lung ventilation

This is a relatively uncommon problem and often the anesthetist is able to compensate (see Chapter 13).

COMPLICATIONS

- Bleeding (discussed above).
- Persistent/progressive pneumothorax.
- The cut surface of lung parenchyma rarely leaks beyond 3–5 days provided the patient is not on positive-pressure ventilation. A longer duration of underwater seal chest drain usually does the trick.
- A persistent large leak usually means a bronchopleural fistula. This will probably require re-exploration and repair.
- Compromised ventilation to the remaining ipsilateral lung.
- In lobectomy or segmentectomy, adjacent normal bronchi might accidentally be included in the stapling line. The stapler must be used with care, especially in small children and infants. In difficult cases, consider suturing of the divided end of the bronchus.

15

Esophageal atresia and tracheo-esophageal fistula

STEVEN S. ROTHENBERG

INTRODUCTION

Esophageal atresia with or without a tracheo-esophageal fistula (TEF) is one of the rarer congenital anomalies, occurring in 1/5000 births. Traditionally these patients have presented shortly after birth because of an inability to pass an oro-gastric tube, respiratory distress, or an inability to tolerate feeds. The condition may be associated with other major congenital anomalies (VATER syndrome) or may be an isolated defect. Improvements in maternal–fetal ultrasound have now resulted in prenatal diagnosis in a number of cases. This allows the surgeon to plan for delivery and eventual surgery. Patients with a TEF require emergency surgical intervention to prevent aspiration of gastric acid and over-distension of the intestines. Those with pure atresia can be dealt with electively as long as the infant's oral secretions are controlled by continuous or intermittent suction.

Indications

- All patients with esophageal atresia and/or TEF require repair.

The decision to use an endoscopic approach in these patients depends on a number of different factors, the most important being the stability of the infant and the surgeon's and anesthesiologists' experience with thoracoscopy in neonates. The infant first needs to undergo a thorough evaluation to look for are any other congenital anomalies, the most relevant of which is an echocardiogram to determine the anatomy and function of the heart as well as the location of the aortic arch.

Contraindications

ABSOLUTE

- Severe hemodynamic instability.
- Significant prematurity <1500 g.

RELATIVE

- Congenital cardiac defects.
- Multiple congenital anomalies.
- Size (1500–2000 g).
- Significant abdominal distension.

Congenital heart defects are not an absolute contraindication to a thoracoscopic approach, and repairs have been successfully completed in patients with an atrial septal defect, ventricular septal defect and tetralogy of Falot. However, patients with severe cardiac anomalies may not be able to tolerate even the short periods of single lung ventilation that are required to ligate the fistula. It is also important to determine the side of the aortic arch, as this will determine the surgical approach. A right-sided arch will necessitate a right-sided approach, which can be done with minimal added difficulty.

Other anomalies that may change the surgical approach include intestinal atresias. Imperforate anus or cloacal anomalies are not a contraindication, and a thoracoscopic TEF repair can be combined with a laparoscopic evaluation/repair of these defects. However, a proximal atresia may result in significant early gastric distension, which may cause immediate problems. The surgeon must evaluate each situation separately and determine the most appropriate approach.

Advantages and disadvantages

There are two main advantages to a thoracoscopic approach. The first is the avoidance of a postero-lateral thoracotomy incision and all of its inherent morbidity, including pain and respiratory compromise in the postoperative period, and scoliosis, shoulder girdle weakness, and chest wall asymmetry in the long term. The second is the improved visualization afforded by the endoscopic approach. The scope provides a magnified view superior to that obtained with surgical loops. It also gives the surgeon a superior view of the fistula, upper and lower esophageal segments, the plane between the upper pouch and membranous trachea, the vagus nerve and other vital structures.

The primary disadvantages are the small working space and the fine manipulations, especially suturing the anastomosis, required in this confined area. Also, currently the sutures can only be placed one at a time, creating a great deal of tension on the initial sutures (see 'Technique' below) and increasing the risk of the sutures tearing out. It is also necessary to achieve some degree of single lung ventilation for the procedure, which can create both anesthetic and technical problems.

Some question whether or not the fact that the thoracoscopic approach is transpleural rather then retropleural is a disadvantage. This would assume that the risk of infectious complications (mediastinitis/empyema) is less with the retropleural approach. While this theoretically is true, the use of appropriately placed chest drains and antibiotics should negate any perceived advantage.

EQUIPMENT/INSTRUMENTS

Essential

(Short 18–20 cm in length, 3.0 mm in diameter.)

- Three or four 3.0 mm and/or 5.0 mm cannulae; 5 mm cannulae require a reducer for 3 mm instruments.
- 3–5 mm 30° wide-angle telescope; should be approximately 20 cm in length.
- Curved dissector (Maryland).
- Curved scissors (insulated).
- Needle driver.
- 5 mm endoscopic clip applier.
- 4-0 polydioxanone surgical (PDS) suture on a TF needle.

Optional

- Hook cautery.
- LigaSure™ 5 mm dissector.
- Knot pusher.

PREOPERATIVE PREPARATION

Preparation does not differ from that for the open procedure. A suction catheter should be placed in the upper blind pouch and the patient should be placed in a head-up position to prevent reflux of gastric contents through the fistula. Broad-spectrum antibiotics should be given and the work-up for other congenital anomalies completed. Mechanical ventilation should be avoided until induction of anesthesia if at all possible. This will minimize the amount of abdominal distension caused by air passing through the fistula. Once the baby has been stabilized, surgery should be performed as soon as possible to minimize the risk of aspiration. In the case of pure atresia, surgery can be performed in a more elective manner. Often it will be necessary to place a gastrostomy tube first. The decision to proceed with the esophageal repair will depend on the gap between the two segments. If this is not clear, thoracoscopy may offer a less invasive way of evaluating the two ends and the gap between them.

TECHNIQUE

General endotracheal anesthesia is administered but low peak pressures should be used until the fistula is ligated to prevent over-distension of the abdomen. Local anesthetic (0.25 percent marcaine) is inserted at the trocar sites. An attempt should be made to obtain a left mainstem intubation by blind manipulation of the endotracheal tube. However, if this cannot be achieved easily, the endotracheal tube should be left in the trachea just above the carina. Time should not be wasted trying to manipulate the tube down the left side, as excellent right lung collapse can be achieved with CO_2 insufflation alone. Wasting even minutes trying to place a bronchial blocker or other manipulations can compromise the eventual success of a thoracoscopic approach. A urinary catheter is optional.

Positioning

Once the endotracheal tube is secure, the patient is placed in a modified prone position with the right side elevated approximately 30–45°. If there is a right-sided arch, the right side is approached. This positioning gives the surgeon access to the area between the anterior and posterior axillary line for trocar placement while allowing gravity to retract the lung away from the posterior mediastinum. This arrangement gives excellent exposure of the fistula and esophageal segments without the need for an extra trocar for a lung retractor. Generally, small rolls are sufficient to provide stabilization for positioning or a small beanbag can be used. **(See Figure 15.1)**

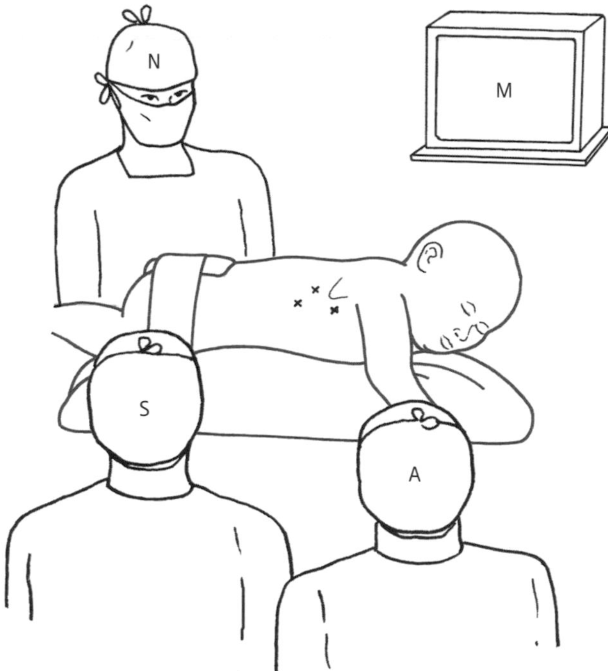

Figure 15.1

The surgeon and the assistant stand at the patient's front and the monitor is placed at the patient's back. This allows the surgeon and the assistant to work in line with the camera towards the point of dissection. The assistant should not be placed on the opposite side of the table, as this will place him at a paradox with the telescope. The scrub nurse can be on either side of the patient, depending on the room layout.

Port placement

Port placement is extremely important because of the small chest cavity and the intricate nature of the dissection and reconstruction. The procedure can be performed with three ports, but occasionally a fourth port is necessary to retract the lung.

The initial port (3–5 mm) is placed in the fifth intercostal space at approximately the posterior axillary line. This is the camera port and gives the surgeon excellent visualization of the posterior mediastinum in the area of the fistula and eventual anastomosis. As mentioned, a 30° lens is used to allow the surgeon to 'look down' on the instruments and avoid 'dueling'.

The two instrument ports are placed in the mid-axillary line one to two interspaces above and below the camera port. The upper port is 5 mm to allow for the clip applier and suture. The lower port is 3 mm. Ideally these ports are placed so that the instrument tips will approximate a right-angle (90°) at the level of the fistula. This positioning will facilitate suturing the anastomosis. A fourth port can be placed either higher or lower in the thoracic cavity to help retract the lung, but this is not necessary in the majority of cases.

Step 1: Ligate the fistula

- Once the chest has been insufflated and the lung collapsed, the surgeon must identify the fistula. In most cases the fistula is attached to the membranous portion of the trachea just above the carina. This level is usually demarcated by the azygus vein.
- After the azygus vein has been identified, it should be mobilized for a short segment using a curved dissector or scissors. The vein is then cauterized and divided. It is often easiest to do this with a small hook cautery, although bipolar cautery or other sealing devices can be used. Ties or clips are generally not necessary and could interfere with the dissection of the fistula.
- With the vein divided, the lower esophageal segment is identified and followed proximally to the fistula. Because of the magnification afforded by the thoracoscopic approach, it is easy to visualize exactly where the fistula enters the back wall of the trachea. A 5 mm Endoclip® can then be applied safely. Care should be taken to avoid the vagus nerve. A single clip is usually sufficient. The fistula can then be safely divided with scissors. The distal segment may retract, making it difficult to visualize: therefore it may be preferable to wait until the upper pouch is dissected out before completely dividing the fistula. The fistula may also be suture ligated, but this requires delicate suturing at a time when an air leak from the divided fistula may be causing increased respiratory compromise. **(See Figure 15.2)**

Step 2: Mobilize the upper pouch

- Attention is now turned to the thoracic inlet. The anesthesiologist places pressure on the nasogastric tube to help identify the upper pouch. The pleura overlying the pouch is incised sharply and the pouch is mobilized with blunt and sharp dissection. In some cases it is helpful to place a stay suture in the tip of the pouch to aid in applying traction. The plane between the esophagus and trachea can be seen well, and the two should be separated by sharp dissection. Mobilization of the upper pouch is carried on up into the thoracic inlet. **(See Figure 15.3)**
- Once adequate mobilization is achieved, the distal tip of the pouch is resected. This should be an adequate section so that there is a sufficient opening to prevent later stricture formation.

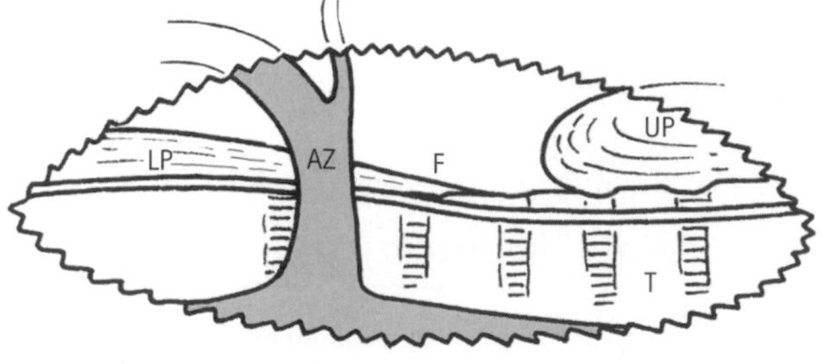

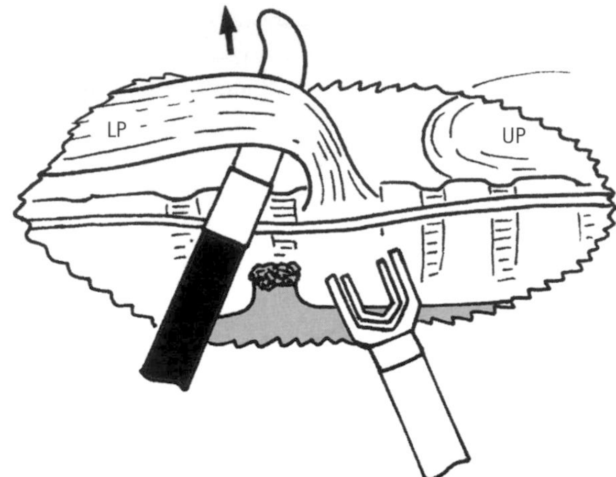

Figure 15.2

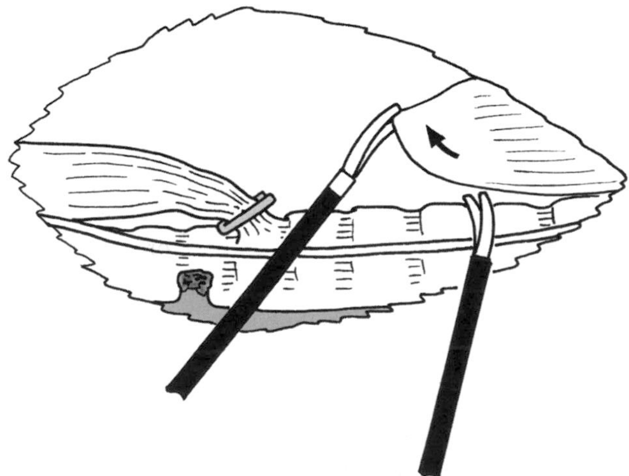

Figure 15.3

Step 3: The anastomosis

- With the two ends mobilized, the anastomosis is performed. The first stitch (4-0 PDS on a TF needle) is placed in the center of the anterior (patient's) wall. The suture is placed from inside out on the upper pouch and from outside in on the lower segment. This leaves the knot intraluminal but allows better visualization of

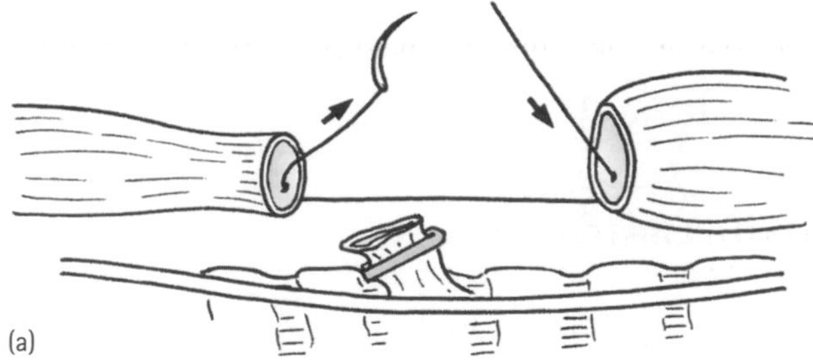

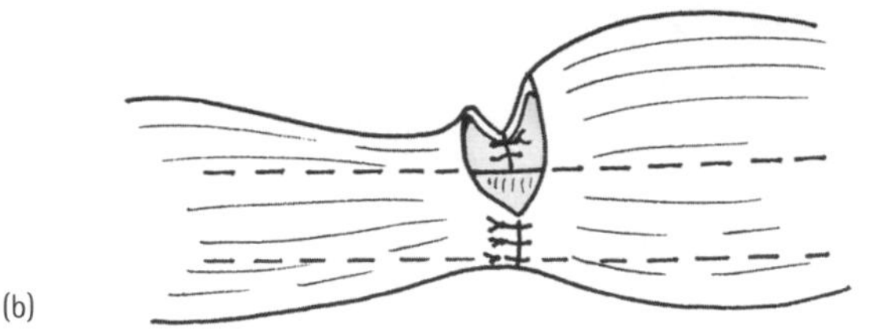

Figure 15.4

the anastomosis and mucosa-to-mucosa approximation. Adequate bites should be placed to prevent the sutures from tearing out. The knot is then tied extracorporeally using a knot pusher. This allows the two ends to be brought together with slow, steady tension under direct vision. Conversely, the suture can be tied intracorporeally, but the small working space and tension make this more difficult. With this suture tied, two to three more sutures are placed on the anterior wall in the same fashion.
- With the anterior wall complete, the anesthesiologist applies gentle pressure to the nasogastric tube, allowing the surgeon to pass it into the lower segment. This insures patency of the lower esophageal segment and acts as a stent to prevent compromise of the lumen while the anastomosis is completed. The surgeon then completes the back wall with three to four more sutures, this time placing the knots extracorporeally. Care should be taken with each bite to ensure that the mucosa is incorporated. The anastomosis generally requires only seven to eight sutures. Once the two ends are brought together and the tension is removed, the knots can be tied intracorporeally if desired. The nasogastric tube is left in place in the stomach. **(See Figure 15.4)**
- A chest tube is then placed through the lower trocar site and the tip is placed near the anastomosis (under direct vision with the endoscope). The other ports are removed and the sites are closed with absorbable suture. Steri-strips are applied and the chest tube is secured with a 3-0 Prolene® or silk suture.
- The patient is placed supine and the endotracheal tube is pulled back into the trachea if a left mainstem intubation was achieved. The chest tube is connected

to a Pleurovac and 15–20 cmH_2O suction is applied. If a large air leak is present, the surgeon must determine if the fistula ligation is secure.

POSTOPERATIVE CARE

The patient is left intubated and sedated for the first 12–24 hours. If the anastomosis is tenuous and under significant tension, it may be necessary to keep the infant intubated and paralyzed for a number of days (3–7) to diminish stress on it. Care should be taken to avoid early extubation, as the need to re-intubate the infant could result in disruption of the anastomosis.

If there is no significant chest tube drainage, it can be placed to water seal on the second postoperative day. On the fourth or fifth day a contrast study is obtained while withdrawing the nasogastric tube through the anastomosis to ensure there is no leak. Conversely, the surgeon may elect to start feeds without a study. Once feeds are started, the chest tube is removed if there is no evidence of any leak or increased drainage. Feeds are advanced as tolerated and the child is discharged usually on the seventh to eighth postoperative day.

The majority of patients will have significant reflux and it is generally wise to give H2 blockers and prokinetic agents as a precaution.

PROBLEMS, PITFALLS AND SOLUTIONS

Inadequate visualization

- If a left mainstem intubation cannot be obtained, it is necessary to use insufflation to collapse/retract the lung. Usually a pressure of 4 mmHg and a flow of 1 L/min are adequate to keep the lung deflated once it is collapsed, but a higher pressure of 7–8 mmHg may be needed to obtain complete collapse.
- Positioning is critical: if the patient is not placed far enough in the prone position, the lung will obscure the view of the posterior mediastinum.
- If adequate visualization cannot be obtained, place a fourth port for a small lung retractor; however, this may crowd the small operative field.

The patient does not tolerate single lung ventilation

- There will usually be a brief period of desaturation after the lung is collapsed. However, this will generally improve after a few minutes as the patient compensates by shunting blood away from the collapsed lung.
- The anesthesiologists should use low pressures with small tidal volume and frequent rate until the shunting has corrected.
- A retractor may be necessary to compress the lung locally rather then relying on CO_2 insufflation.
- If the patient does not tolerate any of the above manipulations, the surgeon may want to abandon a thoracoscopic approach and convert to an open thoracotomy.

Inability to identify the fistula

- Examine closely the area anterior to the mid/lower thoracic spine.
- Look for distension of the lower esophageal segment with ventilation.
- Identify the vagus nerve and trace it as it runs adjacent to the lower esophageal segment.

Bleeding

- Bleeding is generally not a problem once the azygus vein is safely ligated. This can be achieved with monopolar or bipolar diathermy or the LigaSure™.

Dissection of the upper pouch

- Constant pressure on the nasogastric tube helps define the upper pouch. This part of the dissection is relatively straightforward. The esophagus is separated from the trachea using sharp dissection.
- A good portion of the tip of the upper pouch should be resected transversely to allow for good visualization of the mucosa and avoid later stricture formation.

The anastomosis

- The greatest difficulty is approximating the two ends. Make sure the initial suture has an adequate bite of both the upper and lower segments.
- Apply slow, constant pressure while bringing the two ends together.
- If the ends cannot be completely approximated with the first stitch, secure it leaving a small gap. Then place the second suture to complete the approximation and decrease the tension on the first suture.
- If more than two or three sutures tear out while attempting the anastomosis, the gap may be too great to close. In these instances it is probably safest to convert to an open procedure to assess the situation. This is likely to happen only in cases of long gap pure esophageal atresia.

- If the anastomosis is completed but there has been a partial tear of the esophageal wall, a pleural flap can easily be mobilized and used to re-enforce the anastomosis. An approximately 1 cm width flap can be stripped off the chest wall laterally and draped around the esophageal anastomosis. This can be secured in place with just two sutures, one at each corner.

COMPLICATIONS

Operative complications are rare in this procedure and most issues revolve around obtaining adequate exposure and approximating the two ends of the esophagus. Anesthetic issues and sutures tearing out are the most commonly encountered problems. It should be remembered at all times that the end result should not be compromised and at no time should the patient's safety be placed at risk to accomplish the procedure thoracoscopically.

Postoperative complications include stricture and anastomotic leak. If adequate drainage was performed at the time of surgery, the leak can generally be handled conservatively with time, antibiotics and nothing by mouth. Drainage should be continued until there is no longer evidence of anastomotic leak (saliva in the drain). Then a contrast study should be obtained prior to starting feeds. Once feeds have been started and there is no evidence of a leak, the drain can be pulled. Only in cases of near-complete disruption of the anastomosis or inadequate drainage resulting in sepsis should the chest be re-explored. Stricture formation is dealt with in the same way as with the open procedure.

FURTHER READING

Bax KMA, Van der Zee D. Feasibility of thoracoscopic repair of esophageal atresia with distal fistula. *Journal of Pediatric Surgery* 2002; 37:192–6.

Louvorn HN, Rothenberg SS, Remberg O, et al. Update on thoracoscopic repair of esophageal atresia with and without tracheo-esophageal fistula. *Pediatric Endosurgery Innovative Techniques* 2001; 5:135–40.

Rothenberg SS. Thoracoscopic repair of tracheo-esophageal fistula and esophageal atresia in newborns. *Journal of Pediatric Surgery* 2002; 37:869–72.

16

Thoracoscopic sympathectomy

Z. COHEN

INTRODUCTION

Operative interruption of the thoracic sympathetic pathway is indicated in the treatment of a variety of sympathetic disorders, e.g. hyperhidrosis (commonest), facial blushing, Raynaud's disease, splanchnic pain, and reflux sympathetic dystrophy. In children, however, palmar hyperhidrosis is the only disorder in which sympathectomy is indicated.

Primary palmar hyperhidrosis is a pathological condition in which perspiration occurs in excess of that required for thermal regulation and is diagnosed when underlying causes have been ruled out. It is a very distressing and embarrassing condition, causing psychological, social and occupational disturbances. Surgical intervention – 'upper thoracic sympathectomy' – offers immediate and permanent relief. In theory, there is no age limitation for the procedure. In practice, however, hyperhidrosis is rarely a problem under the age of 6 years.

Contraindications

- Hyperhidrosis secondary to underlying pathology, e.g. hyperthyroidism and phaeochromocytoma.
- Suspected significant pleural adhesions (previous major thoracotomy or empyema).

EQUIPMENT/INSTRUMENTS

Essential

- 10 mm cannula.
- 10 mm 0° operating thoracoscope.
- Standard 45 cm curved, double-jaw action, grasping forceps to fit the 10 mm operating thoracoscope.

Optional

- Two additional 5 mm cannulae.
- 5 mm 0° telescope.
- 5 mm curved grasping forceps.

PREOPERATIVE PREPARATION

A chest X-ray is usually necessary to exclude any lung pathology and/or signs of major pleural adhesions. Routine blood count and cross-match are advisable.

TECHNIQUE

The procedure is performed bilaterally in a sequential manner under general anesthesia using ordinary endotracheal intubation. The patient is placed in a supine position, slightly elevated at the shoulders, with both arms abducted to 90° and a 45° reversed Trendelenburg position. A wide area, often the entire chest and axillae, is prepped. **(See Figure 16.1)**

A 10 mm incision is made in the anterior axillary line in the fourth or fifth intercostal space. The mechanical ventilation is discontinued for a few seconds while the Veress needle is inserted into the pleural cavity. (Conversely, an open technique thoracoscopy can be used.) A pneumothorax is created using CO_2 to a pressure of 12 mmHg in adolescents and 10 mmHg in younger children. The Veress needle is then removed and a 10 mm cannula is inserted, through

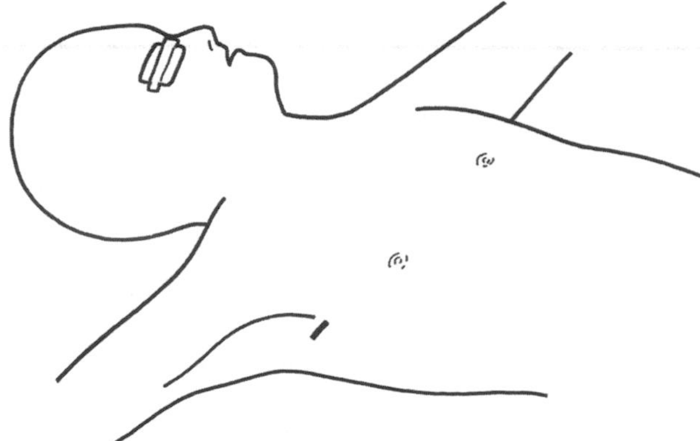

Figure 16.1

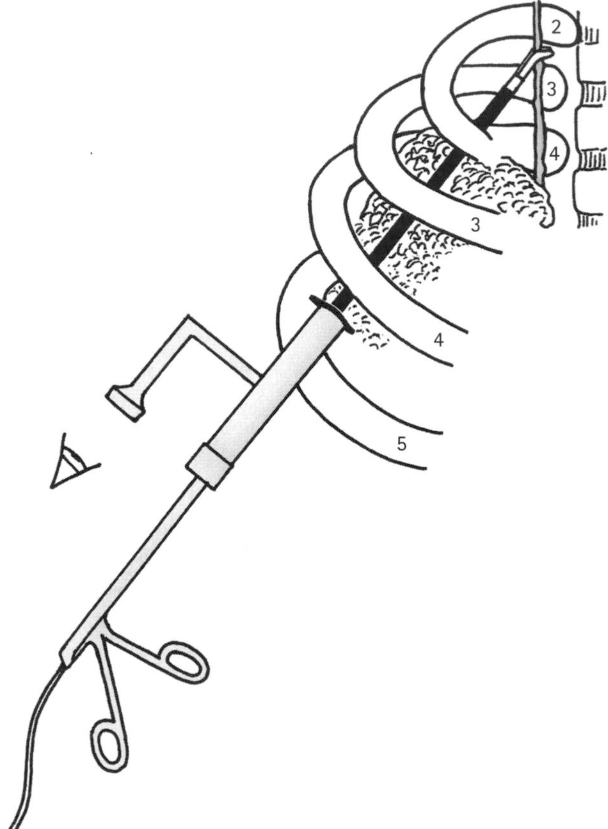

Figure 16.2

which the operating thoracoscope is introduced. A pair of 45 cm grasping forceps connected to electrocoagulation is now introduced through the working channel of the operating thoracoscope. The ribs are counted from above using the tip of the grasping forceps. Usually the first rib is not seen, but can be felt by pushing the grasping forceps gently against it. The second and third ribs are easily seen. The sympathetic chain is usually easy to identify under the parietal pleura running vertically over the neck of the ribs in the upper costo-vertebral region. **(See Figure 16.2)**

The sympathetic chain is then grasped at the inferior border of the second rib, elevated over the rib and completely

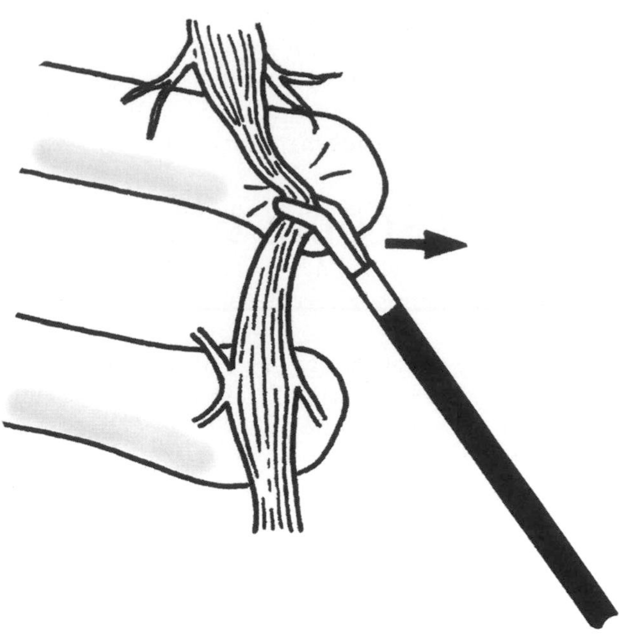

Figure 16.3

resected to the inferior border of the third rib using coagulation only. This allows resection of the second and third ganglia. If severe axillary hyperhidrosis is also present, the T4 ganglion can be resected as well. Formal mobilization of the chain and/or incising the overlying pleura are usually unnecessary, although a bipolar device is preferable to avoid retrograde propagation of coagulation (the devices available do not have a grasping effect). A medium-power monopolar coagulation is usually safe and easily achieves complete sympathectomy. **(See Figure 16.3)**

The grasping forceps are removed and the lung is re-expanded under direct vision. The thoracoscope is removed and the skin is closed promptly. A brief spell of positive-pressure ventilation immediately prior to skin closure minimizes the incidence of residual/postoperative pneumothorax. A chest drain is usually unnecessary. The same procedure is repeated on the contralateral side.

POSTOPERATIVE CARE

A chest X-ray is performed immediately after surgery to ensure complete lung expansion. Oral non-steroidal analgesia may be necessary for the first 24 hours and the patient is usually ready to leave the hospital the day after surgery.

PROBLEMS, PITFALLS AND SOLUTIONS

- Occasionally the sympathetic chain is difficult to visualize, but it can be identified by rolling the chain/ganglia under the grasping forceps.

- Sometimes the apex of the lung obstructs the operating field. In this situation, the operating thoracoscope may be used to push the lung downwards and away from the sympathetic chain. Alternatively, the insufflation pressure may be increased to 14–15 mmHg.
- Occasionally adhesions can be found between the parietal pleura and lung. Adhesiolysis may be necessary using an additional 5 mm cannula and scissors. Dense chronic adhesions may require conversion to an open technique.
- Minor bleeding can disturb the view. To avoid bleeding, grasp and then lift the chain from its bed before it is being coagulated and disrupted completely.
- The satellite ganglion is usually not seen endoscopically as it is covered by a characteristic fat pad. Caution must be taken during coagulation of the second ganglion to avoid retrograde propagation of coagulation to the satellite ganglion.

COMPLICATIONS

- Horner's syndrome is very rare and preventable. Avoid extending the dissection above the second rib, high-power coagulation and prolonged coagulation.
- Major bleeding from intercostals vessels is rare. Additional cannulae and suction irrigation may prove helpful. An open thoracotomy is seldom required.
- Intra-operative air leak from the lung parenchyma and significant postoperative pneumothorax necessitating intercostal drainage for 24–48 hours postoperatively are rare. Compensatory hyperhidrosis is relatively common. The patient usually has increased perspiration of the feet and/or trunk and, less commonly, the face. The incidence ranges from 30 percent to 50 percent and its mechanism is unknown. All patients and parents must be made aware of the possibility of this side effect, although most patients are able to tolerate it.

17

Empyema

STEVEN S. ROTHENBERG

INTRODUCTION

Empyema has traditionally been treated by antibiotics and varying degrees of chest drainage, including pleurocentesis, tube thoracostomy, mini-thoracotomy and formal thoracotomy. More aggressive intervention has often been delayed because of the perceived morbidity associated with surgical intervention. This has often led to days, weeks or even months of antibiotics and pulmonary compromise as these infections were allowed to resolve without adequate surgical drainage. Thoracoscopic debridement offers an opportunity to provide early intervention to diminish the morbidity and recovery period associated with an empyema while limiting the surgical trauma. Very advanced or late empyemas are much more difficult to deal with surgically because the fibrous peel is much harder and fixed. Thoracoscopic treatment of this later stage of disease is possible but more difficult and associated with greater morbidity. This is another argument in favor of early intervention.

Indications

- Large amount of pleural fluid with evidence of loculations, significant pleural peel and/or lung collapse.
- Persistent fever, elevated white blood cell count or C-reactive protein (CRP), despite intravenous antibiotic therapy $\pm$ drainage.
- Evidence of trapped lung with respiratory compromise.
- Thick pleural fluid not adequately drained by pleurocentesis or thoracostomy tube.

Thoracoscopic decortication is a minimally invasive way of obtaining early surgical debridement and drainage with minimal morbidity. Through two or three small incisions, the pleural space can be widely debrided and completely drained and all loculations can be broken down. Early intervention is encouraged, as the pleural peel is less fibrous and easier to debride. The decreased surgical morbidity and quicker overall recovery should encourage both the surgeon and the chest physician to intervene earlier rather than later.

Contraindications

ABSOLUTE

There are no real contraindications to a thoracoscopic decortication. If the patient's condition is deteriorating, surgical debridement is indicated. If the patient is too unstable for surgical intervention, a chest tube should be placed under local anesthetic and surgical debridement performed as soon as the patient can tolerate a general anesthetic.

RELATIVE

- A previous thoracotomy may make access to the pleural cavity more difficult because of adhesion formation.
- Evidence of necrotizing pneumonia or a large intraparenchymal abscess. This may cause concern about the development of a bronchopleural fistula following debridement.
- Late or advanced empyema with very thick, fibrous peel.

It is rare that thoracoscopic decortication is not an appropriate first step. Even if there is significant lung necrosis, debridement of the infected and injured tissue may be adequate for resolution, without creating a bronchopleural fistula. If formal resection is required at a later date, the surgeon can evaluate the lung parenchyma visually, which may help in a decision for more aggressive surgery if the patient fails to improve clinically.

Advantages

- Provides access to the entire pleural cavity through limited incisions. Allows the surgeon to verify visually that all loculations and fluid collections are removed or broken down.
- Decreased postoperative pain and therefore decreased splinting following surgery as compared to a standard or mini-thoracotomy. This allows for more aggressive chest physiotherapy and facilitates deep breathing and lung expansion by the patient.
- A chest tube can be placed to the most dependent or involved area under direct vision.
- Allows the surgeon to inspect the lung for necrosis.

Disadvantages

- Limited access and port size can make it difficult to remove all infected tissue.
- The patient may not tolerate the lateral decubitus position.
- Significant or mature pleural peel can make access to the pleural cavity difficult, increasing the risk of lung injury.

EQUIPMENT/INSTRUMENTS

Very few specific instruments are necessary because the procedure does not require any fine dissection. The size of the instruments depends on the size of the child. For children weighing less than 10 kg, 3 mm instruments may be used, with 5 mm instruments used in larger children. Because of the smaller thoracic cavity, short (20 cm) shaft length is preferable.

Essential

- Two or three ports: these may range from 3 mm to 10 mm. It is often necessary to put in at least one large (10 mm) port in order to facilitate removal of the infected tissue. These ports should be 50–70 mm in length, depending on the size of the child and the thickness of the chest wall.
- 4 mm or 5 mm 30° angled telescope.
- 3 mm or 5 mm blunt grasper. Often an atraumatic bowel clamp works best: it has a large surface area and can be used to grasp and strip out the infected peel.
- 5 mm or 10 mm suction/irrigation device.
- A chest tube.

Optional

- 5 mm fan retractor to retract the lung and expose all areas of the thoracic cavity.
- 5 mm peanuts for breaking down adhesions and loculations.
- Pressure bag for irrigating fluid.

PREOPERATIVE PREPARATION

These patients are often septic with compromised pulmonary and hemodynamic status. The patient's condition should be optimized with fluid resuscitation, aggressive pulmonary care and antibiotics. It is helpful in many cases to have a preoperative computerized tomography (CT) scan. This will help in making the decision to proceed with thoracoscopy by determining the amount of loculated fluid, inflammatory peel, and evidence of parenchymal injury. Ultrasound examination may also be used to determine the amount, location and degree of loculated fluid.

This information can then be used in the operating room to aid in the placement of the initial ports. The site with the greatest fluid collection can be chosen for the initial port placement to avoid injury to the lung, which maybe adherent to the chest wall in some areas.

Although it is unusual to have significant blood loss during the procedure, the patient should be typed and cross-matched for a unit of blood as a precaution. Many of these patients are anemic, and preoperative transfusion may be necessary to help with preoperative stabilization.

TECHNIQUE

The procedure is performed under general endotracheal intubation. Single lung isolation with either a double-lumen endotracheal tube or mainstem intubation of the contralateral side is preferable but not mandatory. Single lung isolation may help in preventing cross-contamination of the airways during manipulation of the affected side. It will also aid in maintaining working space by preventing inflation of the trapped lung as the peel is removed. However, carbon dioxide insufflation is usually adequate to maintain lung collapse until attempts are made to re-expand the lung actively with positive pressure. The patient's respiratory

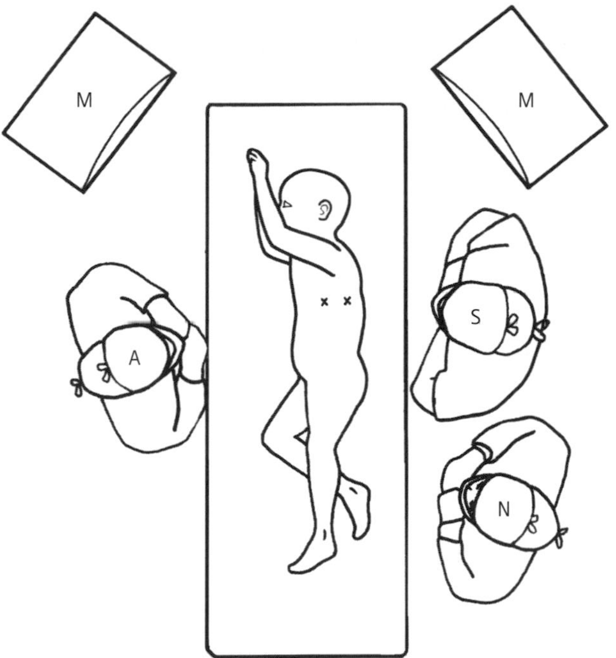

Figure 17.1

status should not be compromised further and excessive time should not be spent trying to get single lung isolation.

The procedure is best performed with the patient in a formal lateral decubitus position. This allows the greatest access to the entire pleural cavity. The patient is supported on a beanbag or with rolls. As with all procedures performed in a lateral decubitus position, it is important to place an axillary roll and sufficient padding at all pressure points. Tape or a strap can be used to support the patient's position. Patients with severe pulmonary compromise may not tolerate having their good lung compromised by being in a dependent position. In these cases a modified supine position can be used, with the affected side elevated 25–30°. **(See Figure 17.1)**

In this case the surgeon and the assistant are positioned on either side of the patient. This facilitates the procedure, as the entire pleural cavity needs to be explored and it allows the surgeon and the assistant to work the camera and instruments from whichever side is better for access to a particular area. The scrub nurse may be positioned towards the feet on whichever side is convenient. Monitors should be placed on both sides at approximately the level of the shoulders.

Port placement

Port placement can be somewhat variable, depending on the size of the patient and the area of the chest cavity most involved. In general, the procedure can be performed with just two ports. These are placed in the anterior and posterior axillary lines at the fifth or sixth interspace. If necessary, a third port can be placed to reach an area not readily accessible by the other two or if retraction is required. Placement is dependent on the findings at thoracoscopy. If the chest wall is large enough, one of the ports should be a 10 mm to facilitate removal of the infected peel. However, it is important to remember that the larger the port size, the more limited the range of motion will be at that site because of the restriction of the rib cage.

The primary goals of the operation are to remove as much of the infected fluid and fibrous peel as possible, break down any septa, allow for re-expansion of the lung and provide adequate drainage. All of this should be accomplished in an efficient manner without taking excessive time. With this in mind, the following steps should be followed.

Start the procedure by inserting a needle or the Veress needle into a space that appears to contain fluid. Aspirate the area. If free-flowing fluid is obtained, it is safe to insert a trocar in this area without causing injury to the lung, which can be adherent to the chest wall. Alternatively, a small cut down can be made, similar to that used for putting in a chest drain, to gain initial access.

Insert a 5 mm trocar and make a quick visual survey. Then insert the suction device and remove as much fluid as possible. If there is limited space, use the telescope or the suction device as a blunt probe to break down adhesions and create more space. Keep the scope or instrument next to the chest wall as you sweep with it: this will avoid inadvertent injury to the lung parenchyma. Breaking down the adhesions allows the lung to collapse and improves visualization. Insufflating with CO_2 can also help with this.

Once an adequate space has been made, the second trocar should be inserted. This can now be done under direct visualization with the telescope.

With two ports in, mobilization of the fibrous peel can now start in a systematic method under direct vision. Depending on where the largest area of involvement is, a larger (10 mm) port should be placed at this site. The blunt grasper is used to grasp some of the peel and then a sweeping motion is used to strip as much as possible off the lung surface or chest wall. The more fibrous the peel, the more effective this is. The tissue can almost be removed in strips. If the peel is newer and less fibrous, much of it may be able to be broken up and removed with the suction device alone. **(See Figure 17.2)**

Work should proceed in a clockwise direction to ensure that all areas are addressed. When an area becomes difficult to reach, the scope and grasper are exchanged, which usually gives a better view and exposure to the area. If the surgeon is now working out of the smaller port and the peel cannot be easily brought out through it, it can simply be mobilized and left in the pleural cavity and then removed through the larger trocar when convenient.

The monitors may also need to be repositioned to try to keep the surgeon in line with the camera and the area being worked in. However, because the field of dissection is constantly changing, it is acceptable at times for the surgeon to be operating out of a partial paradox, as the stripping of the peel does not require fine motor movements.

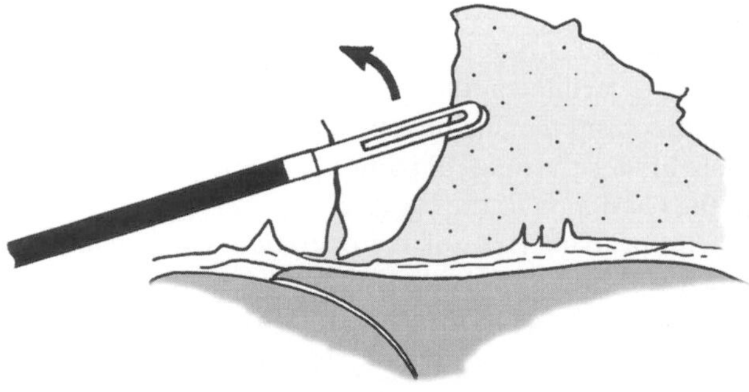

Figure 17.2

Once the majority of the peel is removed and all loculations are broken down, the chest cavity is irrigated with copious amounts of saline (1–2 L, depending on the child's size). Antibiotics may be added if desired.

The desired effects of the procedure are to remove the majority of infected fluid and tissue, break down all loculations, free and re-expand the trapped lung, and establish adequate drainage. It is not necessary to remove every piece of the peel. The time of the procedure should be kept to a minimum to avoid prolonged anesthesia. It should last no more than 60 minutes and, in most cases, takes significantly less. If adequate drainage and lung re-expansion are achieved, the residual infected peel will be reabsorbed as long as the patient's clinical picture improves.

If the fibrous peel is so organized and hard that it cannot be stripped away bluntly, the disease may be beyond the range of a thoracoscopic approach. It is extremely difficult to try to surgically cut and remove a hardened peel thoracoscopically because of the mechanical disadvantage of the small instruments and the limited visibility associated with any bleeding.

After irrigation, the trocars are removed. A single chest tube is placed through the anterior port site and placed posterior so it lies in a dependent position. The sites are closed in layers with absorbable suture and the chest tube is placed to suction.

If the patient is stable, it is best to extubate him or her at the end of the procedure. The limited surgical trauma allows aggressive postoperative physiotherapy. Spontaneous breathing and coughing should help keep the lung expanded and the airway clear.

POSTOPERATIVE CARE

Postoperative analgesia is administered in the form of intravenous morphine for the first 24–48 hours. Epidural or spinal anesthesia is rarely needed. The chest tube should be left to suction for at least the first 24 hours and then until the drainage falls below 25–50 mL for an 8-hour period, depending on the size of the patient. It is then placed to water seal and checked by chest X-ray after 12–24 hours. If the chest X-ray shows no pneumothorax or increased effusion, the chest tube can be safely removed. This is usually possible 2–4 days after surgery. The patient is kept on intravenous antibiotics until afebrile for 24–48 hours, after which, depending on the clinical course and the organism involved, a final course of oral antibiotics may be given.

PROBLEMS, PITFALLS AND SOLUTIONS

Difficult access to the pleural cavity

- If adhesions between the lung and chest wall make visualization/access difficult, blind blunt dissection must be carried out. This can be accomplished with the telescope, suction device or any blunt instrument.
- At times it may be necessary to choose an alternative initial site. If so, the pleural cavity should be probed with a needle to aspirate for fluid, and a CT scan should be done to confirm the findings.
- Widen the trocar site to allow the insertion of a single finger for digital manipulation to create an intrathoracic space. A port may then be secured at this site, or standard instruments can be inserted through the small incision.
- Increase CO_2 insufflation pressure.

Bleeding

- Some bleeding is to be expected as the inflammatory peel is mobilized. This can usually be dealt with by using the irrigating fluid to clear the field. However, as in all endoscopic cases, bleeding will decrease visibility because it absorbs the light.
- Monopolar cautery can be used in some cases if the site of bleeding is relatively localized and discrete.
- If vigorous parenchymal bleeding is encountered, there are very few maneuvers available to the surgeon. The best course is to remove the ports, place a relatively large-bore chest tube and re-expand the lung. This should allow for tamponade. If the bleeding persists at an aggressive rate after a few hours, it may be necessary to perform a formal thoracotomy.

Air leak

- Parenchymal injury is not uncommon. Most parietal pleural injuries are superficial tears that will seal after a few days of lung expansion and chest tube drainage. If there was significant lung necrosis and/or abscess, a significant air leak or bronchopleural fistula may result. However, the majority of these leaks will also seal.
- If there is a persistent large air leak, the surgeon should suspect significant lung necrosis. A CT scan may help

evaluate the degree of lung injury. Fibrin glue, blood, and chemical pleurodesis can be attempted, but are likely to fail in this scenario. Re-exploration with possible formal lobectomy may be required.

Inability to mobilize the fibrous peel

If the pleural peel is too fibrous or thick to be removed with thoracoscopic instruments, the procedure should be converted to an open thoracotomy. This is likely to be a long and bloody procedure. The best way to prevent this is to encourage early intervention whenever possible.

COMPLICATIONS

The major complications of bleeding and persistent air leak have already been discussed. The only other major issue is the possibility of incomplete drainage and/or recurrent effusion. This is a rare complication if an adequate debridement is performed at the first surgery. One option is percutaneous drainage under CT or ultrasound guidance if there is a single, isolated fluid collection. The other option is repeat exploration thoracoscopically or via open thoracotomy if necessary. Lytic therapy with urokinase can be considered as an adjunctive therapy but is rarely necessary.

The decision to perform a more aggressive debridement/resection in the case of necrotizing pneumonia should be made based on the patient's clinical course, findings at the time of the initial thoracoscopy, CT scan results, and the degree of air leak (if any) present.

FURTHER READING

Klena JW, Cameron BH, Langer JC, et al. Timing of video-assisted thoracoscopic debridement for pediatric empyema. *Journal of the American College of Surgeons* 1998; **187**:404–8.

McGahren ED. Use of thoracoscopy for treatment of empyema in children. *Pediatric Endosurgery & Innovative Techniques* 2001; **5**:117–24.

Merry CM, Buffo AJ, Shah RS, et al. Early intervention by thoracoscopy in pediatric empyema. *Journal of Pediatric Surgery* 1999; **34**:178–81.

Rothenberg SS, Chang JHT. Thoracoscopic decortication in infants and children. *Surgical Endoscopy* 1997; **II**:93–4.

18

Thoracoscopic clipping of patent ductus arteriosus

EMMANUEL VILLA, THIERRY FOLLIGUET AND FRANÇOIS LABORDE

INTRODUCTION

Patent ductus arteriosus (PDA) was the first congenital heart lesion to undergo surgical intervention and the first in which a trans-catheter approach was performed. In children, video-assisted thoracoscopic surgery (VATS) is becoming increasingly popular.

We started thoracoscopic ligation of PDA in 1991. Since then, the technique has undergone minor modification and become highly standardized.

Indications

- Low birth weight neonates/premature infants with a significant shunt.
- Older children with persistent PDA.

Contraindications

ABSOLUTE

- Ductus diameter >8 mm.
- Patient size (lower limit 1 kg).
- Presence of calcifications.
- Active infection, or aneurysm.

RELATIVE

- Significantly high pulmonary hypertension.
- Previous thoracotomy.
- Failure of previous interventional techniques.

Advantages

- Avoids the morbidity of thoracotomy.
- Allows an excellent visualization of the ductus and recurrent laryngeal nerve.

Disadvantages

- Small working space in neonate.
- Difficulty controlling bleeding (major vascular injury).
- The duct is not formally divided.

EQUIPMENT/INSTRUMENTS

Essential

- Thoracoscope 4–5 mm.
- Titanium clips (9 mm).
- Angled hooks (blunt hooks or rods to use as retractors).
- 2.5–5 mm trocars.
- Hook cautery.
- Scissors.
- Dissector.
- Suction device.

Optional

- Lung retractor.

PREOPERATIVE PREPARATION

Standard pre-surgical laboratory analysis and chest X-ray are performed on an outpatient basis. Transthoracic echocardiography is repeated on the admission day for complete cardiac re-evaluation and determination of ductus size. Angiography and cardiac catheterization are not routinely employed if accurate anatomical and functional definition is obtained with ultrasonography.

TECHNIQUE

The procedure is carried out under general anesthesia. A central line is placed via the jugular vein and an arterial line is usually not necessary. Electrocardiogram monitoring, oximetry and capnography are routine.

After the induction of general anesthesia and standard intubation, the patient is positioned on his or her right side, as for a postero-lateral thoracotomy. The surgeon and the scrub nurse stand on the left side of the patient, the assistant on the right. The monitor is placed on the right side of the patient. **(See Figure 18.1)**

Two small incisions are made in the left hemithorax using a No. 11 blade. The first incision is made just posterior to the scapula in the third intercostal space, for the videothoracoscope introduced via a 5 mm cannula. A second incision is made in the fourth intercostal space just below the angle of the scapula for the electrocautery hook, which is introduced via a 5 mm cannula. Two or three 60° angled hooks, 1 mm in diameter, are introduced directly through the third intercostal space (mid region) just in front of the scapula, for lung retraction.

The upper lobe of the left lung is retracted inferomedially using the angled hooks. The PDA is identified and the mediastinal pleura is opened carefully with the electrocautery hook. The PDA is carefully dissected and released from the surrounding tissues and its junction with the aorta is freed completely. The pericardium is dissected on the pulmonary side to protect the recurrent laryngeal nerve from any traumatic injury. It is essential to dissect on both sides of the PDA to allow adequate ligation. The clip applier is then introduced without any trocar through the fourth intercostal space cannula site. A first titanium clip (9 mm) is placed as distal as possible from the aortic junction on the pulmonary side of the PDA and a second clip is applied on the side close to the aorta. After visual confirmation that both clips are in place, the lung is inflated and a 2 mm diameter chest drain is placed. The wounds are closed using absorbable suture. **(See Figure 18.2)**

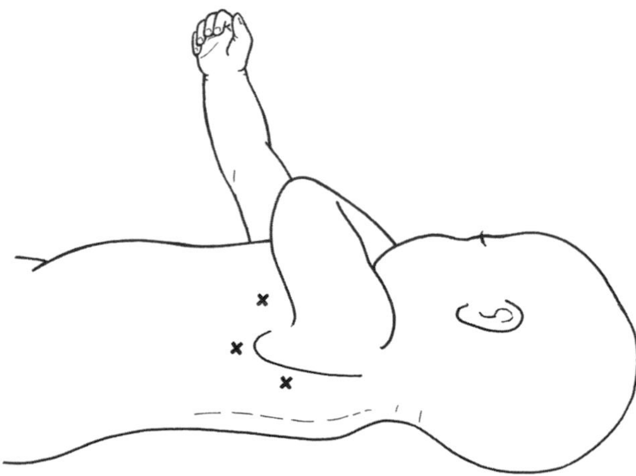

Figure 18.1

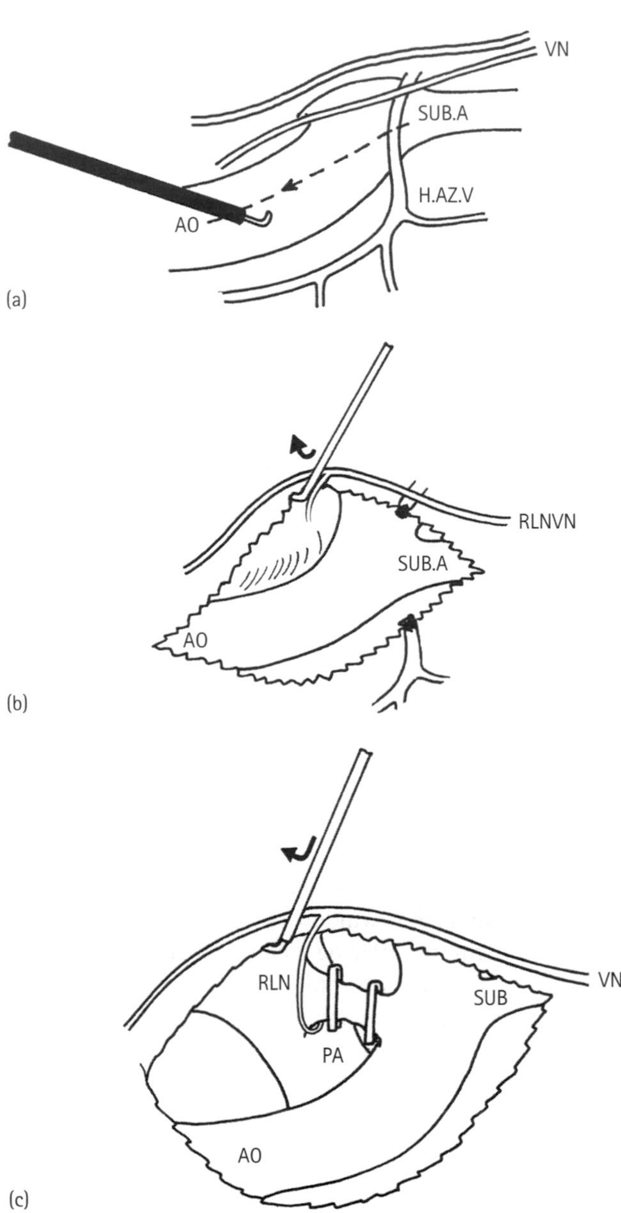

Figure 18.2 *(a) Incision through the pleura overlying the aorta; (b) division of the hemiazygous vein and exploration of the PDA; (c) clipped PDA.*

POSTOPERATIVE CARE

Color-flow Doppler echocardiography is performed in the operating room or in the recovery room before extubation to assess the completeness of closure of the PDA. If there is a persistent shunt, the patient is taken back immediately to the operating room for re-application of a new clip by VATS. Otherwise, the patient is extubated and transferred back to either the intensive care unit or pediatric ward, depending on his or her condition and age. The pleural suction catheter is removed a few hours after extubation. A routine chest X-ray and a transthoracic echocardiogram are performed before the patient is discharged from the hospital 12–24 hours postoperatively. All patients are then regularly followed up by their own pediatric cardiologist. Prophylactic antibiotics may be required in the presence of residual shunt.

PROBLEMS, PITFALLS AND SOLUTIONS

Inability to visualize the ductus

This can happen for a number of reasons. The anesthesiologist may be using high vent pressures, making collapse of the lung difficult. This can be overcome by inserting a low flow of CO_2 to help compress the lung (1 L/min, 4–6 mmHg). A selective right mainstem intubation may also be performed. Most patients are able to tolerate this short period of single lung ventilation. The patient may be placed in a more prone position so that the lung is retracted by gravity.

Incomplete occlusion of the ductus

This is a difficult problem to recognize. Establishing the size of the ductus preoperatively with echocardiography helps ensure that it is not larger then the available clip. Performing an echocardiogram in the operating room prior to extubation can ensure that no significant flow is left prior to awakening the patient. If necessary, a second clip can be applied. A 'window'-type ductus may also cause difficulty accurately placing a clip. If there is only a small amount of residual flow, this will probably occlude with time and no further manipulation should be necessary. Because we are not dividing the ductus, we routinely perform a rigorous echographic evaluation immediately after surgery and before discharge. This protocol has allowed us to detect 1–4 percent of incomplete closures. Each of these patients underwent additional surgery and the second procedure was unsuccessful in one-quarter of patients re-operated on using VATS. Therefore it seems wise to rectify incomplete occlusion by open surgery if the first VATS operation fails. This would allow shortcomings in clip size, anatomic anomalies and difficult visualization to be more easily overcome.

The ductus tears

This is a disastrous, but fortunately rare, problem. If the ductus tears during dissection, an atraumatic dissector should be used to try to occlude the ductus and stop the bleeding. If this works, it is likely that the clip, when applied, will also stop the bleeding. The clip applier should always be test fired once before using it on the ductus to ensure it is working properly and not scissoring. If the bleeding starts after application of the clip, a second adjacent clip can be applied to try to occlude the tear. Because of the small size of these patients, there is very little room for error. Therefore, a tray of conventional instruments for open surgery and 1 unit of cross-matched blood should be available to use in case of emergency.

Occlusion of the wrong structure

This is also a rare problem but must be avoided at all costs. The key is meticulous dissection to identify all structures adequately. If the anatomy is not clear, an intraoperative echocardiogram should be preformed. Also a pulse oximeter should be placed on a lower extremity, distal to the ductus, and test clamping should be performed prior to placing the clip to ensure that flow to the distal extremity is not interrupted.

COMPLICATIONS

In our series, complications occurred in 6.8 percent of patients (48/703) and the incidence of a complicated course in low birth weight infants was 22.7 percent (5/22). Suboptimal outcomes were recorded in 17.9 percent of the Down's syndrome group (5/28; $p = 0.036$, relative risk 2, confidence limit 1.2–7.5). **(See Tables 18.1–18.3)**

Table 18.1 *Incidence of complications**

	%	(No.)
Recurrent laryngeal nerve dysfunction:	3.0	(21)
transient	2.6	(18)
persistent	0.4	(3)
Pneumothorax	1.3	(9)
Transfusion	0.1	(1)
Chylothorax	0.6	(4)
Thoracotomy:	1.0	(7)
for hemostasis	0.3	(2)
for incomplete closure	0.7	(5)

*Incidence of residual patency is reported analytically in the text. Patients $n = 703$.

Table 18.2 *Complications according to body weight repartition*

LBWIs % (number)	Non-LBWIs	p	Relative risk LBWI vs non-LBWI	95% Confidence limits	
				Lower	Upper
Recurrent laryngeal nerve dysfunction					
13.6 (3)	2.6 (3)	0.025	5.1	1.4	16
Long-lasting recurrent laryngeal nerve dysfunction					
4.5 (1)	0.3 (2)	NS (0.09)	11.1	2.1	58.1
Pneumothorax					
9.1 (2)	1.0 (7)	0.026	7.7	2.1	28.2
Transfusion					
4.5 (1)	0	0.031			
Chylothorax					
0	0.6 (4)	NS (1)			
Immediate residual patency					
0	1.4 (10)	NS (0.7)*			
Residual patency at discharge					
0	1.0 (7)	NS (0.8)*			
Residual patency at follow-up					
0	0.6 (4)	NS (0.9)*			
Thoracotomy					
4.5 (1)	0.9 (6)	NS (0.2)	4.7	0.7	30.5
Overall complicated course					
22.8 (5)	6.3 (43)	0.013	4.1	1.5	10.4

LBWIs, low birth weight infants.
*One-sided.

Table 18.3 *Sub-analysis of residual patency and thoracotomy*

LBWIs	2.5–25 kg % (number)	>25 kg % (number)	p*
Immediate residual patency			
0	1.4 (9)	2.5 (1)	NS (0.7)
Residual patency at discharge			
0	0.8 (5)	5 (2)	0.006
Residual patency at follow-up			
0	0.3 (2)	5 (2)	0.001
Thoracotomy			
4.5% (1)	0.6 (4)	5 (2)	0.006

LBWIs, low birth weight infants.
* significance at value 0.025.

Residual patency of the ductus

This may be treated by a repeat VATS or standard thoracotomy. If the residual shunt is small, it may occlude on its own without further intervention. Chylothorax was managed conservatively, with the exception of one patient who required thoracoscopic treatment. In this group, mean postoperative stay was 10 ± 6.7 days (range 6–20).

Recurrent laryngeal nerve dysfunction

This is best avoided by meticulous dissection, avoiding direct contact with the nerve, and making sure the nerve is not entrapped by the clip. This injury is often transient and may improve with time.

Pneumothorax

This is usually due to residual air or CO_2 in the pleural cavity and should resolve spontaneously.

Bleeding

As already discussed.

FURTHER READING

Burke RP, Wernosky G, van der Velde M, Hansen D, Castaneda AR. Video-assisted thoracoscopic surgery for congenital heart disease. *Journal of Thoracic and Cardiovascular Surgery* 1995; 109:499–508.

Gross RE, Hubbard JP. Landmark article February 25, 1939: Surgical ligation of a patent ductus arteriosus. Report of first successful case. *Journal of the American Medical Association* 1984; **251**:1201–2.

Laborde F, Folliguet TA, Etienne PY, Carbognani D, Batisse A, Petrie J. Video-thoracoscopic surgical interruption of patent ductus arteriosus in 332 pediatric cases. *European Journal of Cardio-thoracic Surgery* 1997; **11**:1052–5.

Le Bret E, Papadatos S, Folliguet T et al. Interruption of patent ductus arteriosus in children: robotically assisted versus videothoracoscopic surgery. *Journal of Thoracic and Cardiovascular Surgery* 2002; **123**:973–6.

Mavroudis C, Backer CL, Gevitz M. Forty-six years of patent ductus arteriosus division at Children's Memorial Hospital of Chicago. Standards of comparison. *Annals of Surgery* 1994; **220**:402–9.

19

Endoscopic-assisted correction of pectus excavatum

KLAUS SCHAARSCHMIDT

INTRODUCTION

Pectus excavatum (funnel chest) is the most common congenital hereditary chest wall deformity. The incidence rate is 1 in 1000 live births, with a 3:1 male:female predominance. Although most cases are sporadic, familial (autosomal dominant) and acquired cases (secondary to cardiac surgery) have also been reported. In 20 percent of cases, signs of deformity are evident within the first year of life and symptoms such as dyspnea, cardiac dysfunction and reduced physical performance develop at the onset of puberty.

Pectus excavatum was first reported by Bauhinus in 1594, described by Eggle in 1870 and first surgically corrected by Meyers in 1911 and then by Sauerbruch in 1913. Ravitch described excision of all deformed cartilages with anterior Kirschner wire and suture fixation of the sternum in 1949. Rehbein and Hegemann described sternal stabilization by axial costal re-anastomosis and metal struts in 1965. Recently, Nuss popularized thoracoscopy in the management of chest deformity and laid the foundation for the present techniques employed worldwide.

The aims of surgery in general are:

- adequate retrosternal mobilization,
- elevation and possibly restoration of the sternum,
- lowering the everted and often concaved ribs of prominent costal arches,
- to ensure minimal morbidity,
- to improve cardiorespiratory performance and cosmesis.

Indications

- Patients must be at least 10, preferably 12, years of age.
- Symmetric and asymmetric deformities.
- Girls with significant breast asymmetry (sunken breast).
- Symptomatic patients (breathlessness and limited physical performance).
- Recurrent deformity following previous surgery.
- Secondary deformities following median sternotomy, e.g. cardiac surgery.
- Patients who are affected psychologically.

Contraindications

- Acute respiratory infection.
- Uncorrected hemorrhagic disease.
- Lack of patient motivation.

EQUIPMENT/INSTRUMENTS

Essential

- A funnel chest set of instruments including large and extra large pectus introducer, bar flipper, two bar benders and an anvil bar bender rather than the hand-operated pectus bender.
- Two monitors on each side of the patient.

- 5 mm cannula and 5 mm 30° angled telescope.
- Different sizes of straight and angled luer bone pliers.

Optional

- Straight and angled monopolar diathermy hook and thoracoscopic Satinsky clamp.
- Bipolar diathermy.

PREOPERATIVE PREPARATION

Full coagulation status is investigated in all patients. Contact allergies to metals, particularly nickel, must be excluded and, if doubtful, skin tests are performed. Alternatively, tailor-made tetanum bars (computerized tomography (CT) base) are used. Three to five routine CT sections through the deepest point of the funnel, respiratory function tests and electrocardiographs (ECGs) are obtained in all patients. In those who have associated syndromes such as Marfan or Romano–Ward, echocardiography, long-time ECG and fundoscopy by an ophthalmologist are required. Self blood donation (usually 1 unit) is prepared 2–4 weeks prior to surgery.

TECHNIQUE

An epidural catheter at T6 or T7 level and/or peri-operative intravenous analgesia for 5 days provide excellent analgesia. A double shot of cephalosporin prophylaxis and 24 hours of urinary catheter are given to all patients. The patient is positioned supine with the thorax elevated 5–10 cm on a soft bolster and the arms adducted. The procedure is conducted from both sides of the patient, with the monitors being placed towards the patients' shoulders. **(See Figure 19.1)**

The procedure includes the following steps.

- Small incisions and adequate sub-muscular pockets are made for access.
- Bar ends plus stabilizers are placed into the sub-muscular pockets directly on the ribs.
- Each bar including stabilizer is fixed to all adjacent ribs by 8–14 pericostal figure-of-eight sutures under thoracoscopic view.
- Stabilizers are jammed on the bent bar by a bone hammer and not fixed with wires (because wires usually break quickly).
- In older patients (over 16 years of age) with severe deformity, a second or third shorter bar is inserted through the same incisions.
- The bars are placed extrapleurally whenever possible.
- Incisions are closed in layers to ensure complete muscle cover for all metals.
- An extrapleural bar position is feasible in more than 90 percent of patients.
- Longer bars without stabilizers may provide an advantage.

Bilateral 2.5–4 cm transverse skin incisions are made directly over the fifth ribs in the anterior axillary line and wide subcutaneous pockets are created. The muscles (serratus anterior and external oblique) are split, and generous sub-muscular pockets to accommodate the bars and stabilizers (if necessary) are created directly over the fifth ribs. Bilateral 5.5 mm cannulae are placed in the seventh intercostals space and the anterior axillary line. Bilateral pneumothorax is created using CO_2 at 8 mmHg. **(See Figure 19.2)**

Under direct thoracoscopic views, small extrapleural pockets are created in the fourth intercostal space using conventional blunt forceps through the previously created right sub-muscular space/incision. An external pleural tunnel is then created along the fourth intercostal space and fifth rib towards the pleuro-pericardial fold. Care is taken to stay on the pleural side of the internal mammary vessels. The forceps are then replaced by the Lorenz dissector, which is carefully and gradually advanced, pushing the pericardium away from the sternum until it becomes visible under the left mediastinal pleura.

The right dissector is held by an assistant while an identical corresponding extrapleural tunnel is developed from the left side. Once the two instruments meet, the left is gradually withdrawn while the right follows through the tunnel and emerges through the left intercostal site of entry. During this maneuver, care must be taken to maintain

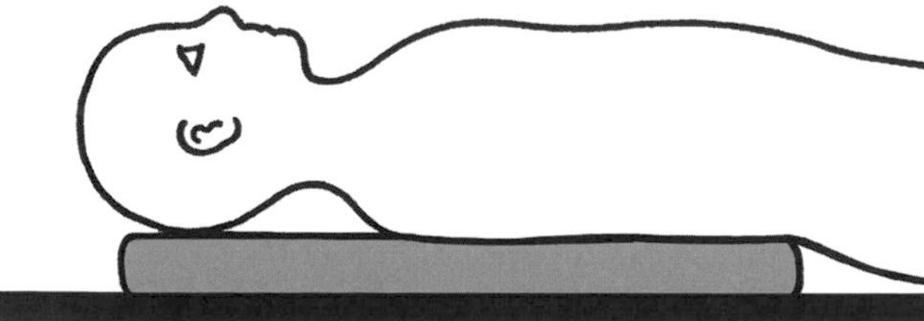

Figure 19.1

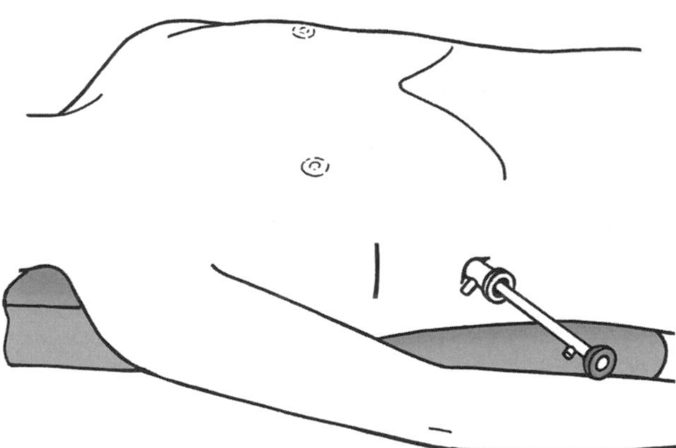

Figure 19.2

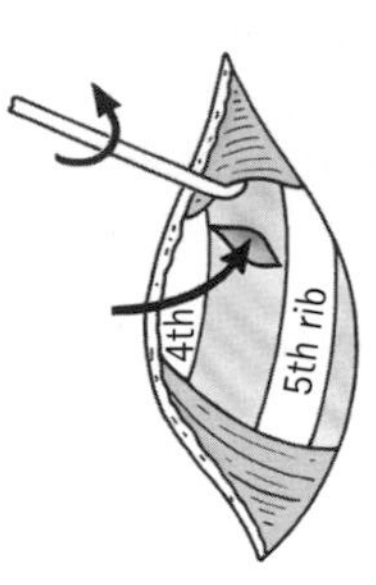

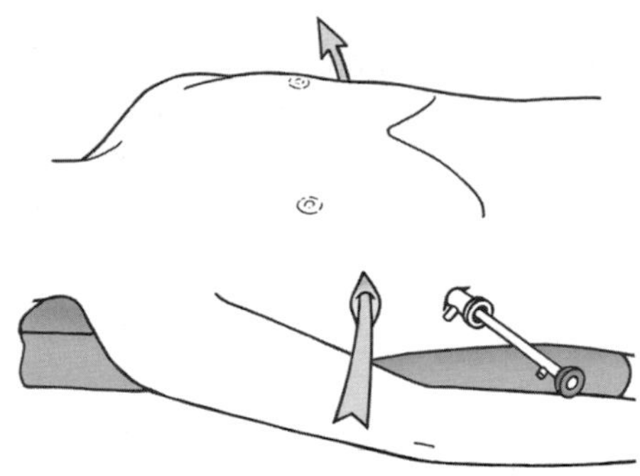

Figure 19.3

contact between the two instruments. The tunnel is made wide enough to allow for turning of the bar. (**See Figure 19.3**)

If more than one bar is required, identical tunnels are created two intercostal spaces higher or one to two spaces lower using the same maneuver through the same but probably extended skin incisions.

The bars are fixed to every rib they cross using strong figure-of-eight braided polyglactin sutures under thoracoscopic view. The sutures are passed from outside around the rib and out through the next intercostal space. A minimum of ten pericostal sutures per bar is usually required. The fulcrum of rotation is the point where the bar enters the thorax, whereas the ends of the bar and the sternal section of the bar may move. Therefore, fixation close to these entry points gives the maximum protection against bar rotation.

If necessary, multiple sternal and costal partial ventral osteotomies are carried out using bone pliers through the skin incision and sub-muscular tunnels created during the early stages of the procedure (this may require extended incisions). (**See Figure 19.4**)

Sub-muscular suction drains are usually necessary to prevent seroma and hematoma formation. Intercostal chest drains, which can be placed through the site of the thoracoscopic cannulae, are usually not necessary. The wounds are closed in layers.

POSTOPERATIVE CARE

Epidural analgesia and/or morphine infusion may be required for up to 5 days. Oral analgesia may be administered for 4–6 weeks. Sub-muscular suction drains and/or chest drains are removed after 1–3 days postoperatively. The hospital stay is usually about 7–10 days; however, the older adolescent with multiple bars and extensive repair may need to stay longer.

Plain chest X-ray and repeat ultrasound scan are used to detect postoperative pneumothorax and effusion soon after surgery and maybe prior to discharge of the patient from the hospital.

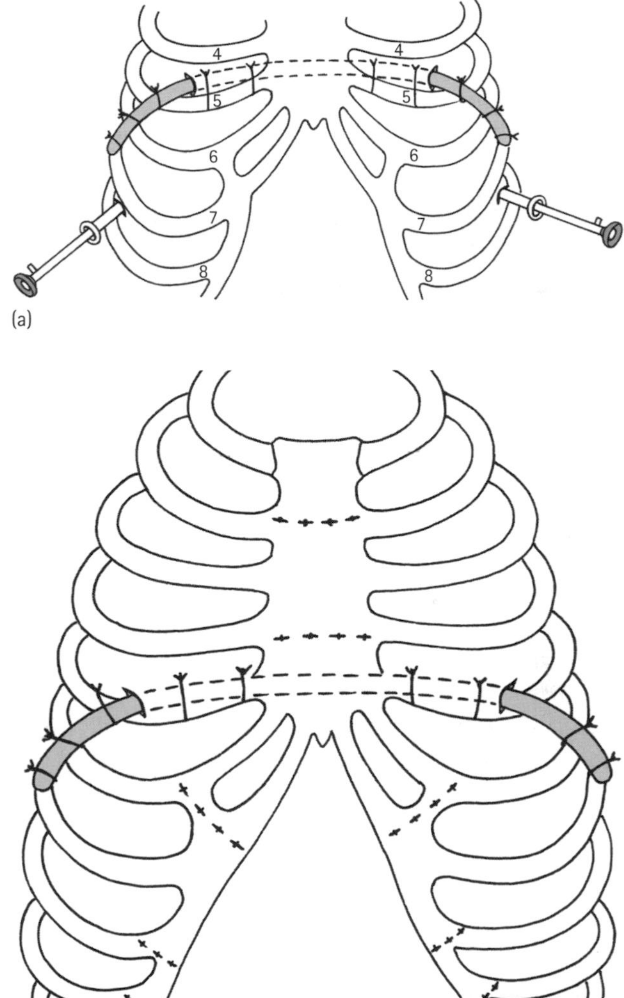

Figure 19.4

An elastic compression bandage is worn on the thorax for 4–6 weeks, especially when prominent costal arches are corrected. The patients are allowed mild exercise after 2 weeks and full activity after 8 weeks postoperatively.

PROBLEMS, PITFALLS AND SOLUTIONS

- Female breasts must always be palpated thoroughly to exclude benign lesions preoperatively.
- Bleeding from ruptured internal mammary and intercostal vessels is usually not a serious problems. However, it can be a nuisance and increase the likelihood of postoperative pleural effusion and wound hematoma. Meticulous technique cannot be over-emphasized.
- Bar stability may be jeopardized by:
  - improper technique,
  - major disruption of the intercostal spaces during the operation,
  - inadequate fixation,
  - postoperative seroma, hematoma and infection.

Meticulous technique, appropriate fixation of the bar, and sub-muscular suction drain minimize the risk.

COMPLICATIONS

- Pneumothorax is usually not a problem. The lungs are expanded fully prior to removal of the thoracoscopic cannulae using positive-pressure ventilation. Chest drains are usually unnecessary.
- Postoperative pleural effusion greater than 300 mL usually requires needle aspiration and/or chest drain with or without general anesthetic.
- Bar instability (as above).
- Infection requires early removal of the bar.

FURTHER READING

Hosie S, Sitkiewicz T, Peterson C et al. Minimally invasive repair of pectus excavatum – the Nuss procedure. A European multicentre experience. *European Journal of Pediatric Surgery* 2002; **12**:235–8.

Nuss D, Kelly RE Jr, Croitoru DP et al. A 10-year review of a minimally invasive technique for the correction of pectus excavatum. *Journal of Pediatric Surgery* 1998; **33**:545–52.

Schaarschmidt K, Kolberg-Schwerdt A, Dimitrov G et al. Submuscular bar, multiple pericostal bar fixation, bilateral thoracoscopy, a modified Nuss repair in adolescents. *Journal of Pediatric Surgery* 2002; **37**:1476–80.

Schaarschmidt K, Kolberg-Schwert A, Lempe M et al. Extrapleural, submuscular bars placed by bilateral thoracoscopy – a new improvement in modified Nuss funnel chest repair. *Journal of Pediatric Surgery* 2005; **40**: in press.

Section C: Gastrointestinal

20

Rigid endoscopy of the esophagus – basic technique

DAVID A. LLOYD

INTRODUCTION

Endoscopic inspection of the esophagus is an integral part of its evaluation for disease and functional disorders, and in some cases for management. Before the introduction of fiberoptic endoscopes, esophagoscopy was performed using rigid open tubes illuminated by a battery-powered bulb at either the proximal or distal end of the tube. Although the flexible fiberoptic endoscope has replaced the rigid esophagoscope for routine endoscopy, the latter still has important applications in pediatric surgical practice, notably the removal of foreign bodies.

Indications

DIAGNOSTIC

Flexible endoscopy is the method of choice for routine diagnostic esophagoscopy. However, larger biopsies may be taken through the rigid esophagoscope, which may be an advantage. More importantly, the rigid esophagoscope is advanced without the need to insufflate air into the esophagus. This is important if a traumatic injury to the esophagus is suspected because air will not egress through a perforation. In the case of caustic injury, the purpose of esophagoscopy is to confirm that the esophagus has been damaged. In the acute phase, no attempt should be made to pass the endoscope through the damaged segment because of the risk of perforation.

Rigid esophagoscopy in the newborn will confirm the presence of esophageal atresia and also allow measurement of the length of the upper esophagus. Combined rigid esophagoscopy and bronchoscopy may be useful for identifying or excluding an H-type tracheo-esophageal fistula in an infant with recurrent respiratory infections.

THERAPEUTIC

The main value of the rigid endoscope in contemporary pediatric surgical practice is as a tool for therapeutic esophagoscopy.

- Dilatation of esophageal strictures. The commonest causes of esophageal strictures in children are peptic (secondary to reflux oesophagitis), anastomotic (post-repair of esophageal atresia) and caustic (following ingestion of sodium hydroxide). The rigid esophagoscope enables dilatation under direct vision using bougies in graduated sizes.
- Foreign body removal. A range of instruments can be passed down a rigid esophagoscope to manipulate and grasp foreign bodies in the esophagus.
- Sclerotherapy. Sclerotherapy for esophageal varices may be performed through the open rigid endoscope. An adapted Negus instrument is available with a slot at the distal end into which the varix is manipulated and stabilized for injection. Following injection, the endoscope is rotated to compress the varix and control bleeding at the injection site. Note that the bleeding from a gastric varix may be impossible to visualize

with a rigid esophagoscope, and therefore fiberoptic endoscopes are preferred by many surgeons (see Chapter 24).

Contraindications

ABSOLUTE

- Child not fit for general anesthesia.
- Lack of expertise and facilities.

EQUIPMENT/INSTRUMENTS

Essential

- Esophagoscopes in a range of sizes.
- Light source and cable.
- Suction equipment, including catheters.
- Foreign body grasping forceps.
- Biopsy forceps.
- Saline for irrigation, with syringes.
- Bougies for dilatation.
- Fogarty balloon embolectomy catheters.

Desirable

- 3.0 mm Storz rigid bronchoscope for esophagoscopy in neonates.

A number of types of rigid open tube esophagoscope are suitable for use in children. The Chevalier–Jackson design has a circular cross-section and the Negus design has a slightly larger oval cross-section. The distal end of the esophagoscope expands in diameter and is beveled, with an anterior lip designed to open up the esophageal lumen by elevating the anterior wall of the esophagus. Illumination is from either the proximal or distal end of the esophagoscope; the latter generally provides brighter illumination. The original electrical light source has been replaced by a fiberoptic light transmitted through an optic rod inserted along a channel on the inside of the esophagoscope. **(See Table 20.1)**

The Storz solid endoscope uses a fiberoptic light source transmitted through an optical telescope that locks into the metal sheath. This instrument provides excellent visualization of the esophagus. However, the working channel is smaller than that of the Negus and Chevalier–Jackson instruments and this instrument is of limited value for therapeutic esophagoscopy.

Before commencing an esophagoscopy it is essential to ensure that all the equipment is present and compatible. Ensure suction catheters and operating instruments can be passed through the esophagoscope and that they are of sufficient length to extend beyond the distal end of the endoscope.

Table 20.1 *Negus esophagoscopes*

Negus esophagoscope	Dimensions
Infant small (or neonatal bronchoscope)	20 cm length, 6.6 mm diameter
Infant	20 cm length, 8.6 mm diameter
Child short	25 cm length, 10 mm diameter
Child	35 cm length, 10 mm diameter
Adolescent/adult	35 cm length, 11.6 mm diameter

PREOPERATIVE PREPARATION

Rigid esophagoscopy is performed under general anesthesia, and routine anesthetic preparation is necessary. The presence and position of any loose teeth should be recorded and, if necessary, permission sought for their removal. If a stricture is suspected, a contrast swallow should be performed prior to endoscopy. If a swallowed foreign body is suspected, a preoperative chest radiograph should be obtained.

TECHNIQUE

Rigid esophagoscopy requires general anesthesia with endotracheal intubation and muscle relaxation. The endotracheal tube minimizes the risk of aspiration and prevents tracheal compression during esophagoscopy.

The child is positioned supine on the operating table with the head and neck aligned and the neck extended. The endotracheal tube is taped to the left side of the mouth, leaving the right side free for endoscopy. A gum shield or pad of gauze is used to protect the upper teeth. The eyes should be taped closed. A pillow is placed under the upper thorax. This straightens the cervico-thoracic spine and hence the esophagus, facilitating passage of the esophagoscope. Ideally the head should rest on an adjustable anesthetic table to allow the position of the cervical spine to be adjusted if necessary. **(See Figure 20.1)**

For right-handed operators, the esophagoscope is held between the thumb and index finger of the right hand, with the left thumb resting on the upper teeth and the left middle finger on the lower teeth, thus protecting them from direct contact with the instrument. The right hand is used to guide the esophagoscope, holding it as one would a pencil. The situation is analogous to holding a snooker cue with the left hand while playing the shot with the right hand. As the esophagoscope is inserted, it rests on the thumb and middle finger of the surgeon's left hand and not on the child's teeth. During insertion, the lower lip may roll into the mouth and become crushed against the teeth; this must be avoided by everting the lip with the fingers of the left hand.

The esophagoscope is lubricated and, with the beveled lip anterior, is held in a vertical position as it is inserted into the mouth. It is slowly advanced along the hard and

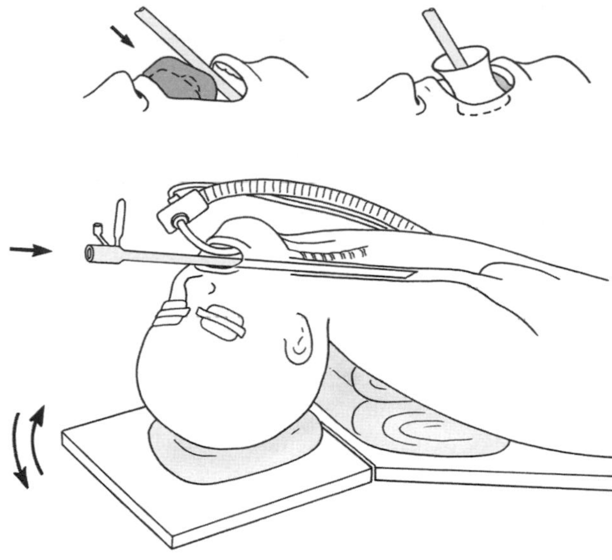

Figure 20.1

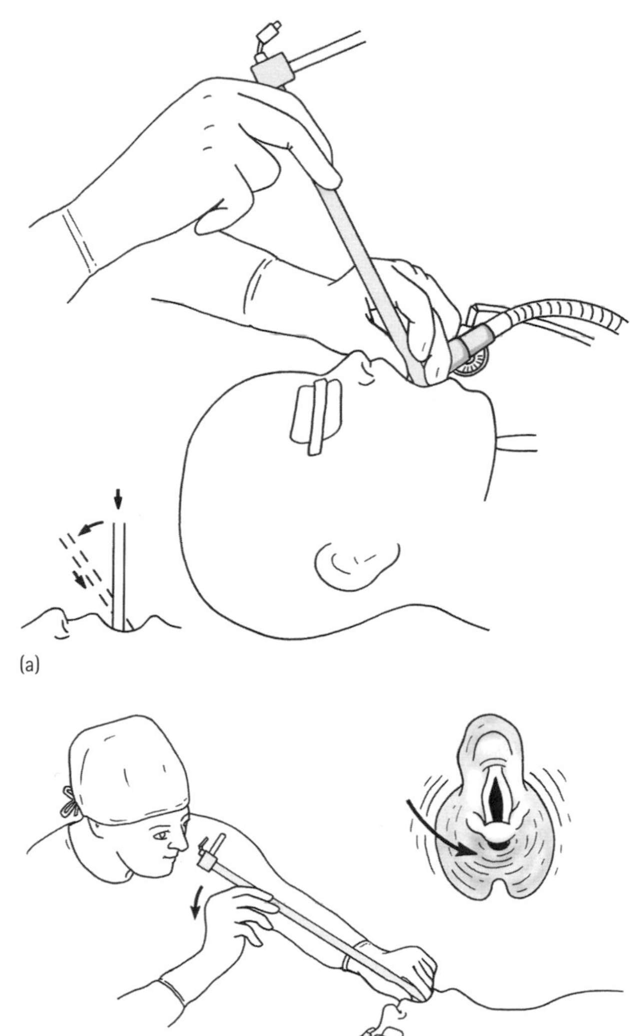

(a)

(b)

Figure 20.2

soft palate through the oral cavity into the pharynx, keeping to the midline, using the uvula as a landmark. During this phase the esophagoscope is moved from a vertical to a near-horizontal position, ensuring that the fulcrum is on the surgeon's left thumb and not on the patient's teeth. The lip on the distal end of the esophagoscope is used to elevate the larynx and reveal the cricopharyngeus muscle, which marks the beginning of the esophagus. Alternatively, at the level of the epiglottis, the esophagoscope is passed to one side to enter the piriform fossa and then returned to the midline to see the cricopharyngeus. (**See Figure 20.2**)

Once the upper esophagus is entered, the endoscope is gently advanced using the thumb and middle finger of the left hand to protect the patient's teeth. The lumen must be visible at all times while the instrument is advanced to minimize the risk of perforation. In the thorax, the esophageal lumen opens and closes with respiration. The thumb of the left hand is used to elevate the distal end of the esophagoscope to obtain a clearer view and to avoid damage to the posterior wall of the esophagus by the leading edge of the instrument. Further extension of the patient's neck may be necessary. Secretions must be cleared regularly by suction. During progression down the esophagus, the pulsating indentation of the aorta is seen anteriorly, followed by the indentations of the left main bronchus and then the heart. It may be necessary for an assistant to raise the lower thoracic spine to enable the distal esophagus to be seen clearly.

At the esophago-gastric junction, the lower esophageal sphincter may be closed. This will yield to gentle pressure, allowing the esophagoscope to enter the stomach. The distance of the esophago-gastric junction from the incisor teeth should be noted. The transition from the flat, pale-pink esophageal mucosa to the velvet-like bright-pink/red gastric mucosa should be apparent.

Careful examination of the esophagus as the esophagoscope is withdrawn is essential, because lesions or foreign bodies may have been missed during insertion. The esophagoscope is removed slowly, keeping it in the midline all the way, protecting the teeth and adjusting the degree of neck extension as necessary.

POSTOPERATIVE CARE

Following esophagoscopy, fluids are allowed as soon as the child is awake, followed by free access to food provided there are no clinical contraindications. A mild analgesic may be required if the throat is particularly painful, but this is unusual.

PROBLEMS, PITFALLS AND SOLUTIONS

- Often the cricopharyngeus is contracted when viewed down the esophagoscope. The endoscope cannot be advanced into the upper esophagus until the sphincter relaxes and the lumen can be seen. Usually the cricopharyngeus will relax in response to gentle pressure from the esophagoscope. It may be necessary to extend the neck further during this phase. If the cricopharyngeus repeatedly fails to relax, the lumen may be identified by first passing a bougie or catheter into the esophagus and then passing the esophagoscope over the bougie.
- In infants, a 3 mm rigid bronchoscope may be preferred for esophagoscopy. This instrument is narrower and the distal end not widened, making it easier to pass through the relatively narrow pharynx into the esophagus. However, the bronchoscope may not be sufficiently long to reach the esophago-gastric junction.
- The esophageal lumen must remain in view at all times and this can be difficult, particularly if the esophagus is diseased. Altering the degree of neck extension and gently raising or lowering the patient's shoulders may help. If these measures fail, a soft catheter may be passed down the endoscope and used to find the direction of the lumen.
- Careless handling of the esophagoscope risks damage to the esophageal wall. Minor bleeding may be encountered when dilating an esophageal stricture or negotiating an esophagus damaged by caustic injury or peptic ulceration. Irrigation with ice-cold saline injected down the esophagoscope with a syringe and then aspirated by suction may clear the view. If a satisfactory view of the lumen cannot be obtained, the procedure should be terminated.

COMPLICATIONS

Esophageal perforation

The risk of perforation during esophagoscopy is greatly reduced when the procedure is performed in a controlled manner under general anesthesia. In particular, the lumen must be in view while the instrument is passed, and pressure on the posterior esophageal wall by the advancing end of the esophagoscope must be avoided by lifting the distal end of the instrument anteriorly. A risk still exists when the esophagus has been injured, as with caustic injury or severe reflux esophagitis, or as a result of dilating a tight fibrous stricture.

Evidence of perforation includes supraclavicular crepitus, pleuritic chest pain, fever and tachycardia, progressing, if untreated, to septic shock. A chest X-ray must be obtained and may show air in the neck or mediastinum, which may be widened, or a left pneumothorax. A water-soluble contrast esophagogram is required to confirm and localize the perforation. Management depends on the site and extent of the perforation. A minor perforation confined to the mediastinum may heal with antibiotics and intravenous feeding. Direct repair is required for a major leak and for perforation into the pleural cavity.

Dental damage

The risk of damage to the teeth by the endoscope and of loss of loose teeth has been discussed.

FURTHER READING

Pearson FG, Cooper JD, Deslauriers J et al. (eds), *Esophageal Surgery*, 2nd edn. New York: Churchill Livingstone, 2002.

21

Upper gastrointestinal endoscopy – basic techniques

DAVID C.G. CRABBE

INTRODUCTION

Fiberoptic endoscopy is the standard method for examination of the upper gastrointestinal (GI) tract in infants and children. Reliable endoscopes are now available to permit upper GI endoscopy in children of all ages, from premature infants to adolescents, and complete inspection of the esophagus, stomach and duodenum can be performed rapidly and safely.

Indications

DIAGNOSTIC UPPER GI ENDOSCOPY

- Persistent upper GI symptoms, e.g. pain, dysphagia, hematemesis, vomiting.
- Suspected chemical (caustic) injury.
- Biopsy of the esophagus, stomach or duodenum, e.g. diagnosis of celiac disease from distal duodenal biopsy.

THERAPEUTIC UPPER GI ENDOSCOPY

- Dilatation of esophageal strictures.
- Injection sclerotherapy of esophageal varices.
- Percutaneous endoscopic gastrostomy and percutaneous endoscopic gastro-jejunal tube placement.
- Removal of foreign bodies in the esophagus or displacement of foreign bodies from the esophagus into the stomach.

Contraindications

- Uncorrected hypoxia.
- Uncorrected bleeding diatheses.

EQUIPMENT/INSTRUMENTS

Essential

- Fiberoptic gastroscope(s):
  - premature infant–infant: 5 mm outer diameter (OD) gastroscope,
  - child 1–7 years: 8 mm OD gastroscope,
  - child 7+ to adult: 10 mm OD gastroscope.
- Light source (high-intensity xenon or halogen).
- Suction apparatus and connecting tubing.
- Pulse oximetry, electrocardiogram (ECG) monitoring, oxygen.
- Equipment and skills for endotracheal intubation and mechanical ventilation of the lungs if procedure not performed under general anesthesia.
- Biopsy forceps, guide-wires, brushes etc.
- Mouthguards in a variety of sizes if endoscopy is to be performed under sedation.

Desirable

- Imaging equipment, including camera, television screen and video recorder/printer.
- If advanced interventional work such as stricture dilatation or placement of gastro-jejunal tubes is contemplated, an image intensifier is required and assistance from an experienced radiologist is highly desirable.

- If an esophageal foreign body is suspected, it is prudent to have a range of rigid esophagoscopes and grasping forceps available in case the object cannot be retrieved using the fiberoptic endoscope.

Endoscope controls

The body of the endoscope contains controls to direct the tip of the instrument, insufflate air, wash the lens and aspirate air or fluid. The inner, larger, steering control angles the tip of the instrument upwards/downwards and the smaller, outer, control angles the tip from side to side. These controls can be locked into a fixed position individually with braking levers. Occasionally the controls will need to be locked to facilitate biopsy of a lesion but for general use, and certainly during insertion and withdrawal of the endoscope, the direction controls should be allowed to move freely. The valves for insufflation (proximal) and suction (distal) are operated by the surgeon's index and middle fingers. Control of air insufflation is achieved by occlusion of the valve. The suction valve has two positions. Partial depression applies suction. Complete depression directs a jet of water backwards onto the lens on the endoscope to wash away mucus or debris.

TECHNIQUE

The child should be fasted for 4 hours prior to upper GI endoscopy, whether the procedure is performed under local anesthesia with sedation or under general anesthesia. The presence and position of any loose teeth should be noted. Continuous ECG and oxygen saturation monitoring is essential for both.

General anesthesia offers many advantages for upper GI endoscopy: the anesthetist assumes responsibility for sedation and maintenance of the airway, and recovery from anesthesia is predictable and rapid. Anesthesia for upper GI endoscopy does, however, require endotracheal intubation. The endotracheal tube should be taped in place down the left side of the mouth, leaving the right side for insertion of the endoscope.

When local anesthesia and sedation is being used, the child is sedated with intravenous midazolam 0.05–0.1 mg/kg plus meperidine 1 mg/kg. Mucosal anesthesia is achieved with lidocaine up to a total dose of 3 mg/kg. If upper GI endoscopy is performed under sedation, it is essential to have equipment available and the expertise to intubate the airway and ventilate the child in the event of excessive sedation and hypoxia. Topical anesthesia of the pharynx can be achieved using 10 percent lidocaine spray solution (note high concentration).

If endoscopy is to be performed under sedation, the child should be swaddled tightly in a sheet or blanket to prevent movement of limbs once the procedure starts. The child should be placed on the operating table left side down, head on a small pillow and neck in a neutral position. A mouthguard should be inserted carefully over the upper incisors to prevent bite damage to the endoscope. The endoscopy nurse should stand behind the patient's head to prevent movement, to keep the mouthguard in place and to assist with handling the endoscope. The surgeon stands opposite.

If endoscopy is performed under general anesthesia, the child can be positioned either in the left lateral position or supine on the operating table. The child's eyes should be held closed with adhesive paper tape to prevent corneal abrasion. If the supine position is adopted, the neck is held in a neutral position with a head ring or sandbags on either side. The surgeon stands above the head of the patient with the scrub nurse to his or her left. A mouthguard is not necessary, although the nurse should take care to protect the child's lips from abrasion by the gastroscope. (**See Figure 21.1**)

The body of the gastroscope is held in the surgeon's left hand, using the thumb to operate the control wheels and the index finger to operate the insufflation/suction buttons as necessary. Rotation of the larger control wheel will angle the tip of the gastroscope upwards and downwards and rotation of the small control wheel angles the tip laterally.

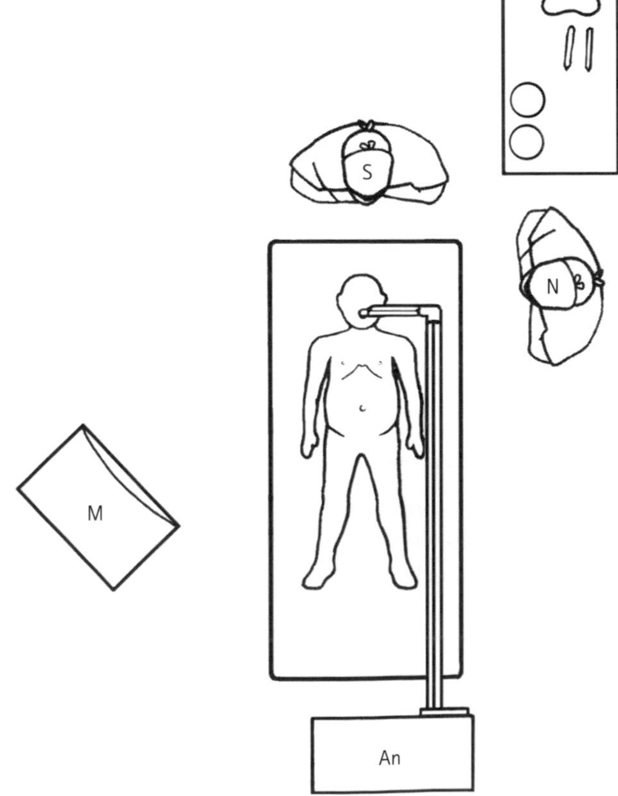

Figure 21.1

The surgeon's right hand guides, advances and rotates the shaft of the gastroscope. (**See Figure 21.2**)

The insufflation and suction controls should be checked prior to insertion of the gastroscope and the distal 10 cm of the instrument lubricated with aqueous gel. The steering control locks should be released so that the tip of the instrument is free to move.

Whether sedation or general anesthesia is employed, upper GI endoscopy involves gentle passage of the instrument down the esophagus into the stomach and duodenum. Whatever the original indication for the endoscopy, it is good practice to perform a complete survey of the upper GI tract. It is down to personal preference whether this starts at the top of the esophagus and ends with the duodenum or whether the endoscope is advanced to the duodenum first and the examination performed from duodenum backwards.

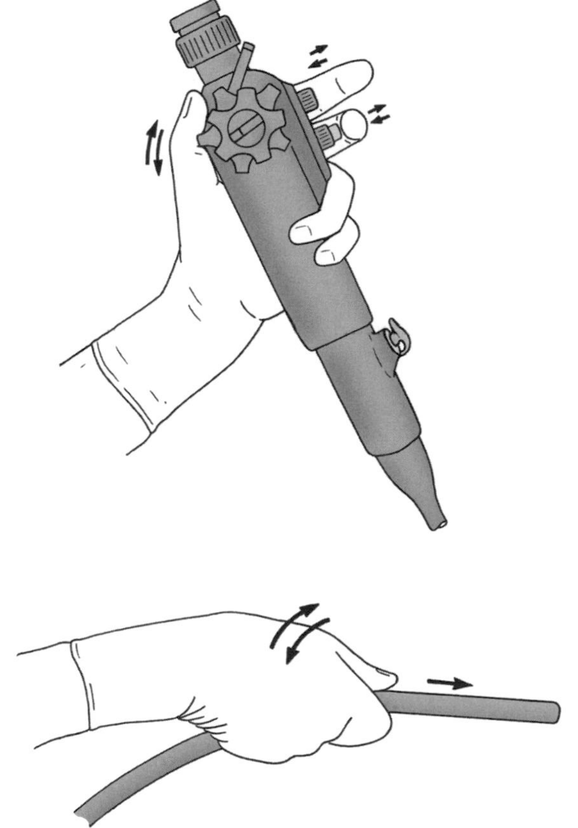

Figure 21.2

The initial phase of the endoscopy involves passage of the endoscope through the pharynx and cricopharyngeus into the upper esophagus. This can be difficult, particularly in a restless child, and a number of techniques have been developed. The safest method involves steering the endoscope through the pharynx into the esophagus under direct vision. The shaft of the gastroscope is held in the right hand about 20 cm from the tip and inserted through the mouthguard. The endoscope is advanced over the back of the tongue, following the midline raphe by direct vision. As the endoscope is advanced, the epiglottis will come into view.

The tip of the gastroscope is then angled slightly to permit the instrument to pass behind the larynx to one side or the other, rather than in the midline. At this point the tip will be at the level of the cricopharyngeus, which may be closed. Air should be insufflated and the endoscope advanced gently through the sphincter. In the sedated child this should be co-ordinated with spontaneous swallowing movements. In the anesthetized child the anesthetist can lift the mandible forwards, which tends to open the cricopharyngeus and aid passage of the endoscope.

The endoscope should be advanced down the esophagus carefully, visualizing the lumen at every stage. This can be achieved by cautious insufflation of air and direction of the endoscope tip to ensure it remains concentric with the lumen. The lumen of the esophagus distends as air is insufflated and this should provide a clear view ahead. If the lumen fails to distend, the possibility of a stricture is immediately raised. The endoscope should not be advanced blindly, especially if resistance is encountered. If the way forward is not immediately apparent, the endoscope should be withdrawn slightly and a little air insufflated to identify the lumen. The esophago-gastric junction is visible clearly as an irregular junction between the pale esophageal mucosa and the darker gastric mucosa (the Z-line). This distance should be recorded from the measurements on the endoscope – about 20 cm in an infant. (**See Figure 21.3**)

Abnormalities in the esophagus are commonly encountered during pediatric endoscopy. The presence of esophagitis should be noted and the proximal extent (distance) recorded. The earliest signs of esophagitis are mucosal edema and congestion. Ulceration, contact bleeding and inflammatory exudate will be apparent in more severe cases and ultimately a stricture may develop. If endoscopy is performed after repair of esophageal atresia, the site of the anastomosis will be visible in the mid-esophagus at around 15 cm from the teeth. Esophageal varices are usually obvious as 'varicose

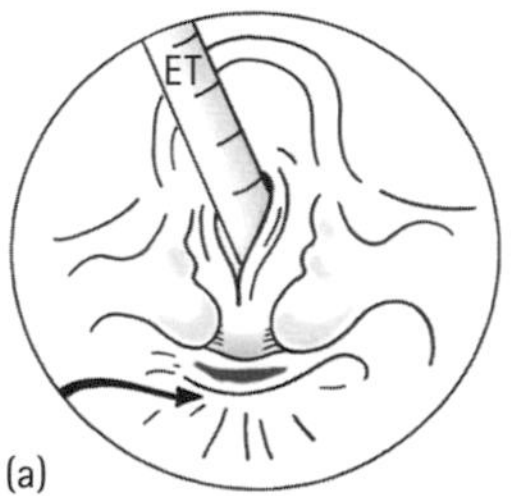

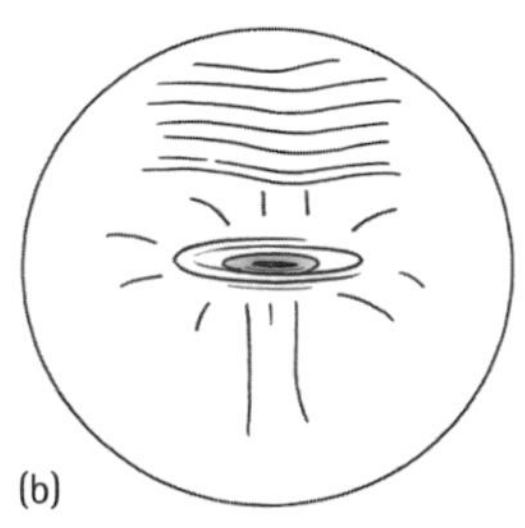

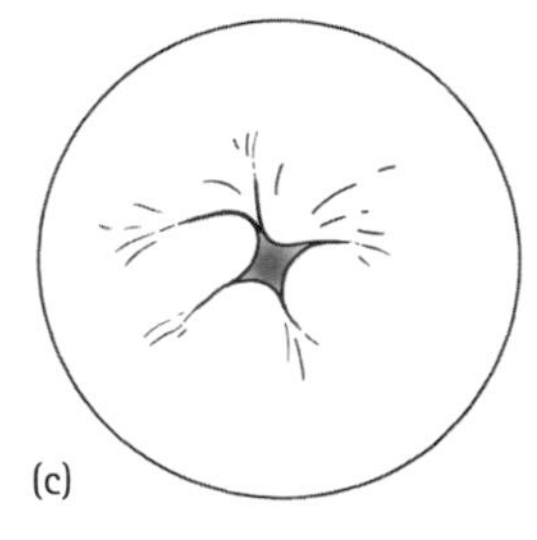

Figure 21.3 *(a) View of the epiglottis; (b) cricopharyngeus sphincter; (c) esophago-gastric junction.*

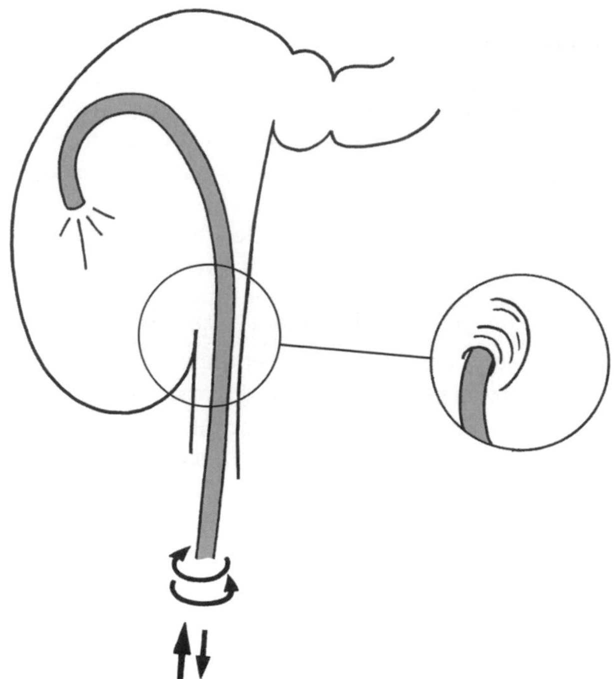

Figure 21.4

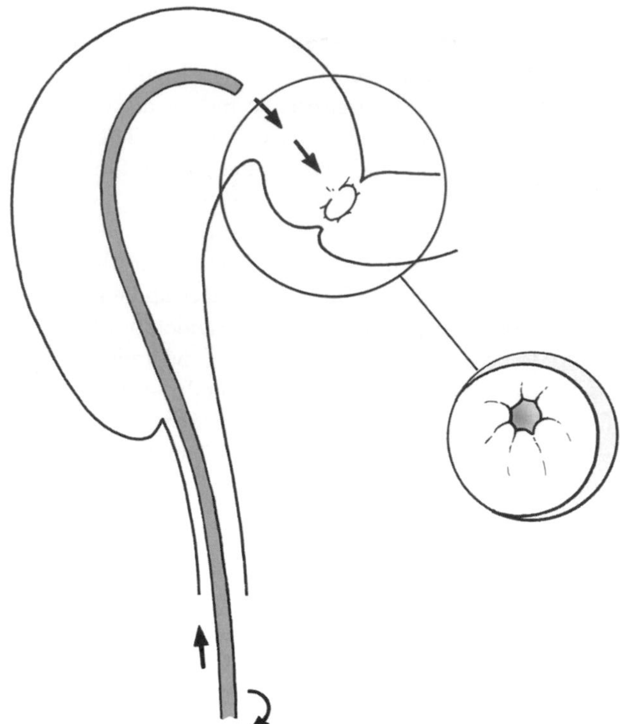

Figure 21.5

veins' in the lower esophagus, just above the Z-line. The esophagus appears dilated in achalasia and often contains food debris. In this condition the endoscope will pass through the cardia without resistance.

As the endoscope is advanced further it will fall into the stomach. The stomach should then be inflated sufficiently to permit visualization of the antrum and pylorus. Over-distension of the stomach may compromise ventilation, particularly in an infant. The mucosa should be examined systematically to include all surfaces. This will necessitate retroflexion of the endoscope to examine the fundus and the esophago-gastric junction from below (the J-maneuver). It is convenient at this point to aspirate any residual fluid in the stomach that pools in the fundus.

The J-maneuver is performed by rotating both direction control wheels to the limit of their range. **(See Figure 21.4)**

The endoscope is straightened and the surgeon must then apply a clockwise torque on its shaft to rotate it through approximately 90°. This will align the endoscope with the long axis of the stomach and permit inspection of the body and antrum of the stomach. **(See Figure 21.5)**

Gastric ulcers are rare in children but, as in adults, are usually found on the incisura angularis. Hyperemia of the antral mucosa is common but there is a poor correlation between macroscopic and microscopic appearances, although a follicular appearance is commonly seen in association with *Helicobacter* infection. Biopsies should be taken from at least three separate points in the antrum. To bring the pylorus into view, the tip of the endoscope is elevated slightly (by anti-clockwise rotation of the large control wheel). Further advancement of the endoscope will be necessary and it is almost inevitable that a loop will form along the greater curvature of the stomach. The pylorus should be observed from within the antrum and the endoscope advanced in time with a convenient wave of peristalsis, which will culminate in opening of the sphincter.

Once the tip of the endoscope is within the duodenal bulb, frequently withdrawing the instrument will result in a paradoxical advancement as the redundant loop along the greater curve of the stomach is taken up.

Examination of the duodenal bulb is frequently difficult because the endoscope tip falls back into the antrum. A thorough examination is important to detect peptic ulcers. Further passage of the endoscope into the second part of the duodenum often requires a combination of rotation, advancement and elevation/depression of the tip with a corkscrew-type motion. Once into the second part of the duodenum, the duodenal papilla will come into view. Further advancement of the endoscope is not usually possible because the redundant loop reforms in the stomach. **(See Figure 21.6)**

As the endoscope is withdrawn at the end of the examination, care should be taken to empty the stomach of air. This will make the postoperative recovery more comfortable for the child.

Biopsies

Endoscopic cup biopsy forceps are available for all the pediatric endoscopes. Cup forceps with a central spike facilitate biopsies from the esophagus and duodenum,

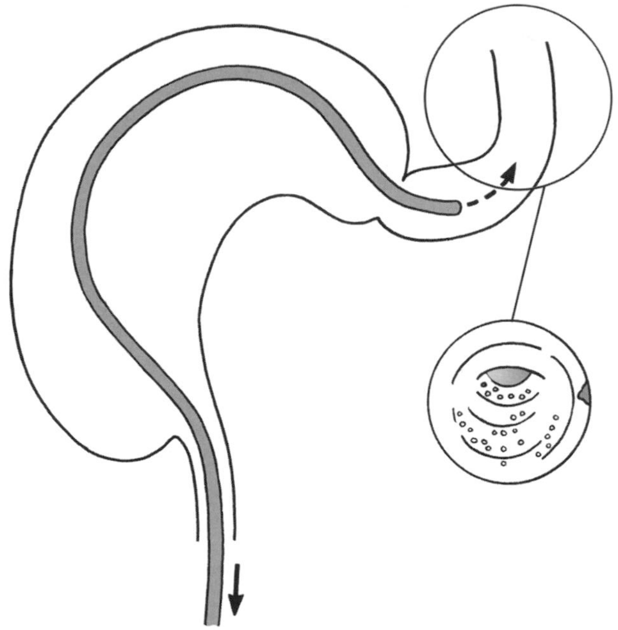

Figure 21.6

where any lesion has to be approached tangentially. Cup forceps without a central spike should be used to biopsy lesions in the stomach, which can be approached face-on. At least three biopsies should be taken from each site. Endoscopic biopsies are small and they should be teased out of the forceps carefully using a hypodermic needle and placed on to filter paper or into a biopsy cassette to prevent loss. The biopsies should be submerged in formalin and the containers labeled carefully, especially if multiple biopsies are taken from the same patient.

If biopsies are taken from the esophagus, the distance above the esophago-gastric junction should be recorded. A common reason for the erroneous diagnosis of Barrett's change is that biopsies are unwittingly taken from the esophago-gastric junction. Biopsies to confirm or exclude *Helicobacter* infection should be taken from at least three separate sites in the gastric antrum. Bedside urease testing kits can be used for rapid diagnosis of *Helicobacter*, but the diagnosis should always be confirmed by histology. Biopsies from the second part of the duodenum can be taken to confirm the diagnosis of celiac disease. It is important that multiple biopsies are taken from as far round the second part of the duodenum as can be reached. These biopsies should be handled with particular care, as the diagnosis of villous architecture can be difficult to determine if the specimens have been traumatized.

POSTOPERATIVE CARE

Postoperative recovery following fiberoptic upper GI endoscopy is usually smooth and uncomplicated. If topical anesthesia of the pharynx is employed, it is important to keep the child fasted for 2 hours postoperatively to prevent aspiration. Oxygen saturation should be monitored in the early postoperative period by pulse oximetry. Endoscopy under sedation or general anesthesia can be performed safely as a day-case procedure provided the child is otherwise fit and well.

PROBLEMS, PITFALLS AND SOLUTIONS

- Hypoxia is a potential complication of upper GI endoscopy performed under sedation. Supplemental oxygen should be administered. Temporary withdrawal of the gastroscope may be necessary.
- Endoscopy performed under sedation in children requires great patience, particularly during the initial insertion of the instrument. Discomfort and distress can be minimized by gentle manipulation of the endoscope and avoiding excessive insufflation of air. Occasionally additional sedation is required and it is usually better to administer further opiate.
- Loss of anatomical bearings: the endoscope should be advanced only if the lumen is clearly visible. If the view is lost, the instrument should be withdrawn until the view is restored, often after further insufflation of air.
- Blurred vision: this is usually due to mucus, food debris or blood fogging the end of the gastroscope. The tip of the instrument can be cleaned by fully depressing the insufflation button, which will direct a jet of water back on the lens of the endoscope. If this is not effective, water or saline can be flushed down the biopsy channel using a 20 mL syringe.
- Food residue in the stomach indicates either that the patient has not been starved properly or that there is gastric outlet obstruction. Attempts to aspirate food residue will block the suction channel. Food debris in the esophagus is an important sign of achalasia. If it is not possible to steer round food debris, the examination should be terminated because there is a significant risk of aspiration. The endoscopy should be rescheduled for another occasion when the child is appropriately fasted. The anesthetist should be aware of the risk of aspiration during emergence from anesthesia and the child recovered in the lateral position with head-down tilt on the operating room table.
- Minor bleeding is common after biopsies are taken. This will invariably cease spontaneously in the absence of a serious coagulopathy. If upper GI endoscopy is performed to identify the cause of acute upper GI bleeding, blood is likely to be present in the stomach or duodenum. Copious irrigation and suction will be necessary, with water or saline injected down the biopsy channel. If a clot is adherent to the wall of the stomach or duodenum, this should be irrigated away

to view the underlying mucosa because a bleeding ulcer with adherent clot that has bled significantly will invariably re-bleed.

COMPLICATIONS

Upper GI endoscopy is a safe procedure in children. Problems are only likely to be encountered with serious underlying medical diseases. Perforation of the upper GI tract during a diagnostic fiberoptic endoscopy is vanishingly rare. The upper esophagus is most vulnerable if a blind intubation is performed. If endoscopy is performed in the presence of a caustic injury or to dilate a stricture, the risk of perforation is considerably increased. If a perforation is suspected, the endoscopy should be abandoned immediately. The perforation should be confirmed with an upper contrast study as soon as possible and appropriate treatment commenced.

FURTHER READING

Cotton PB (ed.). *Practical Gastrointestinal Endoscopy: The Fundamentals.* Oxford: Blackwell Science, 2002.

22

Esophageal dilatation

NIYI ADE-AJAYI, DEREK ROEBUCK AND LEWIS SPITZ

INTRODUCTION

The aim of dilating an esophageal stricture is to improve swallowing. Traditionally this has involved bougienage, but more recently balloon dilatation has become popular. The choice of technique is based on previous individual and institutional experience as well as the equipment available. For long asymmetric strictures, balloon dilatation under radiological control offers a number of advantages. The stricture is traversed by a flexible guide-wire, positioned under fluoroscopic control, which reduces the risk of creating a false passage, and balloon inflation results in a controlled radial dilatation of the stricture. The chief disadvantage of balloon dilatation is the loss of tactile feedback perceived by the surgeon during passage of a bougie. The progress of a balloon dilatation is monitored instead by assessing the pressure exerted on the inflating syringe and fluoroscopic screening of balloon inflation. Widespread use of balloon dilatation is limited by the lack of essential expertise and the relatively high cost of the disposable equipment.

Recurrent stenosis is a problem after any type of esophageal dilatation. Steroids, *Botulinum* toxin and mitomycin have all been injected into esophageal strictures to reduce this tendency, with limited success. Indwelling stents can be used to maintain the esophageal lumen. However, problems with stent migration, erosion and trauma associated with removal limit their widespread use in children. Biodegradable stents are being developed which may have a major impact on the management of esophageal strictures in the future. However, for practical purposes, the majority of strictures in children have to be managed by repeated dilatation unless esophageal replacement is considered.

Indications

CONGENITAL

- Cartilaginous (intramural) esophageal rings.
- Esophageal web.
- Fibromuscular dysplasia.

ACQUIRED

- Gastro-esophageal reflux.
- Caustic, foreign body and drug ingestion.
- Postoperative:
  - anastomotic – following repair or replacement of the esophagus,
  - tight fundoplication.
- Epidermolysis bullosa.
- Achalasia.

Contraindications

- Recent perforation of the esophagus.
- Complete occlusion of the esophagus.
- Previous unsuccessful attempts at dilatation:
  - very recent esophageal perforation should be considered an absolute contraindication.

PREOPERATIVE PREPARATION

A contrast swallow should be performed before dilating an esophageal stricture. The esophagogram will identify the position, extent and caliber of the stricture. Our preference is to perform esophageal dilatation under general anesthetic. The experience is less unpleasant for the child and cooperation is guaranteed, which may reduce the likelihood of complications. Standard pre-anesthetic preparation is mandatory.

Many children undergo repeated esophageal dilatations. It is important to have clearly defined objectives and these include symptomatic improvement, measured increase in esophageal diameter and weight gain. It is also important to ensure that the underlying cause of the stricture is corrected. If the stricture does not respond to repeated dilatations over a period of 3–6 months, esophageal replacement should be considered.

EQUIPMENT – BOUGIENAGE

Essential

- Equipment for rigid esophagoscopy.
- High-intensity light source.
- Lubrication gel.
- Appropriate esophageal dilators.

Several types of dilator are available in sizes suitable for use in children. Eder–Puestow and Savary–Gilliard dilators run over a guide-wire. Follower bougies follow a filiform guide. Tucker's dilators are controlled by a transesophageal string. Gum elastic bougies, or the more modern plastic equivalent, are passed through an esophagoscope under direct vision, or blind down the esophagus. **(See Table 22.1)**

The choice of dilator depends on the age of the patient, the experience of the surgeon and the underlying pathology. Filiforms and followers may be suitable for a baby with an early stricture following repair of esophageal atresia, while Savary–Gilliard or Eder–Puestow dilators may be preferable for an older child with a peptic stricture. Tucker's bougies work well for children with caustic strictures who require repeated dilatations.

Table 22.1 *Examples of esophageal dilators*

Dilator	Features
Chevalier–Jackson	Gum elastic or polythene. Designed for passage through a rigid esophagoscope. Flexibility increased by warming the tips.
Savary-Gilliard	Hollow core polyvinyl chloride.
Eder–Puestow	Graduated metal olive-shaped dilators on solid shaft, which are passed over a guide-wire.
Filiform and followers	Gum elastic or polythene. Fine filiform guides the follower bougie through the stricture.
Tucker's dilators	Sausage-shaped silicone rubber dilators with a loop at either end to tie onto a transesophageal string.

Desirable

- Fiberoptic upper gastrointestinal endoscope.
- Image intensifier and suitable operating table.

TECHNIQUE – BOUGIENAGE

The procedure is performed with the child in the supine position, under general anesthesia with endotracheal intubation and muscle relaxation. The endotracheal tube is secured to the left side of the mouth, leaving the right side free for instrumentation. Antibiotic prophylaxis should be given to infants, immunocompromised children and those at risk of infective endocarditis.

Esophagoscopy should precede the first dilatation. A detailed description of the technique of rigid esophagoscopy is provided in Chapter 20. It is imperative that the precautions to protect the patient's teeth and eyes described in that chapter are followed. The purposes of the esophagoscopy are to identify the upper limit of the stricture, inspect the esophageal mucosa and retrieve any food debris lying above the stricture.

The surgeon stands at the head of the patient with the anesthetist and anesthetic machine to his or her left. The scrub nurse stands to the right side of the patient. The esophagoscope is manipulated with the surgeon's right hand whilst the left thumb and index finger are used to open the mouth and protect the teeth and lips from the endoscope. The rigid esophagoscope is passed under direct vision through the cricopharyngeus into the esophagus, taking care to ensure the lumen is in view at all times.

With the esophagoscope in place, resting on the thumb and index finger or the surgeon's left hand, a bougie of the appropriate size is selected and held close to the distal end by the thumb and index finger of the surgeon's right hand. This 'pen' position allows careful control of the amount of force applied to dilate the stricture. The dilator is advanced through the esophagoscope to the upper level of the stricture, which is then entered under direct vision. With larger bougies, confirmation that the dilator has entered the stomach is evident from inspection and palpation of the abdomen. It is important to appreciate the caliber of the bougie, which first appears tight in the stricture. This dimension should be recorded in the operation note. Passage of sequentially larger bougies provides gradual dilatation of the stricture. As a general rule, rupture of the stricture is very unlikely if dilatation is limited to three sizes of dilator above the initial caliber of the stricture. Useful guides to the size of dilator ultimately required include the size of the patient's thumb and the diameter of the esophagus proximal and distal to the stricture on a contrast swallow, provided the films are not magnified. **(See Figure 22.1)**

It is sometimes necessary to pass a dilator larger than the esophagoscope. The trajectory should be established with a dilator that passes through the endoscope. The esophagoscope is then removed and the larger dilator(s) are passed blind along the same trajectory. Tactile feedback as the dilator passes through the stricture is important and if more than slight resistance is felt, great caution should be exercised passing larger bougies.

This general technique is suitable for gum elastic bougies. If the filiform and follower system is used, the stricture should first be cannulated with the filiform under vision through the esophagoscope. Dilatation is then accomplished by attaching serial followers to the filiform and guiding them down the esophagoscope through the stricture.

The Savary–Gilliard and Eder–Puestow dilators run over a guide-wire. The guide-wire can be passed through the stricture under vision with a rigid esophagoscope or alternatively through the biopsy channel of a fiberoptic endoscope. Confirmation that the end of the guide-wire is in the stomach should be obtained by fluoroscopy unless the stricture is mature, not particularly tight and has been dilated successfully before. Once this position is confirmed, the endoscope is slid backwards off the guide-wire, which has to be grasped at the lips by an assistant as soon as it appears. The dilator is then fed over the guide-wire and down the stricture.

There is considerable debate, and no consensus, about the length of time a dilator should be left in a stricture. In our practice, once the largest dilator to be used is down, the anesthetists prepare to reverse the anesthetic. We leave the dilator in place until immediately prior to extubation and do not routinely carry out endoscopy post-dilatation.

Tucker's technique for esophageal dilatation involves leaving a permanent thread, or string, through the esophagus which is taped to the cheek and the abdominal wall. This involves creating a gastrostomy. A length of heavy silk or linen thread is attached to the tip of a small dilator. The dilator is run through the stricture and retrieved through the gastrostomy. This end of the string is tied securely to the gastrostomy tube. The proximal end of the string is tied to a shirt button and taped to the child's cheek. **(See Figure 22.2)**

Tucker's dilators are sausage-shaped silicon rubber dilators with a loop of string at each end. Dilators are sequentially tied on to one end of the string and pulled through the esophagus. Dilatation is performed under general anesthesia. Dilatation can be performed in an antegrade manner, releasing the string from the cheek and tying on a dilator. The gastrostomy tube is removed and traction applied to the gastric end of the string, pulling the bougie through the esophagus. Dilatation can also be performed in a retrograde manner, reversing the above procedure and tying the bougie on to the gastric end of the string. The size of the gastrostomy limits the size of dilator if retrograde dilatations are performed.

The string can be bought out through a nostril and taped to the cheek, which is more comfortable for the child. This is accomplished easily by passing a fine Tucker's bougie through the nostril and retrieving the end through the mouth with a pair of McGill forceps. The string is tied to the end of the bougie and then pulled through the nose. This procedure has to be reversed and the string retrieved through the mouth before dilatation can begin.

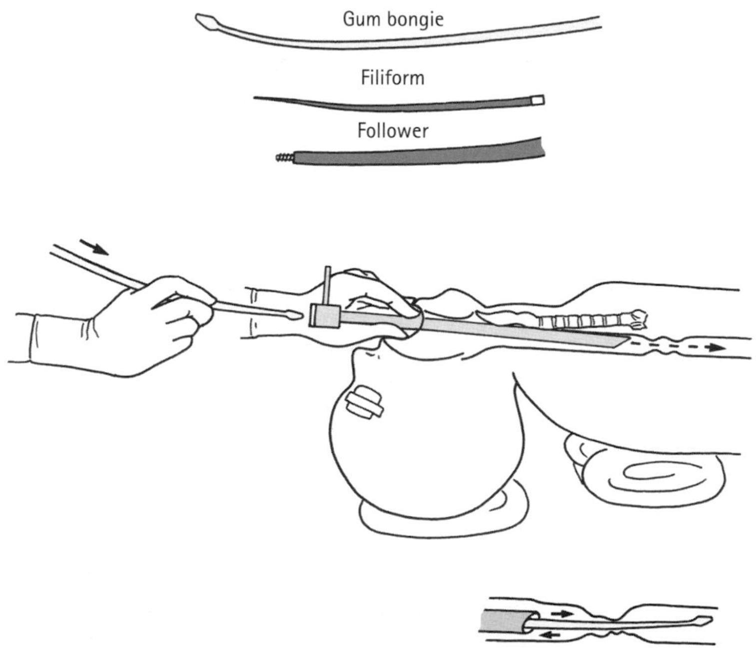

Figure 22.1

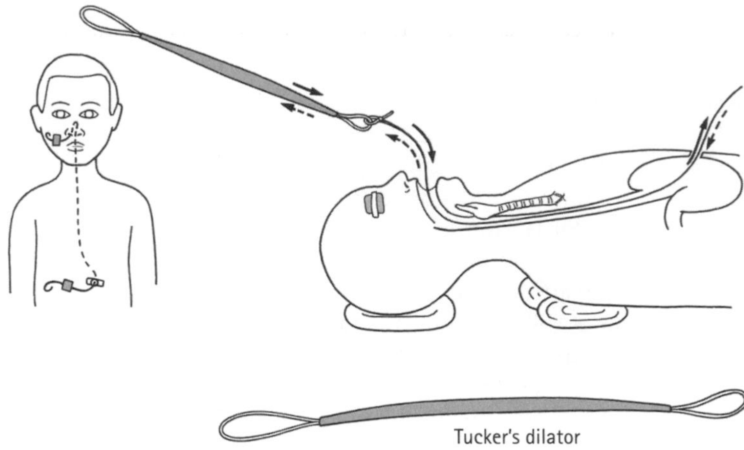

Figure 22.2

EQUIPMENT – BALLOON DILATATION

Essential

- Single plane X-ray screening table with image intensifier.
- Lead body suits and thyroid shields for all theatre staff.
- Radiation film badges for staff regularly involved with radiation exposure.
- 5 Fr curved-tip guiding catheter.
- 0.89 mm (0.035) guide-wire, straight floppy tip.
- Balloon catheters.
- Water-soluble iodinated contrast medium.
- 0.9 percent sodium chloride.
- Laryngoscope.

Desirable

- Biplane screening facility (interventional radiology suite).
- Option for image capture.
- Adjustable radiological table.
- Hydrophilic guide-wires, including 0.46 mm (0.018) diameter.
- Equipment for rigid or flexible esophagoscopy.

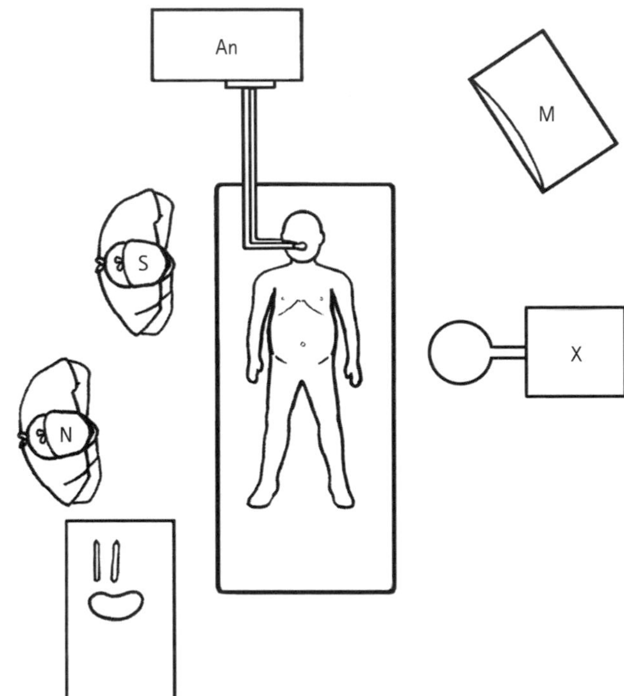

Figure 22.3

TECHNIQUE – BALLOON DILATATION

Balloon dilatation is best performed in the radiology department, where the fluoroscopy equipment is superior. In some circumstances, particularly where anesthetic facilities are not available in radiology, dilatation can be performed in the operating room with a mobile image intensifier. The configuration of most radiology suites means that it is easier for the operator to stand to the right of the patient's head (instead of at the head of the table) in order to see the imaging monitors. The scrub nurse stands to the right of or opposite the surgeon. **(See Figure 22.3)**

The first step is to traverse the stricture with a guide-wire. The guide-wire should be long enough to allow attachment and removal of the balloon dilator whilst maintaining a safe length of wire through the stricture into the stomach. In children, guide-wires 145 cm or 180 cm long and 0.89 mm (0.035) diameter are appropriate. Hydrophilic guide-wires are more expensive than standard wires but they are very smooth and available with very soft tips, which are probably less traumatic. We do not routinely use J-tipped guide-wires. The guide-wire should be moistened with saline prior to use.

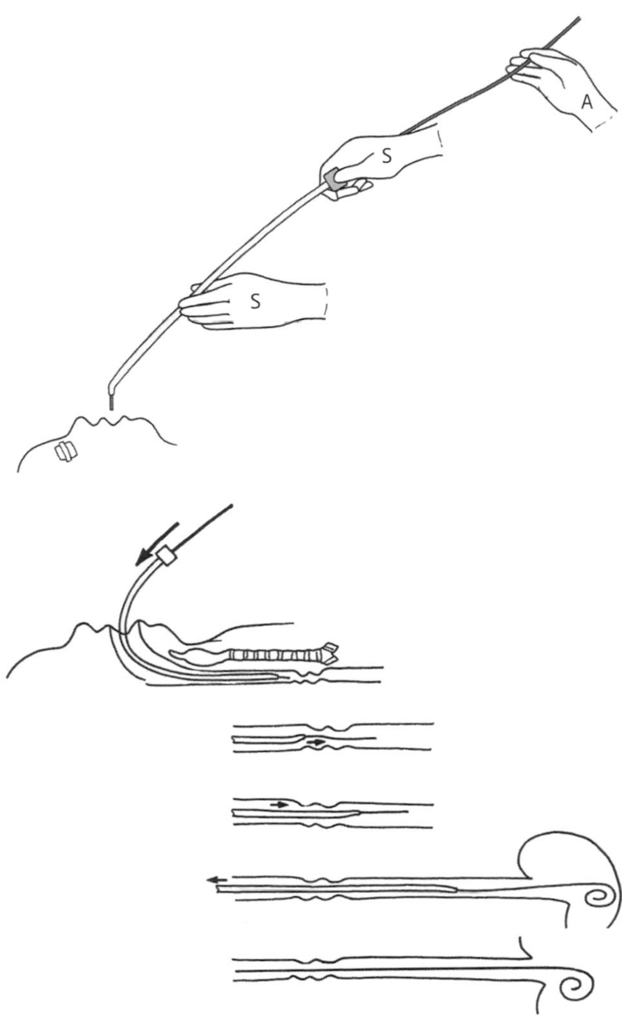

Figure 22.4

The flexible end of the guide-wire is first fed through a 5 Fr curved-tip guiding catheter. This facilitates passage of the guide-wire down the esophagus and through the stricture. The right-handed surgeon holds the tip of the guiding catheter in the left hand while the end of the catheter is held in the right hand. The assistant steadies the rest of the guide-wire. The catheter is introduced through the right side of the mouth into the pharynx. The curve at the tip of the guiding catheter aids steering. The tip of the wire tends to coil up in one of the piriform fossae. To avoid this, the catheter should be directed towards the midline, and this can be done with fluoroscopy in the frontal plane. If difficulty is encountered entering the upper esophagus, the catheter can be inserted under direct vision using a laryngoscope. It is easier to follow the progress of the guide-wire and catheter down the cervical esophagus if the image intensifier C-arm is rotated into the left anterior oblique position, because this projects the wire away from the endotracheal tube. **(See Figure 22.4)**

If a contrast esophagogram has not been performed preoperatively, the guide-wire should be withdrawn at this stage and water-soluble contrast medium injected through the catheter to determine the position and length of the stricture. The guide-wire is then re-inserted. The guiding catheter is advanced until it is in a suitable position to direct the tip of the guide-wire into the mouth of the stricture. Neither the guide-wire nor the catheter should be advanced in the face of resistance. The guide-wire and guiding catheter are then negotiated through the stricture under fluoroscopic control. Once the guide-wire is safely coiled in the stomach, the guiding catheter can be removed.

On occasions, it is impossible to cross an esophageal occlusion with the catheter and guide-wire. The esophagus above the occlusion is usually very dilated and it may be impossible to find the entrance to the stricture to advance the guide-wire. If the child has a gastrostomy, the guide-wire can be inserted from below. Contrast in the stomach will identify the esophago-gastric junction and facilitate crossing of the occlusion from below.

A 260 cm long guide-wire may also be inserted through the stricture under vision using a flexible endoscope. The floppy end of the wire is threaded down the biopsy channel and then directed into the stricture under vision. Subsequent progress is monitored by fluoroscopy. The endoscope is slid back off the guide-wire, which must be grasped by an assistant as it appears at the patient's mouth.

With the guide-wire safely in position, the balloon catheter can be attached. The choice of balloon is based on the age and size of the patient, the underlying disease and the length and diameter of the stricture (as assessed from the contrast swallow). The ultimate aim is to dilate the stricture to the same diameter as the healthy esophagus. This will range from about 8 mm to 18 mm. *It is recommended that dilatation to the final size is achieved in two or more separate procedures in children with tight strictures to reduce the risk of perforation. This is particularly important for caustic strictures.* A larger balloon (up to 30 mm) may be used across the esophago-gastric junction for achalasia. The length of the balloon must be sufficient to ensure a stable position is maintained during inflation (see below).

The position of the balloon on the catheter is indicated by two radio-opaque markers. The catheter should be advanced so that the markers straddle the stricture. Two 5 mL or 10 mL Luer-Lok™ syringes are connected to a three-way tap, which is attached to the side arm of the balloon catheter. The use of small syringes allows for greater inflation pressure than one larger syringe. The balloon is inflated with water-soluble contrast medium diluted 50:50 with water (approximately 150 mg/mL iodine concentration). This permits faster balloon inflation and deflation than full-strength contrast, which is very viscous. If the balloon is too short, or incorrectly centered across the stricture, it will tend to slide proximally or distally as it is inflated. Inflating the balloon gradually, under fluoroscopic control, so that the 'waist' of the stricture lies in the middle of the balloon will prevent this. Balloon inflation syringes are available with an integral pressure gauge. Although these devices may be

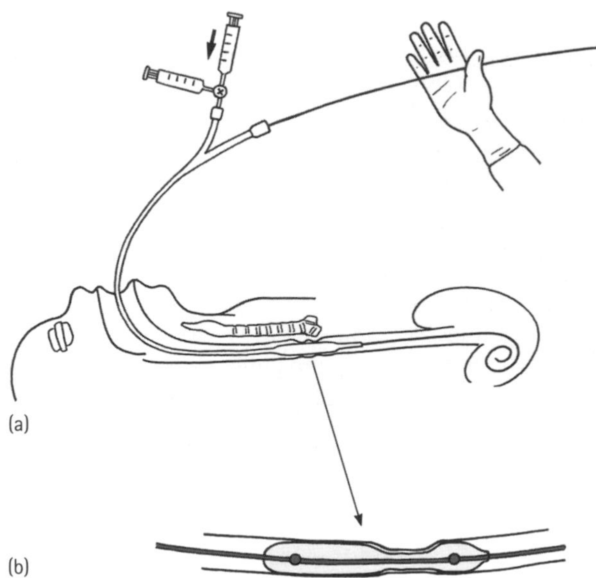

Figure 22.5

useful for very fibrotic strictures, when a high inflation pressure is required, they are expensive and do not have the same 'feel' as hand inflation. If there is more than one stricture, the distal one should be dilated first and then the balloon deflated and withdrawn to dilate the proximal narrowing. **(See Figure 22.5)**

There is no consensus on how long the balloon should be left inflated. Our practice is to maintain inflation for 10–30 seconds. Progress is monitored by fluoroscopy and the amount of pressure the surgeon has to exert on the inflating syringe. Abolition of the waist on the balloon indicates successful dilatation. It is important to ensure there are no air bubbles in the balloon inflation channel, as they reduce this tactile feedback.

The balloon will take longer to deflate than to inflate. It should be deflated completely before withdrawal to reduce mucosal injury. This is particularly important for children with epidermolysis bullosa. It is common to see a small amount of blood on the balloon when it is removed. A completion esophageal contrast study can be performed, either through the lumen of the balloon-carrying catheter or by re-inserting the original guiding catheter over a guide-wire. This will confirm that there has been no esophageal perforation, but is not useful for establishing the effectiveness of the dilatation. Mucosal swelling renders the post-dilatation esophagogram little different from the pre-dilatation images.

Recording the level of the esophageal stricture(s) is important for children who require repeated dilatation. Radiological landmarks on screening which help to gauge the level of the stricture include cervical and thoracic vertebrae, the carina, diaphragm and esophago-gastric junction. The fixed bony landmarks are the most reliable.

POSTOPERATIVE CARE

The length of time the child spends in hospital after dilatation depends on age, diagnosis, tightness of the stricture and ease of dilatation. For infants at risk of postoperative airway obstruction and children who have had a tight stricture dilated for the first time, an overnight hospital stay is prudent. Subsequent dilatations may be carried out on a day-case basis. Unless perforation is suspected, it is generally safe to offer clear fluids by mouth when the child is fully awake and then soft diet as tolerated.

Some children complain of chest or throat pain after dilatation, but this is usually minor and soon settles. More significant pain indicates the need for a chest X-ray and contrast swallow to exclude perforation.

PROBLEMS, PITFALLS AND SOLUTIONS

Esophageal bougienage

- If the proximal esophagus is dilated and the stricture tight, it can be very difficult to find a way into the stricture. A preoperative contrast study is imperative and the opening should be sought under direct vision with an esophagoscope. If the lumen can be found, dilatation with filiforms and followers should be tried. If the lumen cannot be found, retrograde dilatation from the lower esophagus through a gastrostomy should be tried. If the problem persists, Tucker's technique should be used.
- Loss of vision as a result of secretions or blood. Regular suction down the endoscope should keep the lumen clear. The lumen should always be in view as the dilator is passed. The procedure should be abandoned if a good view cannot be obtained.
- Creation of a false passage is dangerous and difficult to recognize. The risks of perforation are high and the procedure should be abandoned.
- If perforation is suspected, dilatation should be abandoned. The diagnosis should be confirmed immediately with a contrast study. Management of a perforation is discussed below.

Balloon dilatation

- Difficulty negotiating the guiding catheter or guide-wire through the pharynx is common. Altering the head position may help. An intubating laryngoscope may be useful to guide the catheter through the cricopharyngeus. Alternatively, the guide-wire can be passed fluoroscopically with the C-arm in a left anterior oblique position.

- A dilated proximal esophagus can make it difficult to find the way into the stricture with the guide-wire. Contrast should be injected through the guiding catheter to define the lumen. Altering the curve of the guide catheter may help. If all else fails, a retrograde approach through a gastrostomy should be tried.
- The risk of creating a false passage is minimized by using a floppy tipped guide-wire and gentle handling.
- Dislodgment of the endotracheal tube during manipulation is well recognized. To prevent this, the anesthetist should have access to and control of the endotracheal tube at all times during the procedure. Inadvertent displacement mandates immediate suspension of the dilatation to allow airway control to be re-established.
- If tracheal occlusion or vagal stimulation with bradycardia occurs, the procedure should be suspended until cardiorespiratory stability is restored.

COMPLICATIONS

Perforation is the most serious complication of esophageal dilatation. The underlying disease process is important and caustic strictures require particular caution. Despite the utmost care, perforation may still occur. The surgeon should be involved in the management of these patients. Immediate management involves resuscitation with attention to airway, breathing and circulation. Intravenous fluids and broad-spectrum antibiotics should be commenced. An urgent contrast study should be arranged to document the site and extent of the perforation. Intercostal chest drainage may be necessary to treat an effusion or a pneumothorax. Definitive treatment of the perforation will depend on the underlying cause of the stricture and the magnitude of the perforation. Conservative treatment is appropriate for the majority of cases. A water-soluble contrast swallow should precede re-introduction of oral fluids. If further dilatation is necessary, this should be deferred for 6–8 weeks unless there are compelling reasons to do otherwise.

FURTHER READING

Earam R, Cunha-Melo JR. Benign oesophageal strictures: historical and technical aspects of dilatation. *British Journal of Surgery* 1981; **68**:829–36.

Pearson FG, Cooper JD, Deslauriers J et al. (eds), *Esophageal Surgery*, 2nd edn. New York: Churchill Livingstone, 2002.

Yeming W, Somme S, Chenren S, Huiming J, Ming Z, Liu DC. Balloon catheter dilatation in children with congenital and acquired esophageal anomalies. *Journal of Pediatric Surgery* 2002; **37**:398–402.

23

Foreign bodies in the upper gastrointestinal tract

JOHN C. CHANDLER AND MICHAEL W.L. GAUDERER

INTRODUCTION

The simple curiosity of young children or the neurologically impaired can lead to the ingestion of foreign bodies. These objects may become lodged at one of any number of locations in the gastrointestinal (GI) tract. The bowel wall then becomes subjected to mechanical, chemical and inflammatory changes, eventually leading to ulceration and possibly perforation.

Anatomical narrowings of the upper GI tract include the cricopharyngeus muscle (upper esophageal sphincter), impingements due to the aortic knob and the left mainstem bronchus, the lower esophageal sphincter, the pylorus and the curves of the duodenum. Pathologic anomalies which may predispose to the lodging of foreign bodies include anastomotic strictures following repair of esophageal atresia, fundoplication, vascular rings, esophageal webs, duplication cysts, cartilaginous rests, achalasia, reflux strictures and duodenal webs. A foreign body impaction may be the first indication of a congenital abnormality. **(See Figure 23.1)**

The patient or caregiver may not be able to relate a history of ingestion. A high index of suspicion should therefore be maintained in the face of otherwise unexplained choking, refusal to eat, vomiting, drooling, wheezing, bloodstained saliva or respiratory distress. It is not uncommon for the patient to carry a misdiagnosis of an upper or lower respiratory tract infection. When such an 'infection' fails to resolve, a foreign body should be considered. Foreign bodies should always be included in the differential diagnosis for such an initial presentation in the pediatric age group.

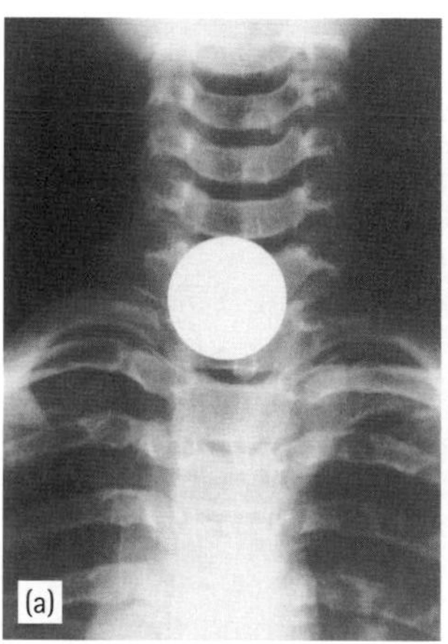

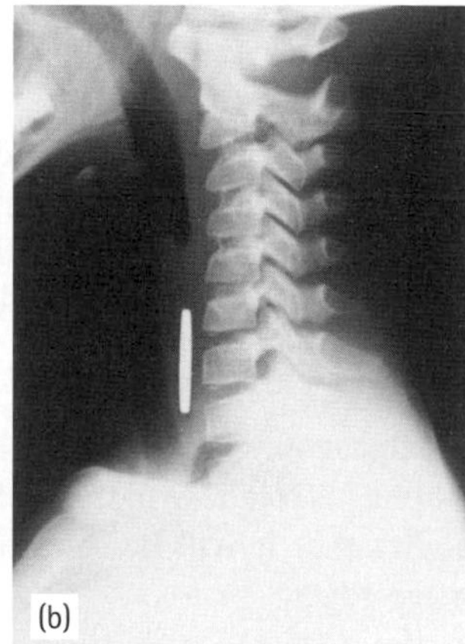

Figure 23.1

Indications

- Foreign bodies in the hypopharynx, esophagus, stomach and proximal small bowel that, due to their size, are unlikely to pass spontaneously or are producing symptoms.
- Sharp or ulcerogenic objects that fail to advance from the stomach or duodenum over 12–24 hours. For such items in the esophagus, observation after localizing by radiograph is unwarranted.
- Smooth, non-obstructing objects lodged in the esophagus for any length of time, in the stomach for

a few days to a month, and in the proximal small bowel for a few hours.

Contraindications

- Clinical indications or radiographic evidence of perforation requiring an open surgical procedure.

Advantages

- Endoscopic techniques provide minimal additional trauma and should not violate the integrity of the GI tract.
- The patient may be discharged shortly after the procedure.

Disadvantages

- The maneuvers for extraction may be technically difficult.
- Perforation may be missed.

Alternative methods

Observation is a valid option under certain conditions. Smooth, round objects that make it to the stomach are very likely to pass through the entire GI tract, and therefore 3–4 weeks should be allowed for this to happen. If the object has not been seen in the stool during that time, a radiograph is obtained.

Glucagon, given as an i.v. bolus, can be used to relax the esophagus to allow passage of food impactions and foreign bodies that it will be safe to pass (coins, objects without sharp edges).

Bougienage, with the intent of pushing the offending object distally, should be used with great caution. Underlying pathology may be missed, and such pathology would increase the inherent risks associated with this maneuver.

Proteolytic enzymes such as papain have been associated with hypernatremia, erosion and esophageal perforation, and cannot be recommended.

EQUIPMENT/INSTRUMENTS

Essential

- Appropriate-size laryngoscopes.
- McGill's forceps.
- Pediatric-sized flexible endoscope.
- Tools for the flexible endoscope:
  - rat-tooth and alligator forceps
  - polypectomy snare
  - Dormier basket
  - retrieval net.
- Assorted rigid esophagoscopes.
- Tools for the rigid endoscope:
  - biopsy forceps
  - alligator forceps
  - Fogarty catheter.

Additional tools

- 'Penny pincher'.
- Catheter with magnet.
- Over-tubes for larger children.

PREOPERATIVE PREPARATION

Although the cricopharyngeus muscle has been identified as the narrowest portion of the entire GI tract, it is certainly *not* true that objects that pass through it will necessarily traverse the entire GI tract. That sphincter may indeed relax enough to permit passage of an object large enough subsequently to become lodged at the level of a non-distensible portion of the esophagus, such as the aortic arch or left main bronchus. In fact, an object is more likely to be located at one of these junctures. Therefore, plain radiographs are recommended for confirmation and localization. Images should include at least two views in order to obtain a three-dimensional conception of the foreign body and to ensure that multiple foreign bodies are not missed in silhouette. Judicious use of enteral contrast has been suggested for radiolucent objects, but we are more inclined to perform endoscopy directly owing to the concern for aspiration and because coating the esophagus and foreign body with the contrast agent may compromise endoscopy.

TECHNIQUE

Laryngoscopy

Objects that are impacted in the hypopharynx may require extraction aided by the use of a laryngoscope and McGill's forceps or other grasping instrument. Positioning for this maneuver is best supine, with the bed height such that the surgeon maintains an erect posture (either standing or sitting). The orientation of a flat object will probably be coronal and the McGill's forceps should be oriented accordingly. **(See Figure 23.2)**

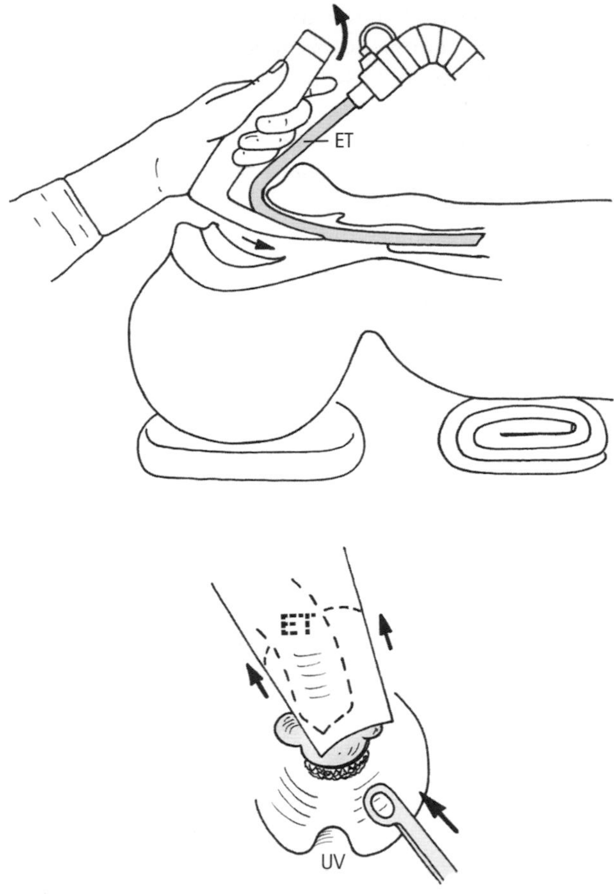

Figure 23.2

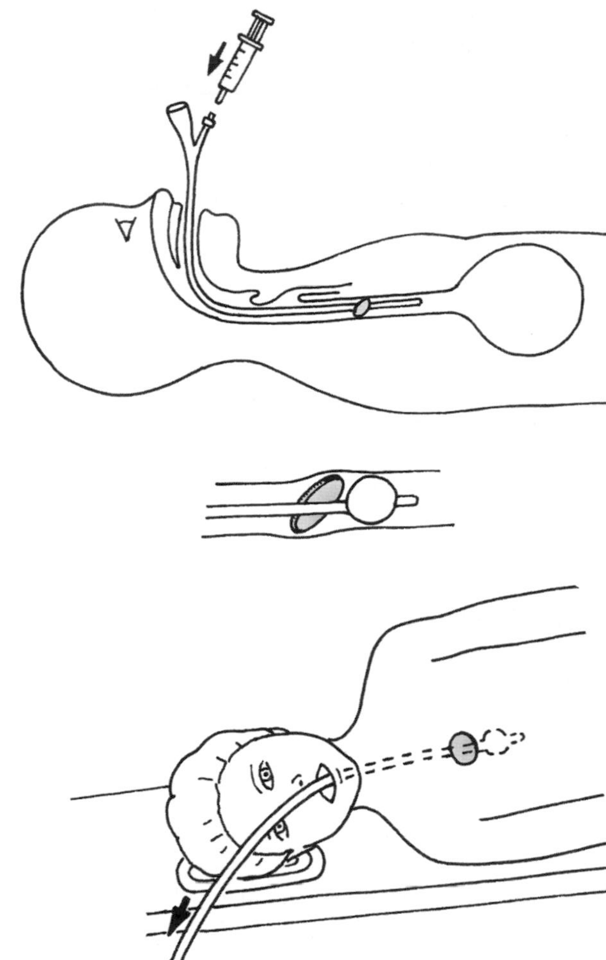

Figure 23.3

Balloon catheter

A number of surgeons and radiologists utilize a balloon catheter (i.e. Foley) with or without fluoroscopic guidance for extraction in conscious patients, especially when the object is a coin (as are the great majority). Caution must be used with this technique, as control of the object is lost as it enters the oropharynx, predisposing to airway occlusion or laryngospasm. Positioning of the balloon distal to the object may be accomplished in any position, but the final stages of extraction should probably be performed with the child in a lateral decubitus or Trendelenburg position. **(See Figure 23.3)**

Penny pincher

This is a minimally invasive technique developed for the extraction of the most common esophageal foreign body – a coin. The penny pincher is an endoscopic grasper placed within a rubber catheter. It is positioned such that the grasper tips reside just within the catheter, and extend outward when deployed. **(See Figure 23.4)**

We find that no sedation is required for this technique. Small children who cannot cooperate may be wrapped in a blanket, papoose-style. At least two assistants should be present to help position the child.

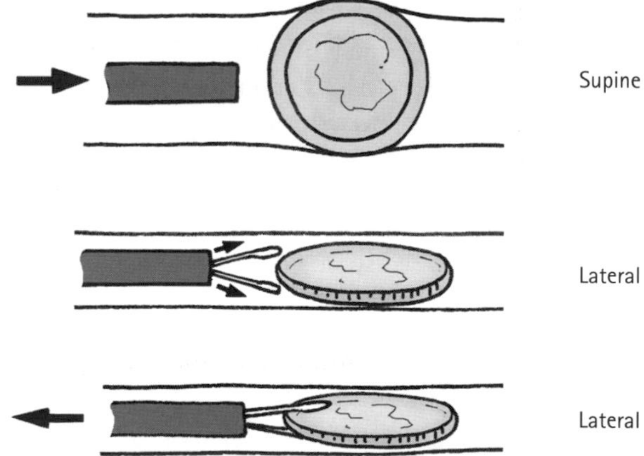

Figure 23.4

The patient is placed supine on a fluoroscopy table. A scout film is taken to re-confirm the location of the coin. A bite block is placed. The penny pincher is inserted into the oropharynx in the closed position, then advanced into the esophagus and positioned just above the coin. The position of the patient should be changed to lateral decubitus at this

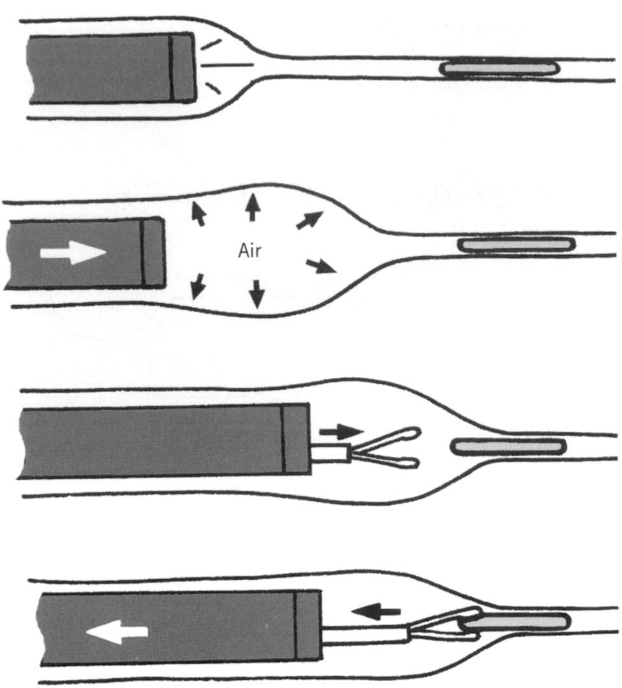

Figure 23.5

point, as the relationships of the prongs to the object are best determined in this position. The coin should be grasped with minimal forward advancement of the device in the open position. The penny pincher is then withdrawn with the coin in tow, under fluoroscopic visualization. Control of the coin must be maintained until it exits the mouth.

Flexible esophagoscopy

Flexible esophagoscopy may be used when it is expected that the object can be retrieved in one or a few maneuvers. General anesthesia is preferred, but not essential. If general anesthesia is not used, moderate sedation is suggested, along with a topical anesthetic for the pharyngeal mucosa (such as benzocaine). **(See Figure 23.5)**

The patient is placed supine or in the lateral decubitus position. The endoscope is inserted into the oropharynx through a bite block with a slight curve to facilitate passage through the hypopharynx. If difficulty passing the scope into the esophagus is encountered, ensure that the child does not have a cuffed endotracheal tube occluding the esophagus (see Chapter 21).

Excessive pressure should never be placed on the endoscope in order to advance it, owing to the risk of perforation. The scope should be able to be advanced, however, with slight pressure, as long as there appears to be mucosa sliding by the lens, indicating advancement. Care should be taken to avoid dislodging the object as the endoscope is advanced. If it is inadvertently advanced into the stomach, it could become harder to extract.

A variety of tools exists to place down the operating channel of the endoscope, allowing a grasp of the object. Once grasped, the entire scope, with the object in tow, can be withdrawn from the esophagus.

It is often wise to re-insert the endoscope to visualize the esophageal mucosa following extraction, especially if the object has been lodged for a considerable time, has sharp edges, or otherwise has the potential to cause significant injury. The stomach can be decompressed at this time.

Flexible endoscopy is the preferred minimally invasive method of foreign body extraction in the stomach and first portion of the small bowel. Items such as marbles and disc batteries can be difficult to grasp with available tools. A basket or positioning the object near the pylorus may be helpful.

Rigid esophagoscopy

General anesthesia is used, due to the need to control the airway during the introduction and manipulation of instruments in the hypopharynx. The patient is positioned supine with a generous shoulder roll permitting hyperextension of the neck. The surgeon sits at the head of the table, which has been rotated 45–90° from the usual orientation. A video tower is positioned at the foot of the table. Although endoscopy can be performed without camera hook-up, visualization by the operating team facilitates other team members performing their roles without the need for constant direction (see Chapter 20).

The rigid esophagoscope is introduced into the hypopharynx following a sweep of the tongue to the side with a laryngoscope (to the left if the surgeon is right-handed and introducing the scope from the right lateral aspect of the mouth, as in endotracheal intubation). Attention must be paid to the teeth, lips and gums to ensure that these structures are not injured. As in flexible endoscopy, the entire lumen may not be visible during advancement, but gentle, continuous pressure may be used for advancement as long as mucosa appears to be sliding by. **(See Figure 23.6)**

Upon visualization of the object, a decision can be made regarding which instrument to use for extraction. The instrument is inserted into the open sheath of the esophagoscope. The object, especially if it has sharp edges, may be partially or wholly drawn into the scope sheath prior to retracting in order to limit further injury.

Once the object has been removed, the scope should be introduced once more to evaluate the extent of any injury. Consideration should be given also to treatment of stricture if present.

POSTOPERATIVE CARE

In the recovery room, the patient may be permitted to drink if there is no respiratory compromise. If drinking is

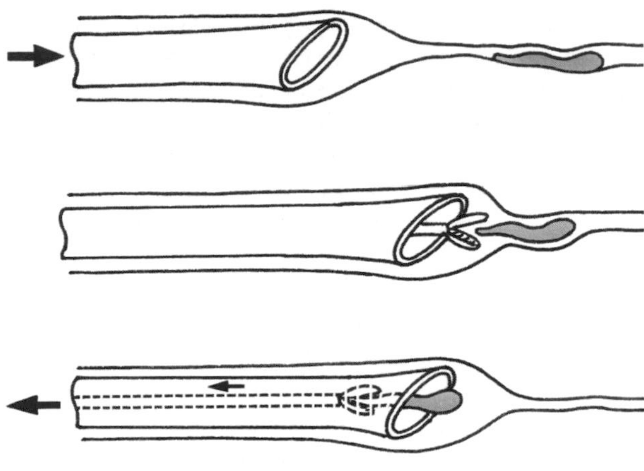

Figure 23.6

tolerated, he or she may be discharged from the recovery room. If it is not tolerated, perforation or other injury should be suspected (see below).

PROBLEMS, PITFALLS AND SOLUTIONS

- The use of these instruments requires knowledge of the equipment, dexterity and, ideally, experience. While attempting extraction maneuvers, the airway must remain patent to permit ventilation by the anesthesiologist while protecting other structures (teeth, lips) from injury. This is facilitated by 'dry runs', especially to identify equipment problems.
- An object just distal to the cricopharyngeus may not be able to be grasped with a flexible scope because, as the scope is withdrawn just enough to allow opening of the forceps placed down the operating channel, the sphincter closes. It is best to use rigid endoscopy in this situation.
- A thickened tracheo-esophageal interface (stripe) with an associated focal narrowing of the trachea has been predictive of failure of Foley balloon catheter extraction. This may be extrapolated to other minimally invasive techniques performed without visualization (e.g. the penny pincher).
- Organic matter and some other objects will often fragment upon grasping. In these cases, use of the rigid scope would be preferred, allowing multiple passes of the extracting instrument. Alternatively, upon fragmentation, the matter can be carefully advanced into the stomach, either by bougienage or with the endoscope.
- Attempts endoscopically to extract bezoars, whether of hair or vegetable matter, are not likely to meet success. Consideration can be given to the use of papain (with the complications mentioned above), but operative intervention is probably required.

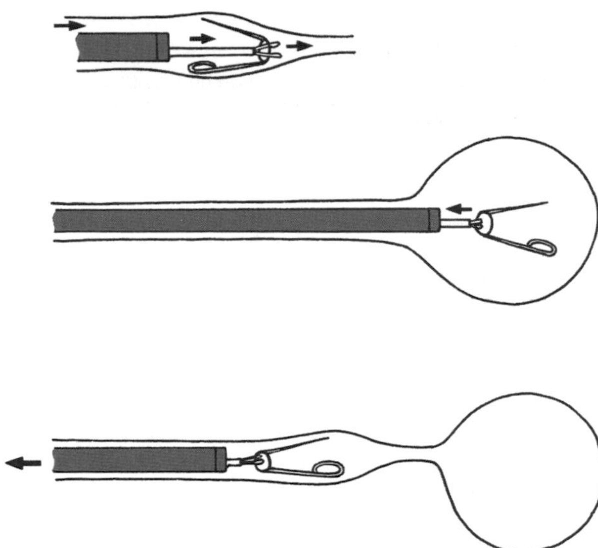

Figure 23.7

- Disc batteries, whether live or expended, cause liquefaction necrosis and, if they become lodged, can give rise to perforation. Batteries in the esophagus should be promptly recovered. A stone retrieval basket or retrieval net is most often successful. Alternatively, a balloon may be placed through the scope. The balloon is passed through the working channel of the endoscope, distal to the foreign body, inflated and then withdrawn to trap the battery between the balloon and the scope. The balloon, battery and endoscope are then removed as a unit. If the battery cannot be directly retrieved from the esophagus, consideration should be given to advancing it into the stomach, where it can usually be retrieved with a basket.
- Although sharp objects that enter the stomach are likely to pass through the GI tract uneventfully, the complication rate can be as high as 35 percent. Therefore, an attempt should be made to extract sharp foreign bodies in the stomach or duodenal sweep. Retrieval forceps or polypectomy snares are good tools to use in this setting. While extracting, orient the object so that the sharp point trails.
- Flexible endoscopy would be the preferred method of extraction of an open safety pin or similar hinged object in the esophagus. Whereas simply removing the object retrogradely may induce more trauma, the hinge or corner may be grasped and advanced to the stomach. Upon withdrawing the endoscope with the object in tow, the object should rotate 180° as it encounters the gastro-esophageal junction, allowing it to be dragged through the esophagus in a retrograde fashion without inducing trauma. **(See Figure 23.7)**
- Large, sharp or irregularly shaped foreign bodies may lodge in the hypopharynx, where they can trigger severe respiratory distress. The object should be extracted

expeditiously. The maneuvers taught in cardiopulmonary resuscitation courses should be considered – Heimlich maneuver or back thrusts in the smaller child. 'Crash' intubation may need to be carried out.

COMPLICATIONS

- The symptoms and signs of perforation should be recognized. Perforation should be suspected in the event of persistent discomfort and the inability to tolerate liquids. Other signs include fever, cervical swelling, erythema, tenderness or crepitus for oropharyngeal or proximal esophageal perforations. If there is any concern, a water-soluble contrast fluoroscopic study should be obtained. Perforation may not be appreciated on endoscopy.

Diagnosis of perforation of the esophagus must be pursued aggressively. Traditional methods called for aggressive operative intervention, with thoracotomy, debridement and irrigation, followed by repair and possible cervical esophagostomy. However, there are studies demonstrating safety of less aggressive, less invasive management with placement of tube thoracotomy, broad spectrum antibiotics and frequent imaging studies.

- Bleeding, especially as the presenting symptom, may be an ominous sign of erosion into the aorta or the pulmonary artery, or of a broncho-esophageal fistula. Maintain a high index of suspicion in such unusual circumstances.
- Aspiration of either the foreign body or pooled secretions is a significant risk, predisposing to laryngospasm, croup or pneumonia. From the initial encounter, vigilance to the child's airway should be maintained.

FURTHER READING

American Society for Gastrointestinal Endoscopy. Complications of upper GI endoscopy. *Gastrointestinal Endoscopy* 2002; **55**(7):784–93.

American Society for Gastrointestinal Endoscopy. Guidelines for the management of ingested foreign bodies. *Gastrointestinal Endoscopy* 2002; **55**(7):802–6.

Truax C. Surgery of the esophagus – removal of foreign bodies. In: *The Mechanics of Surgery*. San Francisco: Norman Publishing, 1899 (historical interest).

24

Esophageal varices

MARK D. STRINGER

INTRODUCTION

Bleeding from esophageal varices is the commonest cause of serious gastrointestinal hemorrhage in children. Esophageal varices develop in response to increased porto-systemic collateral blood flow which is secondary to portal hypertension. Portal hypertension in children may be due to:

- primary venous obstruction at a *prehepatic* (e.g. portal vein obstruction), *intrahepatic* or *posthepatic* (e.g. Budd–Chiari syndrome) level,
- intrinsic liver disease (e.g. cirrhosis, fibrosis), which is associated with increased portal venous flow and vascular resistance,
- rarely, an arterio-portal venous fistula in an unobstructed portal venous system.

Chronic liver disease is the commonest overall cause of portal hypertension, but portal vein occlusion is the most frequent cause of extrahepatic portal hypertension. Patients typically present with hematemesis and/or melena, splenomegaly, or other features of chronic liver disease.

The risk of bleeding does not bear a linear relationship to the portal pressure, but rather to the size of the varix and the thickness and integrity of its wall. Varices are most likely to bleed if they project into the esophageal lumen, if the overlying mucosa is blue and particularly if there are 'red signs' such as cherry-red spots on the varix. **(See Figure 24.1)**

The junction between mucosal and submucosal varices in the lower 2–5 cm of the esophagus is the usual site of bleeding.

Endoscopic treatment of bleeding esophageal varices is a highly effective therapy, associated with a low mortality

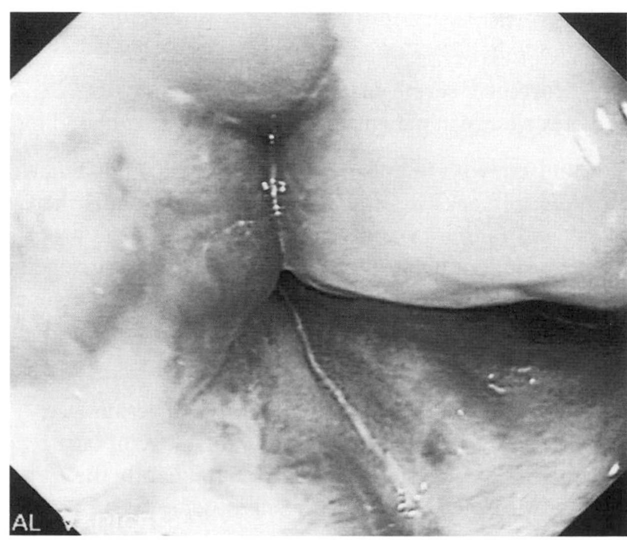

Figure 24.1

from bleeding (approximately 1 percent) and a re-bleeding rate of <10 percent. It is the treatment of choice for the primary management of bleeding esophageal varices in most children. However, primary surgical treatment of extrahepatic portal hypertension (meso-portal bypass) is possible in some patients. Porto-systemic shunting is reserved for children with variceal bleeding unresponsive to sclerotherapy and bleeding from gastrointestinal varices. Devascularization, esophageal transection or direct suture can be performed for the same indication in the non-shuntable child. Symptomatic hypersplenism may require porto-systemic shunting, splenic embolization or splenectomy. Liver transplantation is the procedure of choice for children with complications of portal hypertension secondary to severe underlying liver disease.

The *advantages* of endoscopic methods of treating esophageal varices are that they are minimally invasive, effective and applicable to all age groups. The main *disadvantage* is that endoscopic therapy treats only one manifestation of portal hypertension (albeit a life-threatening one) rather than the underlying cause.

Indications

- Variceal bleeding.
- Prophylaxis against variceal bleeding in a child who is returning to an environment where facilities for treating esophageal varices are inadequate. Primary prophylaxis against bleeding from esophageal varices is controversial and cannot currently be recommended as a routine procedure.

Contraindications

There are few absolute contraindications to the endoscopic treatment of esophageal varices.

- Lack of expertise and facilities.
- Uncorrected severe coagulopathy.
- Latex allergy in patients scheduled for variceal banding.

Children with esophageal varices demand a detailed multidisciplinary assessment with specialist pediatric hepatology and radiology and surgical expertise. The appropriate management of bleeding esophageal varices will depend on the etiology of the portal hypertension and the general condition of the child. Thus the relative contraindications to endoscopic treatment include the following.

- Varices complicating end-stage chronic liver disease: endoscopic therapy can provide valuable temporary control but liver transplantation is frequently the optimum definitive therapy. Sclerotherapy is best avoided immediately prior to transplantation because there is a risk of delayed esophageal perforation.
- Varices secondary to arterio-portal hypertension: treatment of the arterio-portal fistula should be the aim.
- Where an alternative treatment of portal hypertension is deemed more appropriate, e.g. a meso-portal (Rex) bypass, a porto-systemic shunt or excision of a caval web causing hepatic venous outflow obstruction.

EQUIPMENT/INSTRUMENTS

- A fiberoptic endoscope, preferably a videoscope, of suitable caliber for the child and for endoscopic instruments (sclerotherapy needle or variceal ligation equipment). A small and large endoscope to treat all ages is preferable. The author uses a gastrointestinal videoscope (7.7 mm outer diameter, 2.2 mm instrument channel) for injection sclerotherapy in infants and small children, and a gastrointestinal videoscope (10.2 mm outer diameter, 2.8 mm instrument channel) for variceal banding at all ages beyond infancy.
- Injection sclerotherapy needle: a 25 G × 5 mm sclerotherapy needle delivered in a 1.8 mm × 200 cm catheter is suitable for all children.
- A variety of sclerosants can be used, e.g. 5 percent sodium morrhuate, 1 percent polidocanol and bovine thrombin, but most experience has been with 5 percent ethanolamine oleate, which is readily available in most countries. Ethanolamine oleate is supplied in glass ampoules and should be warmed to 37 °C prior to use to facilitate injection.
- Endoscopic variceal ligation device: the 4 or 6 shooter Saeed multi-band ligator is currently used by the author for variceal ligation in children. The device fits an endoscope with a 9.5–13 mm diameter and requires a minimum endoscope channel diameter of 2.8 mm. **(See Figure 24.2)**
- The multi-bander avoids the need to reload and re-insert the endoscope during the application of multiple bands.
- An appropriate-sized pediatric Sengstaken-type tube to provide temporary balloon tamponade in the rare circumstance in which variceal bleeding cannot be controlled endoscopically. A 14 Fr four-lumen pediatric Sengstaken tube is suitable for most children. The tube should be kept in a refrigerator because cooling to 4 °C increases rigidity and facilitates intubation.

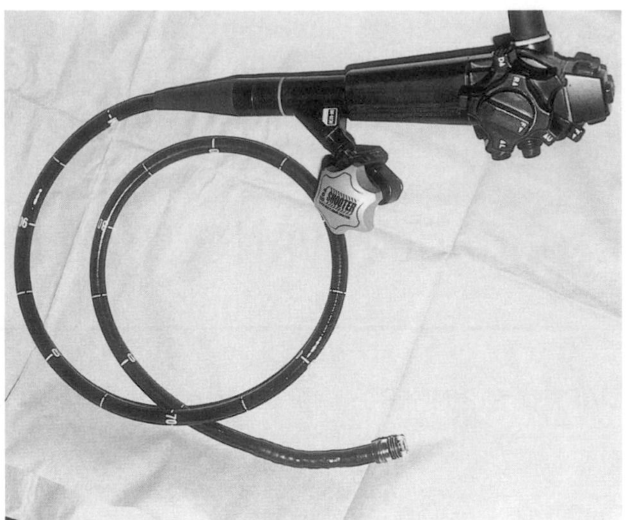

Figure 24.2

The operator should be familiar with the manufacturer's operating instructions for each piece of equipment. There is no longer any place for rigid endoscopes in the management of esophageal varices in children. Overtubes are hazardous and unnecessary.

Box 24.1 Emergency management of bleeding esophageal varices

Resuscitation

- Airway (must be secure).
- Breathing (give O_2 if shocked).
- Circulation: insert two i.v. cannulae (22 G or larger) and commence i.v. fluids (5% dextrose if well perfused, colloid if poorly perfused).

Investigation

- Blood count, coagulation studies, urea, creatinine, electrolytes, liver function tests.
- Blood cultures, cross-match (at least 2 units packed red blood cells).
- Monitor and maintain blood glucose.
- Accurate monitoring of (a) fluid balance, (b) cardiorespiratory status.
- Watch for encephalopathy.

Treatment

- Transfuse packed red cells *slowly*, aiming for Hb ~10 g/dL (avoid over-transfusion).
- Give vitamin K 1–10 mg slowly i.v. and correct coagulopathy with fresh frozen plasma and platelets.
- Start octreotide infusion: bolus dose of 1 μg/kg i.v. (maximum 50 μg) over 5 min followed by an infusion at 1–3 μg/kg per h (maximum 50 μg/h) via dedicated i.v. line; continue infusion until 24 h after bleeding ceases and wean slowly over 24 h.
- Keep nil by mouth initially.
- Give gastric protection: ranitidine 1 mg/kg i.v. t.d.s. and oral sucralfate.
- Start i.v. antibiotics if evidence of sepsis.
- Ensure appropriate-sized pediatric Sengstaken-type tube is available to provide balloon tamponade if necessary.
- Consider prophylaxis against encephalopathy if poor liver function.
- Urgent upper GI endoscopy within 24 h to confirm source of bleeding and to begin treatment of varices by banding or sclerotherapy, if appropriate.

Stringer MD. Pathogenesis and management of esophageal and gastric varices. In: Howard ER, Stringer MD, Colombani PM (eds), *Surgery of the Liver, Bile Ducts and Pancreas in Children*. London: Arnold, 2002.

PREOPERATIVE PREPARATION

Acute variceal bleeding is managed by a combination of general resuscitative measures, cautious blood transfusion, octreotide or vasopressin infusion to reduce splanchnic blood flow and portal venous pressure, optimization of clotting parameters and, rarely, balloon tamponade. Endoscopy is carried out within 24 hours of admission under general anesthesia with endotracheal intubation. **(See Box 24.1)**

In patients readmitted for ongoing endoscopic treatment of esophageal varices, biochemical liver function tests, a full blood count and clotting profile should be checked, and blood grouped and saved prior to the procedure.

TECHNIQUE

Esophageal varices in children may be treated by endoscopic injection sclerotherapy (EIS) or endoscopic variceal ligation (EVL). Injection of sclerosant into the esophageal varix results in venous thrombosis, localized chemical esophagitis and mucosal ulceration. With ligation (also known as banding), the varix is aspirated into a transparent cylinder fitted to the end of the flexible endoscope and an elastic band is released by a trip-wire passing through the biopsy channel. **(See Figure 24.3)**

Strangulation of the varix causes it to thrombose and slough.

Whilst EVL and EIS are similarly effective, EVL offers more rapid eradication with fewer treatment sessions and lower complication rates. Esophageal ulcers caused by banding are more superficial and resolve more quickly than those induced by sclerotherapy and the incidence of esophageal stricture and systemic complications is less. The two techniques may be used in combination. With currently available equipment, the limiting factor for EVL is whether the loaded apparatus can be safely negotiated past the cricopharyngeus. With the ligator fitted, the external diameter of the scope tip is close to 12 mm and often this cannot be utilized safely in small children (<10 kg).

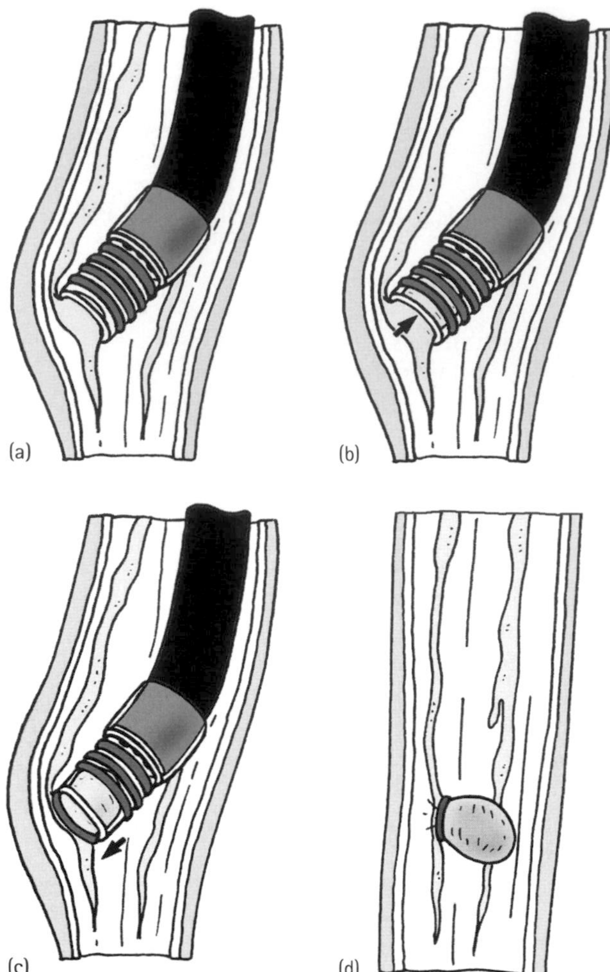

Figure 24.3 *Banding.*

Variceal eradication is usually achieved within two to four sessions of EVL, whereas EIS typically requires five to six injection sessions. Varices may not appear dramatically different during the first few interventions.

In children EIS and EVL are both best performed under general anesthesia with endotracheal intubation. Adequate intravenous access is essential. Cross-matched blood should be available during initial treatments. Antibiotic prophylaxis is recommended for children at risk of bacterial endocarditis, those with ascites, and the immunosuppressed. Endoscopy can be performed with the child positioned supine or in the left lateral position. An experienced endoscopy nurse is an invaluable assistant.

Prior to intubation, the endoscope suction and irrigation are checked, together with the injection/banding equipment. The endoscope is carefully introduced into the upper esophagus, which can be facilitated by gentle extension of the neck. The shaft of the endoscope should be lubricated.

Assessment of esophageal varices should include their location, extent, size, color and the presence of 'red signs'. A grading system can be useful. Large varices may show 'red signs' of recent or impending variceal hemorrhage. These stigmata include 'cherry-red spots' and 'varices on varices'. Care should be taken to avoid excessive air insufflation, which will flatten the varices and minimize their appearance. **(See Box 24.2)**

Box 24.2 Grading of esophageal varices

Grade 1 – varices present but small and collapsible (usually lower 5 cm).
Grade 2 – tortuous veins filling less than one-third of the esophageal lumen.
Grade 3 – tortuous veins filling more than one-third of the esophageal lumen.
Grade 4 – varices with 'red signs' or active bleeding.

'Red signs', e.g. cherry-red spots, varices or varices appearance.

Provided there is no active bleeding, the remainder of the upper gastrointestinal tract is assessed, looking particularly for (a) portal gastropathy characterized by mucosal hyperemia and dilated submucosal veins, (b) discrete fundal varices, (c) duodenal varices, (d) other sources of upper gastrointestinal bleeding such as peptic ulceration, and (e) any coexisting pathology. If there is a large amount of blood in the stomach, repeated suction and water irrigation together with repositioning of the patient should allow inspection of the underlying mucosa.

Endoscopic variceal ligation (banding)

After the initial survey, the endoscope is removed from the patient and the banding device assembled. The multi-band variceal ligator handle is inserted into the accessory channel of the endoscope and the loading catheter is inserted through the handle until it exits the tip of the endoscope. The trigger cord is attached to the hook on the end of the loading catheter, which is then withdrawn up through the endoscope and out through the multi-band ligator handle.

The transparent cylinder with preloaded bands and trigger cord is attached firmly to the end of the flexible fiberoptic gastroscope.

With the endoscope straight, the trigger cord is secured to the handle of the multi-band ligator and wound onto the spool until taut. **(See Figure 24.4)**

The outer aspect of the endoscope and transparent cylinder are lubricated and re-introduced into the esophagus. The selected varix is aspirated into the transparent cylinder by applying suction and, whilst maintaining suction, the band is deployed by rotating the multi-band ligator handle. **(See Figure 24.5)**

Care should be taken to aspirate only the relatively mobile varix and not the deeper esophageal wall. The suction button is released and a little air is insufflated to release the ligated varix. Treatment begins with ligation of the

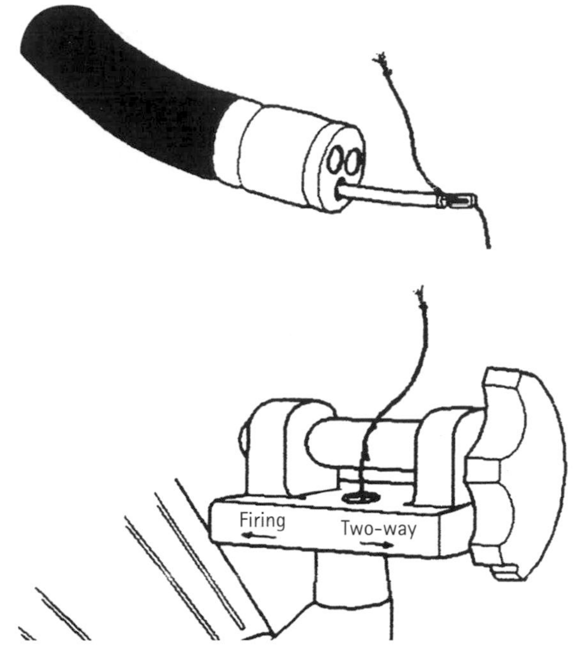

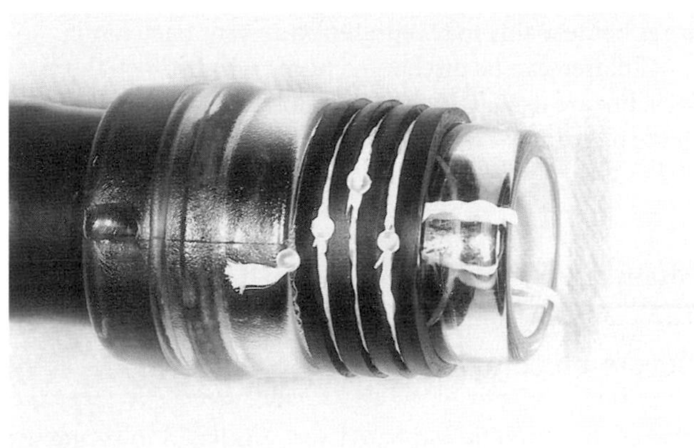

Figure 24.4

most distal varix in the esophagus just above the cardia. Subsequent bands are applied proximally to variceal columns in the lower 5 cm of the esophagus. In younger children, up to four bands are applied to the varices at each session, but up to six can be used in teenagers. The endoscope should be withdrawn gently with the transparent cylinder still attached to its tip. The treatment is repeated after 1–2 weeks and then monthly until the varices have been obliterated. Surveillance endoscopy is performed after 6 months and then at 6–18-monthly intervals.

Endoscopic injection sclerotherapy

After assessment of the varices and the upper gastrointestinal tract, the endoscope is withdrawn into the lower esophagus and the sclerotherapy catheter advanced into the accessory channel of the endoscope. Keeping the needle tip sheathed

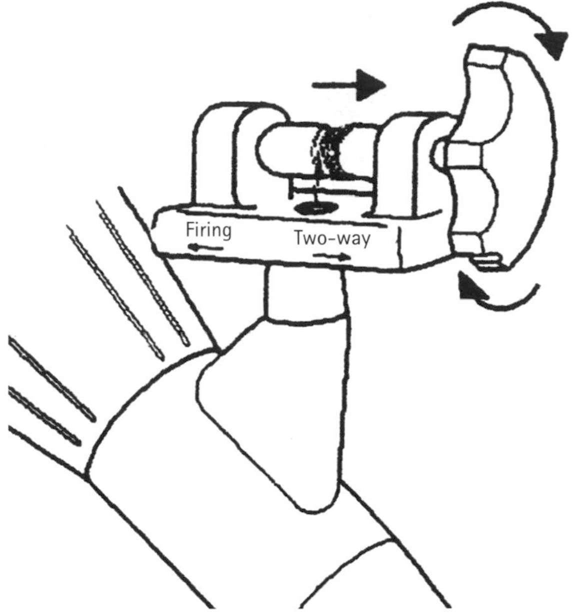

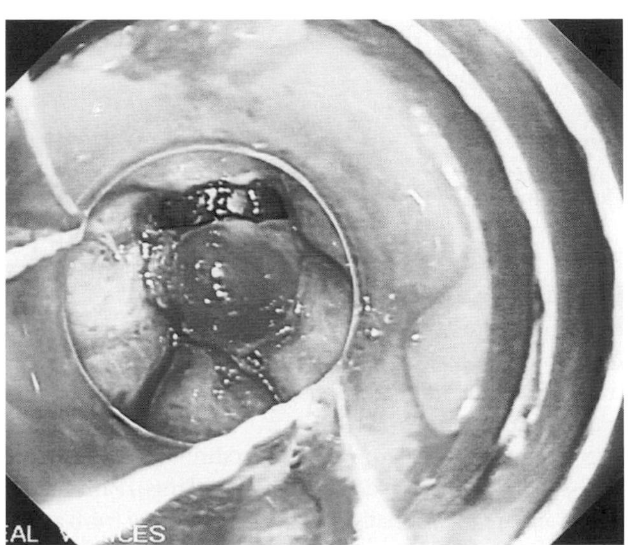

Figure 24.5

in the sclerotherapy catheter, the tip of the catheter is slowly advanced so that it is just visible through the endoscope. The catheter is then primed with sclerosant. The selected varix is aligned with the sclerotherapy catheter tip and the needle is slowly advanced into view. Since advance and withdrawal of the needle (and later the injection of sclerosant) are performed by the endoscopy nurse, a good understanding between the endoscopist and nurse assistant is important. Prior rehearsal of the technique outside the patient can be useful. With the needle projecting from the sclerotherapy catheter, the endoscopist advances the catheter and punctures the varix, which often requires a gentle stab. **(See Figure 24.6)**

The nurse is then instructed to inject the sclerosant and to call out the injected volumes in 0.5 mL aliquots. Successful

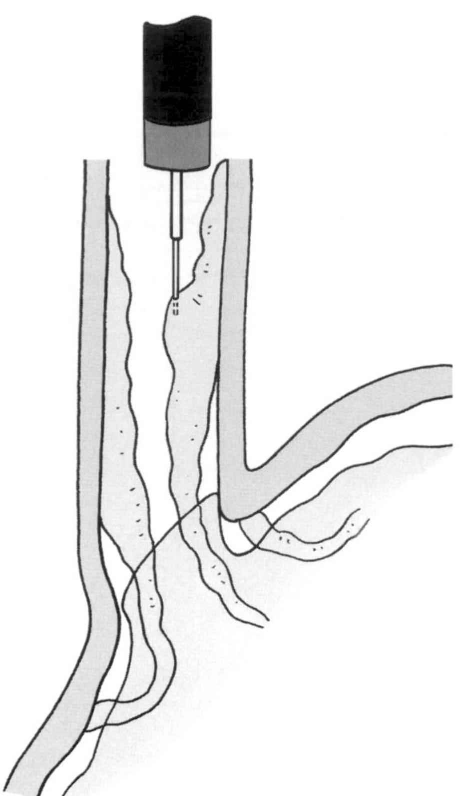

Figure 24.6

injections produce mucosal swelling and blanching. Injections are concentrated on varices at the cardia and in the lower 5 cm of the esophagus and are predominantly intravariceal. Approximately 1–3 mL of sclerosant is injected into each variceal column to a maximum of 10 mL per endoscopy session (maximum 5 mL in infants). Paravariceal injections are occasionally used to stop bleeding from a needle puncture site. Temporary tamponade by passing the endoscope through the cardia and pressing it against the varix can be used to control minor oozing. At the end of the procedure the stomach is aspirated of air and the varices are inspected for hemostasis.

Various sclerosants can be used. The author prefers 5 percent ethanolamine oleate, which is stored in glass ampoules and should be warmed to facilitate injection. Tissue adhesives such as cyanoacrylate have been used as an alternative sclerosant in adults but there is little experience in children. This liquid preparation transforms into a solid after injection into a varix, thereby inducing thrombosis.

Varices are initially injected every 1–2 weeks and then at monthly intervals until sclerosis is complete. Sclerotherapy may need to be deferred for 1 week if significant esophageal mucosal ulceration is present. Endoscopic review is undertaken after 6 months and then annually, but only large recurrent varices require treatment.

POSTOPERATIVE CARE

The patient should be observed regularly with measures of temperature, pulse, blood pressure, pulse oximetry and fluid balance, with quarter-hourly observations for 1 hour, then half-hourly for 2 hours, then hourly for 4 hours etc.

Oral fluids are allowed once the child has recovered from the anesthetic, provided there are no signs of continuing hemorrhage. If the patient remains hemodynamically stable and has tolerated fluids, a soft solid diet can then be given. Oral sucralfate should be administered for 48 hours post-sclerotherapy or banding and intravenous/oral H2-blockers or omeprazole prescribed for 2 weeks to reduce complications from ulceration.

Transient retrosternal discomfort is common after EVL or EIS and usually resolves within 48 hours. A standard dose of oral liquid paracetamol (acetaminophen) can be given. After EIS, fever may occur but typically subsides within 48 hours. A pyrexia >38 °C should be treated with intravenous antibiotics pending the results of blood cultures because this may represent transient bacteremia.

Children can be discharged home within 24–48 hours if well, but are usually observed for longer after treatment for acute bleeding.

PROBLEMS, PITFALLS AND SOLUTIONS

Severe bleeding

The child should be intubated and ventilated to secure the airway and good intravenous access obtained. If the bleeding is not massive, endoscopy should be performed. A combination of suction and irrigation will often expose the dominant bleeding varix, which can then be treated by injection/banding. If the bleeding is rapid, insertion of a Sengstaken-type tube allows temporary control. The uninflated tube is lubricated, introduced into the mouth and passed down into the stomach. This maneuver is facilitated by prior cooling of the tube to 4 °C, which increases its rigidity. The gastric balloon only should be inflated with air in 50 mL increments and its position confirmed radiographically. Bleeding is controlled by moderate traction on the balloon, obtained by taping the tube to the child's cheek or chest. Excessive traction leads to esophageal ulceration or potentially catastrophic balloon displacement. The balloon should be deflated after 12–24 hours, immediately prior to endoscopy. Uncontrolled bleeding from esophageal varices (not responding to at least two sessions of banding or sclerotherapy) in children with reasonable liver function is an indication for surgery (e.g. porto-systemic shunting) or another intervention (e.g. transjugular intrahepatic portosystemic shunt [TIPS]).

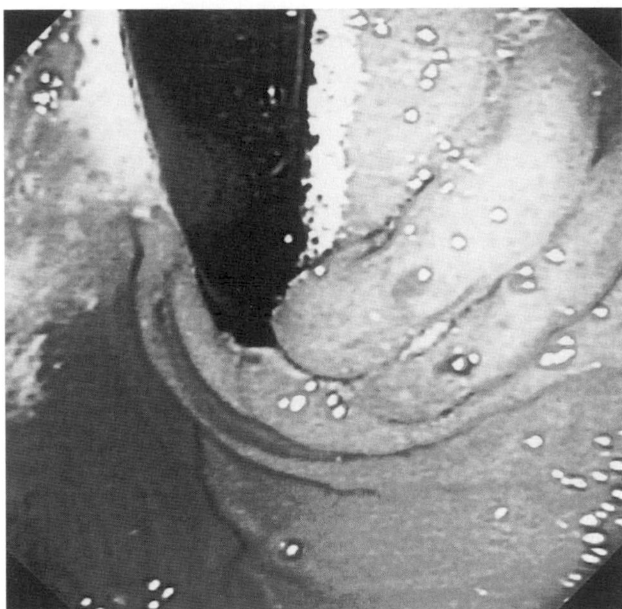

Figure 24.7

Bleeding from fundal varices

Fundal varices contiguous with esophageal varices often respond to endoscopic treatment of the esophageal varices. (**See Figure 24.7**)

Alternative sclerosants, such as bovine thrombin and cyanoacrylate, have been used successfully in adults but have not been formally evaluated in children. Banding of gastric varices is associated with a high re-bleeding rate. Gastric varices are much less likely to respond to endoscopic treatment if they are isolated and not contiguous with esophageal varices. If endoscopic treatment is ineffective or inappropriate, porto-systemic shunting or a local devascularization procedure should be considered in those with satisfactory liver function.

Varices slow to respond to endoscopic treatment

Esophageal varices frequently require several treatment sessions to achieve obliteration. If there is little progress after three or four treatments, the overall treatment strategy should be reconsidered, e.g. those with severe underlying chronic liver disease may require liver transplantation.

Difficulties with variceal banding

- The endoscope is difficult to insert after loading the banding equipment. In small children, make sure that the smallest endoscope compatible with the band ligator is used. Consider the alternative strategy of variceal injection.
- Bleeding after banding. This is uncommon but can usually be controlled by applying a further band to the bleeding point.
- The transparent cylinder becomes dislodged during withdrawal of the endoscope. This should not happen if the multi-band ligator and the endoscope are compatible. If it does, the cylinder can be removed with endoscopic grasping forceps or a Foley catheter through the mouth. The cylinder must never be left in the esophagus. Pushing the cylinder through into the stomach beyond the variceal bands is also potentially hazardous.
- The varices are too small to band safely. If they need treatment, EIS is a better alternative in such cases.

Difficulties with injection sclerotherapy

- Resistance to injection. Check the needle is not blocked. If the needle is patent, this usually means that the injection is too deep and slight withdrawal of the needle corrects the problem.
- Bleeding after needle withdrawal. A small amount of bleeding always occurs and usually stops within minutes. Persistent oozing can often be controlled by a small mucosal injection adjacent to the original puncture site and by temporary tamponade with the shaft of the scope.

Severe esophageal mucosal ulceration

It may be better to defer further endoscopic treatment until this has healed. The patient should be treated intensively with anti-reflux medication including acid suppression.

Esophageal stricture

This complication is now rarely encountered. It responds to simple esophageal dilatation.

COMPLICATIONS

Endoscopic variceal ligation is associated with fewer complications than EIS. Sclerotherapy-related problems in children are much less common than previously reported, probably as a result of using smaller volumes of sclerosant. With both techniques, reported complications have included intercurrent bleeding (usually due to a non-thrombosed varix or an injection ulcer, especially between early treatment sessions), esophageal perforation (very rare), esophageal stricture and recurrent varices.

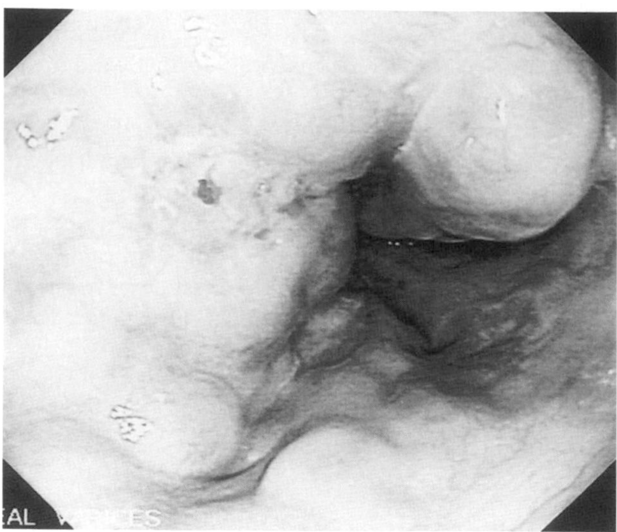

Figure 24.8

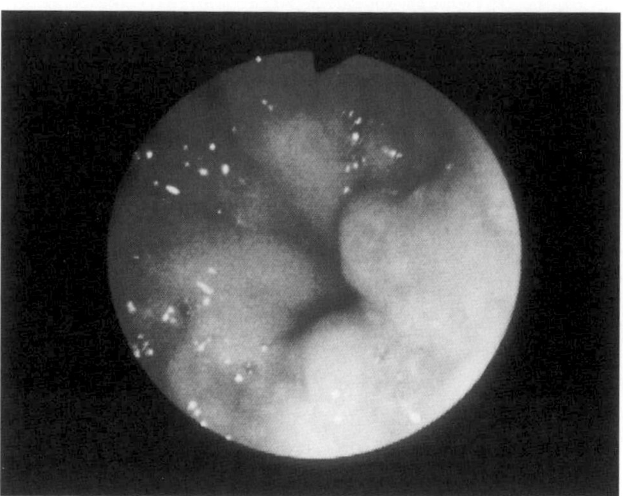

Figure 24.9 *Mucosal tag.*

Sclerotherapy/ligation ulcers

Most sclerotherapy/ligation ulcers are asymptomatic and an inevitable temporary consequence of the treatment. They tend to be deeper after sclerotherapy, particularly when larger volumes of sclerosant are injected. The incidence of sclerotherapy ulcers can be reduced with prophylactic H2-blockers. (**See Figure 24.8**)

Esophageal stricture

An esophageal stricture probably arises from a combination of chemical esophagitis (after EIS), ulceration and acid reflux. After sclerotherapy, the esophageal mucosa heals, leaving residual mucosal tags, and the esophageal wall becomes more rigid. (**See Figure 24.9**)

This may lead to esophageal dysmotility, gastroesophageal reflux and stricture formation. Affected children may experience intermittent dysphagia and heartburn. Dissemination of the injected sclerosant causing a variety of rare distant complications, including peripheral gangrene, paraplegia and renal failure, has been reported. The potential long-term risk of neoplasia after EIS is a concern, but there are few reports of this potential association and systematic studies have so far failed to establish a definite link.

Bleeding after variceal obliteration

This may be due either to other pathology such as peptic ulceration or to recurrent esophageal or gastric varices.

FURTHER READING

Howard ER, Stringer MD, Colombani PM (eds). *Surgery of the Liver, Bile Ducts and Pancreas in Children.* London: Arnold, 2002.

McKiernan PJ, Beath SV, Davison SM. A prospective study of endoscopic esophageal variceal ligation using a multiband ligator. *Journal of Pediatric Gastroenterology and Nutrition* 2002; 34:207–11.

Stringer MD, Howard ER. Long-term outcome after injection sclerotherapy for oesophageal varices in children with extrahepatic portal hypertension. *Gut* 1994; 35:257–9.

25

Percutaneous endoscopic gastrostomy

SPENCER BEASLEY

INTRODUCTION

Gastrostomy is a technique that enables the delivery of enteral nutrition directly into the stomach. It was originally performed as an open procedure. With advances in endoscopy, percutaneous endoscopic gastrostomy (PEG) has become the procedure of choice. Improvements in gastrostomy tube technology mean that current tubes are made of materials that are more durable, softer, easier to use and cause less irritation of the surrounding tissues than their predecessors.

Indications

A gastrostomy may be indicated in any situation in which the oral route is compromised or unavailable for enteral nutrition, and is likely to remain so for an extended period of time. In clinical practice, the indications are varied.

- Inability to swallow adequately:
  - neurologically impaired children.
- Inadequate caloric intake:
  - congenital heart disease with cardiac failure,
  - cystic fibrosis (occasional),
  - children with malignancies or chronic renal failure (occasional).
- Unpalatable diet and medication:
  - eosinophilic colitis,
  - children with chronic disease who are dependent on large quantities of medication (occasional).

Contraindications

There are few contraindications to the placement of a gastrostomy tube without laparotomy or laparoscopy; the choice of minimally invasive technique usually relates to surgical preference and the expertise available. Contraindications include the following.

- Previous laparotomy and adhesions (relative contraindication) – provided the stomach can be opposed to the ventral abdominal wall this need not be of concern.
- In some severely neurologically impaired children or those with marked scoliosis, the stomach cannot be transilluminated endoscopically below the costal margin – in this situation the endoscopic technique should be discontinued and a laparoscopic-assisted gastrostomy (see Chapter 33) or open gastrostomy performed.
- In any other situation in which transabdominal illumination of the stomach and gastric wall indentation cannot be seen clearly.
- Inability to perform endoscopy safely, such as a tight esophageal stricture or non-availability of a gastroscope of appropriate size for an infant.

Advantages over open gastrostomy

There are few controlled studies comparing PEG insertion with the traditional open Stamm gastrostomy. However, it does appear that PEG has a number of advantages over the open technique, including the following.

- It is a short procedure involving no laparotomy incision.
- It is relatively easy to perform, i.e. technically simple.
- There is little postoperative discomfort.
- It can be used immediately after the completion of surgery.
- It involves a shorter hospital stay.
- There is no laparotomy scar, i.e. improved cosmesis.

The frequency of complications reduces with increasing experience. The most serious reported complications of colonic perforation and esophageal injury occurred mainly during the early years of PEG, and are now rare (<3 percent). The procedure can be converted to a laparoscopic one where there is difficulty accessing the stomach.

Disadvantages over open gastrostomy

- It cannot be used in all children (see 'Contraindications'), particularly where close opposition of the stomach to the ventral abdominal wall cannot be achieved with certainty.

EQUIPMENT/INSTRUMENTS

Essential

- Flexible gastroscope of a size appropriate to the size of the infant or child.
- Endoscopic grasping forceps or polypectomy snare.
- Percutaneous endoscopic kit which includes: needle and trocar, scalpel blade, 5 mL syringe for local anesthetic, gastrostomy tube, looped retrieval guide-wire, tube attachments (external flange and feeding ports), scissors.
- 0.25 percent plain Marcain.
- Aqueous lubricating gel.

Choice of gastrostomy device

There are numerous types of PEG tubes available commercially. The choice of tube should be determined by:

- the size of child: a neonate may be well served by a 9–12 G tube, whereas an older child may require a 14–16 G tube;
- the purpose for which it is being placed: a tube of as large a caliber as possible is best for full-volume enteral feeds (improves flow rates and reduces the likelihood of occlusion), whereas one being placed for medication alone can be smaller in caliber.

PREOPERATIVE PREPARATION

Check that all endoscopic equipment and a suitable PEG kit are available. Ensure equipment is also available for laparoscopic guidance or open gastrostomy, in case trocar access to the stomach is unsuccessful.

TECHNIQUE

The procedure is best performed in an operating room under general anesthesia. It is easiest with two surgeons: one to control the gastroscope, the other to place the gastrostomy. A single dose of intravenous flucloxacillin is given at induction to reduce the incidence of postoperative peristomal infection. The patient is in the supine position.

Insertion of gastroscope

The flexible gastroscope is inserted into the stomach and the stomach insufflated. Excessive insufflation should be avoided, as the proximal small bowel also becomes dilated, which pushes the transverse colon over the anterior surface of the stomach and compromises direct percutaneous access to the stomach.

Identification of the anterior gastric wall

The tip of the gastroscope is directed anteriorly to transilluminate the ventral abdominal wall. Bright localized transillumination provides evidence that the stomach is adjacent to the ventral abdominal wall, with no intervening loops of small bowel or transverse colon. Further confirmation of direct apposition is gained from digital pressure at the proposed gastrostomy site where the area of transillumination is brightest; this is seen endoscopically as clear indentation of the anterior wall of the stomach. **(See Figure 25.1)**

Selection of site of gastrostomy

The site of gastrostomy corresponds to the area of brilliant transillumination of the skin and maximal localized indentation as seen on endoscopy. The site chosen should not be right on the costal margin as this may be more uncomfortable for the child and may make any subsequent fundoplication more difficult. It is usually several centimeters to the left of the midline. At this point, 1–2 mL 0.25 percent bupivacaine is injected into the skin, subcutaneous

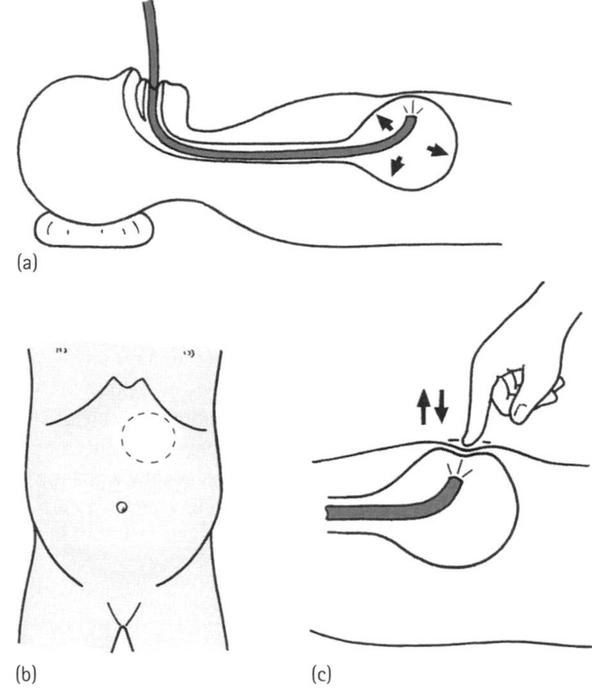

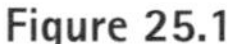

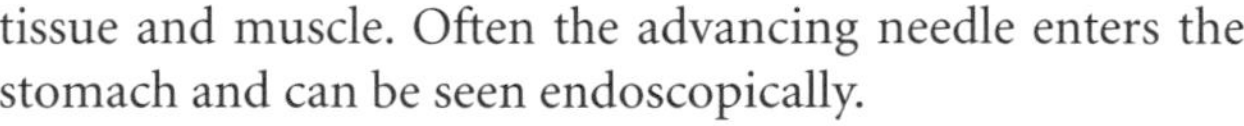

Figure 25.1

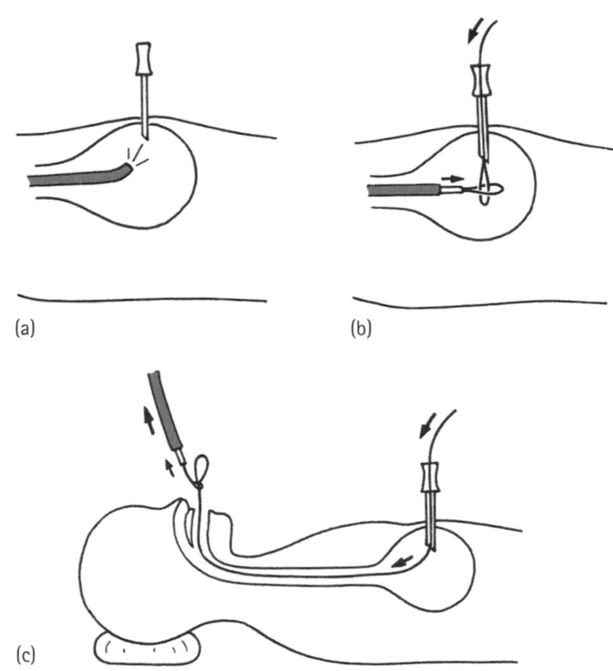

Figure 25.2

tissue and muscle. Often the advancing needle enters the stomach and can be seen endoscopically.

Insertion of needle and trocar

A 5 mm incision is made through the skin with a scalpel. The PEG needle and trocar are introduced through this incision into the stomach with short, firm pushes. Resistance is felt at the level of the anterior rectus sheath and on entering the stomach. Ensure that the needle and trocar are not positioned too close to the pylorus; otherwise, the internal cusp of the PEG tube (once it is inserted) may obstruct the gastric outlet.

On entering the stomach, care is taken to ensure the needle does not damage the tip of the gastroscope or the back wall of the stomach. Once confirmed within the stomach by endoscopy, the needle is removed and the surrounding trocar left in situ.

Retrieval of the wire

A set of endoscopic grasping forceps or a polypectomy snare is introduced down the working port of the gastroscope. The wire (often a plastic loop) of the PEG set is passed through the trocar into the stomach, where it is grasped by the polypectomy snare or endoscopic forceps. Once grasped, the endoscope and the looped wire are withdrawn through the mouth. **(See Figure 25.2)**

Introduction of gastrostomy tube

The tapered end of the gastrostomy tube has a loop that is interlocked with the loop of the guide-wire. The gastrostomy tube is lubricated with aqueous lubricating gel and gently introduced through the mouth by pulling firmly on the abdominal end of the guide-wire. **(See Figure 25.3)**

The tapered end of the tube appears at the abdominal wall site. Traction is continued until the distal flange (gastric retaining flange, cup or crossbar) of the gastrostomy tube has passed through the mouth and esophagus into the stomach, where it can be felt abutting on the abdominal wall. This is achieved with continuous but firm traction.

Fixation of tube

The external flange (usually a disc or crossbar) is slipped over the lubricated tube (use aqueous lubricating gel) until it sits loosely at skin level. The tube is cut at the desired length, but if it is uncertain as to the preferred length, it is better kept long – it can be shortened later, if desired. The feeding port is attached to the tube once the wire extension and tip of the tube have been cut off with scissors.

Check position of internal flange

The gastroscope is re-inserted to check the position of the internal flange against the anterior gastric wall prior to stopping the anesthetic.

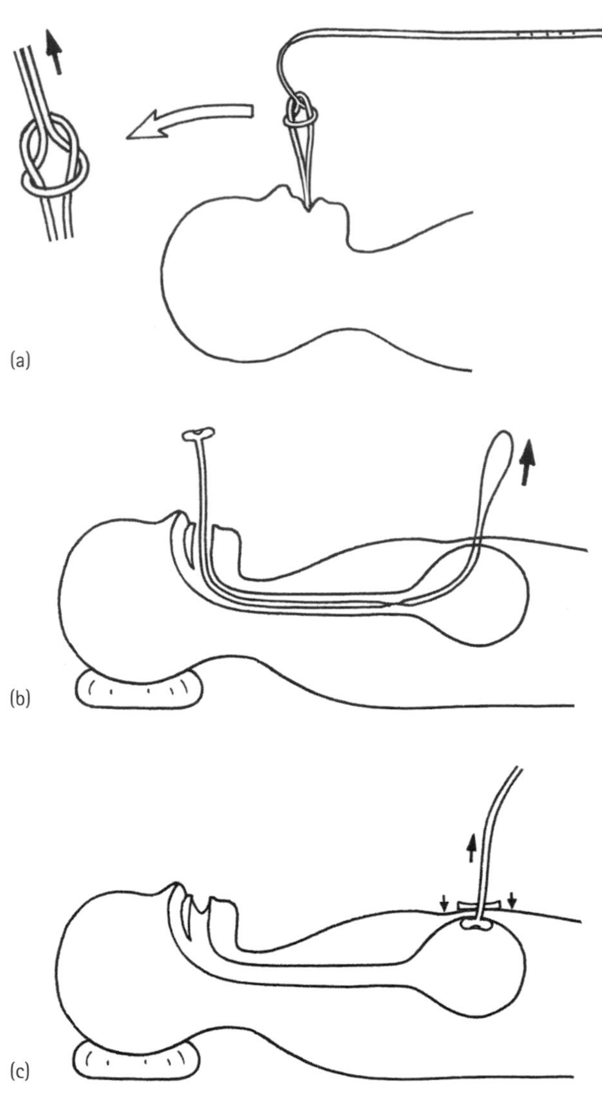

Figure 25.3

POSTOPERATIVE CARE

No specific dressings are required, although a gauze square can be placed beneath the external flange. The external flange should not be applied too tightly to the abdominal wall in the immediate postoperative period. Tube feeds are usually commenced after 12 hours, initially with water and then with other fluids or oral medication. Most children can be discharged within 48 hours. Many gastrostomy tubes last for months or even years. However, they may need to be changed for various reasons (**Table 25.1**).

Elective change of tube (e.g. to a button low-profile gastrostomy tube) should be deferred for at least 3 months after initial gastrostomy placement, although with care most tubes can be replaced after 6 weeks. The procedure can normally be done under sedation, but in some children it is easier and kinder to do it under a short general anesthetic.

Table 25.1 *Reasons for changing a gastrostomy tube*

Problem	Comment
Accidental removal of existing tube	Caused by excessive traction on tube
Occlusion or obstruction of lumen	Caused by failure to flush the tube after use
Deterioration of tube	Due to corrosion – the tube splits and leaks
Fixed flange too tight	Growth of child with improved nutrition increases abdominal wall thickness
Excessive uncontrolled leakage	Sometimes an alternative tube may be helpful
Altered requirements	Circumstances may dictate preference for a different type of tube, usually a change to button low-profile type

Removal of existing tube

Tubes with a fixed internal bar or flange can usually be removed by placing two fingers of one hand on either side of the tube to push downwards while the tube is grasped firmly and pulled out with the other hand. This is best performed under a short general anesthetic. The tube should be held close to its entry point through the skin. If firm pulling fails to remove the tube, it can be cut flush with the skin and the internal component would be expected to be passed per rectum after several days without symptoms. Many clinicians prefer to remove the internal component endoscopically because of the small risk of it becoming impacted at the pylorus or small bowel, particularly in infants or children who have undergone previous abdominal surgery. (**See Figure 25.4**)

Measuring the thickness of the abdominal wall

Most low-profile gastrostomy tubes have a fixed shaft length and the choice of correct tube is determined by the thickness of the abdominal wall. These tubes have a measuring device that consists of a tube shaft marked in centimeters and an inflatable balloon near the tip. The device is lubricated and inserted through the gastrostomy opening. The balloon is inflated when the tip is in the stomach. The device is gently withdrawn until the balloon impacts on the gastric wall, and the abdominal wall thickness is measured on the side of the tube at skin level.

Insertion of new gastrostomy tube though an established track

If the internal retainer on the new tube is a balloon, the tube is simply lubricated and inserted, and the balloon

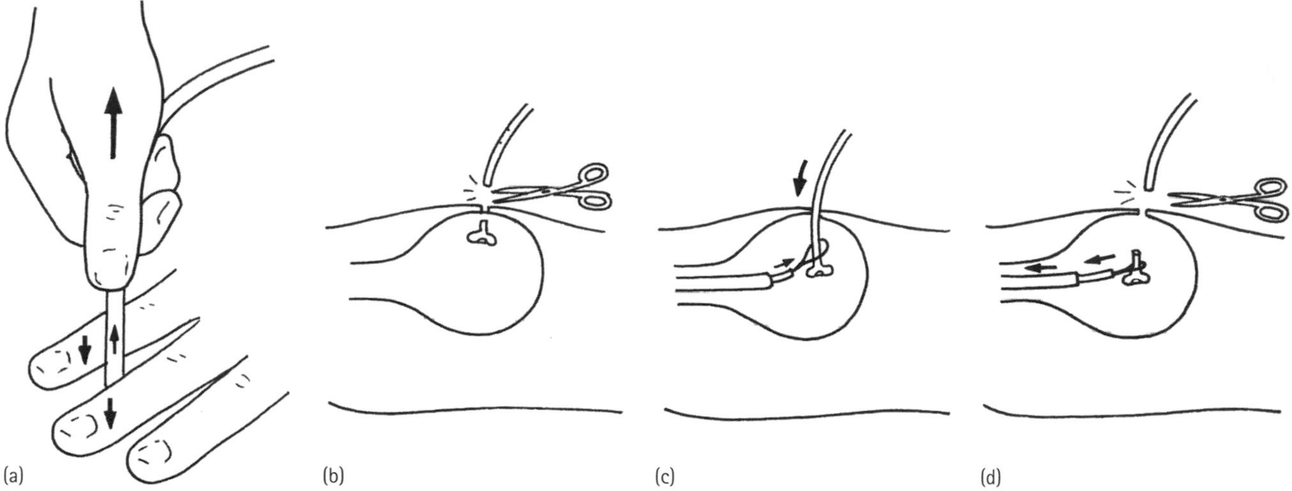

Figure 25.4 *(a) Pulling the gastrostomy out; (b) cutting the flange; (c) and (d) endoscopic removal of gastrostomy.*

inflated. If the external flange is adjustable, it is manipulated down to skin level, but should not be too tight. Other gastrostomy buttons are available with a retaining flange similar in appearance to a de Pezzer catheter. These devices must be inserted with an introducer to straighten the flange, and require moderate force to introduce. Once inside the stomach, the introducer is removed.

PROBLEMS, PITFALLS AND SOLUTIONS

Contact between stomach and ventral abdominal wall uncertain

If transillumination and well-defined indentation cannot be achieved, the procedure should be converted to a laparoscopic-assisted or open one.

Difficulty entering stomach

First check that the stomach is applied to the abdominal wall and good transillumination is present. The needle should be inserted with short, controlled jabs, otherwise it tends to push the stomach away from in front of it. Only insert the needle into the area of illumination. Excessive and prolonged endoscopic insufflation of the stomach will ultimately increase the difficulty entering the stomach because loops of small bowel also become distended with air.

Avoidance of colonic perforation

The transverse colon can lie across the lower part of the stomach, making it vulnerable to laceration during initial needle and trocar insertion. The small bowel can also be injured.

During endoscopic illumination of the abdominal wall, the dark shadow of the colon can sometimes be seen running transversely across the lower third of the illuminated stomach – stay above this line.

The brightness of the gastric illumination and the well-localized indentation of the anterior gastric wall with gentle digital pressure at the intended gastrostomy site provide confirmation that the colon is not between the stomach and abdominal wall.

Avoidance of esophageal injury

Longitudinal injury to the esophagus can occur if a metal guide-wire is grasped too close to its end, such that it is angled proximally and cannot trail in the esophagus during extraction. This complication is rare now that softer, plastic-coated wires are being used.

COMPLICATIONS

Internal flange migration

If the adjustable external flange is too tightly apposed to the skin, pressure from the internal flange or balloon can slowly cause it to erode through the wall of the stomach and cause either local infection (cellulitis, abscess or peritonitis) or catheter extrusion. This problem can be avoided by ensuring that the external flange is not hard up against the skin initially – even a loose flange is secure enough to allow immediate introduction of gastrostomy feeds.

Sometimes the internal flange may enter and obstruct the pylorus, or even advance into the duodenum. This is more likely to happen if the gastrostomy tube is located in the antrum. The chances of this problem occurring can be reduced by positioning the stoma near the most dependent part of the body of the stomach, and by avoiding excessive redundancy in the length of tube between the internal and external flanges. Despite these precautions, prolapse into the pylorus can still occur.

Gastrostomy opening partly closed over or too narrow

If the gastrostomy tube has been accidentally removed and there is delay in replacing it, the stoma will start to close, making replacement of the tube more difficult. If the replacement tube cannot be inserted with ease or safely, the opening can be dilated serially with urethral sounds or a new PEG inserted. All patients should be given a straight tube (e.g. feeding tube), with or without a balloon, usually of the same or smaller caliber, that they can re-insert through the stoma at home until arrangements have been made for a replacement definitive tube to be inserted – this prevents premature closure of the stoma whilst awaiting formal tube replacement.

Excessive granulation tissue around stoma

Granulation tissue around the stoma may become prominent and bleed. This can be controlled by repeated topical application of silver nitrate sticks.

Leakage around the gastrostomy

This is one of the most common and troublesome complications. One of the sequelae of chronic and persistent leakage of gastric acid is peristomal skin excoriation, ulceration and bleeding.

Adjustment of the external flange may help, particularly if it has been too loose, but excessive tightening of the flange is unlikely to be of benefit and may cause skin problems (from pressure) or erosion of the underlying gastric mucosa. Duoderm may help protect the skin.

Replacement of the existing tube with one of larger caliber may help in the short term, but this is rarely a long-term solution.

Decreasing the volume of bolus feeds through the gastrostomy sometimes reduces leakage.

If all these measures fail, the stoma may need re-siting. The old tube can be removed and the stoma allowed to close spontaneously before a new gastrostomy tube is placed endoscopically or laparoscopically. Alternatively, an incision can be made over a new stoma site. A large curved needle is placed through the leaking stoma and back through the new site. The gastrostomy tube follows the tract made by the suture by entering the malfunctioning stoma and exiting through the new one. Once the tube is in place, the leaking stoma is closed extraperitoneally.

Gastro-esophageal reflux

The management of co-existing gastro-esophageal reflux remains unclear and controversial.

The presence of esophagitis on esophageal biopsy at the time of PEG placement has no significant association with the development of clinically significant gastro-esophageal reflux. It is difficult to predict which patients with mild or no symptoms of reflux preoperatively will subsequently develop reflux that requires fundoplication.

On current evidence, it is reasonable to perform a laparoscopic or open fundoplication at the time of gastrostomy in children with symptomatic reflux, esophagitis or recurrent aspiration. When a laparoscopic fundoplication is being performed, the gastrostomy is fashioned laparoscopically at the completion of the fundoplication.

About 10 percent of children require a subsequent fundoplication after gastrostomy alone.

Laparoscopic fundoplication is not compromised by a previous PEG. There will be few, if any, adhesions and the gastrostomy does not have to be disturbed.

FURTHER READING

Beasley SW, Catto-Smith AG, Davidson PM. How to avoid complications during percutaneous endoscopic gastrostomy. *Journal of Pediatric Surgery* 1995; **30**:671–3.

Coughlin JP, Gauderer MWL, Stellato TA. Percutaneous gastrostomy in children under 1 year of age: indications, complications and outcome. *Pediatric Surgery International* 1991; **6**:88–91.

Davidson PM, Catto-Smith AG, Beasley SW. Technique and complications of percutaneous endoscopic gastrostomy in children. *Australian and New Zealand Journal of Surgery* 1995; **65**:194–6.

Grant JP. Comparison of percutaneous endoscopic gastrostomy with Stamm gastrostomy. *Annals of Surgery* 1988; **207**:598–603.

Kimber CP, Beasley SW. Limitations of percutaneous gastrostomy in facilitating enteral nutrition in children: review of shortcomings of a new technique. *Journal of Paediatrics and Child Health* 1999; **35**:427-31.

26

Endoscopic retrograde cholangiopancreatography – basic technique and procedures

THEODORE H. STATHOS

INTRODUCTION

The frequency of diagnosis of children with biliary and/or pancreatic lesions is increasing. Whether this is the result of better recognition of disease processes or because of an increasing predisposition of patients to these diseases is unclear. The effect of treatments such as total parenteral nutrition and the ramifications of neonatal resuscitative techniques that have led to smaller and earlier preterm infants surviving have both been suggested as possible reasons for the apparent increased incidence of these diseases. Whatever the cause, there is a growing need for the skilled use of diagnostic and therapeutic pediatric endoscopic retrograde cholangiopancreatography (ERCP).

Endoscopic retrograde cholangiopancreatography allows the doctor to determine the anatomy of the pancreatic and biliary ductal systems and, in many instances, to resolve the problem therapeutically. In 1968, McCune et al. reported the first successful cannulation of the ampulla of Vater using a straight-viewing gastroscope. In 1976, Waye reported the first pediatric ERCP using a side-viewing duodenoscope. With the development of smaller and better equipment, widespread pediatric ERCP has been possible since the early 1980s. In recent years the technique has become a reality in small children and infants. With the use of specialized equipment and with better clinician training, the risks of complications in the pediatric population are now comparable to those in the adult population. The indications for the procedure are very similar to those for adult patients, with the added challenges associated with congenital lesions of the biliary and pancreatic systems.

Indications

Indications for ERCP can stem from therapeutic needs as well, and arise from both the biliary tract and the pancreatic systems. **(See Table 26.1)**

Contraindications

- Hemodynamically unstable patient.
- Acute pancreatitis.

Table 26.1 *Indications for ERCP*

	Diagnostic	Therapeutic intervention
Biliary	Choledocholithiasis	Stone extraction
	Dilated intrahepatic or extrahepatic ducts	Stone lithotripsy
	Stricture	Sphincterotomy
	Sclerosing cholangitis	Stricture dilatation
	Persistent bile leak	Bridging stent placement
	Congenital abnormalities	Draining stent placement
Pancreatic	Congenital anomalies	Lesser sphincterotomy for divisum
	Pancreatic duct stone	Sphincterotomy, stone extraction
	Pancreatic pseudocyst	Transpapillary drainage
	Recurrent acute or chronic pancreatitis	Bridging stent placement
	Pancreatic mass	Draining stent placement

RELATIVE CONTRAINDICATIONS

- Abnormal duodenal anatomy.
- Abnormal esophageal anatomy.

EQUIPMENT/INSTRUMENTS

The instruments and equipment necessary for a successful ERCP are not extensive and most are used in the diagnostic section of the procedure.

Essential

- Appropriately sized duodenoscope and supportive power source.
- Ampullary cannula.
- Fluoroscopic equipment.
- Contrast dye.
- Monitors for patient status during sedation or anesthesia.
- One well-trained assistant.

The cholangiogram and/or pancreatogram are typically the essential components of a diagnostic ERCP, and are almost always essential in therapeutic ERCP. Consequently, the radiological equipment is an integral component of the procedure.

The child with possible therapeutic needs from the ERCP usually requires the procedure to be performed in the operating room. The ratio of alimentary lumen diameter to endoscope diameter is much smaller in the pediatric patient and increases the risk of airway compromise. C-arm fluoroscopic technology has advanced significantly to the point that image quality rivals that obtainable from the fixed fluoroscopic equipment available. The use of specially built ERCP suites, while luxuriant, is not necessary to accomplish the desired procedure. Fluoroscopic equipment should be selected to ensure minimal radiation exposure to the patient and staff. Modern digital equipment is ideal but not essential. A pediatric radiologist should be available to help interpret any unusual findings.

Optional

- ERCP suite.
- Pediatric radiologist.
- Additional assistant(s).

Therapeutic

- Sphincterotome for the ampulla.
- Balloon dilators in multiple sizes to dilate stricture.
- Sweep balloons in 8.5 mm and 11 mm diameters.
- Lithotripter to fragment stones.
- Basket retrieval device.
- Stents of various sizes and types for both biliary and pancreatic ducts to promote drainage and bypass injured ducts.
- Manometry probe to measure pressure within the ductal system.

The patient is placed in a prone position once sedated or when under general anesthesia. Recent data suggest that the risk of post-procedural pancreatitis is greater with the patient in the supine position compared to the prone position. In one study, 80 children between the ages of 3 months and 19 years, nine of 40 (23 percent) of supine patients and two of 40 (5 percent) of prone patients developed post-procedural pancreatitis. Factors that affect the positioning include the child's pulmonary status, weight, concomitant physical abnormalities, etc. It would seem advisable to use the prone position as the default position unless otherwise indicated by additional confounding variables.

There is a wide variety of contrast dyes available. A water-soluble, non-ionic, low-osmolar formula as well as an iodine-based, ionic, high-osmolar formula are available and have been used successfully in children. An optimal dye concentration has not yet been defined, but typically concentrations between 150 and 300 mg/mL are used. The type of contrast medium does not appear to affect the incidence of post-procedural pancreatitis, but low-osmolar formulae may decrease anaphylactic-type reactions.

An appropriately trained endoscopic assistant is essential to ensure a successful procedure. Since many more adult ERCP cases are done, often an assistant with both adult and pediatric experience is an advantage.

PREOPERATIVE PREPARATION

- Check the full blood count.
- Perform a clotting profile including prothrombin time and partial thrombin time.
- Evaluate serum amylase and lipase.
- Evaluate the anatomy with radiologic studies.
- Choose the necessary anesthesia or sedation.
- Choose an appropriate location for the procedure, suitable for children.
- Select an endoscope appropriate to the size of the child.

As in all procedures, any additional risk factors that the child may have will increase the likelihood of an untoward event; these risks need to be addressed in the preoperative period. The very nature of the condition typically requiring the use of ERCP means that decreased liver function is often encountered. Complete evaluation of red blood cells, white blood cells and platelets as well as coagulation studies and other liver function studies are essential. Patients with diseases of the pancreas and/or pancreatic ducts are at additional risk for postoperative pancreatitis, especially if there is active disease. Therefore measurement of serum pancreatic amylase and lipase as well as assessment of the pancreas using ultrasonography (US), computerized tomography (CT) or magnetic resonance imaging (MRI) are important.

Upper gastrointestinal imaging (barium swallow) and endoscopy help towards identifying anatomic abnormalities which may or may not prove contraindications to the procedure. Ultrasound scan is easy, fast and relatively inexpensive, and can be used to evaluate the ducts and parenchyma of liver and pancreas. A CT scan is best used to evaluate the parenchyma of the liver and pancreas and is of limited use in evaluating the ducts. A specially weighted MRI, magnetic resonance cholangiography (MRC), has recently become available and has been used successfully in children down to the age of 2 years. When carried out by a skilled pediatric radiologist on an appropriate patient, the images of the biliary system obtained in MRC rival those from ERCP. However, MRC images of the pancreatic ducts are less useful, the size of ductal lumen being the limiting factor. Information about the duct system in the preoperative period allows the endoscopist to have the necessary equipment available in the operating room and avoids unnecessary risk.

The patient needs to be assessed to determine the size of the endoscope and the best method of anesthesia. Factors that influence the choice of equipment include the size of the patient's esophagus in relation to the endoscope outside diameter and the presence or absence of esophageal abnormalities – whether congenital, due to age, or of an iatrogenic nature. Many endoscopists have shown that pediatric ERCP is safely done with conscious sedation, using appropriate doses of fentanyl, meperidine, droperidol and/or ketamine, amongst others. General anesthesia is the preferred method for more difficult patients or in cases expected to require additional time and/or more intervention, such as sphincterotomy or stent placement.

Risks

As already mentioned, the risk factors are similar to those seen in adults undergoing ERCP:

- infection
- bleeding
- perforation
- respiratory compromise
- pancreatitis.

The risks of a complication during endoscopy are generally estimated to be about 1:1000. These include infection, bleeding, perforation and respiratory compromise. The use of general anesthesia significantly reduces potential untoward respiratory events. In addition to the possible complications from endoscopy, ERCP has the possible complication of pancreatitis, which occurs in 5–7 percent of diagnostic ERCPs and in 16–19 percent of therapeutic ERCPs.

Consent

Consent for the procedure must contain statistics to provide accurate information to the patient and the patient's family. Additionally, as in all procedures, a general description of the procedure is provided and the probable amount of time needed is typically given. Any possible alternative diagnostic and/or therapeutic procedures need to be discussed to complete the information provided and allow the patient or family to give informed consent.

TECHNIQUE

Diagnostic ERCP

Before the patient is positioned on the procedure table for the ERCP, the endotracheal tube is placed and taped to the right side of the mouth in supine patients (and to the left in prone patients) to allow proper ventilation. A mouthguard is placed in position and the patient is then turned prone, if desired. The duodenoscope is inserted into the mouth and a 60° downward deflexion is placed on the head of the endoscope. Either the esophagus is then blindly intubated or the endoscope can be guided into it using a single finger in the mouth to direct the tip of the endoscope. Rarely, the anesthesiologist will need to place the endoscope in the esophagus for the endoscopist. The endoscope is advanced into the stomach. It is typically slid along the greater curve of the stomach until the pylorus can be seen. Often the endoscope will have to be torqued (twisted) right or left to visualize the pyloric channel. Torquing is preferred to turning the endoscope head so the intubation of the pylorus can be done in a straight fashion. If the left–right control wheel is used to direct the endoscope so the pylorus is visualized, it will prevent a straight insertion into the pylorus which is essential for a successful non-traumatic intubation. Once the pylorus is visualized, the endoscope is advanced very close to the opening and the tip is directed downwards by turning the down controller. The tip of the scope then 'pops' into the duodenal bulb and can be advanced further. The endoscope is advanced to the level of the greater ampulla, at which point is in the 'long scope' position. To get the scope in the 'short scope' position, the directional controls are changed to the down and right position and the scope is slowly withdrawn. This takes the large omega-shaped loop out of the endoscope as it is passing along the greater curve of the stomach and creates a more direct passage to the duodenum, which reduces stress on internal structures as well as on the stomach wall and lining. **(See Figures 26.1–26.3)**

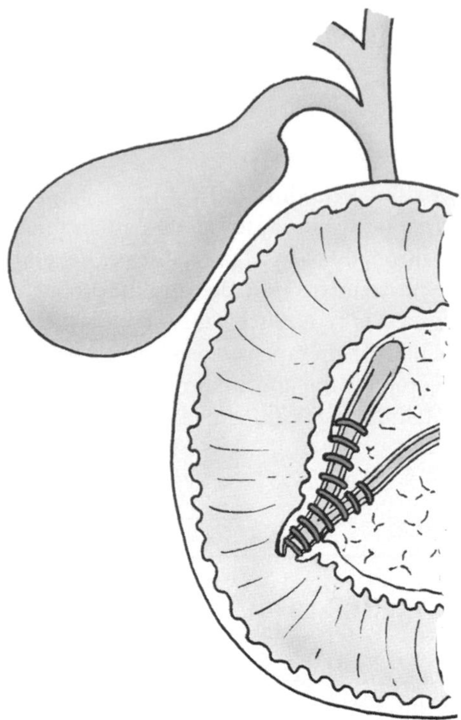

Figure 26.1

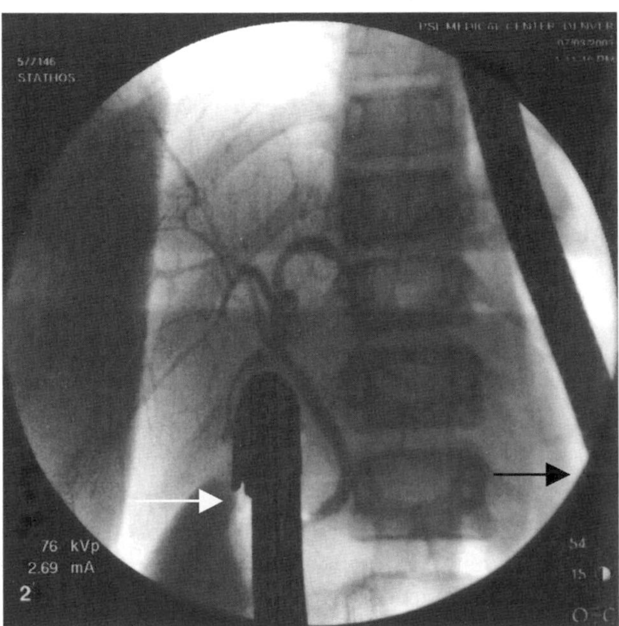

Figure 26.2

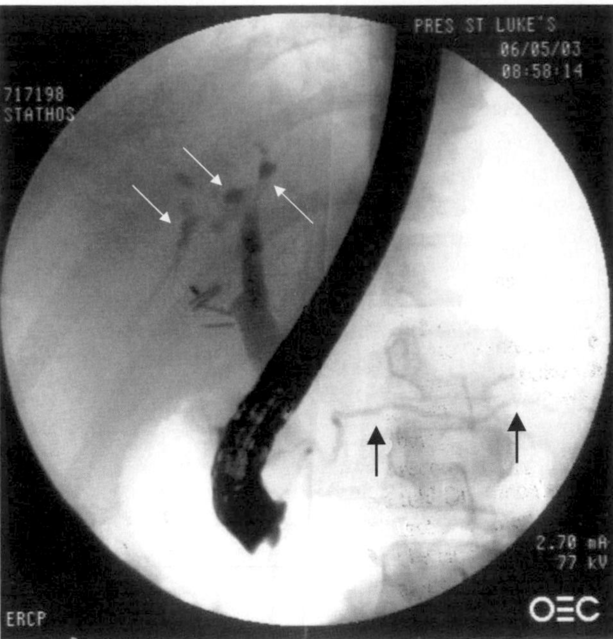

Figure 26.3

Once the greater ampulla is visualized, intubation can be attempted. The cannula is inserted into the lower two-thirds portion of the ampulla to intubate the pancreatic duct. The insertion is done in a straight fashion with little or no upward deflection from the lifter arm on the duodenoscope. Proper alignment is often the key to cannulating the common bile duct successfully. The ampulla needs to be in the 12 o'clock position in the field of view. With the ampulla in this position, the cannula should be inserted into its upper third and deflected upwards. This will optimize the chances of cannulating the common bile duct. The cannula will typically meet some resistance initially and then suddenly slide inward a millimeter or so, indicating likely cannulation of either the common bile duct or the pancreatic duct has occurred. A small amount of dye is then injected through the cannula and the duct is opacified on fluoroscopy. After several tenths of a milliliter has been injected it is often possible to determine which duct has been cannulated. If the dye crosses the patient's midline, it is in the pancreatic duct. The vertebral bodies are a useful landmark by which to recognize the midline during fluoroscopy. If the dye passes straight superiorly, it is likely to be in the common bile duct.

Accessory bile ducts are aberrant ducts that drain individual segments of the liver; they may drain directly into the gallbladder, cystic duct, right and left hepatic ducts, or common bile duct. In rare cases, the right hepatic duct may connect to the gallbladder or cystic duct. These variations and anomalies must be recognized on cholangiography to prevent inadvertent transection or ligation of bile ducts during surgery. The numerous congenital abnormalities of the biliary tree and of the pancreatic ducts can typically be diagnosed with dye injection alone and if diagnosis is the only goal, the procedure is then complete.

Therapeutic ERCP

If therapeutic procedures are to be performed, a 'deep cannulation' will be necessary. Deep cannulation implies that

Table 26.2 *Therapeutic procedures*

Procedure	Indication
Sphincterotomy of the ampullary sphincter	
Greater	Accommodate stone passage, relieve biliary dyskinesia
Lesser	Pancreatic divisum
Balloon dilatation	Biliary or pancreatic duct stricture
Stent placement	Promote drainage through recurrent strictures
	Bypass a traumatized or leaking segment of a duct
Lithotripsy	Crush a stone too large to pass through the ampulla
Balloon sweep	To pull stones from the common bile duct

the cannula is passed well into the common bile duct or pancreatic duct. It is accomplished successfully by an experienced endoscopist in 80–90 percent of procedures where it is indicated. However, it is sometimes only possible using a guide-wire that is inserted into the appropriate duct for guidance or, conversely, if the cannula is deeply inserted into the proper duct, a wire can be inserted and left in the duct for guidance. This is known as a 'deep wire'. After the wire is in place, the instruments can be guided over the wire into proper position to allow a therapeutic procedure to be undertaken. Placement of the guide-wire is verified on fluoroscopy by comparing the wire position to the position of dye previously injected. Stone extraction is common in adult ERCP but much less common in the pediatric population. (**Tables 26.2 and 26.3**)

The following therapeutic procedures are possible during ERCP.

Sphincterotomy of the greater or lesser ampullary sphincter

The sphincterotome is passed over the previously placed deep guide-wire and slid into the ampulla. Once the tome is in place, the wire portion is bowed and electrocautery is passed through the wire. Standard surgical electrocautery regulators are typically used and standard settings employed. In the greater ampulla, a single 5–15 mm cut is made in the superior portion of the ampulla, also referred to as the 12 o'clock position. A typical guideline for the endpoint of the cut is just distal to the juncture where the ampulla meets the wall of the duodenum.

Balloon dilatation

Balloon dilatation of either the ampulla or a stenotic duct is commenced over the deep wire. The balloon size and

Table 26.3 *Conditions associated with cholelithiasis in children according to age*

0–12 months (%)	1–5 years (%)	6–21 years (%)
None (36.4)	Hepatobiliary disease (28.6)	Pregnancy (37.2)
Parenteral nutrition (29.1)	Abdominal surgery (21.4)	Hemolytic disease (5.5)
Abdominal surgery (29.1)	Artificial heart valve (14.3)	Obesity (8.1)
Sepsis (14.8)	None (14.3)	Abdominal surgery (5.1)
Bronchopulmonary dysplasia (12.7)	Malabsorption (7.1)	None (3.4)
Hemolytic disease (5.5)		Hepatobiliary disease (2.7)
Necrotizing enterocolitis (5.5)		Parenteral nutrition (2.7)
Malabsorption (5.5)		Malabsorption (2.8)
Hepatobiliary disease (3.6)		

Modified from Friesen CA, Roberts CC. Cholelithiasis: clinical characteristics in children: case analysis and literature review. *Clinical Pediatrics (Philadelphia)* 1989; **28**:294.

length are carefully chosen based on the particular needs of the patient. Sizes can vary depending on the amount of hydrostatic pressure present in the balloon. The balloon is inflated while centrally positioned across the stricture and is typically left inflated for 1–3 minutes. Various balloon dilators are available that allow dye to be injected both proximal and distal to the balloon. This is very helpful in the detection of biliary stones in the common bile duct.

Stent placement

Biliary stent placement is divided into two categories, permanent stents and temporary stents. The permanent stents are typically used only in patients with a terminal illness associated with an obstructive lesion of the bile or pancreatic ducts and are therefore used rarely in children. Temporary stents are used much more commonly to promote decompression of a dilated duct, to keep a sphincterotomy from closing, or to bridge an area of the duct that may be damaged or leaking. Inserting a deep wire into the appropriate duct starts the stent placement. Next, the stent is guided carefully into place over the wire and left in position.

Lithotripsy

Lithotripsy is done to destroy a biliary or pancreatic duct stone while it is still in the duct. Although this is not a common pediatric occurrence, the procedure is not difficult to perform. After a guide-wire has been placed beyond the stone, the lithotripter is advanced over the guide-wire and the basket is expanded. The basket is then closed around the stone, crushing it in the process. Occasionally, a balloon sweep is necessary to retrieve the debris.

Balloon sweep

A balloon sweep is used to clear the bile ducts or pancreatic duct of any stone or debris that does not easily pass into the intestinal lumen while flushing with dye. This is usually attempted only after a sphincterotomy has been done to accommodate the stone to be removed. A balloon catheter is typically passed over a guide-wire until its deflated portion is beyond the stone. The balloon is then inflated and dye is injected through the catheter proximal to the balloon. If the stone is visualized as a filling defect within the injected dye and the dye does not flush the stone from the duct, the balloon is gently withdrawn from the duct while maintaining the inflation. The stone is typically drawn into the intestinal lumen without having to pull the balloon through the recently cut ampulla.

WIRE BASKET STONE REMOVAL

The wire basket is used to remove especially stubborn stones from the common bile duct or pancreatic duct. The wire basket is very similar to that on the lithotripter but does not have the ability to crush a stone. The basket is expanded around the stone and then closed on it. The stone is then gently removed from the duct. As with the balloon sweep, the patient has usually undergone a sphincterotomy prior to the removal.

POSTOPERATIVE CARE

- Nil orally for 4–6 hours.
- Observe for 6–8 hours.
- Complete blood count (CBC), C-reactive protein (CRP), amylase, lipase measured 4 hours after the procedure.
- Post-sphincterotomy patients should be observed for 12–18 hours.

After an ERCP, the child should be observed for several hours while the sedative or anesthesia wears off. The most common discomfort after the examination is a feeling of bloating from the air introduced during it. Some patients also have a slightly sore throat. Patients should be able to eat 4–6 hours after the procedure.

The child should be hospitalized overnight for observation if a stent is placed into a duct or a sphincterotomy is made into the ampulla.

After discharge from the procedure suite or operating room, symptoms that should be reported immediately are severe abdominal pain, a firm distended abdomen, vomiting, fever, dysphagia or odynophagia, and subcutaneous crepitation.

PROBLEMS, PITFALLS AND SOLUTIONS

Lack of common bile duct cannulation

When the common bile duct cannot be cannulated, additional attention to proper positioning of the tip of the endoscope will often ensure success. If this fails, the position of the endoscope should be changed from the short scope position to the long scope position and the cannulation re-attempted. Ninety to 95 percent of ERCPs are successful.

COMPLICATIONS

Complications of ERCP with or without sphincterotomy are uncommon. The major complications include hemorrhage, perforation, infection and pancreatitis. The relative risks of these complications are not well established in children due to the limited numbers of patients in the studies done to assess complication rates. However, the overall rates appear to be very similar to those established for adults. Another potential risk of ERCP is an adverse reaction to the sedative used. The risks of ERCP vary with the reasons for the test, what is found during the procedure, whether any therapy is undertaken, and the presence of other major medical problems, e.g. heart or lung diseases.

Major complications requiring hospitalization are uncommon. The complication rate of therapeutic ERCP (sphincterotomy, stone removal, dilatation of a stricture, stent or drain placement, etc.) is higher than that for diagnostic ERCP. Often these complications can be managed without surgery.

Bleeding

If there is bleeding associated with the endoscopy not involving a therapeutic procedure, observation is usually sufficient to ensure the problem is not potentially morbid. The endoscope is placed in a position to observe the bleeding to see if it continues actively. Small to moderate lesions are amenable to endoscopic cautery. Occasionally, more major bleeds that do not stop need surgical correction. Bleeding after a therapeutic procedure has been performed is treated in the same fashion, but there is a higher likelihood that ongoing bleeding after a sphincterotomy will require surgery.

Perforation

Perforation from a therapeutic procedure or from the endoscopic portion of the procedure is rare. When it occurs, surgical intervention is usually required. In some circumstances close observation and intravenous antibiotics will suffice for very minor perforations.

Infection or cholangitis

There are no convincing data to suggest that pre-treatment with antibiotics is helpful in preventing cholangitis from occurring in post-sphincterotomy patients. Only rapid treatment after the occurrence is helpful. The antibiotic chosen should be effective against normal enteric flora.

Pancreatitis

The risk of acute pancreatitis in adults and children after ERCP has been reported to be at least 5 percent. Factors include:

- the volume and pressure of contrast material that is injected,
- the number of injections of the pancreatic duct,
- ampullary trauma by multiple attempts at catheterization,
- overfilling of the pancreatic ducts with secondary acinarization of the parenchyma,
- an underlying pathologic process of the pancreatic ducts,
- introduction of bacteria,
- injury associated with sphincterotomy or insertion of pancreatic stents.

The risk of pancreatitis is not increased further by an endoscopic sphincterotomy unless this procedure is performed on patients who have non-dilated pancreatic ducts. The risk is increased when a sphincter of Oddi manometric study is performed, and can be decreased with the use of an aspirating catheter to withdraw as much fluid as possible at the completion of the procedure.

Other methods have also been used in an effort to reduce ERCP-induced acute pancreatitis. Thus far, the use of octreotide (Sandostatin) parenterally, nifedipine orally, and low osmolality and non-ionic contrast has not significantly reduced the incidence of post-ERCP acute pancreatitis. A history of prior acute pancreatitis may ameliorate the clinical outcome of post-ERCP pancreatitis. Patients who have experienced a previous episode of pancreatitis after ERCP are more likely to experience another episode after a second ERCP.

C-reactive protein serum levels may be of significant help in detecting post-ERCP acute pancreatitis.

The treatment of post-ERCP acute pancreatitis is similar to that of other forms of acute pancreatitis but its effects are typically shorter lived. The cessation of oral intake and the use of liberal analgesia for several hours or days are often adequate to ameliorate the process.

FURTHER READING

Adkins RB Jr, Chapman WC, Reddy VS. Embryology, anatomy, and surgical applications of the extrahepatic biliary system. *Surgical Clinics of North America* 2000; **80**:363–79.

Berman L, Harris G, Chawla A, Markowitz J. Magnetic resonance cholangiopancreatography (MRCP): noninvasive visualization of the biliary tree in children. *Journal of Pediatric Gastroenterology and Nutrition* 1997; **152**(25):480.

Celli A, Parsons WP, Perrault J, et al. Therapeutic endoscopic retrograde cholangiopancreatography in children. *Journal of Pediatric Gastroenterology and Nutrition* 1999; **29**(4):497.

Fox VL, Werlin SL, Heyman MB. Endoscopic retrograde cholangiopancreatography in children. *Journal of Pediatric Gastroenterology and Nutrition* 2000; **30**:335–42.

Guelrud M, Mujica C, Jaen D, Plaz J, Arias J. The role of ERCP in the diagnosis and treatment of idiopathic recurrent pancreatitis in children and adolescents. *Gastrointestinal Endoscopy* 1994; **40**:428–36.

27

Proctosigmoidoscopy

RANG N.S. SHAWIS

INTRODUCTION

Sigmoidoscopy is the examination of the sigmoid colon and upper rectum. This can be achieved using either rigid or flexible instruments. Proctoscopy is the examination of the rectum. The aims of proctosigmoidoscopy are to visualize any diseased area of rectum and sigmoid colon from within the bowel lumen, to obtain biopsy samples as required, and to perform the procedure with minimal discomfort and risk to the patient. The recent introduction of small diameter instruments specially designed for children has established proctosigmoidoscopy as an important diagnostic technique. Superficial mucosa lesions of the recto-sigmoid, which are not apparent with conventional contrast studies, can be inspected directly and biopsied.

Although proctoscopy can be performed at the bedside, in practice, satisfactory examinations of children usually need to be done under general anesthesia. Rigid sigmoidoscopy allows the examination of the rectum and sigmoid colon for up to 12 cm in infants and 25 cm in older children. Fiberoptic sigmoidoscopy allows the whole of the sigmoid colon to be visualized with minimal risk when performed appropriately.

Modern sigmoidoscopes have significant improvements in flexibility, providing easier insertion and maneuverability. Video-imaging systems provide high resolution and clear images; in addition, a wide range of endotherapy products can be used without compromising the suction power and above qualities.

Anatomical considerations

The rectum is the terminal portion of the large intestine. It varies in length according to the age and size of the children, and reaches 12–14 cm in childhood. It begins proximally at the level of the third sacral vertebra. The rectum, especially when distended, exhibits a series of shelf-like semicircular folds within the bowel lumen called the valves of Houston.

The shelves divide the rectum into three compartments, the upper and lower compartments are convex to the right whilst the middle is convex to the left. The part of the rectum that lies below the middle valve is called the rectal ampulla and is wider than the rest. The rectum at its distal end becomes continuous with the anal canal (level of pectinate line). The anal canal is less than 1 cm long in neonates and reaches 4 cm in adulthood.

The sigmoid colon measures about 40 cm in adults and because of its mobility it varies in position and shape.

Indications

Proctosigmoidoscopy is performed as part of the initial assessment of a child with the following symptoms: bleeding per rectum, mucus discharge, pain, tenesmus, pruritus, prolapse and peri-anal fistula/sinus. The aim of the examination is to get an unobstructed view of the bowel with the least risk and discomfort to the patient, and to be able to undertake other diagnostic and/or therapeutic procedures as applicable. It is possible to inspect, document (photograph), biopsy and/or treat certain conditions (fissures, hemorrhoids, polyps, ulcers, prolapse and injury) using this approach.

Contraindications

There are no special contraindications; however, in anal stenosis or stricture it may be difficult to perform rigid endoscopy unless the narrowing is dilated first. Particular care is necessary in patients with acute inflammatory bowel disease (IBD) with severe ulceration. In children with constipation or anal pain without other symptoms, the likelihood of finding significant additional pathology on proctosigmoidoscopy is very low.

EQUIPMENT/INSTRUMENTS

Anoscope

The spreadable anal speculum has a particular use for anal examination in the outpatient department. Although most ano-rectal examinations are part of an overall proctosigmoidoscopic assessment, and as such are usually done under general anesthesia in children, there are the occasional instances in which a spreadable anal speculum can be used in the outpatient clinic with satisfactory results both from the child's and family's perspective and from the point of view of adequacy of the examination. Furthermore, in small infants, up to 5 cm of ano-rectum can be inspected by using either a nasal speculum or an auroscope. **(See Figure 27.1)**

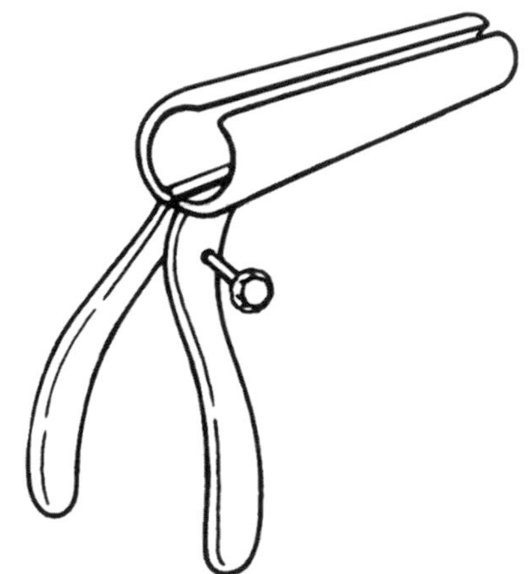

Figure 27.1

Rigid sigmoidoscope and proctoscope

The basic instrument is composed of a straight, hollow tube with an obturator to facilitate insertion. The length is marked on the outside and the inner tube has either a direct or a 90° directional view. The tube can be rotated through 360° and this usually helps in finding the ideal position for treatment or examination. In addition, there is a viewing window and a swivel lens offering two-times magnification, and the tube ends are usually angled. Modern sigmoidoscopes and proctoscopes have fiberoptic illumination. The sigmoidoscope has an insufflation port to which a manual rubber insufflation bulb can be attached. **(See Figure 27.2)**

Various instruments are available and the size varies from a length of 20 to 30 cm with an inner diameter of 11.4 to 20 mm. A scope with an inner diameter of at least 16 mm is needed if polypectomy is considered. It is advisable to use an instrument with distal annular illumination and one insulated end to prevent thermal damage to the rectum during diathermy.

Disposable tubes have superseded the re-usable proctoscope and sigmoidoscope. These are made of thermoplastic materials and the light is usually transmitted through the tube wall. Their major advantage is in the prevention of disease transmission. Illumination is by fiberoptic cable

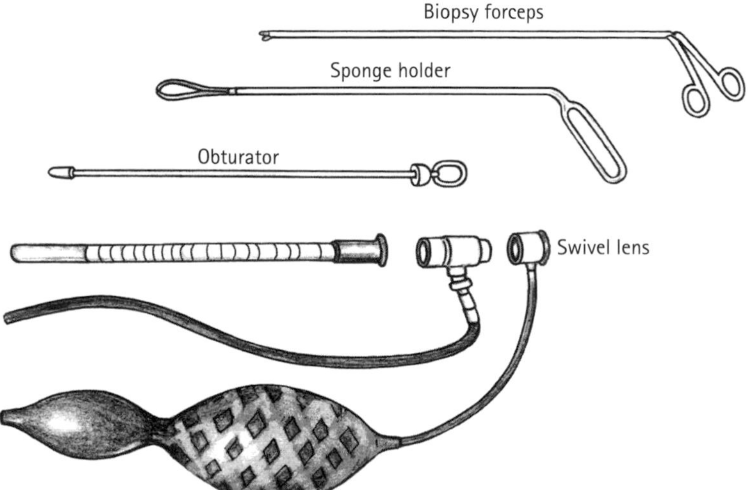

Figure 27.2

and they come in packs in different sizes. The essential set comprises:

- anoscope with proctoscope head
- anoscope/proctoscope tube with straight view
- proctoscope complete with obturator
- sigmoidoscope with obturator
- biopsy forceps with straight jaws
- biopsy forceps with angled jaws
- sponge holder
- suction tube
- insufflation bulb.

In addition:

- plug-in transfomer
- cables
- lights for fiberoptic projector
- battery handles, spare bulb, rechargeable handle (for portable anoscope/proctoscope).

PREOPERATIVE PREPARATION

No special preparation is required for proctoscopy. However, there is evidence of transient bacteremia during the procedure and therefore antibiotic prophylaxis is indicated in children with a cardiac defect, immune compromise or ascites.

Bowel preparation prior to sigmoidoscopy for the majority of patients is adequately covered by a single phosphate enema on the morning of examination. In constipated children only liquids are given 24 hours prior to the examination and a suitable aperient (senna or sodium picosulfate) on the evening before. On rare occasions, bowel preparation similar to that for colonoscopy may be necessary.

TECHNIQUE

Different positions can be used: left lateral, right lateral, supine with legs supported in stirrups (lithotomy) or supine with hips flexed and abducted with legs and thighs supported on pads or towels. The left lateral position is satisfactory in most situations: the patient lies on the left side with the knees drawn towards the chest, and a pillow or protecting pad is placed between the flexed knees. In small infants the supine position with the hips flexed is preferred. **(See Figure 27.3)**

In selected children, a limited examination can be done as an outpatient. Examination usually begins by gently spreading the anal area using a thumb on either side and pushing laterally.

In the majority of children, a more appropriate examination that also allows other diagnostic procedures, such as biopsy, or other therapeutic procedures to be performed involves general anesthesia.

Anoscopy

After inspection and digital examination, a well-lubricated anoscope is introduced directly into the anus. The handle is pointed anteriorly and gently squeezed to open the instrument. The desired position can be maintained by tightening the adjustable screw. The required procedure is then performed before withdrawal, the screw is loosened and the closed anoscope can then be removed.

Proctoscopy

The well-lubricated tube with obturator in place is inserted for 4 cm in a direction towards the umbilicus. When the rectum is entered, the tip is tilted in a posterior direction and introduced fully; next the obturator is removed and the light adjusted. The proctoscope is held in the left hand, leaving the right hand free to carry out manipulations as necessary (enabling excess mucus, liquid/feces to be aspirated or swabbed). The lower rectum is inspected by rotating the tube gently and the whole circumference of the bowel is examined. The tube is then slowly withdrawn and the distal rectum and anal canal inspected. If it is decided to re-advance the scope, it should be withdrawn completely and only re-introduced with the obturator in situ.

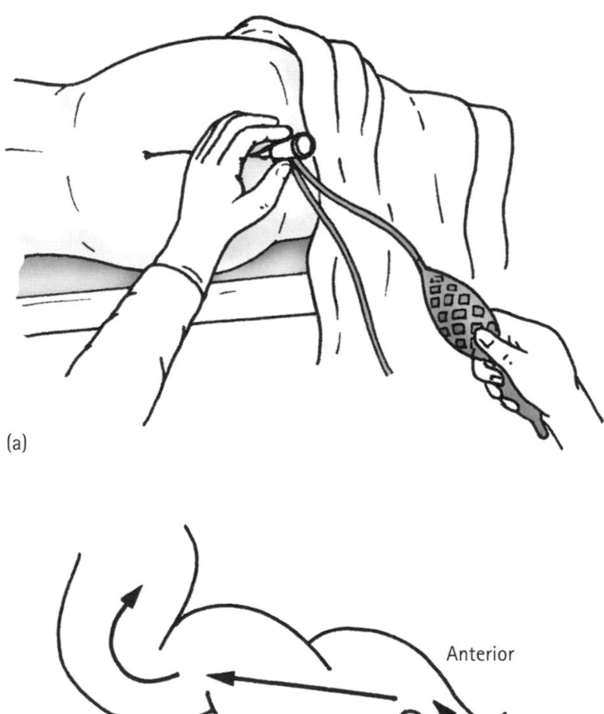

Figure 27.3 *(a) Rigid sigmoidoscope in position; (b) directions in sigmoidoscopy.*

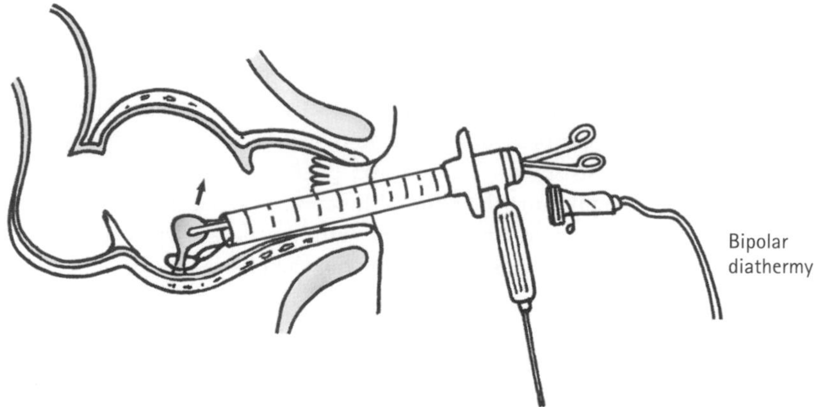

Figure 27.4

Rigid sigmoidoscopy

Following inspection of the peri-anal area and digital examination including bimanual examination, the well-lubricated instrument is introduced for 4 cm (or less in smaller children) in a direction towards the umbilicus. When the rectum is entered, the instrument is advanced in a posterior direction by tilting the advancing end backwards. The obturator is removed, the light adjusted and any mucus or liquid/feces aspirated or swabbed. When there is a good view of the lumen, the instrument can be advanced; if not, it can be withdrawn slightly and the rectum insufflated by squeezing the insufflator and at the same time observing the bowel continuously. The rectum only needs to be distended slightly to reveal the lumen.

The sigmoidoscope is usually held in the left hand and the right hand is free for maneuvering and using endotherapy instruments as required. The upper rectum and proximal sigmoid colon can be inspected circumferentially, and biopsies and other procedures carried out as indicated. If at any time the lumen is not in view, the instrument should not be advanced blindly; rather, it should be withdrawn slightly and minimal insufflation used. As the lumen appears, the sigmoidoscope should be advanced slowly. Up to 25 cm can be examined with minimal risk. However, biopsies – especially using punch forceps – can cause bleeding and perforation.

Polypectomy

Pedunculated polyps situated in the lower rectum can usually be hooked out by the examining finger and removed after ligating or transfixing the stalk with an absorbable suture. However, they often avulse and cause bleeding. These polyps can be dealt with directly with the anal speculum in situ by applying a ligature or suture to the base of the lesion. A polyp high in the rectum is best dealt with by snaring. **(See Figure 27.4)**

With the rigid sigmoidoscope inserted, a diathermy snare is introduced to the site of the polyp through the lumen. The grasping forceps are introduced and passed through the snare. The polyp is grasped firmly and gentle traction applied. Most of these polyps have a stalk; the snare is passed over the polyp and on to the stalk.

The snare is then tightened and coagulation current is applied as it is closed. The coagulation process eventually severs the stalk, with no risk of bleeding. Small polyps may be removed through the scope. Larger ones are held in grasping forceps, and the polyp, forceps and scope are removed together. The area is then inspected. A diathermy ball may be used to achieve hemostasis if there is ongoing bleeding. If too much traction is applied to the polyp, there is a risk that the snare might include normal mucosa and this could lead to perforation.

Fiberoptic sigmoidoscopy

INSTRUMENT

The flexible sigmoidoscope has an adjustable tip, channels for irrigation and insufflation and a working channel that can be used for procedures such as biopsy, coagulation, snaring, injection etc. It has a working length of about 60 cm and instruments are available in various diameters (the diameter selected depending on the size of the patient). The smallest fiberoptic sigmoidoscope is 15.4 mm at the tip, with a 13.3 mm shaft.

TECHNIQUE

The patient is placed in the left lateral position, or supine if a small infant. A rectal examination is carried out to exclude a low ano-rectal lesion. In doing so, the anal canal is gently and slightly stretched and lubricated. Irrespective of whether sedation or general anesthesia is employed, sigmoidoscopy involves gentle passage of the instrument into the lower colon and rectum. The instrument is manipulated/advanced through the opening of the lumen by angling the tip, using the adjusting knobs with the left hand and using the right hand to advance the shaft. **(See Figure 27.5)**

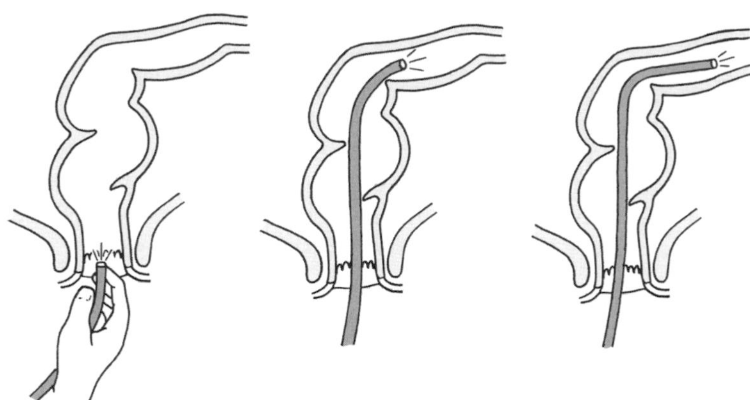

Figure 27.5

The well-lubricated tip of the instrument is inserted 'sideways' for 4–5 cm. Initial inspection may reveal a red blur as the tip is in direct contact with the mucosa – gently insufflate the rectum and withdraw the instrument, slightly adjusting the flexible tip until the lumen comes into view. After aspirating excessive fluid and mucus, the sigmoidoscope can then be advanced along the rectum with the lumen in full view as far as the recto-sigmoid junction.

Negotiation of the recto-sigmoid junction must be attempted with minimal insufflation of air and under direct vision. This will be aided by angling the instrument to follow any angulation at the junction. The junction's distance varies according to the size and age of the child. At times, especially when there is acute angulation of the sigmoid colon, the lumen will be difficult to visualize. In these cases the scope should be advanced along the bowel wall, taking care that the mucosa is not blanched and that the movement is smooth and progressive. Otherwise, withdraw the sigmoidoscope slowly until the lumen is visible again and re-angle the tip of the instrument towards the lumen. It may be helpful to twist the shaft of the sigmoidoscope rather than attempting to redirect it using the adjusting knobs to achieve this maneuver. Insufflating excessive air may lead to increased acuteness of the angle and should therefore be avoided. By careful manipulation of the tip and twisting the shaft of the instrument, the sigmoid colon should be reached in most children.

If a large loop is forming, a combination of gentle withdrawal and clockwise rotation of the shaft will straighten the loop and the sigmoid colon, making further advance possible.

Short withdrawal and advancement will fold the colon over the instrument, permitting visualization of a greater length of colon. This maneuver is often helpful, but excessive friction between the instrument's shaft and the colon wall should be avoided.

Although inspection of the colon up to the splenic flexure is possible in some children, in most the lumen is only partially visible during instrument advancement, and insertion is only possible as far as the descending colon. Thorough examination is conducted during slow withdrawal of the instrument with the lumen in full view. Biopsies and sampling should be undertaken at this stage. Areas of interest can be cleaned with water using the irrigation channel for better viewing and photographic documentation. Previously insufflated air must be aspirated during withdrawal to prevent discomfort to the patient in the postoperative period.

POSTOPERATIVE CARE

After a routine procedure, apart from the usual post-anesthetic recovery care, no special observation is necessary and most children can go home fully awake. If a patient has had a biopsy or polypectomy, the passage of a small amount of old blood with the first stool should be expected. Nevertheless, the family should be warned to report back if there is significant bleeding, as this may require medical attention and even blood transfusion.

PROBLEMS, PITFALLS AND SOLUTIONS

- Advance the scope only when the lumen is visible.
- Insufflate only small amounts of air.
- If there is no progress, withdraw slightly, twisting the shaft of the instrument in a clockwise direction.
- Reserve full inspection and procedures for the withdrawal stage.
- It is important to appreciate the anatomy and limitations of the technique.
- Perseverance in difficult cases, particularly in small infants, increases the possibility of complications.
- The presence of severe ulceration in IBD increases the risk of complications.
- Negotiation of the recto-sigmoid junction can be technically difficult.
- Excessive insufflation increases the angulation of the sigmoid colon, increasing the risk of perforation, and prevents advancement of the instrument.

- Punch biopsy of the upper rectum and sigmoid colon through a rigid scope carries a higher risk of perforation.
- Applying excessive traction on polyps may lead to inclusion of bowel wall within the snare and can cause perforation and/or bleeding.
- Diathermy snaring of wide-based polyps may cause thermal injury and lead to immediate or delayed perforation of the relatively thin wall of the bowel in children.

Lack of progress/inadequate view

- Inadequate view. Withdraw slightly; if the lumen becomes clear, advance the scope; otherwise, insufflate a small mount of air – if the view is still not adequate, twist the shaft of the flexible scope and repeat these maneuvers until the lumen is clearly seen.
- Excessive mucus/feces. Aspirate or swab. If the bowel is not properly prepared, manual evacuation plus washout with warm normal saline may be necessary.
- Blood. Gentle aspiration alternating with saline irrigation can help to enhance the view.

Inadequate examination

- If technically difficult and no further information can be obtained safely without increasing the risk to the child, the procedure should be terminated.
- Depending on the indication for the procedure, a contrast study may be indicated as an alternative; otherwise, re-admission at an appropriate future date, with adequate bowel preparation and proper discussion with the family, may be needed.

COMPLICATIONS

Perforation

Although perforation is very rare, it is a serious complication and the family must be warned of the possibility. It may occur in technically difficult procedures, especially when performed on a child suffering from acute IBD with severe ulceration. A plain abdominal film can usually identify intraperitoneal free air where perforation is suspected because of abdominal pain or abdominal distension. Laparoscopy/laparotomy is usually needed. If there is minimal contamination, over-sewing of the perforation is usually sufficient. When there is gross contamination and/or delay in diagnosis, a de-functioning colostomy may be necessary.

Bleeding

Bleeding may occur because of rough handling in technically difficult procedures, or following biopsy or polypectomy. If observed during the procedure, direct pressure to the bleeding point with a cotton swab (rigid sigmoidoscopy/proctoscopy) or diathermy of the bleeding area may be necessary. If excessive, blood transfusion may be required.

Fecal incontinence/soiling

Incontinence has been reported following aggressive anal dilatation prior to instrumentation; it is usually transient.

CARE OF INSTRUMENTS

A nurse/assistant must be trained and be responsible for the care, maintenance and disinfecting of the various instruments according to the manufacturer's recommendations, which usually include the following.

- Debris within the suction, irrigation and working channels must be brushed.
- Instruments should be washed immediately after use.
- All tubes and hollow parts must be flushed with fresh detergent solution.
- Instruments are then placed in an ultrasonic cleaner, rinsed in tap water, and a solution of 2 percent glutaraldehyde used for disinfection.
- The cleaning room/area should be adequately ventilated.
- Staff using the glutaraldehyde solution should wear gloves to protect their skin.

The availability of disposable (rigid proctoscopes and sigmoidoscopes) instruments negates the need for sterilization, with no risk of transmitting infection.

FURTHER READING

Bailey H, Love M. *Short Practice of Surgery.* London: Arnold, 2000.

Cook RCM. Polypectomy, in *Rob and Smith's Operative Surgery*, 4th edn. London: Butterworths, 1988.

Gauderer MW, Decon JM, Boyle JT. Sigmoid irrigation tube for the management of chronic evacuation disorders. *Journal of Pediatric Surgery* 2000; **37**(30):348–51.

Nielsen RG, Fenger C, Pedersen SA, Quist N, Sorensen J, Husby S et al. Diagnostic benefit of gastrointestinal endoscopy in infants under one year of age – a two-year survey. *Ugeskr Laeger* 2001; **163**(80):1074–8.

Ringel Y, Dalton CB, Brand LJ, Hu Y, Jia H, Bangdiwala S, Drossman DA. Flexible sigmoidoscopy; the patients' perception. *Gastrointestinal Endoscopy* 2002; **55**(3):315–20.

28

Colonoscopy – basic techniques and specific procedures

I.D. SUGARMAN

INTRODUCTION

Colonoscopy is an important technique for the investigation of large bowel disease in children. Proficiency at colonoscopy requires time and patience but the dividends for the pediatric lower gastrointestinal (GI) surgeon are many.

There are major differences between colonoscopy in adults and in children. In adults, colonoscopy is most often performed as part of the assessment of colonic malignancy. In children, it is most often performed as part of the assessment of inflammatory bowel disease (IBD) and the management of large bowel polyps. Therefore, full colonoscopy and ileoscopy are imperative. Furthermore, the pediatric surgeon must be capable of performing colonoscopy on children from infancy to adolescence. This requires familiarity with several different endoscopes: a neonatal gastroscope is often the most appropriate instrument to examine the colon of a baby, whereas the pediatric colonoscope or even an adult colonoscope may be appropriate for colonoscopy in an adolescent. With experience, the surgeon will appreciate the effect factors such as endoscope flexibility have on navigation of the flexures of the colon.

Although many surgeons still perform rigid sigmoidoscopy as a first-line investigation of children with lower GI bleeding, colonoscopy offers many advantages. For example, although the majority of children with polyps will have a single juvenile polyp within 15 cm of the anus, not infrequently more than one polyp is found if a full colonoscopy is performed.

Indications

DIAGNOSTIC

- Investigation of symptoms suggestive of IBD.
- Follow-up assessment of IBD management.
- Lower GI bleeding.
- Polyposis syndrome surveillance.
- Chronic diarrhea.

THERAPEUTIC

- Polypectomy.
- Percutaneous cecostomy or distal antegrade continence enema (DACE) tube insertion.
- Foreign body removal (rare).
- Dilatation/stenting of strictures (very rare in the pediatric population).

Contraindications

ABSOLUTE

- Signs of peritonitis.

RELATIVE

- Unprepared bowel.
- Acute colitis.
- Uncorrected bleeding diathesis.

EQUIPMENT/INSTRUMENTS

Essential

- Pediatric colonoscope (working length 133 cm).
- Light source.
- Suction apparatus and connecting tubing.
- 0.9 percent sodium chloride in 20 mL aliquots and syringes.
- Biopsy forceps.

Desirable

- Adult colonoscope (working length 168 cm).
- Various gastroscopes.
- Imaging equipment (including camera, TV screen, digital recorder and printer).
- Carbon dioxide insufflator.
- Magnetic endoscopic imager – see 'Problems, pitfalls and solutions', page 175.

For interventional colonoscopy

- Hot biopsy forceps (diathermy biopsy forceps).
- Ligating loops, applicator and retrieving forceps or Dormier basket.
- Diathermy loop with monopolar diathermy generator.
- Dye (blue/black fountain pen ink or methylene blue 1:20 dilution). Ink is useful to 'spray' onto the colonic mucosa to highlight fine detail (e.g. small adenomas) and to 'tattoo' bowel at a site of previously excised polyp.
- Epinephrine (1:10 000): submucosal injection of epinephrine can be useful to assist hemostasis and if endoscopic removal of sessile polyps is to be attempted.
- Endoscopic clips plus applicator: useful for control of hemorrhage.

Choice of endoscope

The choice of endoscope will depend on the age and weight of the child. The optical definition of video-endoscopes is vastly superior to that of conventional endoscopes. As experience is gained, the surgeon will find the larger, stiffer endoscopes preferable for colonoscopy in younger children. **(See Table 28.1)**

Variable-stiffness colonoscopes offer significant advantages. The ability to stiffen the endoscope after a loop has been removed will prevent recurrence and allow more rapid advancement along 'straight' sections of the colon. This can substantially reduce the time taken to complete a colonoscopy.

Table 28.1 *Endoscopes used by author for colonoscopy*

Age	Weight (kg)	Endoscope
Neonate (<44 weeks' gestation)	<5	Olympus N30 gastroscope Length: 90 cm Diameter: 5.2 mm Channel size: 2.0 mm
1–12 months	5–10	Olympus XP20 gastroscope Length: 100 cm Diameter: 7.9 mm Channel size: 2.0 mm
1–7 years	10–24	Olympus PCF240I colonoscope Length: 130 cm Diameter: 12 mm Channel size: 3.2 mm
8 years +	25+	Olympus CF240AL colonoscope Length: 160 cm Diameter: 12 mm Channel size: 3.2 mm

PREOPERATIVE PREPARATION

Colonoscopy is very difficult if the colon is not empty. Various regimes for bowel preparation have been described. It is important to choose a method that is acceptable to the child, especially if repeat colonoscopy may be necessary. We have found sodium picosulphate (Picolax) effective and well tolerated. **(See Box 28.1)**

A clinical nurse specialist forms an essential part of our lower GI endoscopy team. She visits the child and family at home and explains the procedure and why preoperative bowel preparation is necessary. Bowel preparation takes place at home and children are admitted generally as a day case. Compliance rates are high and the quality of the bowel preparation is excellent.

Preoperative investigations may include a complete blood count, liver function tests, C-reactive protein and coagulation studies. Other investigations may be performed in children with suspected IBD, including abdominal ultrasound (looking for thickened bowel and peristalsis), ^{99m}technetium-labeled white cell scans (focal areas of increased uptake suggest active disease) and barium contrast studies (assessment of small bowel disease, particularly the ileo-cecal region).

If colonoscopy is contemplated in a child with an acute colitis, a plain abdominal X-ray is wise to document the degree of colonic dilatation and to exclude perforation. In this situation the child should be worked up with coagulation studies and a blood group and save in case it is necessary to proceed to immediate laparotomy.

Intravenous antibiotics should be administered at the induction of anesthesia to all children with known or suspected IBD prior to colonoscopy. Children at risk of infective

Box 28.1 Preoperative bowel preparation for children undergoing colonoscopy

- Clear fluids for 24 hours preoperatively.
- Sodium picosulphate/magnesium citrate (Picolax) according to the following schedule.

	Dose of Picolax (g)	
Age (years)	24 hours preop.	18 hours preop.
<2	1.25 (¼ sachet)	1.25 (¼ sachet)
2–5	2.5 (½ sachet)	2.5 (½ sachet)
5–10	5 (1 sachet)	2.5 (½ sachet)
>10	5 (1 sachet)	5 (1 sachet)

- On arrival at the day ward, a phosphate enema is administered if the stool effluent is not clear according to the following schedule.

Age (years)	Dose of phosphate enema
<5	¼ enema
>10	½ enema

endocarditis should also receive prophylactic antibiotics. Our preference is for single doses of ampicillin (25 mg/kg body weight), gentamicin (2.5 mg/kg body weight) and metronidazole (7.5 mg/kg body weight). The routine use of antibiotics in children undergoing colonoscopy is not necessary.

TECHNIQUE

Colonoscopy can be performed in children under general anesthesia or sedation. The author's preference is for the former. Many children require repeat examinations, and unpleasant memories of a previous colonoscopy under sedation may prejudice cooperation for the future.

Before commencing the colonoscopy, the abdomen should be felt for masses and the anus examined for signs of bleeding or Crohn's disease. Digital rectal examination and proctoscopy should be performed because very low polyps may be missed as the colonoscope is inserted. (**See Figure 28.1**)

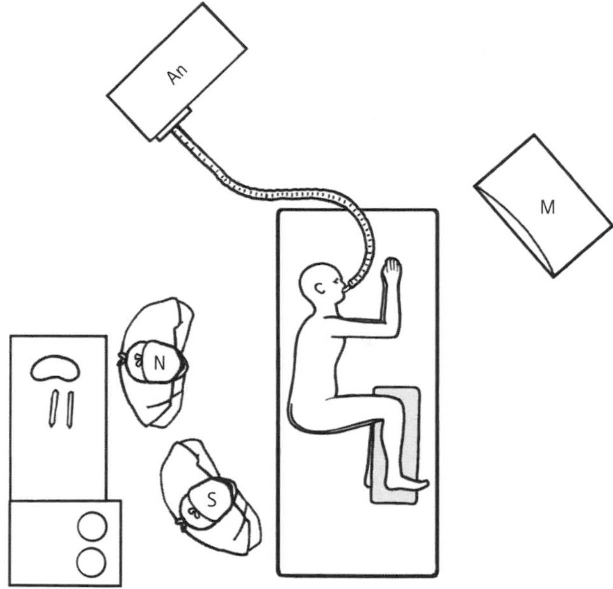

Figure 28.1

The colonoscopy begins with the child in the left lateral position. If the child is particularly small or thin, sandbags can be placed under the hip, under and between the knees and under the ankles to prevent neuropraxia from pressure. The colonoscope is held in the surgeon's left hand. An important skill to acquire early on is the ability to manipulate the direction control wheels (up/down and right/left) with the index finger and thumb of the left hand. This allows the right hand to be free at all times for precise control of insertion, withdrawal and torque of the colonoscope. (**See Figure 28.2**)

The index finger of the surgeon's right hand is inserted into the rectum and the lubricated colonoscope inserted alongside. Air is insufflated to open the rectum and the surgeon then holds the colonoscope about 20 cm from the anal margin with the right hand. The rectum is usually negotiated with relative ease, as the mucosal folds indicate the way forward. (**See Figure 28.3**)

The colonoscope may pass easily into the sigmoid colon, although its tip has to be directed upwards before it can be inserted. Passage along the sigmoid colon is usually straightforward because this part of the colon is open.

The angle between the sigmoid and descending colon can be difficult to negotiate. The colonoscope will tend to form a loop at this stage, which will impede progress (this is

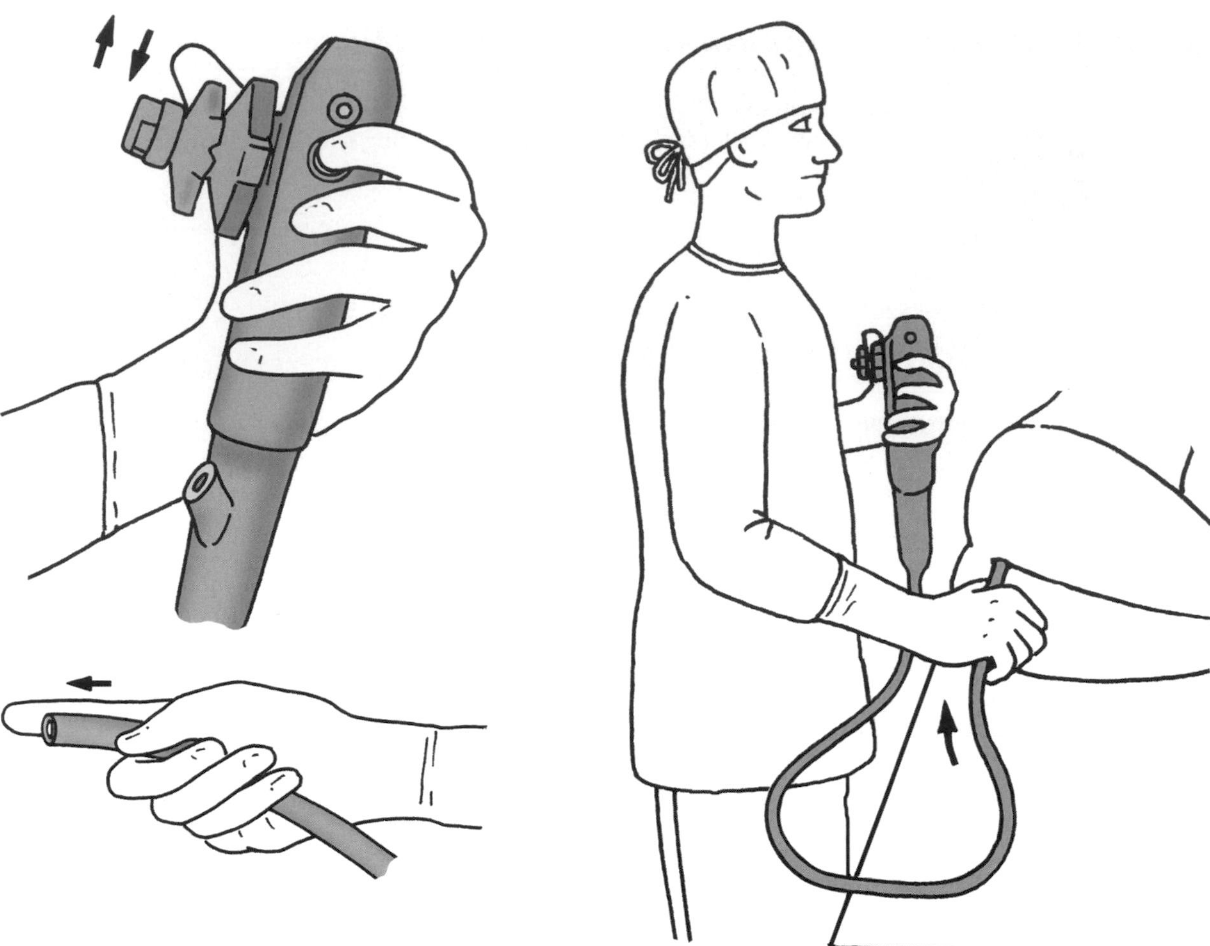

Figure 28.2

discussed in more detail later in the chapter). The descending colon is usually 'closed' and air must be insufflated to visualize the lumen, but once this has been done, passage up to the splenic flexure is relatively easy.

The splenic flexure is the second acute bend encountered during the colonoscopy. In children the angle between the transverse and descending colon tends to be less acute than in adults, making it possible to pass with the endoscope by angling the tip around the flexure. Clockwise torque on the shaft is often required to advance the colonoscope into the transverse colon, which has a characteristic triangular appearance.

Usually it is possible to negotiate the transverse colon quickly, but it can loop if it is long and redundant or if too much air is used. If the colonoscope starts to form a loop, the surgeon will notice what appears to be a bend in mid-transverse colon. Withdrawing the colonoscope slightly and deflating the colon by suction will correct this.

The third true angle encountered during colonoscopy is the hepatic flexure. To the inexperienced, this may appear to be the cecum. However, a blue tinge from the liver seen through the wall of the colon and an impression from the gallbladder will confirm the true position.

Negotiation of the hepatic flexure should be attempted after the colon has been compressed by suction. The tip of the colonoscope is angled around the flexure and often withdrawal of the instrument at this point straightens the transverse colon and results in a paradoxical forward movement of the tip down the ascending colon. The ascending colon is circular and passage down to the cecum is straightforward.

The cecum can be recognized by the appendicular orifice. However, the only certain confirmation is gained by entering the ileum through the ileo-cecal valve. Negotiating the ileo-cecal valve can be difficult because it is often not visible, and if bowel preparation has not been perfect, contamination will occur at this point. The easiest way to identify the ileo-cecal valve is to withdraw the colonoscope from the fundus of the cecal pole into the proximal ascending colon and look for the ileo-cecal ridge. In adults and older children this landmark lies approximately 5 cm from the pole of the cecum. Once the valve, or the raised lip of one edge of the valve, is seen, it is usually possible to angle the tip of the endoscope into it. This may be achieved by advancing beyond the valve, aspirating air and then withdrawing the colonoscope with the tip angled downwards so that it 'falls' into the ileum.

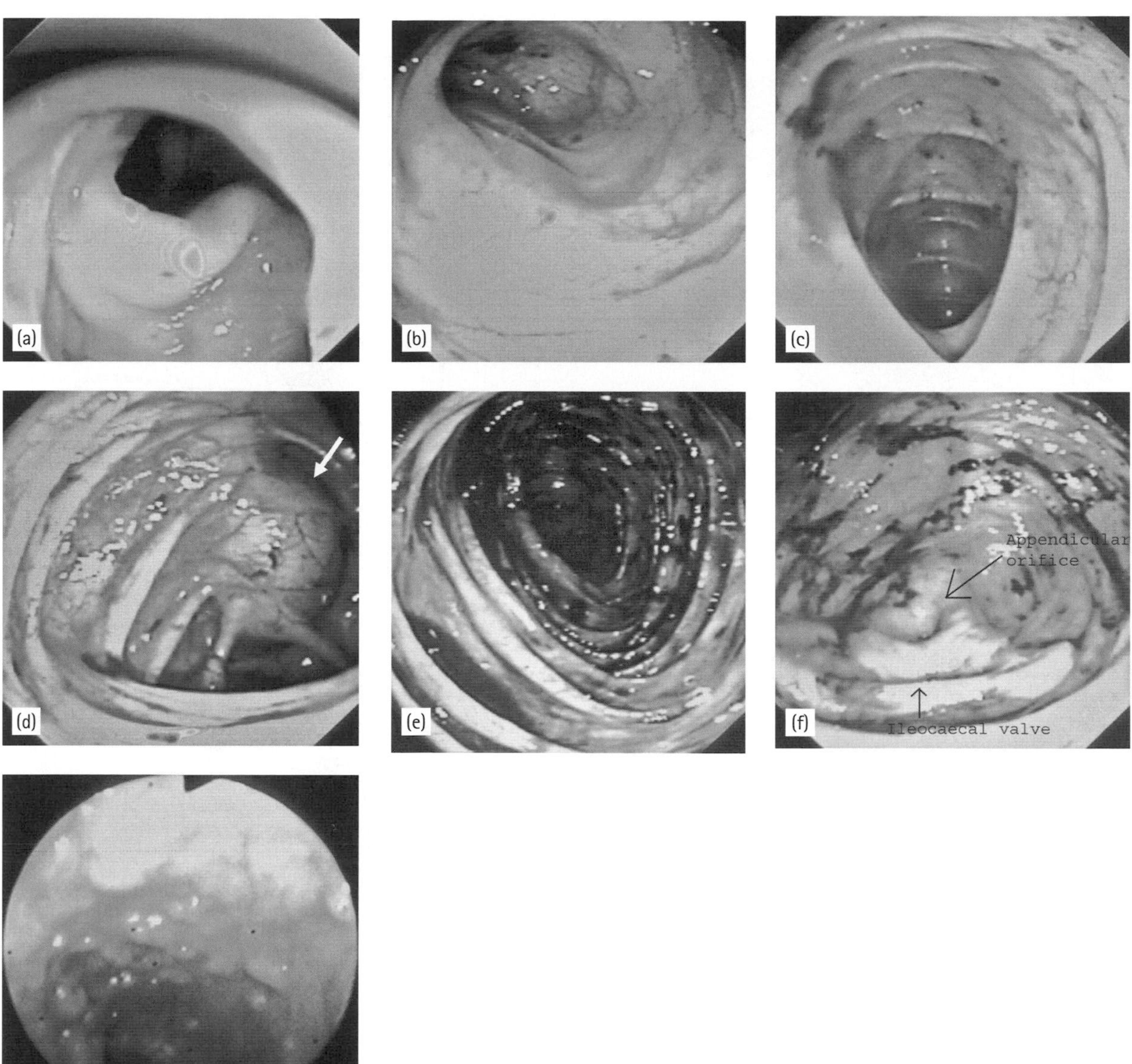

Figure 28.3 *(a) Rectum; (b) sigmoid; (c) transverse colon; (d) hepatic flexure with an impression from the gallbladder; (e) ascending colon; (f) caecum; (g) ileum.*

The appearance of the ileum in children is variable, although lymphoid follicles (Peyer's patches) are usually prominent. The colonoscope can be advanced into the terminal ileum for 5–10 cm to assess the mucosa and take biopsies.

The colonic mucosa must be inspected carefully as the endoscope is withdrawn. Areas of mucosa obscured by stool should be examined after irrigation. It may be necessary to turn the patient to allow circumferential inspection of the mucosal surface. As the instrument is pulled back, air (or CO_2) is aspirated to deflate the colon and minimize postoperative distension and discomfort.

Specific colonoscopic procedures

BIOPSY

This is a standard part of any colonoscopy. An ileal biopsy confirms a full colonoscopy has been performed. If there is obvious pathology, at least two biopsies must be taken. There is some debate about where routine biopsies should be taken. The author's preference is to take two biopsies from the ileum, cecum, ascending colon, transverse colon, descending colon, sigmoid colon and rectum. Biopsies should be taken from the mucosal ridges of the colonic haustra as this minimizes the risk of perforation, particularly in the cecum and ascending colon. Sometimes the haustra can be revealed by deflating the colon slightly. Biopsy site bleeding invariably ceases after a few minutes.

POLYPECTOMY

Small and pedunculated polyps may be removed relatively simply. The treatment of sessile polyps is beyond the scope of this chapter (see 'Further reading' below). Once a polyp is discovered, ensure all the equipment for polypectomy is available and correctly assembled (i.e. ligating snare,

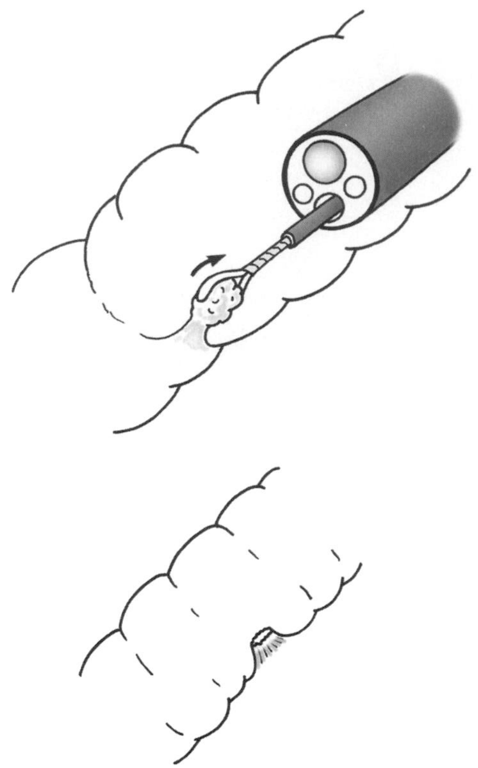

Figure 28.4

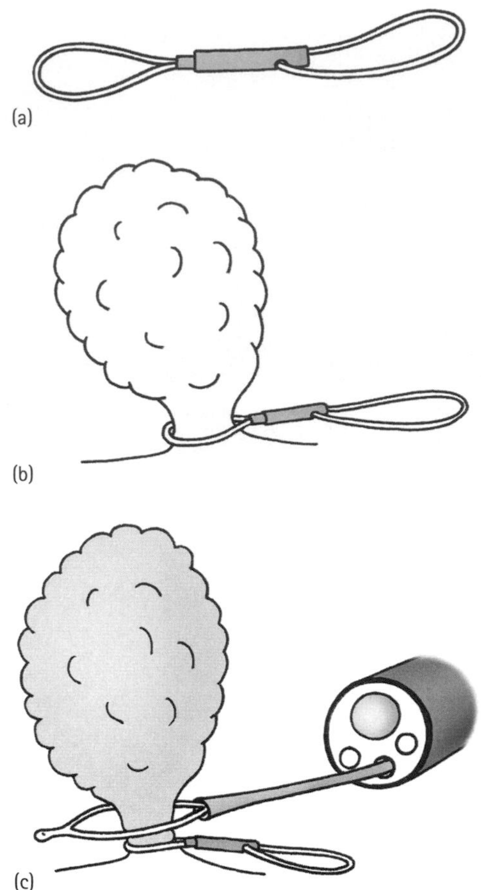

Figure 28.5

electrocautery snare, coagulation setting, diathermy pad and foot pedal).

Small polyps (up to 5 mm in diameter)

- Standard cup biopsy forceps will usually suffice to remove very small polyps (1 mm).
- For larger polyps, the following technique should be used.
  - Grasp the polyp with hot biopsy forceps.
  - Apply gentle traction on the polyp to elevate the surrounding mucosa as a 'pseudo-stalk'.
  - Apply a coagulating current (15 W) for 2–3 seconds. The base of the pseudo-stalk will whiten.
  - Avulse the polyp. A whitened base (termed the 'snow on Mount Fuji' effect) is left behind. **(See Figure 28.4)**

Larger pedunculated polyps

By far the most common polyps seen in children are benign juvenile polyps. Theses are pedunculated and relatively easy to remove with the colonoscope. The safest technique for removing a large polyp involves deploying a detachable snare around its stalk for hemostasis and then using an electrocautery snare for the polypectomy. The ligating snare has to be loaded on to a special applicator (in accordance with the manufacturer's instructions), which is then fed down the colonoscope biopsy channel. **(See Figure 28.5)**

- Encircle the stalk of the polyp with a ligating snare. Ensure that the snare is completely around the polyp. The polyp will change color from bright red to dusky purple as the collar on the ligating loop is tightened. This indicates the snare is tight enough for hemostasis. The snare is then released from the applicator, which is withdrawn from the colonoscope.
- Reload the colonoscope with the electrocautery snare. Carefully maneuver the snare over the stalk of the polyp so that it lies between the ligating snare and polyp itself. Close the snare slowly, ensuring that the polyp does not touch the colonic mucosa, which will short circuit the diathermy.
- Apply coagulation (15 W) continuously whilst *slowly* closing the snare to divide the stalk.
- Retrieve the polyp with either a Dormier basket or tripod grasper. The ligating snare is left behind around base of the stalk of the polyp and will eventually pass per rectum.

COLONOSCOPIC ANTEGRADE CONTINENCE ENEMA (ACE)

This procedure utilizes the principle of percutaneous endoscopic gastrostomy (PEG – see Chapter 23). Standard commercially available 15 Fr PEG tubes are suitable for percutaneous cecostomy. The catheter can be inserted into either the cecum (ACE) or the sigmoid colon (DACE). A PEG tube is inserted initially and after a period of 6–8 weeks can be cut and allowed to pass per rectum, and the track will accept a surface level gastrostomy button device.

- Bowel preparation is per standard colonoscopy.
- In advance of surgery, the optimum site for the cecostomy should be marked on the child's abdomen to ensure this avoids the waistband.
- Prophylactic intravenous antibiotics should be administered at the induction of anesthesia.
- Colonoscopy is performed and the cecum is insufflated until tense. The light from the colonoscope in the cecum can be seen through the anterior abdominal wall and a digital impression on the anterior abdominal wall is seen through the colonoscope.
- The abdominal wall is infiltrated with 0.25 percent levobupivacaine at the site of the cecostomy track.
- A small stab incision is made at the previously marked site and the PEG trocar inserted into the cecum. The guide-wire is inserted and grasped with forceps passed down the colonoscope. Guide-wire, forceps and colonoscope are pulled back through the anus. The cecostomy tube is then attached to the guide-wire and pulled round the colon and out through the track. The tube is secured.
- The washout regimen commences after 24 hours, initially with a small amount of enema solution and washout, increasing daily until the correct combination is found to keep the child clean.
- Six weeks later, the tube can be changed to a surface level gastrostomy button device. This is a simple procedure, which can be performed as a day case under general anesthesia.
  - The PEG tube is cut and the flange pushed into the cecum to pass per rectum. The length of the track through the abdominal wall is measured using a measuring catheter to ensure the correct length of button is inserted.
  - The track may need gentle dilatation to accept a 14 Fr button catheter.
  - A button of the correct length is inserted and the retaining balloon inflated with 5 mL saline.

POSTOPERATIVE CARE

The postoperative recovery should be uneventful. Children may eat and drink after recovery from anesthesia or sedation and may be discharged home the same day. Some children complain of abdominal pain, but this is usually minor and soon settles. Parents should be warned that small amounts of blood may appear in the stools following colonoscopy but that this should settle within 1–2 days. Serious hemorrhage after colonoscopy is exceptionally rare. Sick children with IBD should undergo colonoscopy as an inpatient procedure so that they can commence treatment immediately. Steroids should be avoided prior to colonoscopy as they may hinder histologic diagnosis by their rapid action on mucosal healing.

PROBLEMS, PITFALLS AND SOLUTIONS

The main difficulty encountered during colonoscopy is negotiating the flexures in the colon. Under these circumstances the following maneuvers should be tried.

- Do not push blindly – this causes pain (even in an anesthetized child) and increases the risk of perforation.
- The colonoscope should be advanced by a combination of up/down (left hand on tip direction controls) and torque (right hand on shaft) movements.
  - Clockwise torque is most useful in the sigmoid, descending and distal transverse colon.
  - Anti-clockwise torque is most useful in the proximal/mid-transverse colon.
  - Additional torque (rotating the shaft up to 180°) may help negotiate difficult angles.
- Make movements slowly, especially at the flexures, otherwise the point at which to advance may be missed.
- Consider changing the position of the patient. The shaft of the colonoscope should be held close to the anus to prevent the instrument slipping back down the colon.
  - Begin the colonoscopy with the child in the left lateral position.
  - At the sigmoid–descending colon junction, move the child back to a supine or even right lateral position if the lumen cannot be identified.
  - The splenic flexure may open in the right lateral position.
  - The transverse colon should be easy to negotiate with the patient supine.
  - The hepatic flexure may open in the left lateral position.
  - The ascending colon and cecum will be seen best with the patient supine.
- Use as little insufflation as possible. Gaseous distension will elongate the colon and increase the acuteness of the flexures, making them more difficult to negotiate.
- Keep the shaft of the colonoscope well lubricated.
- The appendicular orifice is often curved and may 'point' to the ileo-cecal valve.
- If not video recording the procedure, take photographs as a record of the findings.

- A thorough examination of the mucosal surface of the colon should be performed as the colonoscope is slowly withdrawn.
- Normal saline should be irrigated down the biopsy channel using a syringe to wash areas of mucosa obscured by stool.
- Colonic spasm can be ameliorated with hyoscine N-butylbromide (Buscopan) 10–20 mg by intravenous injection.
- If a small polyp is seen on insertion, it should be snared immediately and removed because it may prove impossible to locate on withdrawal.
- After completing the colonoscopy, the bowel should be deflated by gentle pressure on the abdomen whilst a finger is holding the anus open. This will minimize postoperative discomfort from colonic distension.

Loop formation during colonoscopy

Loops in the colonoscope tend to occur in the sigmoid and transverse colon. These are problematic for the following reasons.

- A large proportion of the length of the colonoscope shaft will become redundant in the loop, leaving insufficient length to complete the examination.
- It becomes much more difficult to control the direction of the tip of the colonoscope when the instrument is coiled.
- The colon will be stretched by the redundant loop of endoscope, which is painful and increases the risk of accidental perforation.

SIGMOID LOOPS

Two common loops occur in the sigmoid colon – an 'N' loop and an alpha (α) loop.

'N' loops are very common (65 percent in one study) and occur because the sigmoid/descending junction is fixed. If the sigmoid is over-inflated and the stretched, redundant sigmoid colon lifts high out of the pelvis, an 'N' loop forms. To resolve this problem, as soon as the tip of the colonoscope is in the descending colon the endoscope should be withdrawn slowly, ensuring the tip remains in the descending colon. An assistant should then apply pressure with the palm of the hand on the left lower quadrant of the abdomen to prevent the sigmoid colon from lifting into the abdomen. The colonoscope can then be advanced with a clockwise torque to prevent loop recurrence. **(See Figure 28.6)**

Alpha loops often form spontaneously (20 percent in one study). Although an α loop does not hinder the advancement of the colonoscope directly, because there is no acute angulation, it does shorten the functional length of the endoscope and reduce maneuverability of the tip. For this reason it should be removed. With the tip of the colonoscope in the descending colon, near the splenic flexure, the shaft is withdrawn with a clockwise torque applied. This maneuver should be performed slowly, otherwise the tip of the colonoscope is liable to slip back into the sigmoid colon. Once the loop has resolved, the endoscope can be re-inserted maintaining a clockwise torque. If this maneuver fails repeatedly, consider the possibility of a reversed-α loop, which occurs if the descending colon is mobile on a mesentery. The procedure for reducing a reversed-α loop is the same as that for an α loop except that an *anti*-clockwise torque will be required when the colonoscope is re-inserted. **(See Figure 28.7)**

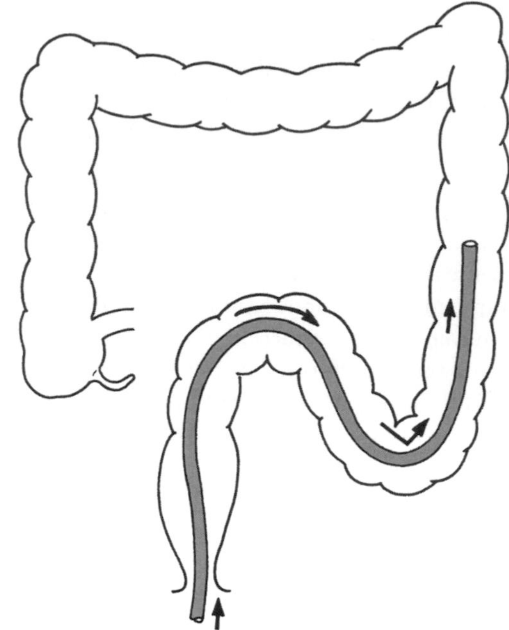

Figure 28.6

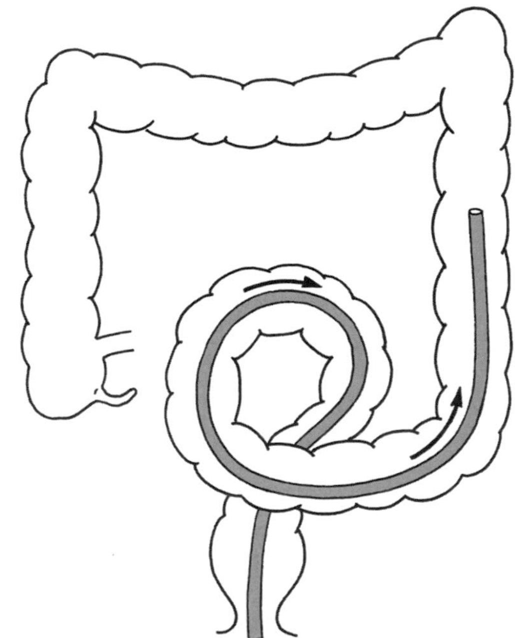

Figure 28.7

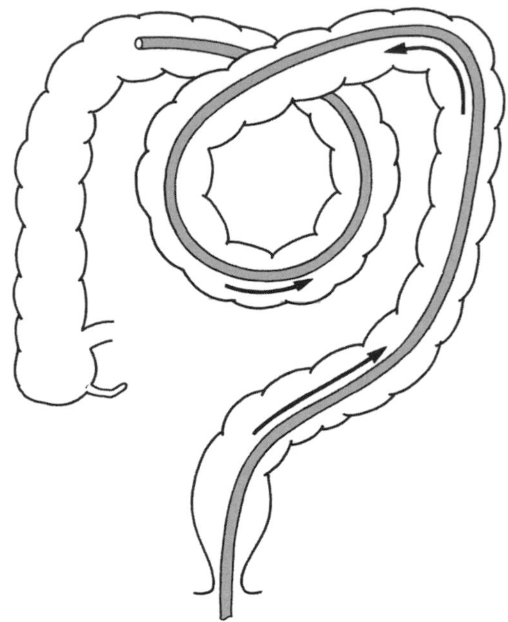

Figure 28.8

TRANSVERSE COLON LOOPS

A long redundant transverse colon will predispose to the formation of either a deep transverse loop or, if this then twists, a gamma (γ) loop (25 percent in one study). **(See Figure 28.8)**

A γ loop may occur spontaneously when negotiating a redundant transverse colon. At the midpoint, the colon descends down towards the pelvis and then twists, forming the loop. A γ loop can be difficult to remove. The colonoscope should be withdrawn slowly with clockwise torque and then advanced after an assistant applies external pressure with a hand in the mid/upper abdomen to prevent the transverse colon descending back towards the pelvis.

Repeated attempts are often necessary to straighten loops encountered during colonoscopy, which may prolong the procedure considerably. There is no doubt that the likelihood of loop formation reduces with experience. The recently developed Olympus ScopeGuide provides real-time electronic imaging of colonoscope position. This improves the frequency and speed of resolution of loops and may be helpful for the trainee colonoscopist. Occasionally it proves impossible to remove a loop. The procedure can be continued provided extreme care is taken and the functional length of the colonoscope is adequate.

Reasons for failure to complete colonoscopy

- Inexperience and persistent loop formation are by far the commonest reasons. Both will improve with practice.
- Equipment failure. This is rare and usually related to light-source failure. It should be remediable and the examination completed.
- Poor bowel preparation. Depending on the degree of contamination of the colon by stool, it may be possible to complete the examination, but the procedure will undoubtedly take longer and there is a higher risk of missing pathology. If the view is inadequate, the examination must be abandoned and the reason for the poor bowel preparation ascertained. If compliance with the purgative is in doubt, the child should be admitted to hospital for supervision of subsequent bowel preparation prior to a repeat colonoscopy.
- Patient discomfort under sedation. The colonoscopy should be rescheduled to be done under general anesthetic.

COMPLICATIONS

Major complications following colonoscopy are rare.

Abdominal distension

Abdominal distension and discomfort are common if the colonoscopy has been particularly difficult and protracted. Minimizing insufflation during colonoscopy is important and scrupulous evacuation of air as the colonoscope is withdrawn will reduce postoperative pain. This problem is reduced if CO_2 is used to insufflate the colon and this also reduces the risk of explosion during diathermy polypectomy.

Perforation

Perforation is the most serious complication of colonoscopy and usually, but not always, occurs after a polypectomy. Perforation should be suspected if the child awakes with severe pain and abdominal distension. A plain abdominal radiograph will confirm the diagnosis. Immediate surgical repair is the treatment of choice, as the bowel is prepared and peritoneal contamination should be minimal. If symptoms develop after discharge from hospital, the child should be re-admitted urgently and investigations undertaken to exclude a delayed perforation. Biopsy in the presence of active IBD carries a higher risk of perforation and requires extra caution when assessing the depth of biopsy.

Bleeding

- Primary – usually post-polypectomy, although it may occur post-biopsy. Hemorrhage can be prevented by performing a polypectomy with a ligating loop around the stalk rather than coagulating the stalk during division. Bleeding may be controlled by re-snaring the stalk, injecting epinephrine (1:10 000) into the surrounding mucosa or applying a hemostatic endoscopic clip to the bleeding point.

- Secondary – may occur 1–14 days post-polypectomy. This usually stops spontaneously, but the patient should be observed until all is well.

Post-polypectomy syndrome

- Secondary to full-thickness heat damage to the colonic wall.
- Occurs following difficult polypectomy, particularly with sessile polyps.
- Symptoms suggest perforation but no free air is seen on abdominal X-ray.
- Treat expectantly with bed rest and antibiotics for 72 hours.

Infection

- Prophylactic antibiotics should be administered to all children at risk of bacterial endocarditis prior to colonoscopy.
- If an acute colitis is suspected or found, it is the author's practice to administer a single dose of intravenous antibiotics (ampicillin 25 mg/kg, gentamicin 2.5 mg/kg and metronidazole 7.5 mg/kg).

FURTHER READING

Cotton PB, Williams CB. *Practical Gastrointestinal Endoscopy*, 4th edn. Oxford: Blackwell Science, 1996.

Saunders BP, Bell GD, Williams CB, Bladen JS, Anderson AP. First clinical results with a real time electronic imager as an aid to colonoscopy. *Gut* 1995; **36**:913–17.

29

Laparoscopy – basic technique

AZAD NAJMALDIN

INTRODUCTION

Laparoscopy is the inspection of the peritoneal cavity by means of a telescope introduced through the abdominal wall after the creation of a pneumoperitoneum.

Laparoscopic surgery is the execution of established and/or new surgical procedures in a way which leads to the reduction of trauma of access, thereby reducing surgical complications, accelerating recovery and improving cosmesis. Surgical procedures are conducted by remote manipulation and dissection within the closed confines of the abdominal cavity or extraperitoneal space under visual control via telescopes, cameras and television screens.

The ability to perform safe and successful laparoscopic procedures relies greatly on the understanding of general and specific principles of surgery, and appropriate application of the equipment and instruments as well as safe access and the creation of a pneumoperitoneum. Failure to do this produces unnecessary complications and puts patients at risk.

This chapter highlights aspects of basic technique in laparoscopy. Further information can be found in Chapters 1 ('Rigid endoscopes'), 3 ('Imaging equipment'), 4 ('Energy used in endoscopic surgery'), 7 ('Instruments in laparoscopy and thoracoscopy'), 8 ('Robotic laparoscopic surgery'), 30 ('Adhesiolysis') and 54 ('Extraperitoneal laparoscopy').

PHYSIOLOGICAL CHANGES

In addition to the usual physiological changes that occur following general anesthesia, drug administration and surgery and the complications of surgery in general, a number of physiological changes can occur as the result of creating a CO_2 pneumoperitoneum/extraperitoneum and of the postural changes involved in patient positioning. These changes may be particularly noticeable in those with pre-existing diseases such as cardiovascular, pulmonary, endocrine and neurological disorders. However, none of the changes is significant if the intra-abdominal pressure is kept below 12 mmHg in newborns/infants and 15 mmHg in older children.

Respiratory changes

- Diaphragmatic displacement will lead to a significant rise in peak airway pressure, increase in physiological dead space, and reduction of lung compliance and functional residual capacity. These and changes in intrathoracic blood volume develop as the result of a pneumoperitoneum, and the Trendelenburg position may lead to atelectasis, shunting and hypoxia.

- During insufflation, CO_2 is readily absorbed into the circulation and removed by the lungs. Inadequate ventilation may lead to significant hypercarbia and acidosis, which in turn causes cardiac dysrhythmia.
- Increased airway pressure helped by the Trendelenburg position may result in pulmonary barotraumas, which may compromise cardiac output.
- Pneumothorax may occur from gas tracking along tissue planes and undetected diaphragmatic hernia. Although mild to moderate pneumothorax is well tolerated, major tension pneumothorax requires immediate abdominal desufflation and a chest drain.
- Gas embolus is exceedingly rare. It is usually caused by accidental intravascular injection of insufflation gas through a misplaced Veress needle or cannula, and forcing of gas into a vein splinted open. Its effects will depend on the rate and volume of gas administered and tend to be less dramatic with CO_2 than with air, as the former is more soluble. Large infusion rates of 3 mL/kg may cause a gas lock at the right atrium and lead to cardiovascular collapse. Cerebral gas embolism may occur in the presence of a right-to-left shunt, e.g. patent cardiac foramen. Gas embolization may be a delayed phenomenon as a result of trapping in the portal circulation.

Cardiovascular changes

A pneumoperitoneum can cause direct pressure on the abdominal arteries and veins and a release of humoral factors, and consequently increased systemic vascular resistance and a fall in cardiac output. These may also lead to a reduction in renal blood flow and urine output.

ANATOMIC CONSIDERATIONS

The principle of endoscopic anatomy is that structures and their relationships to each other are viewed across the television screen in two dimensions instead of the normal three dimensions, with the quality and size altered in accordance with their distance from the telescope as well as with the quality of the camera, light source and monitor in use. Anatomical landmarks and color variations are used to identify structures. Inappropriately planned and placed access cannulae and telescope, technical problems with imaging, adhesions, unexpected enlarged structures and bleeding can greatly hinder the laparoscopic access and view of the anatomical structures. It is important to recognize that in infants and small children, the surface area for access is small, the abdominal wall is thin and highly compliant, the liver margin is below the rib cage, the bladder is largely an intra-abdominal structure, the viscera are close to the anterior abdominal wall and the abdominal cavity is small. In small infants, for example, it may only require 400 mL CO_2 to establish a pneumoperitoneum. The so-called obliterated structures, umbilical vein, arteries and anterior urachus remain relatively large and partially patent in newborns and infants. These anatomical characteristics make access and manipulation in the younger age group more demanding and difficult tasks when compared to older children or adults. On the other hand, young children have well-defined anatomical landmarks due to the lack of excess fat, making the recognition and dissection of structures relatively easy.

PATIENT PREPARATION AND THEATER LAYOUT

The following are important before starting any laparoscopic procedure.

- Informed consent must be obtained for both a laparoscopic and a conventional open approach in case of conversion or emergency use.
- Check that all the required equipment and instruments are available, functioning and compatible.
- The insufflator is set at the required flow and pressure and the display panel is visible to the anesthetist and surgeon.
- The energy power supply (e.g. electrocoagulation or ultrasound) is set at the minimal effective level.
- A conventional set of laparotomy instruments must always be available to use if necessary.
- Inspect and palpate the abdomen for previous scars, enlarged organs, such as liver and spleen, and abdominal masses.

It is important that the urinary bladder is empty before access is obtained through the lower abdominal wall and during lower abdominal laparoscopic procedures. In children, a palpable bladder can be emptied by expression. Catheterization or suprapubic needle aspiration is required if the bladder is palpable but difficult to express, for monitoring renal function and in prolonged lower abdominal procedures. A nasogastric tube is usually necessary to prevent aspiration and to facilitate access to the upper abdomen. A preoperative enema may prove helpful in colonic procedures.

The patient must be properly positioned to facilitate safe access, to optimize exposure and allow for the comfort of the operator. Although laparoscopic surgery can be performed with one monitor, two are preferable so that the surgeon, assistant and scrub nurse can see on either side of the operating table. The monitor should be placed along a straight line with the target organ/operative field in between the operator and the screen. The positions of the operator, assistant and nurse depend on the size of the patient, the procedure to be executed and the surgeon's preference. In upper abdominal procedures, however, the surgeon may find it more comfortable to operate standing between the patient's legs for large patients, or at the foot of

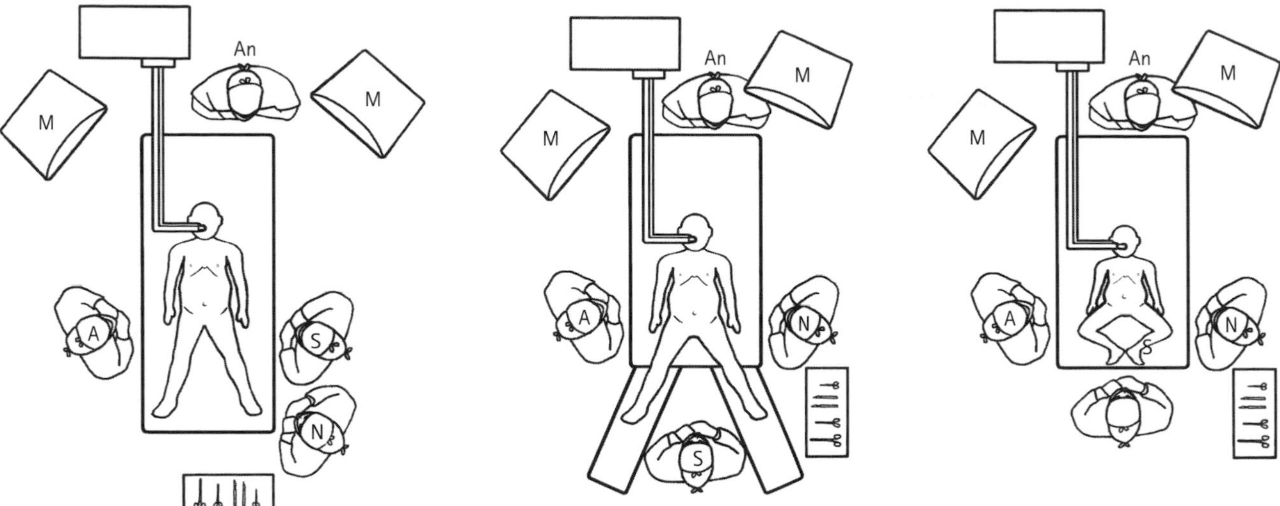

Figure 29.1

the table for infants and small children. A complete lateral or semi-lateral position may be needed for spleen, adrenal and retroperitoneal procedures. Appropriate shoulder and side supports with wedge blocks and strapping secure the patient's position and permit change of position by tilting the table during the procedure. **(See Figure 29.1)**

In pediatric patients, the whole abdomen is usually prepared and draped. This is because the sites of cannulae insertion are often away from the operative field, and an unplanned or additional cannula may be necessary for retraction or manipulation, or wide access may be necessary for conversion to open surgery. The cables and leads are secured to the drapes in such a way that they cause no obstruction to access, the patient and movement around the operating table by the surgeon, anesthetist and theater staff. To prevent interference on the video screen, keep the camera cable separate from that of diathermy. A degree of Trendelenburg position, reversed Trendelenburg or lateral tilt often improves exposure. The heat produced at the end of the light, cable and telescope can be sufficient to burn the drape, patient or internal organs if there is prolonged contact. Further, the high-intensity light can also cause retinal damage if shone directly into the eye. It is therefore important that the light source is switched on, set at the desired intensity, focused and wide balanced when the primary cannula is already in place and the telescope is ready to enter the peritoneal cavity.

CREATING A PNEUMOPERITONEUM AND INSERTION OF THE PRIMARY CANNULA

A pneumoperitoneum may be created by two methods: the closed method (blind technique) using a Veress needle, or the open method (cut-down technique/Hasson's modifications). Whatever method is chosen, it is important to avoid the site of previous abdominal scarring, abdominal wall vessels, major retroperitoneal vessels, large liver and spleen as well as palpable abdominal masses. Carbon dioxide is the insufflation gas of choice because it is safe and rapidly cleared by the lungs, suppresses combustion during coagulation, has no optical distortion and is inexpensive. Oxygen and air support combustion and have a higher risk of embolism. Nitrous oxide has a risk of gas embolism and is hazardous to the theater staff.

Closed method

The Veress needle is usually placed at the site where the primary cannula will be inserted. The most common entry site is just below or above or through the umbilicus. An alternative site along the para-recti, usually left upper or right lower, may be used, especially if the umbilical region is distorted by previous surgical scars or portal hypertension or if there is a large underlying abdominal mass. An initial skin incision to fit the size of the primary cannula is made. A small nick through the linea alba or rectus sheath facilitates the subsequent passage of the primary cannula. First check the needle is sharp, patent and functioning properly. The needle is held in the middle by the thumb and forefingers, the abdominal wall is then grasped and lifted by the other hand below the incision, which stabilizes the abdominal wall and allows the omentum and intestine to fall away from the site of insertion. Carefully insert the needle at an approximately 45° angle (the middle of the pelvic cavity for a needle inserted through the umbilical region). A definite give with a click is usually experienced as the needle passes through the peritoneum. Once the peritoneum is breached, the needle may only be advanced in parallel and on the inner surface of the parietal peritoneum. A properly placed

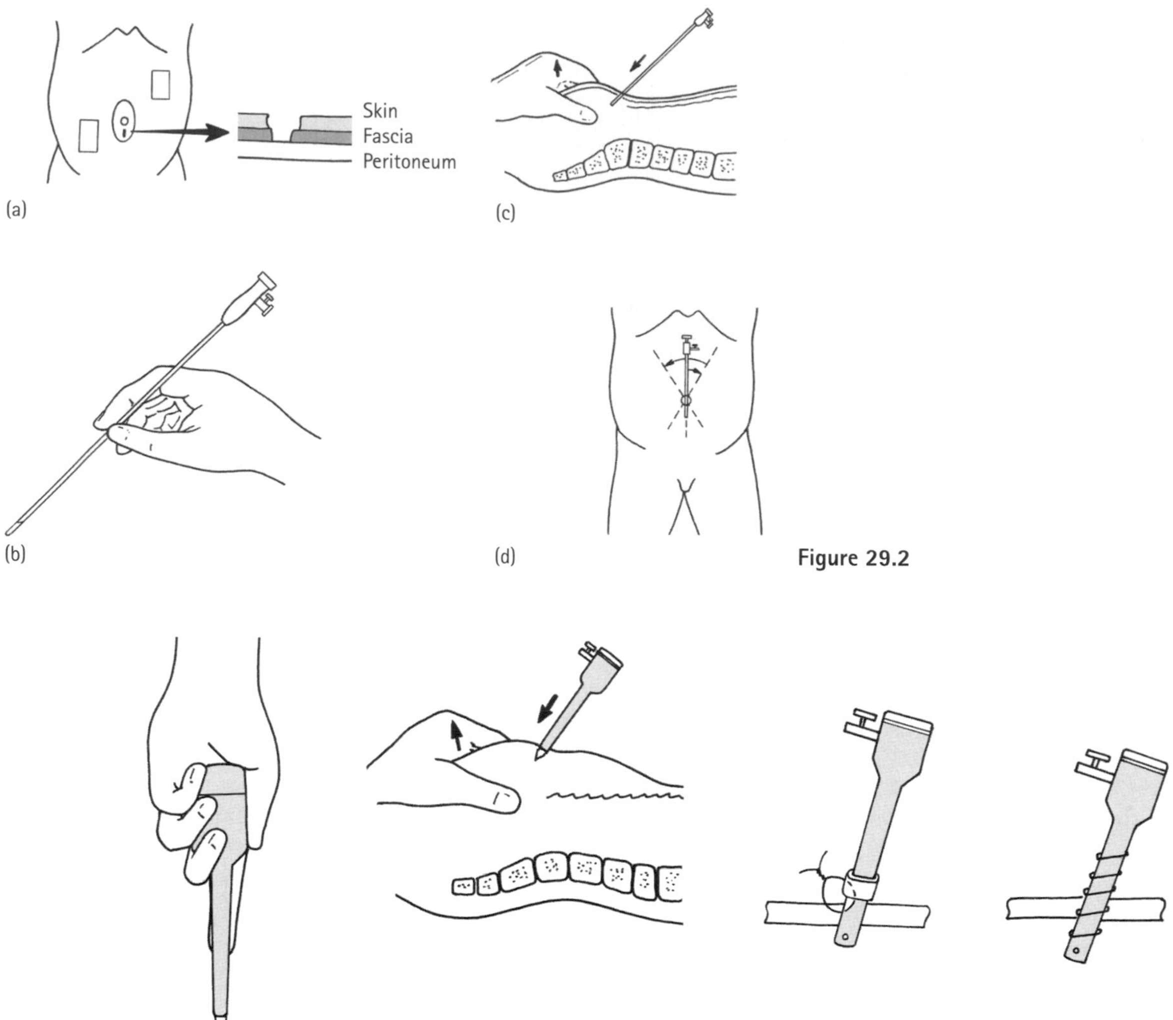

Figure 29.2

Figure 29.3

needle should move freely from side to side on the inner surface of the abdominal wall. **(See Figure 29.2)**

The pneumoperitoneum is established gradually using CO_2 100–1000 mL/min flow and 8–12 mmHg pressure, depending on the size/age of the patient and the procedure to be executed. The pressure should initially be low and rise gradually. High initial pressure (>10 mmHg) indicates that the needle is not in the peritoneal cavity. An established pneumoperitoneum requires approximately 400 mL gas in infants and more than 3 L in adolescents. Throughout the insufflation, the abdomen should expand symmetrically and the patient's ventilation and cardiac output are monitored constantly.

Once the desired pneumoperitoneum has been created, the primary cannula is held in the palm of one hand and the index or middle finger is used along the shaft to act as a stop. The cannula is introduced into the abdominal cavity at an approximately 45° angle through the skin and fascial incisions that were created earlier, while the abdominal wall is grasped and stabilized by the other hand below the site of insertion. A definite give (with an audible click if a cannula with a safety device is used) is experienced as the tip of the cannula passes through the peritoneum. The trocar is then withdrawn and the cannula is advanced 1–2 cm into the abdominal cavity. An initial high pneumoperitoneum pressure (10–15 mmHg depending on the size of the patient) may facilitate a safer insertion of the primary cannula, after which the pressure may be maintained at the desired lower level. For long procedures, a form of cannula fixation (grip-on device or sutures) is advisable to prevent the cannula from falling out and in. The telescope is then inserted and an initial laparoscopy is carried out and the sites of secondary (working) cannulae are selected. **(See Figure 29.3)**

PROBLEMS AND SOLUTIONS

- In a scarred abdomen, a Veress needle may be used a few to several centimeters away from the scar and extreme care must be taken not to injure the viscera. Similar measures are taken if there is a palpable viscera or mass. Here, an open technique laparoscopy maybe considered.

- In an enlarged abdomen, the insertion of a Veress needle may prove difficult secondary to obesity and fluid or gaseous distension of the viscera. A nasogastric tube and/or urinary catheter or even a preoperative enema may prove helpful. The anesthetist should be warned against using anesthetic techniques that might lead to gaseous distension of the stomach and intestinal tract at and after the induction of anesthesia.
- A misplaced Veress needle is the commonest source of complication in laparoscopy but rarely causes significant problems. As described earlier, once the peritoneum is entered, the needle may only be advanced on the inner surface of the abdominal wall, and the inner part of the needle should move freely from side to side. If doubt exists, the following test may be carried out.
  - A 5 mm syringe is used to aspirate blood or visceral content and instil saline, which should flow without resistance and not come back on aspiration. Any saline left in the hub of the needle should disappear rapidly into the peritoneal cavity when the abdominal wall is lifted.
  - The insufflation pressure reading should initially be below 3 mmHg and rise gradually. A high initial pressure or low flow indicates a misplaced needle or an obstructed connection.
  - Asymmetrical expansion of the abdomen indicates a misplaced needle or significant intra-abdominal adhesions.
    - (a) A misplaced needle without aspiration of fluid/blood and insufflation may be repositioned with relative ease. Aspiration of urine is usually not a problem.
    - (b) A misplaced needle with insufflation but without aspiration of fluid or blood usually causes extraperitoneal or omental/mesenteric emphysema. This scenario may hinder subsequent laparoscopy; however, the needle may be withdrawn and repositioned as necessary.
    - (c) A misplaced needle that aspirates bile or visceral content is not necessarily a contraindication for repositioning the needle provided the integrity of the intestinal tract is ensured during the subsequent laparoscopy.
    - (d) A misplaced needle that aspirates blood – see 'Complications' below.
- The primary cannula is too far in. This reduces the effective working space, especially in small infants and in the retroperitoneal space. The cannula may be withdrawn under direct vision through the telescope, which is slightly withdrawn inside the cannula or placed inside a secondary cannula.
- The primary cannula is falling in and out. An anchoring feature built on to the cannula or a specially devised flange or home-made rubber tubing that allows the cannula to be stitched to the abdominal wall prevents cannula displacement.

COMPLICATIONS

- Visceral injury from either the Veress needle or the primary cannula insertion. The former usually causes no significant problems. However, any visceral injury that results from a cannula insertion requires immediate attention, either laparoscopically or through open surgery.
- Vascular injury from Veress needle penetration alone usually results in small or expanding hematomas. The needle should be left in place and insufflation not commenced and, unless the surgeon is an experienced laparoscopist, the procedure should be converted to an open approach to achieve satisfactory hematosis.
- Vascular injury secondary to the primary cannula insertion is potentially lethal. Once suspected:
  - leave the cannula in place to tamponade,
  - do not connect/immediately disconnect insufflation,
  - inform the anesthetist,
  - seek blood for transfusion and help from other surgeons immediately,
  - partially desufflate the abdomen,
  - tip the head of the operating table down,
  - proceed with laparotomy.

COMPLICATIONS OF PNEUMOPERITONEUM

(see also 'Physiological changes' above)

- Gas embolism: this is exceedingly rare and the management should consist of disconnection of the gas flow and desufflation, head-down tilt, general resuscitation and an attempt to aspirate gas from the right cardiac chambers.
- Tension pneumothorax: this is exceedingly rare and requires immediate desufflation and insertion of a chest tube.
- Significant cardiac arrhythmia, hypertension and hypoxia may occur, but exceedingly rarely. They are usually due to a pre-existing pathology or surgical complications.
- Subcutaneous emphysema around the cannula sites is common but requires no active treatment. Emphysema of the head and neck or genitalia may occur from gas tracking along the tissue planes and tends to resolve spontaneously over a short period of time.

Open method

Open technique laparoscopy provides an alternative safe method for insertion of the primary cannula and creation of a pneumoperitoneum. This is particularly so in scarred abdomen, in very young infants and in the presence of intestinal distension or visceromegaly and large intra-abdominal

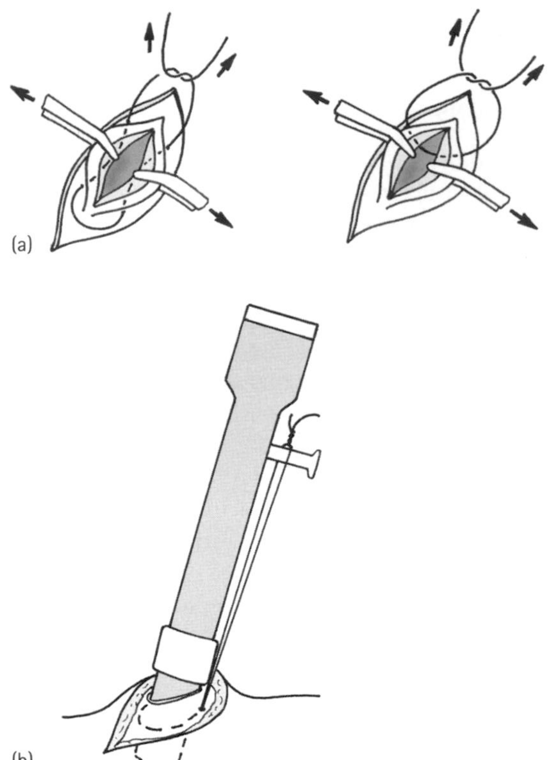

Figure 29.4

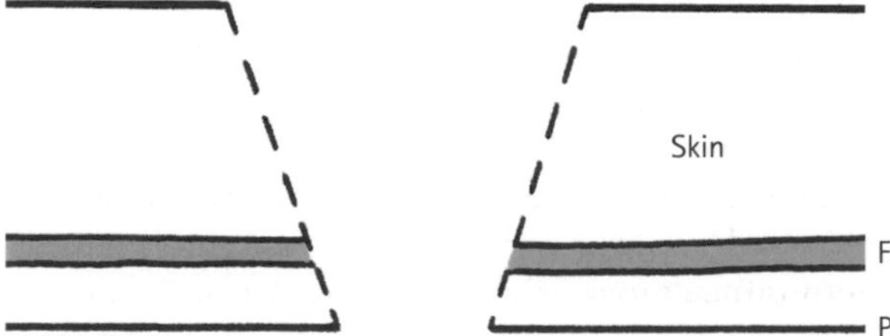

Figure 29.5

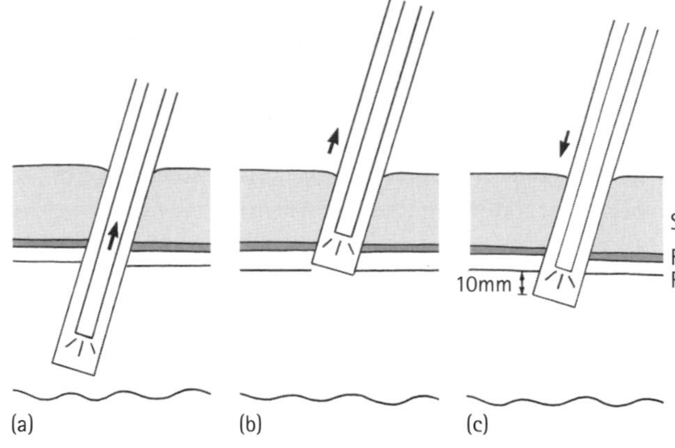

Figure 29.6

masses. It is the technique of choice for extraperitoneal laparoscopy.

The primary cannula may be placed anywhere in the abdominal wall depending on the nature of the procedure to be executed, the size of the patient and the surgeon's preference. A skin crease incision to fit the size of the primary cannula is made usually at or around the umbilical region. The linea alba is exposed and incised longitudinally and the edges are picked up with mosquito forceps. An incision is then made through the peritoneum and a 2-0 either purse-string or simple suture is inserted. Care must be taken to include both the strong fascia and peritoneum with each bite. An ordinary 'primary' cannula is pushed off its trocar through the incision into the abdominal cavity and secured with a single throw of suture, thus allowing snug opposition of the fascia/muscle to the cannula and thereby preventing a gas leak. The suture is then secured around the gas port of the cannula, allowing 1–2 cm of cannula to remain inside the abdominal cavity. A cuff of pre-adjusted rubber tube or a purpose-made phalange on the cannula may be used to prevent the cannula from falling into the peritoneal cavity. Alternatively, a modified Hasson's cannula may be used. **(See Figure 29.4)**

PROBLEMS AND SOLUTIONS

- Access in obese children. The incision should be made larger than usual, with the skin component being cut longer than the fascia. **(See Figure 29.5)**
- Access in scarred abdomen. The peritoneum is incised carefully and the underlying adherent bowels or omentum are released before insertion of the suture and cannula, and, if necessary, the incision is enlarged first before it is closed partially to fit the size of the cannula. In case of difficulty, consider an alternative site. Preoperative assessment including ultrasound scan of the abdomen may help to localize the adhesions.
- Cannula too far inside the abdomen. This is not an uncommon problem in obese children, which reduces the effectiveness of the working space created. Measure the thickness of the abdominal wall against the length of the cannula. If necessary, push the cannula far inside first, then readjust its position, with the telescope being withdrawn slightly inside the cannula. **(See Figure 29.6)**
- Gas leak around the cannula. This is not usually a major source of trouble. Avoid unnecessarily long fascial incision. A tight suture (purse-string or simple) or Hasson's cannula might minimize the risk.

COMPLICATIONS

Poor technique is the only factor that may predispose the open method of laparoscopy to the danger of intestinal injury.

SECONDARY CANNULA INSERTION

The position and number of secondary cannulae depend on the type of surgical procedure to be executed, the size of the patient and the presence or absence of abdominal scarring and coexisting abdominal pathology. The cannulae that are used for the working instruments (manipulation, dissection, suturing etc.) are best sited on either side and in front of the telescope at a 45–125° angle to allow easier eye/hand coordination and manipulation and to keep the instruments in view at all times. Straight-line instruments are very difficult to work with and instruments entering the abdomen against the line of view give mirror imaging and are consequently difficult to manipulate. Avoid placing the cannulae too close to the operative field to allow enough space for the instruments to be manipulated and to avoid cannula/instrument clash. Placing the cannulae close to bony landmarks restricts free cannula/instrument movement.

A small incision that matches exactly the diameter of the cannula and a small nick in the underlying fascia facilitate insertion of the trocar/cannula. As for insertion of the primary cannula (closed method), it is advisable to stabilize the abdominal wall anteriorly with one hand and to proceed carefully with insertion of the trocar/cannula with the index or middle finger acting as a stop, using a gentle continuous pressure and rotating movement. The direction of insertion should be perpendicular through the skin and muscle/fascia, oblique through the peritoneum towards the operative field, and parallel to the abdominal wall as soon as the tip of the trocar becomes visible. The point of entry into the peritoneal cavity must be placed under vision. An oblique route of entry through the abdominal wall is slightly more difficult than the direct 'perpendicular', but has the advantages of reducing the risk of gas leak preoperatively and herniation of viscera through the cannula site postoperatively. Abdominal wall vessels may be avoided by transillumination or viewing from within. It is advisable to fix all busy secondary 'working' cannulae by means of anchoring devices or stitches through the abdominal wall. An instrument that does not require change during the procedure may be introduced into the abdominal cavity without a cannula (e.g. retractor). **(See Figure 29.7)**

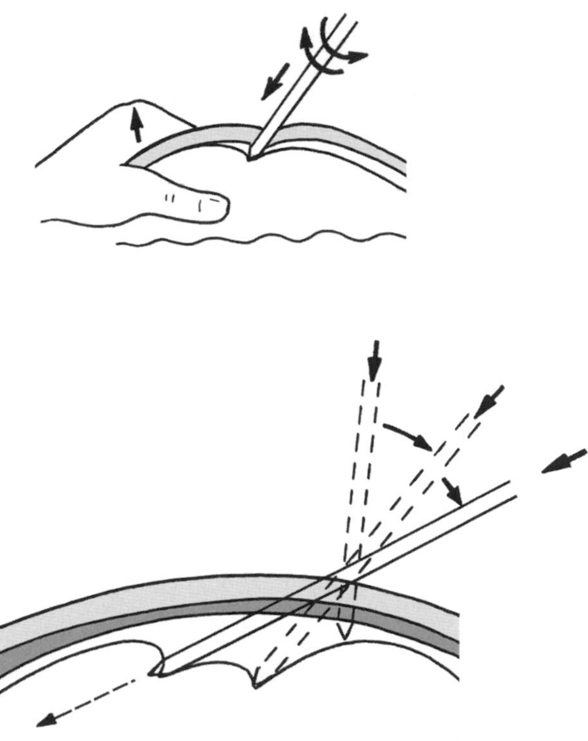

Figure 29.7

PROBLEMS AND SOLUTIONS

- Difficult insertion. In children, the abdominal wall is highly compliant and the peritoneum tends to move ahead of the trocar. This is particularly so with an oblique route of entry, lower abdominal insertion, large trocar/cannulae and low insufflation pressure (below 10 mmHg).
  - Ensure that re-usable cannulae are sharp and that disposable cannulae with safety devices are functioning properly.
  - Stabilize the abdominal wall by grasping it with the hand against the direction of entry. Excessive grasping pressure may cause skin bruising.
  - Use the direct 'perpendicular' route of entry all the way.
  - Direct the trocar/cannula into the primary port, with the telescope being withdrawn sufficiently to avoid damaging the scope, or into another secondary cannula.
  - Remove the trocar and cut the peritoneum with a sharp instrument inserted through the cannula or another secondary cannula.
  - Exert counter-traction using an instrument inserted through another secondary cannula. **(See Figure 29.8)**
  - Consider using Step™ port cannulae, which are probably easier and safer to place.
- Abdominal wall hemorrhage. This is usually minor, but significant hemorrhage from deep epigastric vessels may cause problems. Press the cannula in the direction of the bleed and, if necessary, one or more ligatures inserted either intracorporeally or percutaneously should be sufficient to stop the bleeding. Alternatively, a Foley catheter may be inserted through the cannula site, the balloon inflated and traction exerted until the bleeding stops.
- Cannula dislodgement. As for the primary cannula, anchoring devices and sutures minimize the risk of cannula dislodgement. Replace the trocar and re-advance the cannula as necessary.
- Gas leak or loss of pneumoperitoneum. Ensure the gas supply is adequate, the insufflator is functioning and all connections are tight and patent. Non-compatible instruments/cannula, faulty valves and damaged rubber gas sealant are common the causes of gas leak. A large incision around the cannula may be obliterated by a suture; alternatively, replace the cannula with one of larger diameter. Consider closing the site and placing the cannula at a different location, or use a Step™ port (cannula).
- Adhesions. Adhesiolysis may be necessary to create room for the placement of the secondary cannulae.

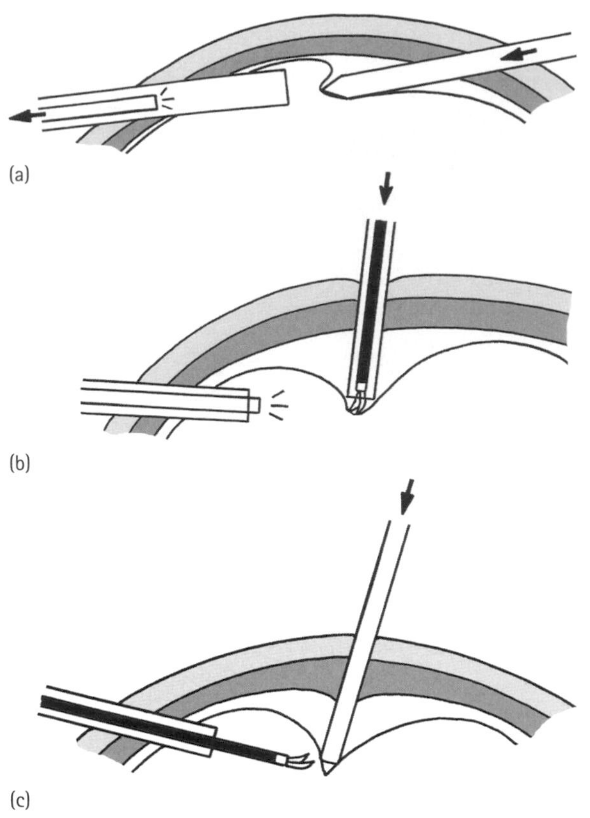

Figure 29.8 *(a) Secondary cannula into the primary cannula; (b) cutting peritoneum within; (c) cutting peritoneum from another cannula.*

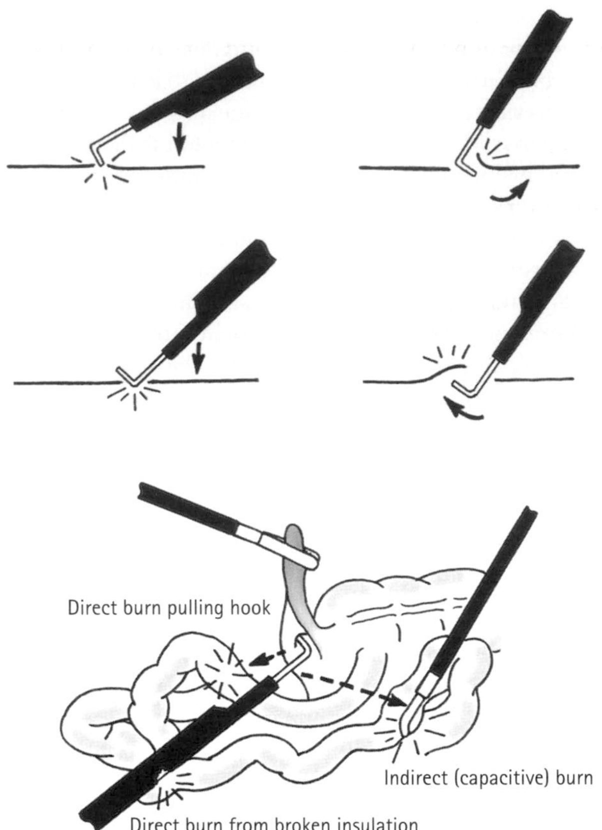

Figure 29.9

MANIPULATION AND DISSECTION

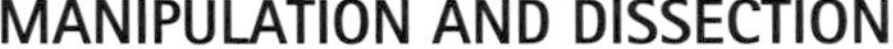

Laparoscopic surgery is a combination of manipulation, retraction, sharp and blunt dissection, hemostasis, suction/irrigation and suturing. As a rule, the tip of all instruments, particularly sharp ones entering, moving or leaving the operative field, must be kept under vision. Tissue planes and structures are exposed by careful manipulation. Access can be improved by gravity shift and retraction. Sharp dissection is achieved by scissors, diathermy energy or Harmonic Scalpel®. Blunt dissection may be carried out by the tip of the scissors and atraumatic grasping forceps as well as by pleglet swabs. Strands of tissue and minor adhesions can be disrupted by careful stripping maneuvers using two sets of atraumatic grasping forceps.

ELECTROCOAGULATION

Monopolar coagulation or cutting current is used commonly, but bipolar coagulation is accepted to be a safer option. With the monopolar system, coagulation is best achieved by grasping the vessel with fine atraumatic and insulated forceps whilst the energy is delivered. Cutting is achieved by either touching or pulling using a fine probe (needle, hook shaped). Alternatively, diathermy scissors may be used, in which case their insulation sleeve should be long enough to reach the blades in order to avoid thermal injury to the surrounding tissues. Care must be taken not to injure other tissues by direct or indirect contact/capacitive coupling. As a rule, the power setting should be minimum, never activate before contact with the tissue and never use a combination of metal cannula and plastic anchoring device, but instead use either all metal or all plastic. After use, the tip of the diathermy instrument remains hot and can easily burn tissue on contact. (**See Figure 29.9**)

The recently developed bipolar-based devices, namely LigaSure™ and plasma kinetic devices, are becoming increasingly popular. They are particularly useful to secure 2–5 mm vessels.

HIGH-ENERGY ULTRASOUND

The ultrasound-activated scalpel/shears deliver energy at 55 kHz vibration and the mechanism for coagulation is similar to that of diathermy. The scalpel produces cutting and coagulation by its sharp edge and flat side respectively. The shears have two blades for cutting and coagulation and are usually applied to vessels less than 2 mm in diameter. Although it produces a slight mist, the device has the advantages of being smokeless and of producing no direct tissue injury beyond the blades.

HEMOSTASIS

During laparoscopic surgery, bleeding is one of the most common causes of conversion to open surgery. Therefore, prevention of hemorrhage by careful manipulation and dissection and appropriate application of cutting and coagulation energy should remain one of the most important principles in laparoscopic surgery. Small vessels may be coagulated by electrocautery or ultrasound. Larger vessels are clipped, ligated or stapled. The new-generation ultrasound shears, LigaSure™ and plasma kinetic energy devices are increasingly used instead of clips and ligatures for 5 mm or even 7 mm vessels. During laparoscopy, minor hemorrhage often appears major because of the magnification. Blood absorbs light and laparoscopic viewing becomes poor in the presence of hemorrhage and a suction irrigation system should always be available for use when bleeding is expected. However, blood clots can be difficult to aspirate via 3–5 mm suction probes.

SUCTION IRRIGATION

A saline drip stand and conventional suction unit connected to a two-way, single-lumen probe that has an easy to operate hand unit (trumpet valve hand unit is the best) is a simple and effective way to achieve suction and irrigation during laparoscopic surgery. If desired, antibiotics/antiseptics or even heparin and anesthetic agents may be mixed with the irrigation fluid. Often omentum, mesentery and intestinal wall are sucked onto the suction probe, and care must be taken to release these before the probe is withdrawn into the cannula. This may be achieved by switching off the suction, transiently switching on the irrigation and gently manipulating the trapped tissue. In general, use a low but adequate suction power and, to avoid rapid loss of pneumoperitoneum, keep the fenestrated end of the probe below the level of fluid to be aspirated.

KNOTTING

Proper knotting is essential in laparoscopic ligation and suturing. External one-way slip knots (Roder) or surgeon's knots (Reef) are less popular than the internal knot.

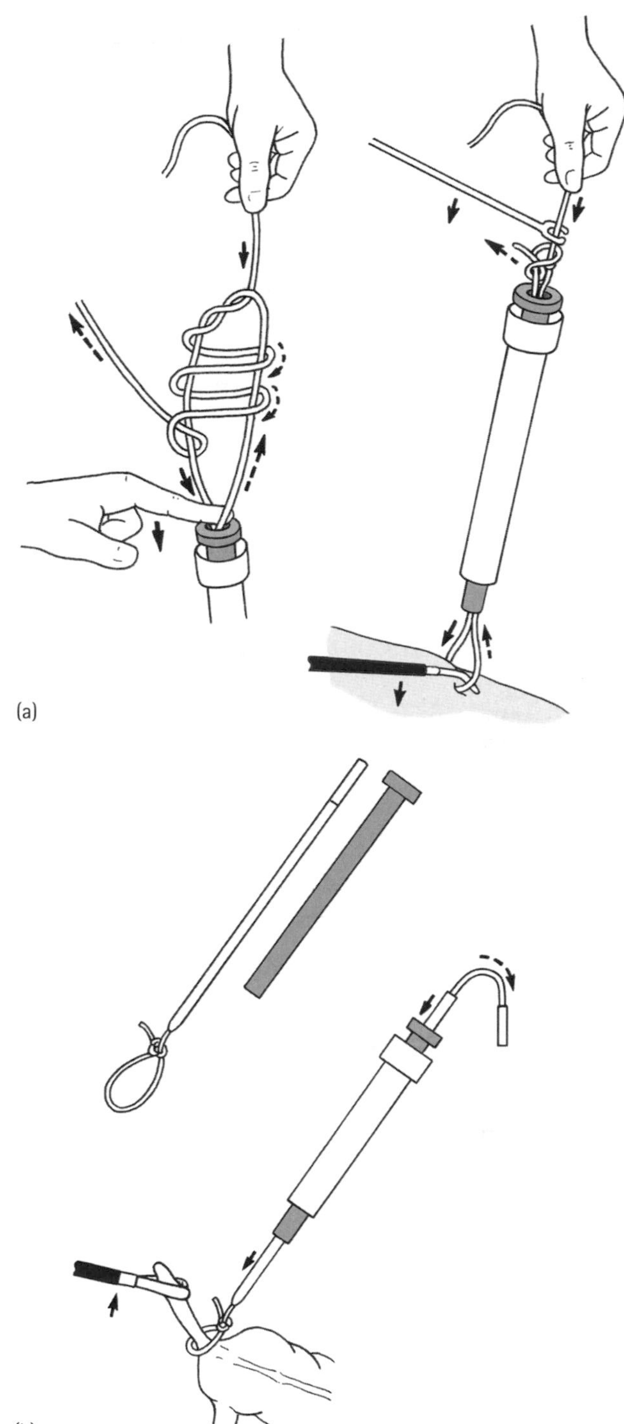

Figure 29.10 *(a) External knotting; (b) a pre-tied loop.*

To tie an external knot, a suture applicator and a knot pusher are required. The disadvantages of external knotting are that it:

- is more cumbersome to perform, at least initially, and requires more length of suture material than internal knotting,
- is unsuitable for continuous suturing,

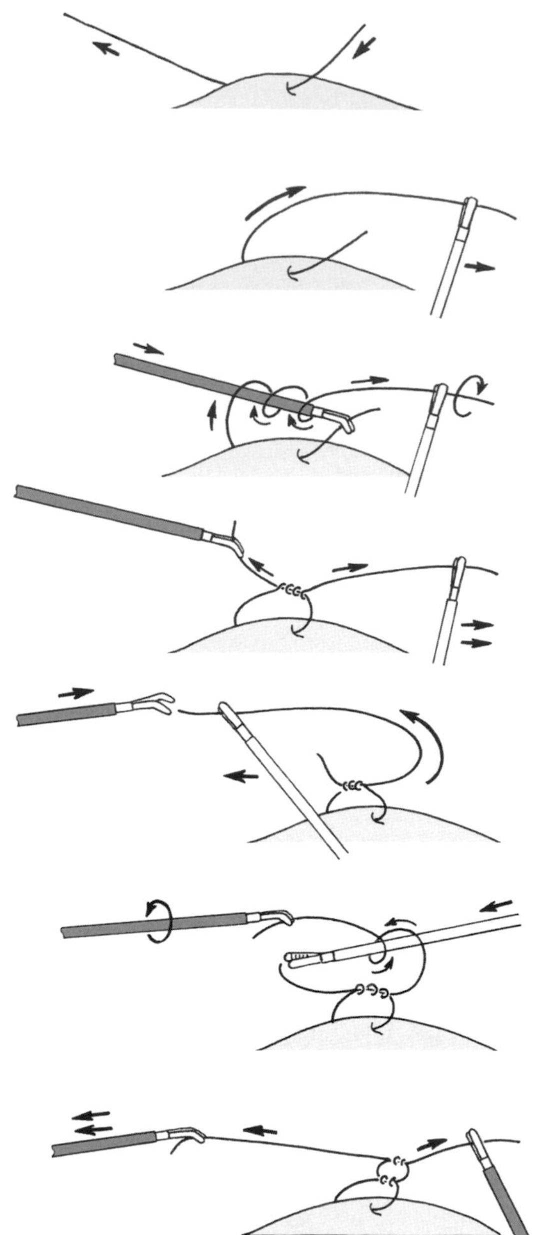

Figure 29.11

- has the potential to damage tissue by serration,
- is unreliable with certain suture materials.

A commercially available pre-tied loop of suture material with a push rod and introducer can be used as a single ligature around most vascular pedicles and tubular structures. (**See Figure 29.10**)

For a beginner, internal knotting is one of the most difficult tasks to perform in laparoscopic surgery. With practice, it can be executed easily, effectively and quickly. The technique suits most suture materials and all purposes. Care must be taken not to weaken or break the suture by rough handling and, until experience is acquired, use a short length of suture, approximately 8–12 cm long, for each individual ligature/suture. (**See Figure 29.11**)

SUTURING

Laparoscopic suturing requires considerable practice and its principle is similar to that of open surgery. Straight, ski or curved needles may be used. However, the size of the curved needle to be used in laparoscopy is dictated by the diameter of the available access working cannula (e.g. a half-circle needle on 3-0 material requires a 10 mm or larger cannula). If desired, an ordinary curved needle may be partly or completely straightened or made into a ski shape. Suturing requires a needle holder to introduce the needle/suture material and a second needle holder or curved or straight atraumatic grasping forceps to assist. It is important that both instruments have boxed-in hinges to allow a smooth glide over the instrument and prevent tangling at the hinge.

First prepare and align the tissue, then introduce the suture by grasping either the needle in the line of the needle holder or the suture near the needle. The point of entry and leaving the abdominal cavity must always be kept under vision. To avoid jamming the needle within small cannulae, it is held head-on in the line of the needle holder. A large ski, straight or partly straightened out needle/suture may be passed percutaneously into the peritoneal cavity.

The second instrument is used to assist in introducing the suture and knotting. Care must be taken not to grasp the suture material hard, thereby weakening or even breaking it. An intracorporeal needle can cause visceral injury and therefore care must be taken when handling needles and their tips must be kept in laparoscopic view at all times. During continuous suturing, a rubber-shod grasper through a third cannula may be used to maintain tension and stabilize the suture. (**See Figure 29.12**)

CLIPS AND STAPLES

The application of a metal or absorbable ligature clip is a simple and effective means of completely occluding small and medium-sized vessels and other ductal structures. It is important that the clip applier approaches the target structure at an angle that allows the surgeon to view the clip as it passes across the structure to be ligated, to ensure safe application and to confirm that no other tissue is trapped within the jaws of the applier. It is advisable to use two clips on the proximal side of structures. Modified, absorbable, self-locking clips are becoming increasingly popular. Metal clips are likely to interfere with radiographic and magnetic imaging, although the titanium clip does not interfere with magnetic resonance imaging.

Adequately prepare the structure to be clipped and hold it in atraumatic grasping forceps. Then insert the loaded

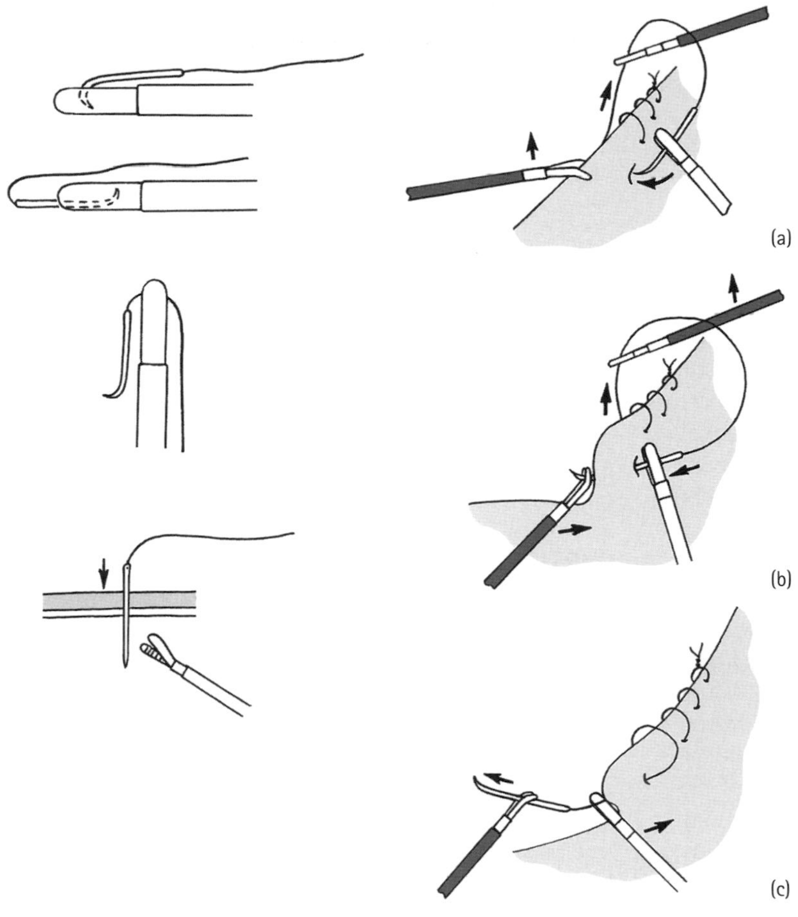

Figure 29.12

applier in full laparoscopic view and place it across the structure. Gently rotate the shaft of the applier to ensure safe and correct positioning of the clip before gently squeezing its handles. Before the grip on the handles is released, move the grasping forceps and re-position to prepare for the application of the second clip.

A linear stapler with a rotatable shaft delivers four to six rows of metal clips while its knife cuts the tissue in the middle. This device allows safe and secure occlusion and division of major vascular pedicles and hollow organs such as the intestinal tract.

IMAGING PROBLEMS

High-quality imaging is critical in laparoscopy. Problems with imaging are a common occurrence and can happen at any time during the procedure. They can be dangerous, time-consuming and very frustrating. The need for quality camera, light source, telescope, connecting cables and television screen cannot be over-emphasized.

- Check that the light cable is compatible with both the telescope and the light source.
- Poor imaging, total blackout and interference on screen can be caused by faulty equipment and/or connections.
- To minimize interference, place the diathermy cable, generator and socket away from the camera system.
- Glare occurs as the result of disturbance of the balance of light intensity by the camera.
- Dark images are usually due to low light intensity secondary to low light output, an old and broken light cable or a camera reaction to high reflection of light from polished metal instruments. Blood in the peritoneal cavity absorbs light, thereby reducing the amount of reflected light, which results in dark images.
- Blurred or poor imaging is usually due to inadequate focusing of the camera, light imbalance, mismatch between camera/light source and telescope, loose connections, moisture and debris at the interfaces (cables, camera and telescope) or a telescope tip contaminated with peritoneal fluid and blood. A quick wipe or rinse inside or outside the peritoneal cavity should restore proper imaging.
- Fogging is often due to a cold telescope and/or cold CO_2 blowing at the telescope from its cannula. Keep the telescope warm before use or use anti-fogging

solutions, and change the port of the gas entry from the telescope cannula to another if possible.
- Smoke and snow storm occur as the result of internal tissue coagulation. Intermittent desufflation via cannula valves clears the space.

EXITING THE ABDOMEN

At the end of the procedure, the operative field and the areas close to the access cannulae are thoroughly inspected for bleeding and signs of inadvertent injury. Hollow viscous perforations may remain unrecognized at the time of operation, but present late with peritonitis, intra-abdominal sepsis or cutaneous fistula. Check for peri-cannula bleeding before and after removing the cannula. At this stage of the procedure, an abdominal wall bleed may require intracorporeal or percutaneously applied simple or square stitches. **(See Figure 29.13)** Remove all instruments and secondary cannulae under vision and ensure omentum is not pulled up into the cannula/cannulae site(s) and evacuate the pneumoperitoneum completely just before or at removal of the last (telescope) cannula. The fascial incisions of cannulae site greater than 4 mm should be sutured with absorbable material. Local infiltration of the wound with an appropriate dose of anesthetic agent may provide adequate pain relief for a few to several hours postoperatively. Some surgeons prefer local infiltration at the time of insertion of laparoscopic cannulae. Skin closure may be obtained using adhesive strips or subcutaneous fine absorbable sutures.

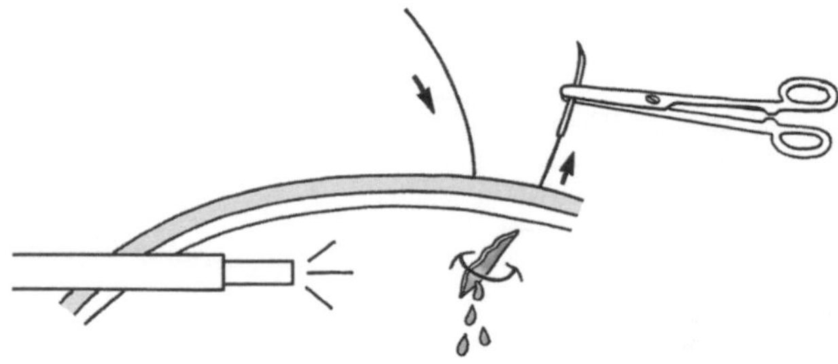

Figure 29.13 *Percutaneous stitch under vision.*

FURTHER READING

Cuschieri A, Buess G, Perissat J (eds). *Operative Manual of Endoscopic Surgery.* Berlin: Springer-Verlag, 1992.

Denziel DJ, Milikan KW, Economou SG, Doolas A, Sung-Tao K, Airan MC. Complications of laparoscopic cholecystectomy: A national survey of 4292 hospitals and an analysis of 77604 cases. *American Journal of Surgery* 1993; **165**:9–14.

Najmaldin A, Guillou P (eds). *A Guide to Laparoscopic Surgery.* Oxford: Blackwell Sciences, 1998.

30

Adhesiolysis

CARROLL M. HARMON AND TAMIR H. KESHEN

INTRODUCTION

Adhesion formation occurs frequently after abdominal and pelvic operations. Approximately 93 percent of patients form postoperative adhesions. These adhesions may lead to acute small bowel obstruction, (partial and complete), recurrent bowel obstruction or chronic abdominal pain. In a study of 1476 children undergoing laparotomy, 2.2 percent had adhesive obstruction, 70 percent of which are caused by a single adhesive band. Classically, open laparotomy has been the method of treatment for intestinal adhesive obstruction. However, over the past decade, exploratory laparoscopy and laparoscopic adhesiolysis have become acceptable, safe methods of diagnosing and treating this disease, with excellent long-term results and minimal morbidity.

Indications

- Acute small bowel obstruction.
- Recurrent small bowel obstruction.
- Chronic abdominal pain.
- Access during other laparoscopic procedures.

Contraindications

ABSOLUTE

- Hemodynamic instability.
- Inability to obtain adequate pneumoperitoneum.

RELATIVE

- Dense, diffuse adhesions.
- Poor visualization (inability to place additional ports under direct visualization).
- Necrotic bowel.

The indications for conversion to laparotomy are discussed later in the chapter.

EQUIPMENT/INSTRUMENTS

Essential

- Three 3–5 mm cannulae (preferably disposable, expandable Interdyne trocar), long or short (depending on patient's body habitus) with reducers.
- Veress needle.
- 4–5 mm, 30–45° angled telescope.
- 3.5–5 mm curved, double-jaw action, insulated scissors with diathermy point.
- Two 3.5–5 mm atraumatic, insulated bowel grasping forceps (non-ratcheted).
- 3.5–5 mm atraumatic, curved, insulated forceps.
- 3.5–5 mm monopolar or dipolar fine hook cautery device.
- 3.5–5 mm needle driver.
- 3-0 silk or Vicryl® suture.

Optional

- Fourth or fifth 5 mm cannula for additional retraction.
- 5 mm Harmonic Scalpel®.
- 5 mm bipolar sealing device (LigaSure™ or equivalent).
- 5 mm clip applicator.
- 5 mm suction/irrigation device.

The size and length of the cannulae depend on the size of the patient and of the available instruments. In an attempt to be as delicate with the tissue as possible, non-ratcheted instruments designed to grasp the bowel are preferred. Both 3.5 mm and 5 mm instruments can perform the procedure well. Other grasping instruments with ends that appose along their entire length (thus distributing pressure evenly along the tissue) are also appropriate when running the length of the small intestine.

The ultrasonic scalpel/shears is an excellent dissecting tool for both blunt and sharp dissection (especially for dense adhesions), but be wary that the tips of the scalpel emit intense heat that may necrose the bowel if touched.

PREOPERATIVE PREPARATION

A complete and detailed history with an emphasis on previous abdominal/pelvic operations and their indications must be obtained. Abdominal X-rays and upper gastrointestinal (GI) contrast study with small bowel follow-through may help pinpoint the area of obstruction. Occasionally, abdominal computerized tomography (CT) scan with oral contrast may help identify both the location of obstruction and the cause. Preoperative ultrasonographic imaging has been reported in adults and children to be beneficial in estimating the degree of visceral immobility secondary to adhesions and assisting in safe trocar placement. In the presence of acute small intestinal obstruction, placement of a nasogastric tube, intravenous infusion of an isotonic solution for rehydration, NPO (nothing by mouth) status and serial abdominal examination are indicated. Broad-spectrum intravenous antibiotics should be administered perioperatively. If free intraperitoneal air is identified, emergency laparoscopy is indicated. In the absence of free air and with no improvement on physical exam or radiographic studies within 24–48 hours of diagnosis, or recurrence of intestinal obstruction requiring more than two hospitalizations, the typical patient should undergo laparoscopy.

TECHNIQUE

General preparation

General endotracheal anesthesia with complete muscle relaxation is the preferred method. It is helpful to discuss with the anesthesiologist the advantages of minimizing gaseous distension of the GI tract during mask ventilation. Nasogastric tube placement with continuous suction facilitates a decompressed stomach and small intestine during the operation. Placement of a Foley catheter (to be removed at the end of an uncomplicated case) is recommended to minimize the risk of bladder injury and to provide more working space.

Place the patient in a supine position. Anchor the patient to the bed and pad pressure points in anticipation of changing bed position several times during the procedure to maximize the visualization of involved tissue. Using alternative bed positions is often critical in successfully completing the laparoscopic operation. If possible, palpate for hepatosplenomegaly and determine where, and how deep, the aortic bifurcation is located. Start the procedure with the surgeon on the patient's right side and the assistant on the left. The scrub nurse and the instrument tray can be on either side of the patient and near the foot of the bed; however, the tray should be far enough away from the foot of the bed to allow it to move into the deep Trendelenburg (feet-up, head-down) position.

Peritoneal access

Attaining pneumoperitoneum may be the most challenging aspect of this procedure. Because of previous adhesions formed as a result of prior operations and lack of knowledge about their positions, knowing how to avoid complications during abdominal access and insufflation is as vital as knowing how to handle complications. Several methods for peritoneal access have been described for use in the setting of re-operative laparoscopic surgery.

An open technique is considered the safest approach by many laparoscopic surgeons for both primary and revision laparoscopic procedures. This approach, however, does not eliminate the possibility of viscus injury, and typically a larger incision is required than for other methods of abdominal access.

The traditional Veress needle approach (closed method) for peritoneal surgery is also used by many surgeons, even in the setting of re-operative laparoscopy. Needle access to the peritoneal cavity can be approached through the umbilicus or at a site distant from previous surgical incisions or cannula sites. After successful peritoneal insufflation, the needle is typically removed and the first cannula is passed blindly. As a first abdominal access approach, this technique has a well-documented incidence of complications, with injury to bowel or vessels from both the needle and the first cannula. The prevalence of these complications can be anticipated to be higher in the settings of re-operative surgery and bowel obstruction secondary to adhesions. Recently, the use of specialized optical trocars following Veress needle peritoneal insulation has been reported to be a safer alternative than 'blind' first trocar placement.

Our preferred peritoneal access technique has been to use a modified open/expandable sheath cannula typically through the cicatrix of the umbilicus for both primary and secondary laparoscopic procedures. The umbilical skin is grasped with toothed forceps on either side, and a vertical incision is made in the cicatrix with a No. 11 blade (with extension of the incision, if necessary, caudad). Using a small curved hemostat to spread and probe the base of the umbilicus usually identifies the position of the umbilical defect. If the umbilicus was the site of a previous surgical incision (open or laparoscopic), limited sharp dissection with a No. 11 blade between the clamps elevating the fascia typically allows access to the peritoneum. Once the umbilical defect has been identified, the expandable sheath over the Veress needle can be gently and safely inserted into the peritoneum at a 45–60° angle from the infra-umbilical skin surface in the direction of the left midclavicular line. A pneumoperitoneum is then created and the needle is removed from the sheath and replaced by a 5 mm cannula. **(see Figure 30.1)**

Through this first cannula, a 30° 3.5–5 mm telescope is inserted. If the bowel or omentum is adherent to the posterior surface of the abdominal wall in such a way that additional trocars cannot be placed under direct vision, attempt a gentle sweeping motion of the telescope along the undersurface of the abdominal wall. It is often possible to 'break through' to a free space in which additional trocars can be safely placed under direct vision.

There is no absolutely 'correct' position for the working ports, because the variable location of adhesions dictates proper positioning of the trocars. What is important is:

- the distance between the two working ports the surgeon is utilizing,
- the distance of the port in relation to the involved tissue,
- the camera position, patient position and the positions of the surgeon and assistant will probably change several times during the course of the operation.

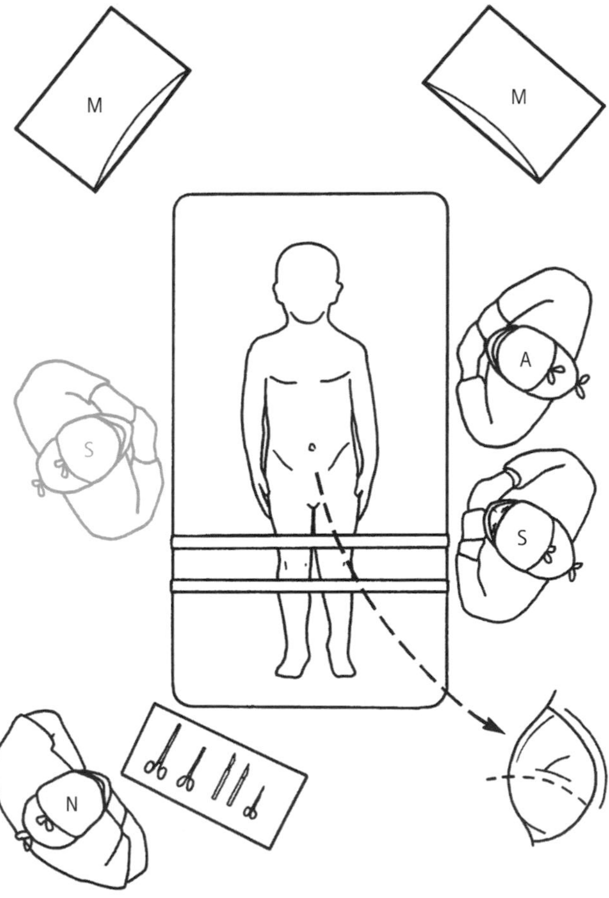

Figure 30.1

It is most desirable to have the camera facing the same direction as the surgeon and his or her instruments; otherwise, it can be quite disorienting. The initial objective is to release all adhesions from the posterior surface of the abdominal wall in order to have maximal visualization of the abdominal cavity. Once this is completed, the easiest way to 'run' the small intestine is by identifying the cecum and ileo-cecal valve and advancing in a retrograde direction back towards the ligament of Treitz (it is more difficult to identify the ligament of Treitz when the small intestine is dilated). With these two points in mind, under direct vision, identify a port position in the suprapubic region (midline) by pressing down and noting an indentation of the abdominal wall cephalad to the dome of the bladder and in between the paramedian umbilical folds. After infiltrating the skin and peritoneum with 0.25 percent Marcain, and making a small transverse incision, a 3–5 mm stepwise expandable trocar can be advanced at a 35–45° angle. Typically, an additional 3–5 mm trocar in the right or left upper quadrant in the midclavicular line provides for a good approach to the left or right side of the abdominal cavity, respectively. Having monitors at the head of the table on either side for approaching adhesions from mid-abdomen to upper quadrants, while positioning the monitors at the foot of the bed, is better for adhesions in the lower abdomen. Ideally, monitors at both the head and foot allow for handling the typical scenario which requires working in both the upper and lower abdominal fields. Attempting to place trocars through previous incision sites, if positionally feasible, maximizes cosmesis.

Adhesiolysis

If adhesions are present on the left side of the abdomen, the assistant should join you on the patient's right side and keep the camera in the umbilical port. Use a non-crushing grasper in your left hand and the curved scissors (with the cautery extension) or hook cautery device in your right hand. Gentle traction of the tissue with your left hand can help identify the adhesions along the posterior surface of the abdominal wall. Identify avascular tissue to incise and cut towards the parietal peritoneum. A combination of gentle, blunt sweeping of either instrument along the abdominal wall can facilitate the adhesiolysis. Rotating the operating table towards you may improve visualization of the adherent tissue. You may have to change positions or instrument sites to optimize the progress of the adhesiolysis. It is important to avoid placing an instrument in a port that would be directly above the tissue you wish to incise. Also, try to keep your working ports far enough away from each other to avoid limiting the range of motion of either instrument (at times, this is easier said than done). It is not a sign of failure to place additional 3–5 mm trocars for additional retraction or incision. **(See Figure 30.2)**

Once the adhesions are divided along the abdominal wall, attention is brought to the ileo-cecal valve. At this time, the surgeon should move to the patient's left side and use the umbilical and suprapubic trocars as the working ports. The assistant should stay on the patient's right, with the camera in the upper quadrant port. Rotating the operating table towards the patient's left and in the Trendelenburg position is helpful. Use the non-crushing bowel forceps to identify and gently elevate the terminal ileum at the level of the ileo-cecal valve. 'Run' the small bowel using a 'hand over hand' technique, pushing the small bowel towards the right paracolic gutter. When resistance is met, the assistant should hold the bowel while you return to the patient's right (rotate the operating table to the right and place it in the reverse Trendelenburg position) and continue 'running' the small bowel in the same fashion, pulling the bowel towards the right paracolic gutter until you reach the ligament of Treitz. When adhesive bands are identified, incise them with the curved scissors. If there are loops of bowel adherent to each other, two graspers may work well to give you the counter-traction necessary to incise the intervening adhesions. **(See Figure 30.3)**

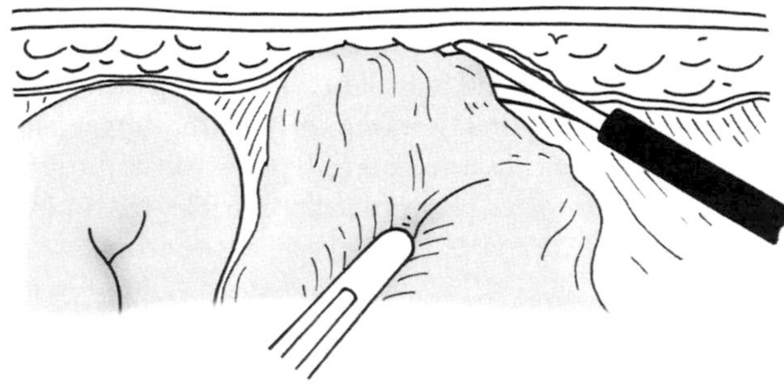

Figure 30.2

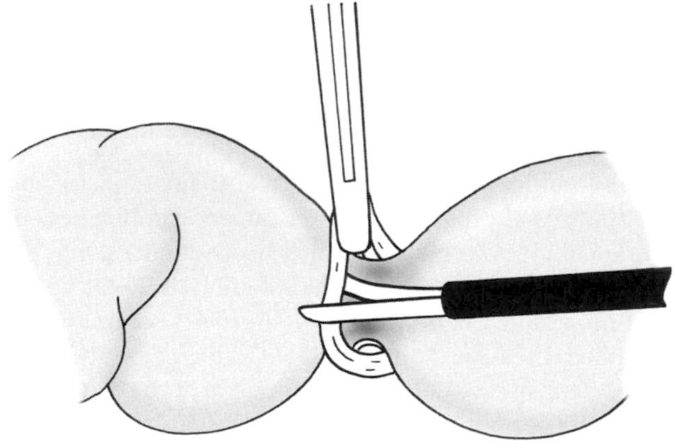

Figure 30.3

Once completed, the pneumoperitoneum is partially evacuated and all trocars (minus the umbilical port) are removed under direct vision to ensure that there is no active bleeding from the sites and to avoid pulling omentum up into the trocar sites. The remaining gas is evacuated and the umbilical trocar is removed. Incisions ⩾4 mm are closed with absorbable, monofilament, subcuticular suture. We utilize a figure-of-eight, buried, absorbable, monofilament suture for the umbilical fascia. To minimize the risk of bowel injury, we use a grooved director to guide needle placement. The skin is then closed, either in the same fashion as at the other trocar sites or with simple, interrupted sutures using 4-0 or 5-0 fast-absorbing Vicryl® (Vicryl Rapide®).

If the case was uncomplicated, the Foley catheter is removed prior to the reversal of anesthesia.

POSTOPERATIVE CARE

Nasogastric decompression and NPO status continue until the ileus resolves. Ambulation should commence soon after operation. A short course of intermittent, low-dose intravenous analgesics, followed by non-steroidal anti-inflammatory medication (either parenteral or enteral, depending on bowel function), is usually adequate for postoperative pain control.

PROBLEMS, PITFALLS AND SOLUTIONS

Difficult access and inadequate view

- To minimize the risk of bowel perforation in the presence of marked dilatation, ensure the umbilical defect is present with gentle probing of the curved hemostat and careful insertion of a trocar. Poor visualization impedes further exploration with laparoscopy. Attempt exaggerated table positioning prior to aborting laparoscopy.
- Dense adhesions or dilated bowel stuck at the undersurface of the usual umbilical access site make probing for the peritoneal cavity with the blunt clamp, prior to trocar placement, dangerous. If the blunt clamp does not pass with relative ease into the peritoneal cavity, an alternative site for the initial trocar should be chosen, such as the upper or lower lateral quadrants. A similar choice may be exercised in the setting of a prior midline laparotomy incision. In difficult cases, consider a laparotomy. Flexibility in the positioning of the operating table, surgeon and assistant and in the number of trocars inserted is very important, as these factors will be dictated by the site of the adhesions.

Strictured bowel

- Often the intestinal obstruction is a result of a single adhesive band, which may leave the bowel wall discolored and contused or having an appearance of narrowing (indentation). Continue with the operation and revisit the site at the end of exploration. Usually viability and luminal integrity are intact and no further intervention is necessary.
- If a stricture is obvious, a strictureplasty can be performed safely using the hook cautery or scissors across the stricture longitudinally and closing transversely.

Bleeding tissue

- Avoid grasping mesentery and only use atraumatic forceps.
- If persistent bleeding occurs, use a clip applicator, LigaSure™, suture LigaSure™ or ultrasonic scalpel.
- When using the scissors, if the adhesions appear vascular, apply diathermy prior to or during the cutting of tissue.

Necrotic bowel

If a segment of necrotic small bowel is present (once the adhesiolysis is completed), divide its mesentery with the Harmonic Scalpel® and then divide the small bowel sharply with the scissors. Laparoscopic anastomosis with an EndoGIA® and sutured enterotomy closure is feasible in older children. A second option is to widen a trocar site to bring the compromised loop of bowel out of the abdomen and to perform bowel resection and extracorporeal anastomosis.

Abscess

Use the suction/irrigator to drain as much of the abscess as possible and pull a Jackson–Pratt (JP) or Blake drain through the closest trocar site (a 7 mm round JP will fit through a 5 mm port).

Cautery injury

Inspect the injury at the end of the procedure. These injuries usually only affect the serosa. If the diathermy device of Harmonic Scalpel® had prolonged contact with the bowel, full-thickness injury may occur. If so, oversew this area with an intracorporeal Lembert suture (3-0 or 4-0 silk/Vicryl®).

COMPLICATIONS

Bowel perforation

Bowel perforation from trocar placement can be avoided by adequate insufflation and visualization. Injuries to the bowel from instrument manipulation often occur because of inappropriate choice of instruments (non-smooth grasping forceps or those that do not distribute equal pressure along the length of the grasping tines) or from over-aggressive tissue handling (lack of experience). Most bowel injuries (serosal tears, small and large bowel full-thickness injuries) can be repaired primarily with interrupted, full-thickness sutures in a single-layer closure. If preferred, a two-layer closure of inner full-thickness sutures, followed by Lembert seromuscular suture closure, can also be done intracorporeally. Irrigation and suction are used for spillage of sucus entericus. If spillage of luminal content is massive and impossible to control, sound surgical judgment may dictate laparotomy.

Vascular injury

- All laparoscopists must be vigilant to avoid major vessel injury, which can be prevented by careful technique and a clear understanding of vessel position (especially during trocar insertion). The occurrence of major vessel injury using a closed trocar placement technique is approximately 0.01 percent.
- The aorta will lie close to the midline, over the vertebral column until L4 level where, in 75 percent of patients, it divides into the right and left common iliac arteries. In 11 percent of patients, it bifurcates just below the L4–L5 disc level. The umbilicus typically lies directly over the L4 vertebra, and in thin patients rests 1–2 cm above the aorta. Palpating the aorta for orientation prior to initial trocar insertion is advised.
- Penetrating a large vessel is usually manifest in the prompt return of blood through the Veress needle (with the valve in the open position). When vascular injury is identified, an immediate lower midline incision is made, with the Veress needle left in position to use as a guide.
- Mesenteric branches can be clipped, grasped and coagulated, or oversewn laparoscopically.
- Inferior and superficial epigastric vessel injury occasionally leads to significant bleeding. Avoid trocar entry along the lines of vessels. In thin patients or neonates, the main vessels are often visualized by transillumination within the abdominal wall. Often the bleeding is manifest in blood dripping along the cannula. If persistent, moving the cannula laterally or medially can aid in identifying the bleeding source, which can be coagulated directly. If necessary,

extending the incision and oversewing the vessel is another option. Replacing the trocar with a Foley catheter and filling the balloon to tamponade the vessel may buy time to complete the case and often permanently stop the bleeding.

Bladder injury

Bladder injury can be easily avoided by placing a Foley catheter for the duration of the operation. It is identified by the appearance of bladder muscularis separated by the trocar or the presence of CO_2 gas in the Foley bag. If a bladder injury is suspected, a retrograde cystogram may be considered. If the injury is intraperitoneal, the cystotomy should be repaired in two layers (laparoscopically or via minilaparotomy). Leave a Foley catheter for 7 days postoperatively. If the injury is extraperitoneal, Foley catheter drainage for 2 weeks is the choice of treatment.

Recurrent obstruction

Delicate handling of the tissue is key. However, adhesions reform regardless of technique. Several studies have been performed to assess the outcome of laparoscopic adhesiolysis, claiming 64–97 percent success with follow-up of 24–62 months. In all the studies, there was only one patient who required re-operation. If obstruction recurs, follow the same steps as described earlier in the chapter.

Ureteral injury

- Careful, gentle dissection and awareness of typical ureteral position will help avoid injury when performing adhesiolysis of small bowel adherent to the lateral pelvic wall.
- Suspected injury can be identified by injecting intravenous methylene blue. Most ureteral injuries present 1–5 days postoperatively with increasing abdominal pain, fever, leukocytosis, ascites or urinoma. Obtain a CT scan and/or intravenous pyelogram for diagnosis and treat accordingly.

Necrotizing fasciitis

There are anecdotal reports of necrotizing fasciitis at trocar sites after laparoscopy, which occurred after leakage of intestinal contents had been identified. Utilization of perioperative antibiotics, careful wound inspection and aggressive diagnosis and treatment can minimize clinical sequelae.

FURTHER READING

Festen C. Postoperative small bowel obstruction in infants and children. *Annals of Surgery* 1982; **196**:580–2.

Keating J, Hill A, Schroeder D, Whittle D. Laparoscopy in the diagnosis and treatment of acute small bowel obstruction. *Journal of Laparoendoscopic Surgery* 1992; **2**:239–44.

Menzies D, Ellis H. Intestinal obstruction from adhesions – how big is the problem? *Annals of the Royal College of Surgeons of England* 1990; **72**:60–3.

Shalaby R. Laparoscopic approach to small intestinal obstruction in children: a preliminary experience. *Surgical Laparoscopy, Endoscopy and Percutaneous Techniques* 2001; **11**(5):301–5.

Sato Y, Ido K, Kumagai M et al. Laparoscopic adhesiolysis for recurrent small bowel obstruction: long-term follow-up. *Gastrointestinal Endoscopy* 2001; **54**(4):476–9.

31

Diagnostic laparoscopy

ALEX C.H. LEE AND RICHARD J. STEWART

INTRODUCTION

Diagnostic laparoscopy has an important and clearly defined role in children. The serosal surfaces of all the solid and hollow viscera of the abdomen and pelvis can be inspected by laparoscopy, but it should not be regarded as a substitute for careful history taking and clinical examination. The procedure is invasive and it should be considered only after appropriate laboratory and radiological investigations have been performed. However, the major benefit of laparoscopy for diagnostic purposes is the opportunity to proceed immediately to treat the pathology using minimally invasive techniques, or at least to guide the placement of an incision for an open procedure.

Indications

- The acute abdomen – including intestinal obstruction.
- Recurrent abdominal pain.
- Evaluation of blunt or penetrating visceral trauma.
- Oncology:
  - tumor biopsy
  - assess operability and monitor progress after chemotherapy.
- Miscellaneous elective procedures.
  - Evaluation of:
    - contralateral processus vaginalis
    - malrotation
    - intersex states
    - impalpable testes
    - other abdominal masses, e.g. duplication cyst or mesenteric cyst.
  - Biopsy in suspected Hirschsprung's disease.
  - Investigation of the jaundiced patient – including biopsy and cholangiography.

Detailed evaluations of intersex and cryptorchidism are given in Chapters 63 and 55, respectively. These subjects are not discussed further in this chapter.

Contraindications

There are few contraindications to diagnostic laparoscopy. Uncorrected hypotension, hypoxia and bleeding disorders are obvious ones. The presence of a previous abdominal incision is a relative contraindication, depending on the expertise of the surgeon and the precise location of the scar.

EQUIPMENT/INSTRUMENTS

Basic diagnostic laparoscopy can be performed through a single cannula. Standard 3 mm, 5 mm and 10 mm telescopes provide an excellent image and are reasonably robust. Operating telescopes with a built-in instrument channel are available that permit simple therapeutic maneuvers. There are also very fine 1 mm telescopes, but the image quality is poor at present and these instruments are very fragile. **(See Figure 31.1)**

The insertion of one or two additional cannulae will permit manipulation of the viscera with atraumatic grasping forceps. For more complex specific diagnostic procedures, further instruments will be required (e.g. cholangiography).

Details of other essential equipment such as insufflator, light source, video camera, monitors and cable/tubing can

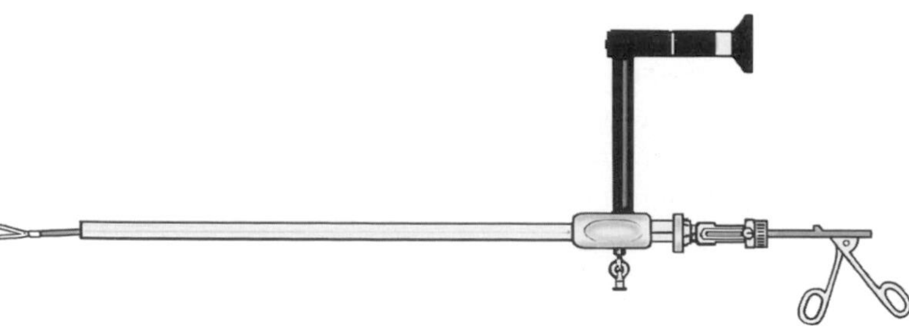

Figure 31.1 *Operating laparoscope.*

be found elsewhere in this book. Media recording in the form of printed photographs, digital still image recordings and digital or analog video recordings is very useful, permitting documentation in the patient notes.

In all cases, full laparoscopy and laparotomy sets should be readily available to allow for therapeutic intervention if indicated.

Essential

- Three trocars (3–5 mm).
- 30–45° telescope (3–10 mm).
- Two pairs of atraumatic insulated grasping forceps (3–5 mm) – without a ratchet.
- Monopolar hook diathermy (3–5 mm).
- Bipolar diathermy (3–5 mm).
- Curved insulated scissors (3–5 mm).
- Suction and irrigation equipment (3–5 mm).

Procedure-specific

- Cup biopsy forceps (3–5 mm).
- Tru-Cut percutaneous biopsy needle.
- Spinal needle for aspiration of fluids (via trocar or transabdominally).
- Cholangiogram needle.
- Tissue removal bag.
- 70° telescope (3–5 mm).
- Laparoscopic ultrasound probe.

Desirable

- Additional standard trocars.
- Atraumatic retractors (3–5 mm).
- 1–2 mm telescopes and cannulae (needlescopic).
- 10 mm 0° telescope with built-in 5 mm instrument channel.
- Babcock forceps (3–5 mm).
- Ultrasound shears (5 mm).
- Atraumatic insulated grasping forceps (3–5 mm) with a ratchet.
- Clips and staples.

PREOPERATIVE PREPARATION

Children should be appropriately resuscitated, fasted and fit for general anesthesia. Hematological and biochemical investigations should be undertaken, with blood grouping or cross-matching if clinically indicated. Preoperative radiological studies should be available. If a diagnostic biopsy is planned, liaison with the pathology service is vital. The indications for preoperative antibiotics are the same as for open surgical procedures.

TECHNIQUE

General anesthesia is required in all pediatric cases. Endotracheal intubation and full muscle relaxation are usually necessary. Nitrous oxide should be avoided to reduce bowel distension. The stomach should be decompressed by a nasogastric tube if distended with air or in children with an ileus or intestinal obstruction. A urinary catheter may be necessary if a palpable bladder cannot be emptied by the Crede maneuver. An empty bladder is essential if pathology is suspected in the pelvis.

The child is positioned supine on the operating table. The entire surface of the abdomen should be prepared. The patient and all anesthetic tubing, intravenous lines, monitoring wires etc. should be secured to allow tilting of the operating table intra-operatively to facilitate examination of the peritoneal cavity.

Depending on the position of the suspected pathology, the main monitor is placed in line with the surgeon and the camera cannula, which is generally umbilical. The operating room should be arranged so that the monitor can be moved according to the position of the pathology found. It is particularly useful to have two monitors, one on either side of the patient, when it is unclear in which quadrant the pathology may be located. In general, the monitor should be placed at the head end of the table for upper abdominal lesions, and at the feet end for pelvic pathology.

Peritoneal access using the open (Hasson) or closed (Veress needle) technique is described elsewhere in this book. The open technique is recommended if there is abdominal distension. The incision is usually placed infraumbilically. Once the first cannula has been inserted,

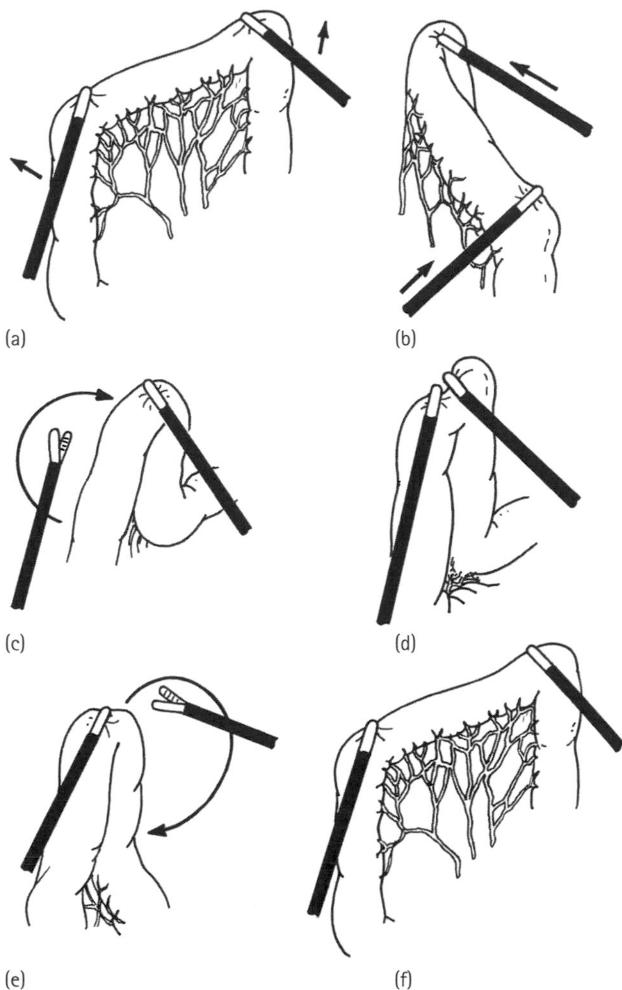

Figure 31.2 *Inspection of mobile intestine using two pairs of atraumatic graspers.*

a pneumoperitoneum is established to a pressure of 8–10 mmHg with a CO_2 insufflator at a flow rate of 0.5–2 L/min.

The operating table may need to be tilted to allow gravity to move the intestine and improve the view and to facilitate further cannula insertion under direct vision if necessary. Optimal triangulation configuration with the primary cannula and working cannulae should be considered, but allowing inspection of the lower and upper abdomen. The optimal positions would allow a manipulation angle of 45–75°, equal azimuth angle and an elevation angle of 60°. It is better to insert additional cannulae rather than struggle with inadequate access.

For routine diagnostic laparoscopy it is essential that a systematic inspection of the abdomen and pelvis is performed. The viscera should be examined using a consistent routine starting with a clockwise inspection from the cecum/appendix, right colon, gallbladder, liver, spleen, stomach, left colon, pelvic organs including uterus, ovaries, fallopian tubes, internal inguinal rings, gonadal vessels and back to the ileo-cecal region. The entire length of the small bowel can be inspected using two pairs of atraumatic grasping forceps until the duodeno-jejunal junction is reached and its position noted. Good communication between the surgeon and anesthetist is essential throughout the procedure as it may be necessary to alter the patient's position or convert to a laparotomy. **(See Figure 31.2)**

The acute abdomen

The child with an acute abdomen is a common diagnostic challenge. The considered use of laparoscopy to aid diagnosis permits early intervention and may avoid an unnecessary laparotomy. In many cases diagnostic laparoscopy will be a preliminary step before a definitive therapeutic procedure, which may also be performed laparoscopically. In some situations, a diagnostic laparoscopy may guide the selection of operative laparotomy incision.

The abdomen should be palpated to assess whether an intra-abdominal mass is present which may determine the location of the initial cannula. If an appendix mass is noted, the surgeon may choose not to proceed and to treat the child with antibiotics. If a mass is present, the initial cannula should be placed at an acceptable distance to enable good visualization. This should be at least the length of the trocar inserted within the abdomen. Otherwise the cannula should be placed at the umbilicus using an open technique.

Lateral tilting of the operating table with the patient either left or right side down may improve visualization by moving the bowel by gravity. In addition, further working cannulae may be inserted to manipulate viscera. When it is unclear which quadrant contains the pathology, working cannulae should be inserted on each side of the umbilical cannula so that both the upper and lower abdomen can be explored. **(See Figure 31.3)**

Ideally, two linked monitors on opposite sides of the patient should be used to avoid difficulties with parallax.

The abdominal cavity should be explored systematically as outlined above. The presence of turbid fluid or serosal inflammation will indicate the presence of peritonitis, and intraperitoneal blood should prompt a search for the source of bleeding following trauma. Dilated proximal bowel with distal collapsed bowel supports a diagnosis of intestinal obstruction and should prompt a search for the cause. Care needs to be taken when handling the dilated bowel, as perforation may easily occur and it can be difficult to identify the obstructive lesion. Laparoscopy for neonatal necrotizing enterocolitis remains a novel application and further experience is necessary to determine the precise role for this technique.

The diagnosis of gastrointestinal bleeding of unknown origin in children can be difficult. Upper and lower gastrointestinal endoscopies are essential diagnostic tools. Laparoscopy can be used to identify a Meckel's diverticulum, a vascular malformation of the bowel or a small-bowel tumor. The patient is prepared as outlined above, with dual monitors. An initial umbilical cannula is inserted and if blood is noted within the bowel lumen, this is a useful

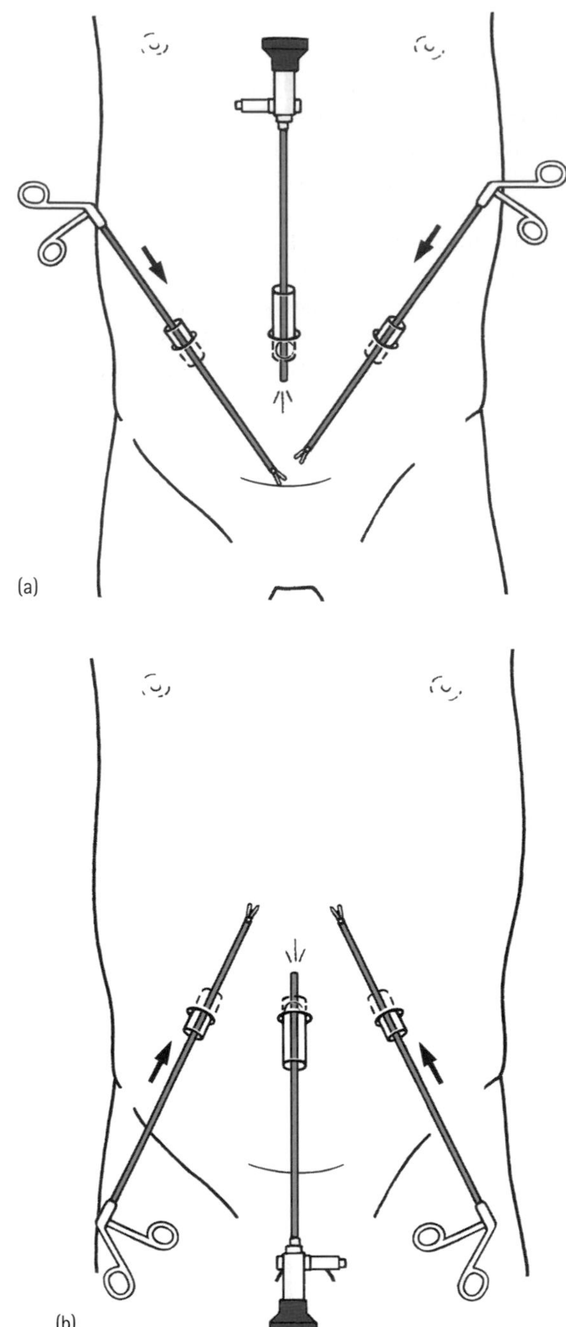

Figure 31.3 *Inspection of the peritoneal cavity. (a) Lower abdomen; (b) upper abdomen.*

guide to a more proximal point of origin. Further working cannulae are inserted as appropriate to perform a detailed examination of the bowel, together with two pairs of atraumatic forceps. If necessary, the entire length from the duodeno-jejunal flexure to the rectum should be examined.

Recurrent abdominal pain

The technique is the same as for acute abdomen. Under general anesthesia, the abdomen should be carefully palpated and the initial cannula inserted by an open technique at the umbilicus. Additional working cannulae should be inserted as described above and the abdomen/pelvis carefully examined. It is crucial to be able to visualize the whole abdomen systematically to ensure pathology is not overlooked. Patience is needed. The presence of an abnormality (e.g. peri-cecal adhesions) does not necessarily mean it is responsible for the symptoms. The resolution of symptoms after treatment of the pathological findings is the best indicator that the treatment was of benefit, although there may be a significant placebo effect from the laparoscopic procedure itself.

Photographic documentation of the laparoscopic findings can be useful to reassure the child and parents that serious pathology was not found during the examination.

Oncology

Diagnostic laparoscopy is a useful tool for the initial assessment and subsequent management of a patient with a suspected abdominal malignancy.

The abdomen should be palpated or a bimanual pelvic examination performed to assess the tumor, and the initial cannula should be placed at a distance, usually in the midline using an open technique. The child may need to be rotated laterally or placed in a head-up/down position to aid visualization of the tumor. If required, additional working cannulae may be inserted to facilitate dissection and mobilization to improve exposure.

Laparoscopy permits a direct visual assessment of the tumor in its anatomical location. Previously unsuspected lesions, including peritoneal secondaries, may be identified. The surgeon can select the most suitable site for biopsy, avoiding major blood vessels and other vital local structures. Tissue for histopathology and cytology can be obtained with a 14 G Tru-Cut biopsy needle or by endoscopic dissection with removal of the sample via a cannula using a tissue retrieval bag or the finger of a surgical glove as a tissue bag, if required. Adequate tissue should be obtained for immunohistochemistry and cytogenetic analysis. Blood loss should be minimal and any hemorrhage can be controlled with Surgicell® or a peanut gauze, as in open access surgery, passed through a cannula at the tip of a pair of dissecting forceps.

Ascitic fluid, if present, should be aspirated and sent for cytology. It may be appropriate to perform a bone marrow aspirate and trephine under the same anesthetic. It may also be appropriate to insert a Hickman or Broviac central venous access catheter for chemotherapy.

Following chemotherapy, laparoscopy may be used to assess operability by evaluating tumor size, location, invasion and metastatic spread. Laparoscopic ultrasonography has become an integral part of the staging of adult upper gastrointestinal and hepatopancreatobiliary malignancies prior to resection, but its use in the pediatric group is limited to cases reports at present. The role of laparoscopic tumor resection, or laparoscopically assisted open resection, in children is undefined at present.

Miscellaneous elective procedures

CONTRALATERAL PROCESSUS VAGINALIS

Contralateral groin exploration in children presenting with an inguinal hernia is controversial. The decision may be aided by inspecting the deep inguinal ring by laparoscopy. Some surgeons perform this procedure routinely, especially in girls and infant boys, in whom the risk of a contralateral hernia is highest. A negative laparoscopy avoids an unnecessary groin exploration. The technique for laparoscopic hernia repair is covered elsewhere in this book.

There are several ways to inspect the deep inguinal ring. A pneumoperitoneum can be established through the hernial sac on the symptomatic side. A 10 Fr nasogastric feeding tube is inserted through the sac into the peritoneal cavity, held in place with a silk tie around the sac and connected to the insufflator. A standard 3 mm trocar and telescope can be inserted through the umbilicus to examine the deep rings. If a 1.2 mm telescope is available, a 14 G cannula can be inserted into the abdominal wall at umbilical level above the contralateral groin. The telescope is passed through the cannula to allow direct in-line visualization of the deep ring. Alternatively, a 70° telescope can be inserted (with or without a cannula) through the open hernial sac, alongside the insufflation tube. The telescope is directed across the lower abdomen to inspect the contralateral deep ring. A positive finding is confirmed when the deep ring is obviously open, as determined by the presence of a patent processus longer than 5 mm, or by obvious crepitus in the groin/scrotum. In these cases, open or laparoscopic contralateral groin exploration is carried out. **(See Figure 31.4)**

Examination of the deep inguinal ring from above allows direct in-line vision that is superior to inspection from the side. There is a significant risk of missing a patent processus due to the partially obscured internal ring when viewed from an angle, even when a 70° telescope is used. Also, when the hernia orifice is small, it can be difficult to insert the feeding tube/trocar into it. Undue force should not be used and it would be safer to abandon this technique in favor of an umbilical approach.

MALROTATION

Abnormalities of intestinal rotation may be identified on upper gastrointestinal contrast studies in children with unrelated symptoms. Assessment of the risk of midgut volvulus can be difficult in these children. Laparoscopy has a definite role in determining the width of the midgut mesentery and evaluating the likelihood of volvulus. The surgeon can then proceed to either laparoscopic or open Ladd's procedure, depending on his or her experience.

The patient is positioned supine with the head slightly raised and secured to allow tilting of the table to raise the left side. An infra-umbilical trocar is inserted, followed by two further cannulae pararectally, one on either side at the level of the umbilicus.

The diagnosis of intestinal malrotation should be considered if the cecum and appendix are lying high in the right upper quadrant of the abdomen. The position of the duodeno-jejunal flexure must be established to confirm the diagnosis. Lifting up the small bowel with a pair of traumatic forceps, possibly with the help of a third instrument inserted through an additional cannula, assesses the width of the base of the midgut mesentery. A decision is then made whether or not to proceed with a Ladd's procedure. Laparoscopic surgery for malrotation is covered in Chapter 39.

PROBLEMS, PITFALLS AND SOLUTIONS

Inappropriate patient selection

Proper patient selection is essential, especially in trauma cases when, despite adequate resuscitation with likely ongoing intra-abdominal hemorrhage, the unstable patient should undergo laparotomy rather than laparoscopy.

Equipment and instruments

Meticulous attention to the preparation and technique is essential. Even though therapeutic treatment may not be carried out, the importance of ensuring all equipment is in working order cannot be over-emphasized. Correct white balancing of the camera is essential. The surgeon must be familiar with the instruments and equipment, and theater staff must be appropriately trained in their use. However, in an emergency situation the surgeon may have to work with staff who are unfamiliar with the laparoscopic equipment. Imaging and recording equipment present particular problems. Particular care is required when handling 1.2 mm telescopes because they are easily damaged.

General or local anesthesia

Although local anesthesia is used for office-based or emergency department diagnostic laparoscopy in adults, general anesthesia is recommended for all pediatric cases.

Difficult access and limited view

The patient must be positioned and secured on the operating table in such a way that the table can be tilted safely during the procedure. The abdomen should be prepared and draped to allow placement of cannulae anywhere within it after the initial survey. Standard theater equipment such

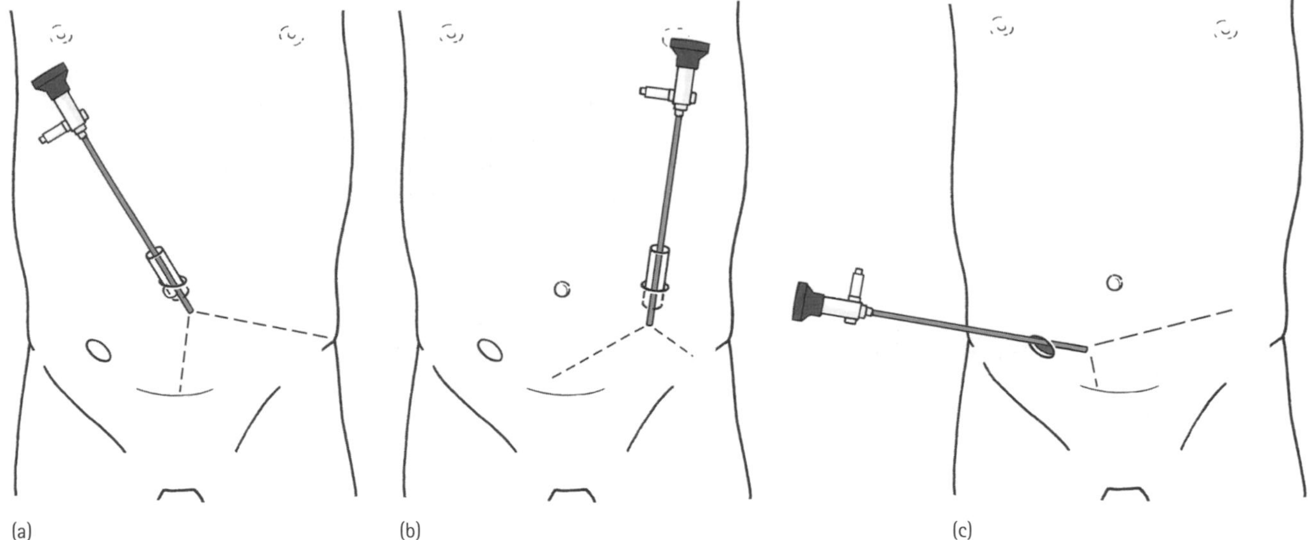

Figure 31.4 *Inspection of contralateral ring. (a) Umbilical trocar; (b) 14G cannula above the contralateral ring; (c) 70° telescope through the open hernia sac.*

as armrests, drip stands etc. should be positioned to avoid restriction of the movement of telescopes and instruments. Additional cannulae should be placed early rather than struggling with limited access and an inadequate view.

Hemostasis has to be meticulous. Even though minor bleeding may not be hemodynamically important, light is absorbed by blood accumulating in the peritoneal cavity and the view deteriorates. The brightness and quality of the image obtained using small telescopes are reduced, and if this hampers the examination, insertion of a larger telescope should be considered.

Abdominal distension

The presence of abdominal distension from an ileus or intestinal obstruction reduces the space available to establish a pneumoperitoneum. Prolonged pre-intubation ventilation by bag and mask should be avoided if possible. Nitrous oxide must be avoided. Increasing the pressure of the pneumoperitoneum will hinder diaphragmatic movement and impair ventilation. Extreme care needs to be taken when the first cannula is inserted, even if an open technique is used. There is an increased risk of accidental perforation of the distended bowel when instruments are being inserted and manipulated. If a safe working space cannot be established, recourse to an open procedure is necessary.

Abdominal mass

The presence of an abdominal mass will usually be noted preoperatively, but it may be apparent only during examination under anesthesia. Care needs to be taken during trocar insertion to avoid damage to the mass or being too close to it, which makes visualization difficult. The mass may distort the anatomy of surrounding structures, exposing them to potential injury. Cannulae should be placed well away from any mass to allow space for the insertion of additional trocar(s) and should be under direct vision at all times. Care needs to be taken when manipulating a large abdominal mass to avoid accidental laceration, especially when finer instruments (2–3 mm) are used. On the other hand, manipulation of a benign cystic mass is usually facilitated by aspiration and decompression. The judicious use of tilting may allow a mobile mass to be displaced and permit better viewing. **(See Figure 31.5)**

Trauma cases

Blood, bile and intestinal contents will obscure the laparoscopic view. If the source of injury is not found quickly, conversion to laparotomy should be undertaken. The threshold and timing to convert will be determined by the experience of the surgeon and the stability of the patient.

The 'normal' Meckel's diverticulum and appendix

Details of the laparoscopic removal of a Meckel's diverticulum can be found elsewhere in this book. If a Meckel's diverticulum is found coincidentally, the surgeon should make a decision about resection. If it could be the source of the patient's problem, resection via the umbilicus

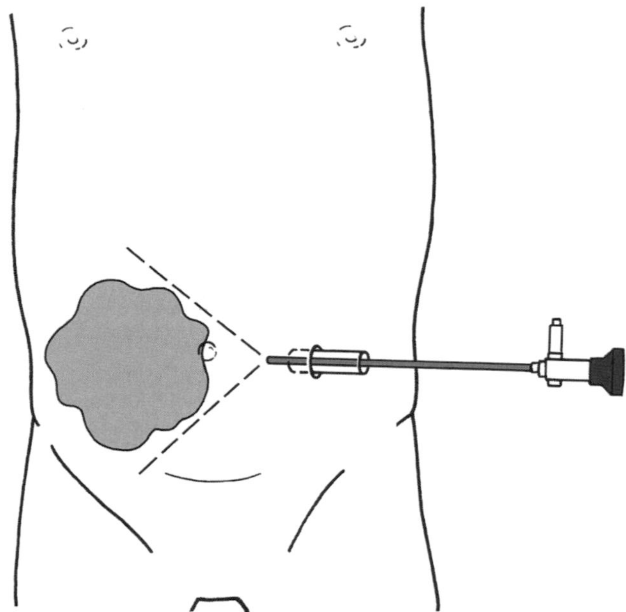

Figure 31.5

extracorporeally can usually be achieved. The risk of adhesions after laparoscopic removal is probably minimal. If a diagnostic laparoscopy is performed for recurrent abdominal pain, a normal appendix should probably be removed. A small appendicolith causing recurrent appendicular colic may not be evident during laparoscopy. Care needs to be taken to ensure the whole appendix is removed because there are reported cases of previous incomplete appendicectomy with recurrent inflammation of the stump.

Laparoscopic surgery for Meckel's diverticulum and the appendix is covered in Chapters 41 and 42.

Tumor seeding

Cannula site contamination of tumor during biopsy or treatment for intra-abdominal tumor cases may worsen the oncological outcome. Removing the tissue with a retrieval bag or within the trocar may minimize this.

Risk of missing potential pathology

A thorough inspection of the abdomen including the pelvis is essential. It is crucial not to rush during the examination, which should be systematic in order to minimize the risk of missing potential pathology. Further trocars should be inserted to aid visualization, which should be planned at the beginning of the case.

COMPLICATIONS

Complications may occur during the creation of a pneumoperitoneum, insertion of trocars/instruments and the diagnostic procedure. Failure to make an accurate assessment of the presence or extent of the intra-abdominal pathology sought can also lead to potential complications. Specific complications depend on the specific diagnostic test (±subsequent therapeutic treatment) performed.

FURTHER READING

Fetko L. Diagnostic laparoscopy for pelvic pain. In: MacFadyen BV, Arregui ME, Eubanks S et al. (eds), *Laparoscopic Surgery of the Abdomen.* New York: Springer, 2004, 490–6.

McMahon RL. Principles of diagnostic laparoscopy. In: MacFadyen BV, Arregui ME, Eubanks S et al. (eds), *Laparoscopic Surgery of the Abdomen.* New York: Springer, 2004, 471–80.

Najmaldin A. Diagnostic laparoscopy. In: Najmaldin A, Guillou P (eds), *A Guide to Laparoscopic Surgery.* Oxford: Blackwell, 1998, 107–10.

Najmaldin AS, Cutner A. Laparoscopic techniques. In: Balen AH, Creighton SM, Davies MC, MacDougall J, Stanhope R (eds), *Paediatric and Adolescent Gynaecology.* Cambridge: Cambridge University Press, 2004, 131–46.

Pryor AD. Diagnostic laparoscopy for suspected appendicitis. In: MacFadyen BV, Arregui ME, Eubanks S et al. (eds), *Laparoscopic Surgery of the Abdomen.* New York: Springer, 2004, 497–506.

Waldschmidt J, Bax NMA. Diagnostic laparoscopy. In: Bax, Najmaldin, Valla, Georgeson KE (eds), *Endoscopic Surgery in Children.* Berlin: Springer, 1999, 137–54.

32A

Anti-reflux surgery – Nissen fundoplication

SPENCER BEASLEY

INTRODUCTION

Laparoscopic fundoplication is an alternative to open fundoplication to correct gastro-esophageal reflux. Like the open fundoplication, it has been shown to increase fasting and post-prandial lower esophageal sphincter pressure and to decrease the rate of transient lower esophageal sphincter relaxation. Mean lower esophageal sphincter pressures increase from about 7 mmHg to 17 mmHg. These changes result in a significant reduction in the time the esophageal mucosa is exposed to acid. Although some studies suggest the motor function of the esophageal body is not affected by laparoscopic fundoplication, there is some evidence that it may decrease esophageal body peristaltic efficiency and the velocity of propagation of peristaltic waves.

There are a number of techniques in common usage for laparoscopic fundoplication, of which the three most widely employed are the Nissen, Toupet and Thal. Each has its proponents, and there is considerable ongoing discussion and controversy over their relative merits. Moreover, for each type of operation, e.g. laparoscopic Nissen fundoplication, there are many variations and refinements that have been proposed. Port placement, the indications for division of the short gastric arteries, the method of crural closure and whether the esophagus should be included in the sutures for the wrap are examples of technical questions for which there is little consensus at this stage. This chapter describes the laparoscopic Nissen fundoplication.

Indications

- Severe and symptomatic gastro-esophageal reflux unresponsive or poorly responsive to standard medication.
- Esophageal stricture caused by esophagitis secondary to gastro-esophageal reflux.
- Anastomotic stricture in infants or children with repaired esophageal atresia and ongoing gastro-esophageal reflux.
- Chronic aspiration or recurrent pneumonia secondary to gastro-esophageal reflux.
- Severe reactive airway disease from asthma exacerbated by gastro-esophageal reflux.
- In conjunction with gastrostomy placement in children with neurological disorders, who have, or are at risk of, exacerbation of their gastro-esophageal reflux. Note that the role of prophylactic fundoplication at the time of gastrostomy in asymptomatic children is controversial. One study of 26 neurologically impaired children without clinical evidence of severe gastro-esophageal reflux prior to percutaneous endoscopic gastrostomy (PEG) insertion found that fundoplication was required in two as a consequence of PEG insertion, although in total 14 developed symptomatic reflux.

Contraindications

While there are no absolute contraindications for laparoscopic fundoplication, there are a number of situations that may make the operation more difficult.

- Hepatosplenomegaly or portal hypertension.
- Short esophagus, including in those with previously repaired esophageal atresia; in addition, children born with esophageal atresia have poor esophageal clearance, a feature that may become more prominent unless the wrap of the fundoplication is made very loose.

- Extensive adhesions from previous upper abdominal surgery (e.g. previous fundoplication, congenital diaphragmatic hernia repair).
- Severe inflammation (esophagitis) of the lower esophagus.
- Pre-existing gastrostomy in situ.
- Very large hiatus hernia.

EQUIPMENT/INSTRUMENTS

Essential

- 5 mm (infants) or 10 mm (older children) ordinary blunt Hasson cannula or equivalent, and a telescope with an adjustable flange.
- 5 mm or 10 mm 30° angled telescope.
- Four 3.5–5 mm ports.
- Needle holders.
- One or two 3–5 mm atraumatic curved insulated grasping forceps without ratchet, with diathermy attachment.
- 3–5 mm atraumatic Babcock or soft grasping forceps with ratchet, with diathermy attachment to hold stomach.
- 3–5 mm toothed grasping forceps with ratchet.
- 3–5 mm double jaw action curved scissors with diathermy attachment.
- Unipolar hook diathermy probe with insulation extending close to end.
- Irrigation and aspiration tubing and sucker.
- Liver retractor and attachments.
- 0 absorbable suture on a tapered needle (2-0 suture if the child is younger than 5 years) for the umbilical port.
- 2-0 non-absorbable sutures for the approximation of the crural fibers and fundoplication wrap.
- 3-0 absorbable suture on a tapered needle for muscle closure.
- 4-0 or 5-0 absorbable suture for skin closure.

Optional

- A second needle holder.
- Ultrasonic shears or bipolar diathermy, for division of short gastric vessels, if needed.
- 5 mm laparoscopic clip applicator, for division of short gastric vessels, if needed.
- Irrigation and aspiration tubing and sucker.

PREOPERATIVE PREPARATION

Most patients will have had confirmation of their gastro-esophageal reflux from a barium study. This study also will have documented the presence of any esophageal stricture, a short esophagus or hiatus hernia, the effectiveness of esophageal peristalsis, whether there is any evidence of gastric outlet obstruction or delayed gastric emptying, and is able to confirm normal rotation of the midgut by identifying the position of the duodeno-jejunal flexure. Twenty-four-hour intra-esophageal pH monitoring documents the number and duration of reflux episodes in a 24-hour period, when they occur in relation to meals and sleep, and the overall length of time the esophagus is bathed in gastric acid (pH < 4).

Esophagoscopy with esophageal biopsy provides both macroscopic and microscopic evidence of esophagitis, and flexible gastroscopy can reveal any gastritis, *Helicobacter pylori* infection or gluten enteropathy. On occasions, and for specific reasons, other investigations may be undertaken; these include technetium-labeled milk scan to detect aspiration, and surface electrogastrography to identify a specific motility disturbance. The place of routine preoperative isotope gastric emptying studies remains uncertain.

Informed consent from parents should include discussion of the following.

- The purpose of the procedure – namely, to correct or prevent reflux.
- The likely outcome, including mention of the potential problems that might occur, and the limitations of the procedure.
- The possibility (albeit rare) of the need to convert to an open procedure for reasons of safety. Up to 5 percent of patients may need conversion to an open procedure, but the rate is probably related to the expertise of the operator.
- Potential short-term and long-term complications of surgery (see below).

Although blood transfusion is rarely required, it is prudent to group and hold blood prior to the procedure. Relevant radiology should be available in theater in case it is required. Many surgeons administer one dose of antibiotic (e.g. cephalosporin) at induction as chemoprophylaxis, although the benefit of prophylactic antibiotics in fundoplication has not been determined.

TECHNIQUE

The child is placed near the foot of the operating table. The legs of smaller children can be supported over the end of the table or in the frog-leg position, taking care of the calves and avoiding pressure points. In larger children the legs are abducted and supported in stirrups so that the main operator can stand between them to operate. The skin is prepared with antiseptic solution from the mid-thoracic level to the pubic area, extending laterally on both sides, particularly on the left. The umbilical port is introduced by the standard open method, making an incision immediately below the umbilicus. After initial inspection of the peritoneal

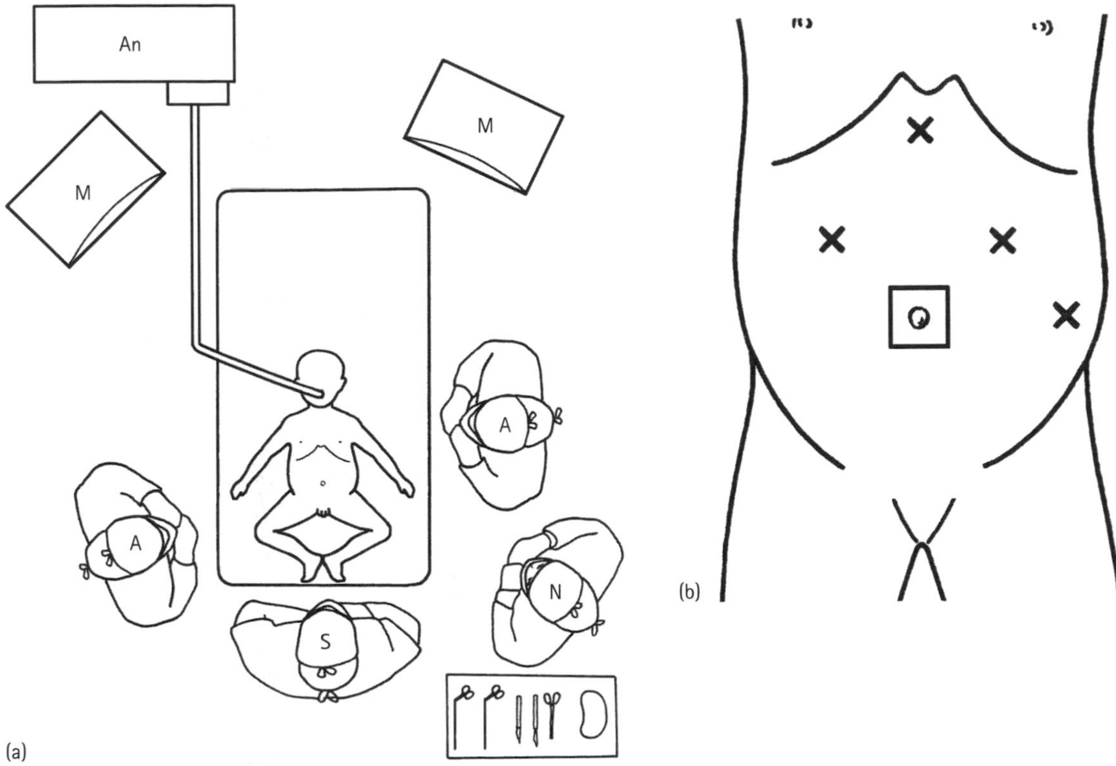

Figure 32A.1

cavity, the remaining cannulae are introduced under vision. The level of the two working cannulae, one on each side of the umbilicus, is determined by the size of the child, i.e. the smaller the child, the lower they will be. The left lower quadrant port is used to control the position of the stomach during mobilization of the lower esophagus and fundoplication. **(See Figure 32A.1)**

The high epigastric port is used to retract the left lobe of the liver upwards. This is best done by the insertion of a liver retractor. Various types of liver retractors are available, including fan and snake retractors. When the 5 mm port is introduced in the epigastrium, it can be removed immediately and the curved snake liver retractor can be introduced through the same track. Alternatively, laparoscopic Babcock grasping forceps can be introduced through the port to grasp the fibers of the anterior edge of the esophageal hiatus, lifting them away from the lower end of the esophagus, and retracting the edge of the left lobe of the diaphragm at the same time.

Atraumatic grasping forceps (Babcock or soft grasping forceps) are introduced through the left iliac fossa port to hold the stomach near the cardia. This allows tension to be put on the stomach and lower esophagus to facilitate dissection of the esophageal hiatus. Through the two working ports, the peritoneum over the phrenico-esophageal ligament is divided. The phrenico-esophageal ligament is incised and dissected using scissors, diathermy dissection or blunt dissection. The initial dissection can be extended either to the left side, or on the right side to the gastrohepatic ligament. Gentle divulsion between the two graspers opens up the plane between the esophagus and crural fibers. The dissection should not be allowed to damage the wall of the esophagus: the forceps may push the esophagus away from the crus, but should not be used to grasp the esophageal wall. **(See Figure 32A.2)**

The sharp and blunt dissection is continued around each side of the lower end of the esophagus and into the esophageal hiatus, taking care to avoid damage to the anterior and posterior vagal trunks, which can be seen clearly coursing over the surface of the esophagus at this point. This part of the dissection is relatively avascular, although small vessels sometimes require control with hook diathermy. The lower end of the esophagus is mobilized. The stomach is retracted towards the left to facilitate dissection on the right side of the esophagus and cardia, and retracted towards the midline to facilitate dissection on the left side, including mobilization of the fundus.

Where the short gastric arteries limit mobilization of the fundus, the upper few vessels are best divided. Grasping forceps introduced through the left lower quadrant port and the right working port can be used to depress the fundus and body of the stomach and retract it medially. A hook diathermy or the ultrasonic shears can then be used to divide the short gastric vessels. The dissection is best commenced from a point cranial to the splenic hilum, and continued upwards beyond the short gastric vessels to include the condensation of the peritoneum over the upper surface of the fundus between the crura and spleen. Care must be

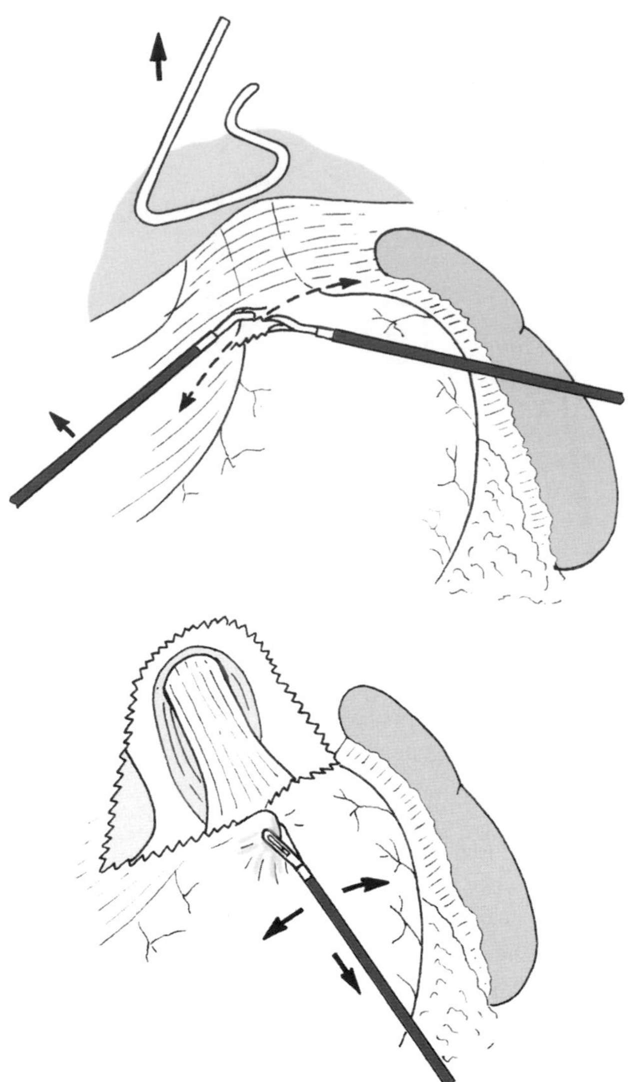

Figure 32A.2

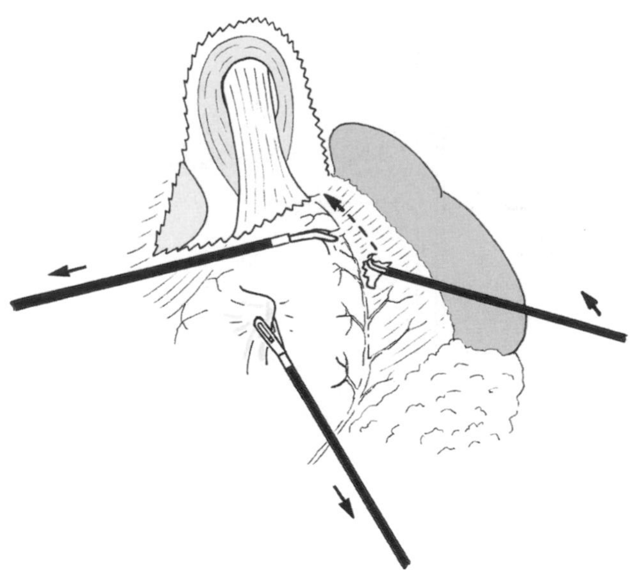

Figure 32A.3

taken to divide the vessels close to the spleen to avoid thermal injury to the stomach, as the short gastric vessels are often very short. There is little agreement as to whether the short gastric vessels should be divided routinely. Although division of the short gastric vessels has not been shown to improve clinical outcome or the physiological parameters of lower esophageal function, it may be associated with a longer operating time, and possibly an increased incidence of gas-bloat syndrome. Most anecdotal experience of surgeons suggests that the fundoplication wrap is more likely to be too tight and placed under excessive tension if the uppermost short gastric vessels are not divided in some patients. Moreover, division of the short gastric vessels also facilitates dissection of the left side of the crus and helps develop the retro-esophageal space. **(See Figure 32A.3)**

A space is developed behind the lower end of the esophagus and below the crural fibers, through which the fundus will be brought. Dissection of this retro-esophageal space is made easier if the stomach-grasping forceps (introduced through the left iliac fossa port) are released from the stomach and repositioned through the right (medial) side of the space, carefully lifting the lower end of the esophagus upwards. This allows the forceps through the two working ports to be used in tandem to enlarge the retro-esophageal space more easily. Rather than lifting the lower esophagus upwards with closed forceps, some surgeons prefer to place a tape or sling around the esophagus, or to grasp it through the gastrostomy site (or toothed grasper from the left iliac fossa port). Whatever technique is used, care must be taken to avoid damage to the esophagus.

Expansion of the retro-esophageal space is done primarily from the right side. The posterior trunk of the right vagus nerve can be seen, and is best retracted anteriorly (upwards) with the esophagus, i.e. the fundus will be brought around through a space posterior to the posterior vagus, rather than between the posterior vagal trunk and esophagus. In general, the space is expanded with blunt dissection until it is large enough to accommodate the fundus comfortably, and does not retract immediately it is released. The ascending branch of the left gastric artery is normally left intact, but the upper part of the lesser omentum may need to be divided in some patients. **(See Figure 32A.4)**

The crural fibers on either side of the esophagus are approximated with one (or occasionally two) interrupted non-absorbable sutures, ensuring there is enough space in the esophageal hiatus for the esophagus to transmit food boluses without obstruction. Some surgeons choose to introduce an esophageal bougie during this part of the procedure to avoid excessive narrowing of the esophageal hiatus as the crural fibers are approximated. Knot-tying during crural approximation is done most easily and quickly extracorporally, but any surgeon performing a laparoscopic fundoplication must have the ability to tie sutures intracorporally if necessary. **(See Figure 32A.5)**

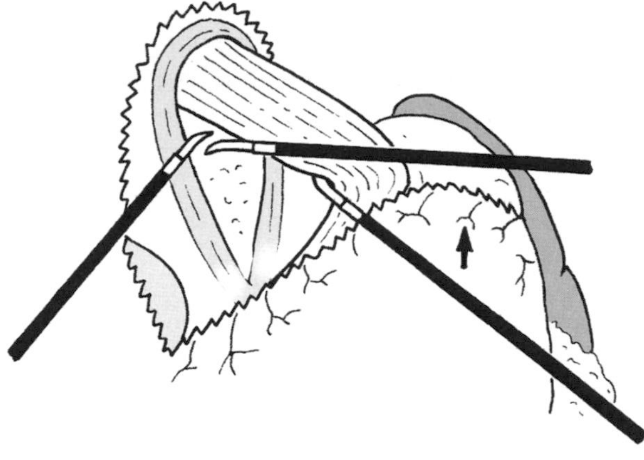

Figure 32A.4

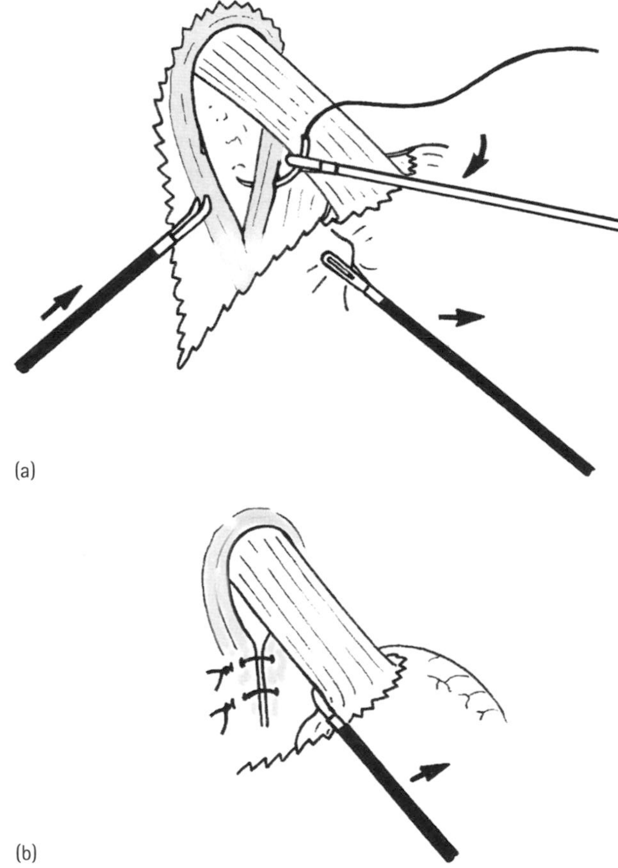

(a)

(b)

Figure 32A.5

The fundus is brought round behind the esophagus using the two pairs of forceps introduced through the working ports. The forceps act in tandem. The wrap must not be twisted, and should lie comfortably as it is brought through the retro-esophageal space. Pulling the wrap backwards and forwards several times while it is behind the esophagus (the 'shoeshine maneuver') provides confirmation that it is not twisted.

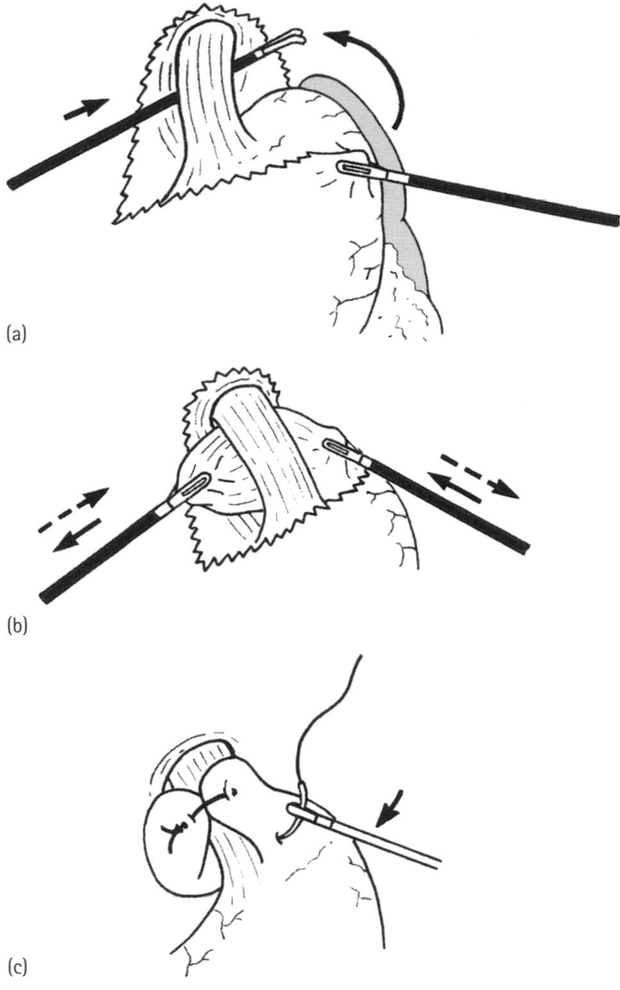

(a)

(b)

(c)

Figure 32A.6

If the fundus immediately 'pulls back' when released, it suggests that it has been inadequately mobilized, i.e. there is insufficient mobile fundus to achieve a loose wrap. In this situation, the upper short gastric vessels may need division or the space behind the esophagus may need enlargement.

The fundus is plicated anterior to the lower end of the esophagus and cardia with two 2-0 interrupted non-absorbable sutures. The two sutures should be 5–10 mm apart. A 'long' wrap is not required (there is no advantage in the wrap being longer than 2 cm), and an excessively long or tight wrap may increase the dysphagic symptoms post-operatively. The sutures of the wrap usually sit at the 10 o'clock position, i.e. the suture line of the fundoplication is slightly to the right of the esophagus. Some surgeons will incorporate the muscle of the anterior wall of the esophagus, or the adjacent inferior surface of the diaphragm, in the fundoplication sutures. **(See Figure 32A.6)**

The wrap should be confirmed as being loose: it should be possible to elevate the completed wrap away from the front of the esophagus by passing dissecting forceps beneath it. To guarantee that the fundoplication wrap will not be too tight and occlude the esophagus, some surgeons

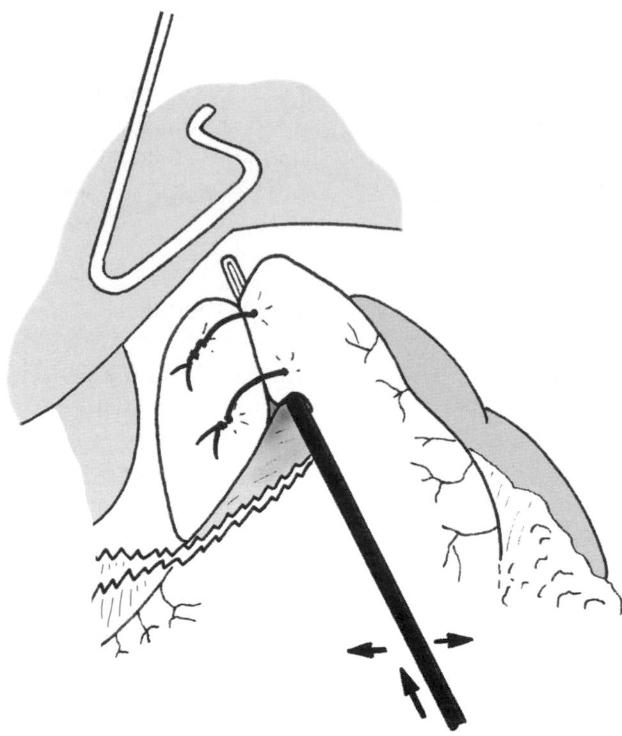

Figure 32A.7

introduce a wide-bore orogastric tube bougie prior to completing it. **(See Figure 32A.7)**

POSTOPERATIVE CARE

A nasogastric tube is left in situ for 18–24 hours to allow decompression of the stomach, unless there is a gastrostomy in place already. Oral feeds (initially fluids and pureed foods) can be commenced at 24–48 hours and increased in volume as tolerated. Postoperative analgesia is not required beyond 48 hours after surgery in 95 percent of patients. Intravenous morphine or epidural analgesia, if used, can usually be stopped after 24–48 hours. Overall, the procedure is well tolerated in children and there is no requirement for routine postoperative high-dependency care, except in those patients with co-morbidities that may require additional support. Most patients stay in hospital for 3–4 days, but a child with multiple other problems (co-morbidity) may have to stay longer.

PROBLEMS, PITFALLS AND SOLUTIONS

Previous abdominal surgery

- Frequently, children requiring anti-reflux surgery have had previous abdominal procedures, most commonly a PEG. Other procedures include ventriculo-peritoneal shunt placement, and gastrostomy for long-gap esophageal atresia. Despite this, laparoscopic fundoplication can be performed safely with minimal morbidity in children with existing gastrostomies or ventriculo-peritoneal shunts.
- Some children have had a previous fundoplication (either open or laparoscopic) that has become unwrapped or a para-esophageal hernia has developed. Laparoscopic Nissen fundoplication is possible in the vast majority (96 percent) of these, although the most likely reason for conversion to an open procedure is the presence of severe adhesions.
- If the view obtained using a 30° telescope (which can be rotated) is satisfactory, a tension-free fundoplication wrap can be performed without taking down a pre-existing gastrostomy – the stoma is best left undisturbed. Otherwise, it is preferable to take down the gastrostomy, perform the fundoplication and refashion the stoma at the completion of the procedure. If the previous site remains a tight fit and healthy, a new gastrostomy device (preferably balloon type) may be placed through the same hole. Otherwise, the previous site is closed and a new one established.

Difficult access

A poor view can result from one or more of the following.

- Inappropriate placement of the camera and instrument ports. Determination of the best position for the ports is based on the size of the child, the presence of scoliosis and the location of pre-existing stomas, e.g. gastrostomy. As a general rule, the smaller the child, the lower in the abdomen the two working ports should be placed.
- The presence of organomegaly, e.g. hepatomegaly or splenomegaly. Careful retraction of the left lobe of an enlarged liver is necessary. When splenomegaly is present, it is more likely that the uppermost short gastric vessels will need to be divided.
- Previous surgery: This may have produced adhesions that require division. In re-do fundoplication, the adhesions are often most severe between the fundoplication and the undersurface of the left lobe of the liver.
- Small operative space in infants. Shorter and smaller (3–3.5 mm) instruments are preferable, and should be introduced through correspondingly small-sized ports. The two working ports should be situated lower in the abdomen at or below the level of the umbilicus. Meticulous technique is required, and extracorporeal knot-tying is an advantage. When intracorporeal knot-tying is required, it is advisable to cut off the needle

and remove it from the abdominal cavity before the knot itself is tied.

- Kyphoscoliosis and limb contractures in neurologically impaired children. These pose specific difficulties in positioning the patient on the operating table. Fixed flexion at the hip may make it difficult to use the working ports (because the leg gets in the way), necessitating modification of the location of the ports. Severe scoliosis may contribute to displacement of the intra-abdominal organs and vertebral column in relation to the usual landmarks.

Large hiatus hernia with or without a short esophagus

Sometimes there is a large hiatus hernia into which the stomach has entered, and it may be adherent to the peritoneum within the hernial sac. The sac does not have to be excised, but the stomach must be mobilized so that it can be reduced into the abdominal cavity below the diaphragm. The distorted anatomy should be recognized and assessed prior to the commencement of dissection. Large hernial defects may be best closed with a synthetic mesh or membrane, particularly in recurrent cases. If the procedure proves extremely difficult, conversion to an open technique may be advisable.

Bleeding

Minor bleeding may occur during dissection of the phrenico-esophageal ligament around the lower end of the esophagus near the cardia, and from the short gastric vessels. Bleeding from the spleen and liver can be avoided by careful instrumentation and positioning of the liver retractor. Prominent lower esophageal veins in portal hypertension tend to be friable, and should be handled extremely carefully and controlled with a Harmonic Scalpel®.

Difficulty creating an adequate 'window' behind the lower end of the esophagus

This is often the most difficult part of the surgery for beginners. Early identification of the crural fibers on either side of esophagus may be difficult, and there is a tendency to shred them during dissection of the esophageal hiatus and to dissect too far into the mediastinum through the hiatus. It is even possible inadvertently to open the pleura; this is most likely to occur in the presence of a hiatus hernia. These problems can be avoided by regular review of the anatomy, use of an angled scope (30°) and retracting the stomach close to the cardia, either to the left or the right, depending on which side of the hiatus is being dissected.

Tearing of the crural fibers with the suture

It is important for the security of the approximation of the crural fibers for reasonably big bites of crura to be included in the suture. Care has to be taken to avoid the suture being directed too far posteriorly, as this may damage the aorta and cause bleeding.

Damage to the posterior vagal trunk

The posterior vagus runs longitudinally on the posterior aspect of the lower end of the esophagus. Sometimes during dissection of the space behind the esophagus it is possible to separate the posterior vagus from the esophagus and create a space that pushes the vagal trunk posteriorly. It is better to ensure that the posterior vagus remains on the surface of the esophagus, and to create a retro-esophageal space posterior to it. When the esophagus is lifted upwards, as described previously, it is important to ensure that the vagal trunk is included with it.

- Need to convert to an open procedure (6 percent).
- Gastric or esophageal perforation (1 percent).
- Pneumothorax (2 percent).
- Splenic injury requiring splenectomy (0.1 percent).

Early postoperative complications are rare but include the following.

- Re-operation for postoperative bleeding (0.2 percent).
- Missed gastric or esophageal perforation (0.4 percent).
- Crural disruption, peri-esophageal herniation or gastric volvulus.
- Ongoing gastro-esophageal reflux.
- Initial dysphagia and poor esophageal clearance: this may result from too tight a wrap, postoperative edema, or pre-existing esophageal dysmotility.

Difficulty with the wrap

There are two main causes of difficulty bringing the fundus of the stomach around behind the esophagus and suturing it anteriorly without undue tension.

- Inadequate space created behind the lower esophagus. This necessitates enlargement of the space by a combination of blunt division with two pairs of forceps pushing in opposite directions. Diathermy dissection may be required to divide the uppermost part of the lesser omentum, including related vessels.
- Relative immobility of the fundus secondary to intact short gastric vessels and the close proximity of the spleen. This necessitates division of one or more of the uppermost short gastric vessels to free the fundus.

Gastric outlet obstruction

There has been little agreement about the objective assessment and significance of gastric outlet obstruction in the presence of reflux. Many surgeons claim it is an extremely rare phenomenon, although there are a few surgeons who perform pyloroplasty frequently or routinely at the time of fundoplication.

COMPLICATIONS

The potential intra-operative complications include the following.

Failed previous fundoplication requiring re-operation

- Re-operative fundoplications can be performed laparoscopically and produce results similar to those of a primary laparoscopic fundoplication.
- Laparoscopic re-operation after a primary open fundoplication can be technically challenging and has a higher incidence of complications, such as inadvertent opening of the stomach, injury to the esophagus, postoperative leaks and pneumothoraces.
- The median length of stay in hospital is about 5 days, significantly longer than that for primary laparoscopic fundoplication.

FURTHER READING

Allal H, Captier G, Lopez M. Evaluation of 142 consecutive laparoscopic fundoplications in children: effects of the learning curve and technical choice. *Journal of Pediatric Surgery* 2001; **36**(6):921–6.

Esposito C, Montupet P, Reinberg O. Laparoscopic surgery for gastresophageal reflux disease during the first year of life. *Journal of Pediatric Surgery* 2001; **36**(5):715–17.

Pimpalwar A, Najmaldin A. Results of laparoscopic antireflux procedures in neurologically impaired children. *Seminars in Laparoscopic Surgery* 2002; **9**(3):190–6.

Rothenberg S. Laparoscopic Nissen procedure in children. *Seminars in Laparoscopic Surgery* 2002; **9**:146–52.

Van Der Zee BC, Bax NM, Ure BM. Laparoscopic refundoplication in children. *Surgical Endoscopy* 2000; **14**(12):1103–4.

32B

Anti-reflux surgery – Toupet procedure

PHILIPPE MONTUPET

INTRODUCTION

Laparoscopic anti-reflux surgery is well established in the treatment of gastro-esophageal reflux disease, and the Toupet procedure provides an alternative to the Nissen fundoplication, particularly in children with significant esophageal dysmotility.

Indications

Although most surgeons use the Nissen technique, there are some situations in which the Toupet operation is considered by some to be more appropriate.

- Dysmotility of the esophagus as demonstrated by a manometric study (neurologically impaired children).
- Previous repair of esophageal atresia.

A partial posterior wrap maintains better anatomical relationships than the 360° wrap of the Nissen fundoplication. It cannot be made too tight, and consequently the risk of postoperative dysphagia is very low (if any), preserves the ability to belch and is easy to reinforce if gastro-esophageal reflux relapses. In this procedure, the gastrosplenic ligament (containing the short gastric vessels) does not need to be divided and the risk of the wrap slipping into the chest is minimal.

EQUIPMENT/INSTRUMENTS

Essential

The umbilical cannula depends on the size of the telescope – 5–10 mm for children, 3–5 mm for infants.

- Three 5 mm (or 3 mm for infants) working ports.
- 5 mm three-finger liver retractor. In infants, all 5 mm instruments can be substituted by 3 mm instruments.
- 5 mm smooth and fenestrated grasping forceps.
- 5 mm hook for dissection and monopolar cauterizing.
- Two 5 mm needle holders.
- Scissors.
- 10 mm 30° angled telescope (in smaller children, a 5 mm 30° telescope can be used).

Optional

- Suction/irrigation device.
- Clip applicator.
- Bipolar diathermy.

TECHNIQUE

The procedure is performed under general anesthesia with endotracheal intubation. The child lies supine in a reverse 15° Trendelenburg position. In smaller children and infants, the legs are folded at the bottom of the table; otherwise, the legs are stretched out and spread open. A handrail is fixed at the right edge of the table in order to lighten the left arm of the assistant holding the telescope. The surgeon faces the patient from the bottom of the table, which can be orientated in front of the monitor.

The video equipment is placed on the right side of the patient's head. All cables are fixed at the level of the right leg. The assistant and the table of instruments are on the right side of the surgeon. The surgeon and the assistant are seated on surgical saddles.

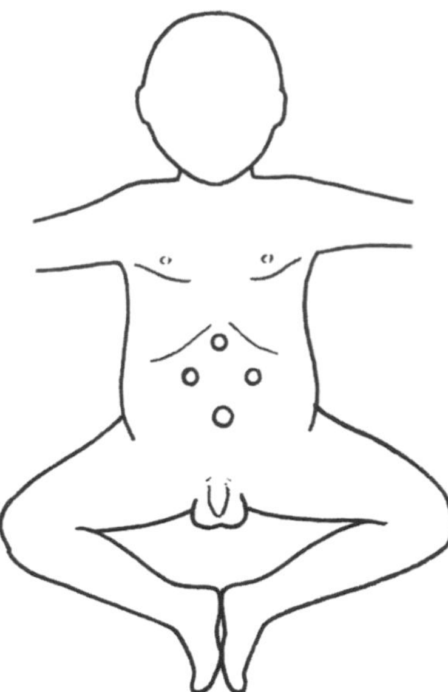

Figure 32B.1

A 10–12 Fr nasogastric tube is inserted. Local anesthesia (0.25 percent bupivacaine) is infiltrated around the umbilicus and the sites of the working ports. The positions of the ports are always the same, even when a gastrostomy is present. The umbilicus is incised at its superior margin, and the three other incisions create a triangle whose apex is below the tip of the xiphoid process, and the lateral points are symmetrical in the upper quadrants. The assistant can hold the telescope and the retractor and therefore a second assistant is not usually required. **(See Figure 32B.1)**

Toupet's procedure consists of two main sequential steps:

1 the dissection
2 the fundoplication (suturing of the valve).

Dissection

The initial dissection is similar to that performed for any type of laparoscopic fundoplication.

- The liver retractor pushes the left and caudate lobes cephalad and to the right respectively, allowing a clear view of the hepatogastric ligament.
- The right crus of the diaphragm is easily located, and the dissection is carried out between the esophagus and the crus using the tip of a smooth atraumatic grasper. Blunt dissection around the esophagus enables identification of the left crus and posterior vagus nerve.
- In the space between the left crus and lower end of the esophagus, the tip of an atraumatic instrument is directed behind the cardia towards the spleen. The ligament is opened, and the window so created is enlarged widely.
- The lower 3–5 cm of esophagus is completely freed. Care must be taken to avoid vagal nerve injury and, if possible, to preserve the main hepatic branches.

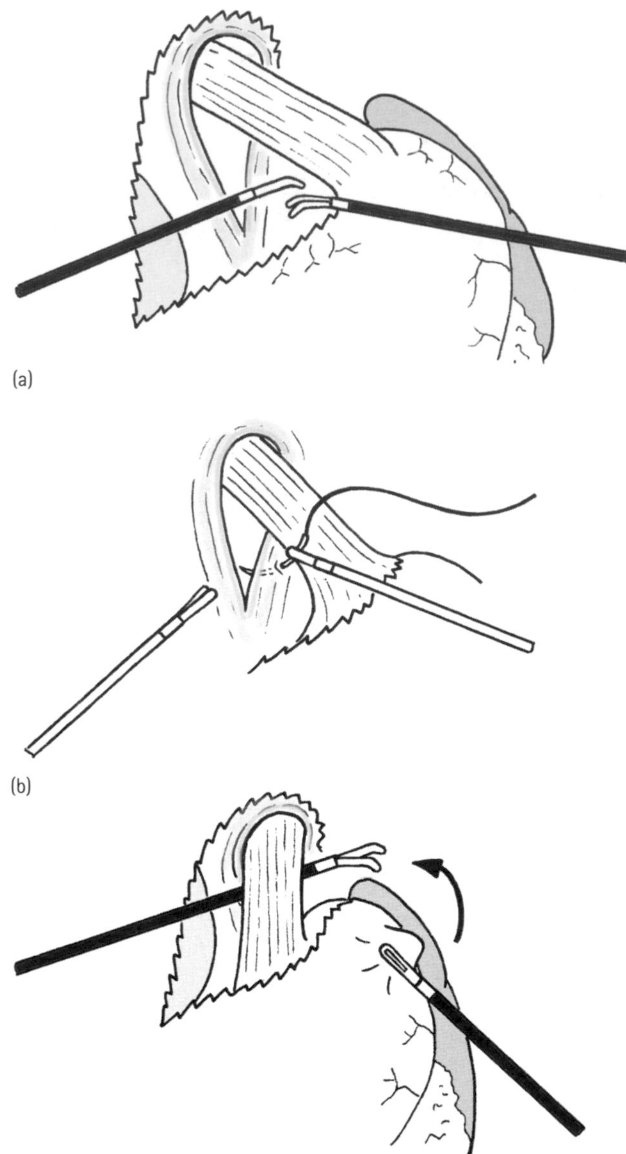

Figure 32B.2

A hiatoplasty is performed by placing one or two nonabsorbable sutures through the crura. The number of sutures is determined by the size of the defect and the nature of the crural fibers (healthy and normal or thin and shredded, or tight and fibrosed). Generous bites are usually necessary and the sutures are tied snug but not tight to prevent ischemic necrosis of the muscle.

The anterior wall of the fundus is grasped through the window behind the lower esophagus and cardia. The fundus is then is manipulated to sit comfortably around the lower esophagus. **(See Figure 32B.2)**

Fundoplication (suturing)

A temporary complete wrap/without tension is now created around the lower esophagus and maintained in position

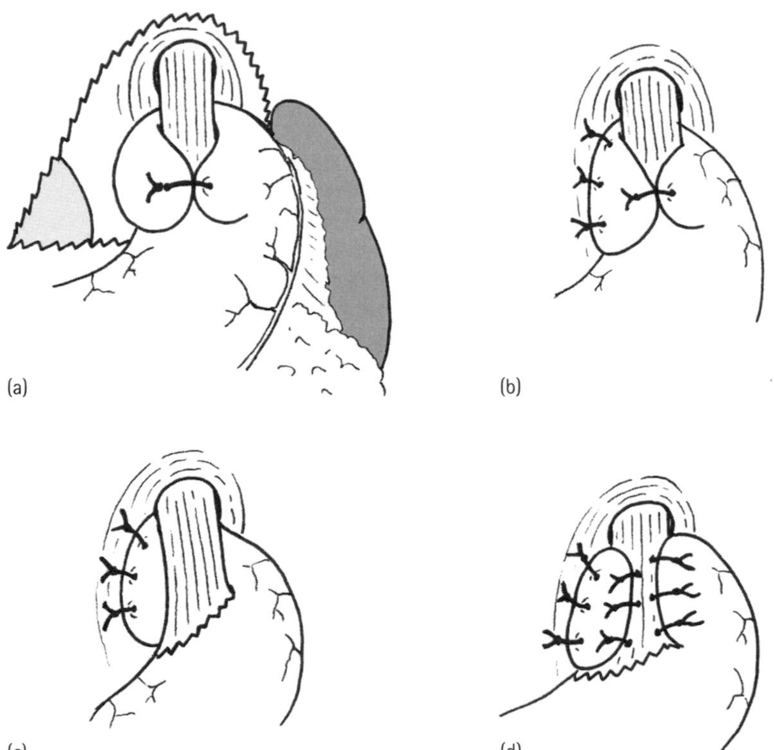

Figure 32B.3

using a single (temporary) stitch called a frame stitch. This maneuver facilitates the final stages of suturing.

The right edge of the fundus is sutured to the right crus with three sutures. The frame stitch is removed.

The telescope is now advanced towards the operative field in order to obtain a clear and magnified view of the surface of the esophagus. The right anterio-lateral surface of the esophagus is opposed to the fundus using three non-absorbable sutures through the muscle layer only. Care must be taken not to allow tension or to incorporate the anterior vagus nerve.

The same maneuver is applied to the left anterio-lateral surface of the esophagus. Once the suturing is completed, a 90° surface area of the esophagus should remain free. **(See Figure 32B.3)**

POSTOPERATIVE CARE

Adequate analgesia, if necessary by morphine infusion, is provided. The nasogastric tube is kept in until the next morning. Oral feeds with liquids and fluid diet are commenced 2 hours after the nasogastric tube has been removed. Normal diet is resumed and the intravenous line is removed on the second postoperative day. Most children are discharged from hospital on the third postoperative day.

It is important to inform the parents about the transient dysphagia that may occur postoperatively. Manometric and upper gastrointestinal contrast studies may be obtained at 4 months and 2 and 5 years postoperatively.

PROBLEMS, PITFALLS AND SOLUTIONS

The problems encountered during the Toupet operation are, more or less, the same as for Nissen fundoplication.

- The assistant should be physically comfortable during the operation. This involves attention to his or her position, provision of a seat, and supporting his or her arm with a handrail. These measures are likely to be translated into better assistance, a better view and increased safety.
- Blind blunt dissection is best avoided as it may damage the spleen and cause bleeding. Minor splenic bleeding will usually stop spontaneously.
- When bleeding occurs, it tends to be relatively minor. It is reasonable to leave the area for a few minutes, after which time it has usually stopped spontaneously. A bloody field should be irrigated with saline and suctioned; this restores better light and facilitates ongoing dissection.
- The posterior vagus nerve is identified in order to avoid damaging it and to provide a landmark to dissection between the crura and posterior wall of the intra-abdominal esophagus.

COMPLICATIONS

The per-operative complications are the same as for Nissen fundoplication.

- Transient dysphagia. This complication is common during the first 3–4 weeks after surgery. It usually improves with time and in our experience has necessitated no early re-operations.
- Re-do Toupet fundoplication. Seven cases of revision fundoplication have been performed in our series of 720 Toupet procedures. Four of them were required during the first year of follow-up, two after 2 years and one after 5 years. In these cases, the re-do surgery was the same, but it necessitated only re-insertion of the sutures of the wrap, because the hiatoplasty was intact.

FURTHER READING

Bensoussan AL, Yazbeck S, Carceller-Blanchard A. Results and complications of Toupet's partial posterior wrap: 10 years' experience. *Journal of Pediatric Surgery* 1994; **29**:1215–17.

De Meester TR, Stein HJ. Minimizing the side effects of antireflux surgery. *World Journal of Surgery* 1992; **16**:335–6.

McKerman JB. Laparoscopic repair of gastro-esophageal disease. Toupet fundoplication versus Nissen fundoplication. *Surgical Endoscopy* 1994; **8**:851–6.

Montupet P. Laparoscopic fundoplication in children. In: Toouli J, Gossot D, Hunter JG (eds), *Endosurgery.* Edinburgh: Churchill Livingstone, 1996, 935–40.

Montupet P, Gauthier F, Valayer J. Traitement chirurgical du reflux gastroesophagien par hemivalve tuberositaire posterieure fixee. *Chirurgia Pediatrica* 1983; **24**:122–7.

32C

Anti-reflux surgery – Thal procedure

KLAUS HELLER

INTRODUCTION

In the original paper of Thal, two different techniques are described. The first is an operation to repair a distal esophageal stenosis. The esophagus and gastric fundus are mobilized, the esophagus is incised longitudinally at the level of the stenosis and the gastric fundus is used to bridge the defect in a manner that prevents gastric reflux. In this process the serosa of the fundus becomes the inner wall of the esophagus.

The second technique is used to repair gastro-esophageal reflux without any stenosis. This is a routine procedure and is often used as a standard technique as well with open and laparoscopic access.

Indications

- Gastro-esophageal reflux with gastrointestinal and general symptoms (vomiting, heartburn, esophagitis, Barrett's dysplasia, failure to thrive, dystrophia, anemia).
- Gastro-esophageal reflux with bronchopulmonary symptoms (recurrent aspirations, recurrent bronchitis and pneumonia, bronchiectasis, asthma-bronchiale equivalent, near-miss sudden infant death syndrome).

Contraindications

ABSOLUTE

- Hemodynamic instability.

RELATIVE

- Severely neurologically impaired children, especially with convulsions or tetraspastics. In these children we prefer the complete Nissen/Rossetti fundoplication, in most cases in combination with a gastrostomy (gastric tube). The 360° cuff is more likely to resist high abdominal pressures.
- In children with severe scoliosis, thoracic access is sometimes preferable as the cardia can be hidden by the costal margin.
- Failed previous fundoplication.
- Previous upper abdominal surgery.

EQUIPMENT/INSTRUMENTS

Essential

- Two 5–10 mm trocars, two 3.5–5 mm trocars.
- 5 mm or 10 mm 30° or 50° telescope with a video camera.
- 5 mm liver retractor.
- Two 3.5–5 mm needle holders.
- 5 mm ultrasonic shears (or a cautery hook).
- 3.5–5 mm scissors.
- 3.5–5 mm dissecting forceps with monopolar diathermy.
- 5 mm suction/irrigation device.
- Non-resorbable sutures 3-0 and 2-0 (Ethibond) with a SH or RB 1-needle.

Optional

- Cautery hook (or 5 mm ultrasonic shears).
- Device to fix the liver retractor.
- Robotic system (Da Vinci or Zeus). This procedure is most suitable for the use of a robotic system. Preparation is carried out with a cautery hook and grasping forceps. All manipulations can be carried out very precisely under three-dimensional vision.

PREOPERATIVE PREPARATION

The diagnosis is based on a barium swallow, 24-hour two-level pH-monitoring, esophago-gastroscopy and esophageal biopsy. Bronchoscopy with bronchoalveolar lavage and detection of lipid-laden alveolar macrophages may add useful information in some children, particularly those with chronic lung symptoms. The gastric scintigraphy with estimation of gastric emptying and registration of aspiration (hot spots in the lungs) or esophageal manometry may prove helpful. Suspected bronchiectasis can be checked by a high-resolution computerized tomography (CT) scan. Bronchopulmonary diseases such as allergy, immunodeficiency, cystic fibrosis, primary ciliary dyskinesia and malformations of the bronchial tree or great vessels are excluded preoperatively. Patients with pre-existing conditions (syndromes) and/or previous surgery suffer more frequently from reflux than normal children. These conditions include: Kartagener syndrome (genetically caused functional and structural deficiency of the bronchial cilia, in which half also have situs inversus), CHARGE-association, congenital microgastria, condition after repair of an esophageal atresia, after gastrostomia and diaphragmatic hernia. Reflux can be a part of Munchausen-by-proxy syndrome. Reflux can induce neurological symptoms in the form of Sandifer's syndrome.

Prior to surgery the author advocates a course of therapy with antacids and propulsive drugs for a minimum of 6 weeks to control local inflammation and evaluate the effect of medication on clinical symptoms. For those who suffer from chronic lung disease, preoperative chest physiotherapy and antibiotics for 3 months or more are thought by the author to be necessary. A blood sample for hematological and biochemical investigation is taken, but cross-matched blood is usually not necessary. An enema to decompress the colon may ease the postoperative course.

TECHNIQUE

The patient is placed in a supine, reverse Trendelenburg position with legs apart and in stirrups. An adequate-sized nasogastric tube is placed. The surgeon stands between the patient's legs, with the camera operator on the right side

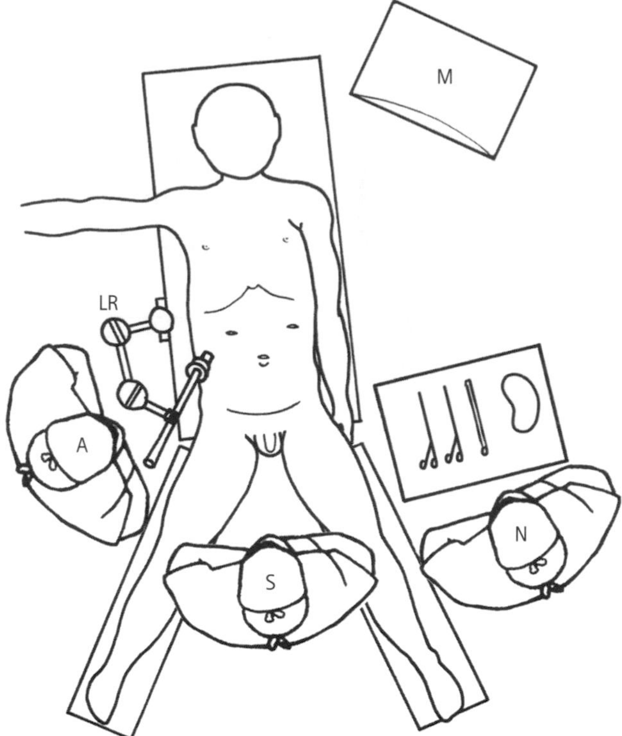

Figure 32C.1

and the scrub nurse on the left. In smaller children the surgeon may stand on the left side. **(See Figure 32C.1)**

Four cannulae are usually required. The first (5–10 mm) is inserted through a mini-laparotomy with a fascial purse-string suture. This suture prevents gas leak and allows fast closure of the abdominal wall at the end of the procedure. A pneumoperitoneum is established using CO_2 at a pressure of 10–12 mmHg. An angled (30° or 50°) telescope is inserted and, under direct vision, two working cannulae are positioned, one on each side (right 3.5–5 mm, left 5–10 mm). A 10 mm cannula allows easy insertion and removal of sutures with SH or RB needles. A fourth cannula is placed lateral to the right working cannula near the subcostal margin for the liver retractor. The retractor is inserted carefully, the left lobe of the liver is lifted superiorly to expose the gastro-esophageal junction. The retractor may be fixed to the side of the operating table with a special device, or held by a second surgical assistant.

The dissection begins at the peritoneal fold at the level of the 'hiatus esophagei' using ultrasonic shears and dissecting forceps. Alternatively, a hook cautery or scissors are used. The peritoneum is divided, and blunt dissection is used at the hiatal margin to separate the right and left crura from the front and the sides of the esophagus.

A window to view the left crus is created behind the esophagus. At this stage the posterior vagus nerve is easily seen. **(See Figure 32C.2)**

Care must be taken to preserve both vagal nerves and avoid injury to the esophagus. Care must also be taken not to

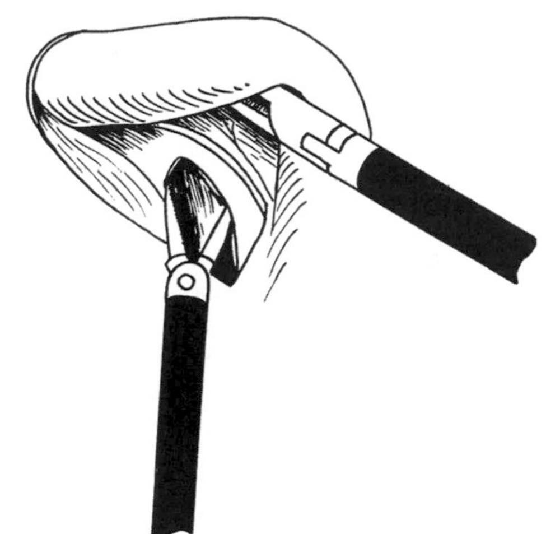

Figure 32C.2

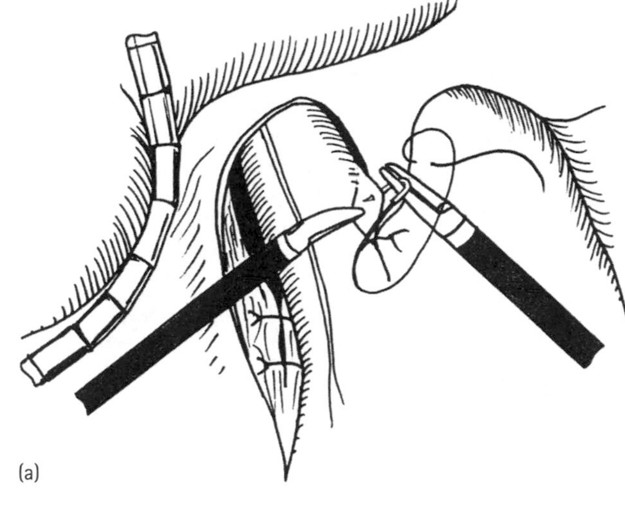

(a)

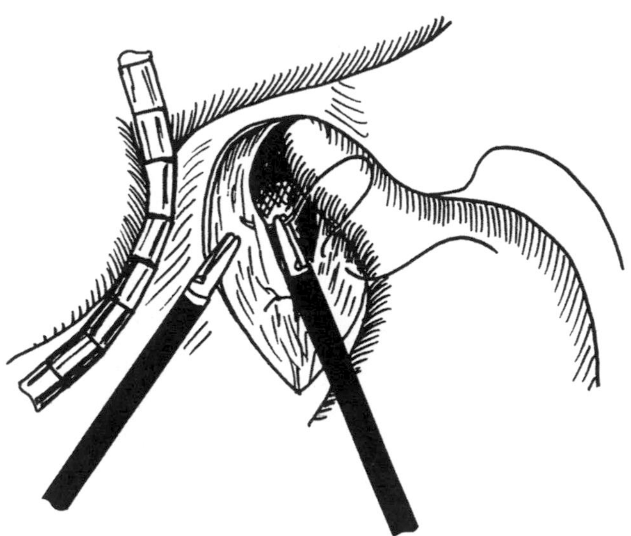

Figure 32C.3

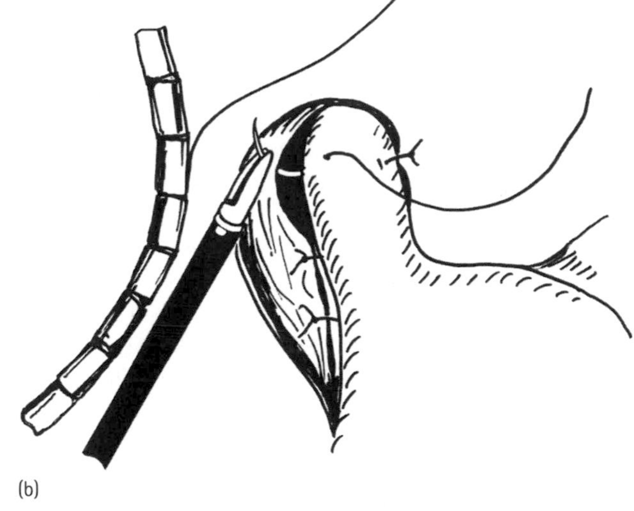

(b)

Figure 32C.4(a) and (b)

dissect deep into the posterior mediastinum behind the left crus. Division of the short gastric vessels is not necessary unless the gastric fundus is very small and/or there is tension on the wrap. Sometimes the spleen is located very close to the distal esophagus and has to be mobilized as necessary.

The retro-esophageal crural approximation (hiatal repair) is then performed using two sutures of 2-0 Ethibond. **(See Figure 32C.3)**

The sutures are introduced through the patient's left-side cannula. They should be about 12 cm long so that they can be used twice. Some surgeons prefer a fifth cannula for an instrument to hold the esophagus antero-caudally. A simple suture, inserted through the abdominal wall, slung around the esophagus and brought out again, can achieve the same end. However, this is generally not necessary. A 22–36 Fr gastric tube is inserted to check and maintain the patency of the esophageal lumen. **(See Figure 32C.4)**

Using Ethibond 3-0, the fundus is sutured to the left side of the esophagus starting at the angle between the esophagus and stomach and is continued cephalad.

The wrap is then completed anteriorly around the esophagus. The sutures are continued anteriorly towards the right and downwards along the right side of the esophagus. In the upper part of the wrap the sutures incorporate the peritoneal cover (not the muscle of the crus) to stabilize the esophageal sutures and to shut off the mediastinum from the peritoneal cavity. **(See Figure 32C.5)**

In all, 10–12 sutures are necessary. We prefer intracorporeal knots. At the end of the operation the operating field is inspected to ensure complete hemostasis. The liver retractor is removed followed by the working cannulae, the trocars and finally the telescope. The previously placed purse-string suture at the site of the cannula is tied and the skin is closed.

In children with a Kartagener-syndrome 'situs inversus', laparoscopic viewing and orientation can be a particular challenge.

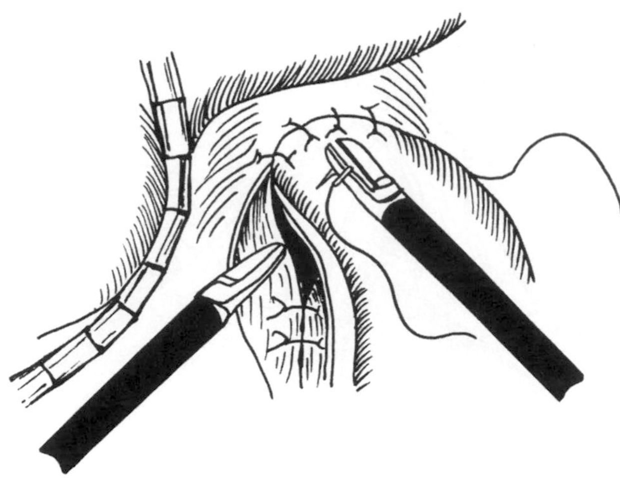

Figure 32C.5

POSTOPERATIVE CARE

All children receive a dose of antibiotics at the start of the operation. However, those who suffer chronic lung disease or infection may continue with antibiotics for 3–5 days postoperatively or even longer. Analgesics are given on demand. The nasogastric tube is removed on the first post-operative day, oral feeding resumes on the second day and the patient is usually ready to leave hospital within a few days. We recommend mushy food for 6 weeks to prevent bolus obstruction in the distal esophagus.

PROBLEMS, PITFALLS AND SOLUTIONS

These are the same as for other anti-reflux procedures (see Chapters 32A and 32B).

COMPLICATIONS

Early

- Esophageal or gastric perforation. Creating a window behind the oesophagus is the most difficult part of the operation. A combined gentle sharp and blunt dissection is mandatory. Dissection should be carried along the crus, not the esophagus, to avoid injuring the posterior wall of the esophagus and vagus nerve. Injuries are rare and can usually be successfully closed endoscopically.
- Pleural injury. There is a tendency to dissect from the right side towards the mediastinum and behind the left crus. Adequate exposure of the left crus from the left will help avoid this problem.
- Vagal nerve injury. Care must be taken to avoid vagal nerve injury during dissection at the level of gastro-esophageal junction.
- Bleeding. Bleeding may occur at and around the lesser curvature and in the retro-esophageal space. Usually the vessels can easily be grasped and hemostasis achieved using ultrasonic shears or diathermy. Suction/irrigation may be necessary.
- Liver injury. If space between the liver and esophagus is tight and/or the liver retractor cannot be placed in an optimal position, liver injury might occur. The safest way to retract the liver is to place the retractor against the diaphragm above the esophageal hiatus. Bleeding usually stops spontaneously, but diathermy may be used if necessary.
- Conversion to open surgery. In routine procedures, conversion is rarely necessary. Inadequate viewing, bleeding and lack of expertise are the usual contributing factors.

Delayed

- Stenosis.
  - This may occur as a result of inadequate mobilization of the stomach or esophagus.
  - The wrap may be too tight.
  - The crural repair may be too tight.
- Recurrent reflux. This is a common occurrence in neurologically impaired patients who persistently gag and retch. Meticulous dissection and attention to the geometry of the wrap will minimize the incidence.
- Gas bloat syndrome. Persistent gastric bloat is relatively rare and may be treated with a modified feeding regimen (small but frequent boluses).
- Dumping syndrome. This is a rare complication unless a pyloroplasty is performed.
- Para-esophageal hernia. This is usually secondary to weak muscle or an inadequate crural repair. It requires re-doing.
- Prolonged dysphagia. This is usually secondary to an improperly constructed wrap or tight repair. A barium swallow should be obtained and esophageal dilatation is considered. In extreme circumstances re-do surgery may be required.

FURTHER READING

Ahrens P, Heller K, Beyer P et al. Antireflux surgery in children suffering from reflux-associated respiratory diseases. *Pediatric Pulmonology* 1999; **28**:89–93.

Esposito C, Montoupet P, Amici G, Desruelle P. Complications of antireflux surgery in childhood. *Surgical Endoscopy* 2000; **14**:622–4.

Kinsbury M. Hiatus hernia with contorsions to the neck. *Lancet* 1964; **1**:1058–64.

Mattioli G, Esposito C, Lima M et al. Italian multicenter survey on laparoscopic treatment of gastroesophageal reflux disease in children. *Surgical Endoscopy* 2002; **16**:1–4.

Thal AP, Hatafuku T, Kurtzman R. New operation for distal esophageal stricture. *Archives of Surgery* 1965; **90**:464–72.

33

Gastrostomy

AZAD NAJMALDIN

INTRODUCTION

Fashioning of a gastrostomy as a means of maintaining enteral nutrition in those unable to feed normally was first attempted in 1837, and it was 40 years later that a patient survived the procedure. Since the initial success, numerous modifications have been reported. Percutaneous endoscopic gastrostomy (PEG) is now a well-established minimally invasive method for fashioning a gastrostomy. Nevertheless, significant complications are still reported, the most feared of all being injury to the viscera, which occurs in up to 3 percent of patients. In recent years, however, laparoscopic insertion or assisted gastrostomy has been introduced as an alternative minimally invasive method with the following advantages.

Advantages

- Precise positioning of any gastrostomy device on the abdominal and gastric walls.
- Minimizes the risk of inadvertent visceral injury. This is particularly so if open technique laparoscopy is used.
- Secure insertion of any gastrostomy tube or button as a primary procedure.
- As an alternative method when PEG is contraindicated.

Disadvantages

The disadvantages of the technique include the following:

- Necessitates laparoscopy (insertion of one or more cannulae and creation of a pneumoperitoneum).
- The procedure takes longer to perform than PEG.

Indications

- Primary insertion of gastrostomy.
- Patients undergoing other laparoscopic procedures such as anti-reflux surgery.
- When PEG gastrostomy is contraindicated:
  - not possible to pass a gastroscope,
  - abdominal scarring,
  - abdominal wall pathology,
  - large hiatus hernia,
  - severe kyphoscoliosis,
  - visceromegaly/large abdominal masses,
  - coagulopathy,
  - large ascites.

The limitations of the laparoscopic insertion or assisted gastrostomy are essentially related to the experience of the surgeon. The technique is contraindicated in patients who cannot tolerate general anesthesia and a low-pressure pneumoperitoneum.

EQUIPMENT/INSTRUMENTS

The types, number and size of instruments and cannulae depend on the exact nature of the procedure to be executed and whether the gastrostomy is inserted during other laparoscopic procedures.

In laparoscopic-assisted PEG, a 3.5–5 mm cannula and telescope are required in addition to the standard PEG kit.

The following equipment is needed for laparoscopic gastrostomy.

- Two/three 3.5–5 mm cannulae.
- 3.5–5 mm, preferably angled, telescope.

- One or two 3.5–5 mm atraumatic graspers.
- 3.5–5 mm needle holder (purse-string technique).
- 2-0 Vicryl® suture on straightened out taper-cut or round or ski needle (purse-string technique), or two strong 2-0-1 polydioxanone surgical (PDS) suture on large, half-circle taper-cut or round needle depending on the size of the patient (U-hitching suture technique).
- Needle, guide-wire, dilator and peel-away sheath (14 Fr gastrostomy requires 18 Fr peel-away). Alternatively, use a diathermy needle or scissors to establish the site of entry for the gastrostomy on the stomach wall.
- Nasogastric tube.
- Gastrostomy device.
- In difficult cases, e.g. scarred abdomen, or in the presence of large intra-abdominal lesions/visceromegaly, additional laparoscopic instruments are required for adhesiolysis, retraction etc.

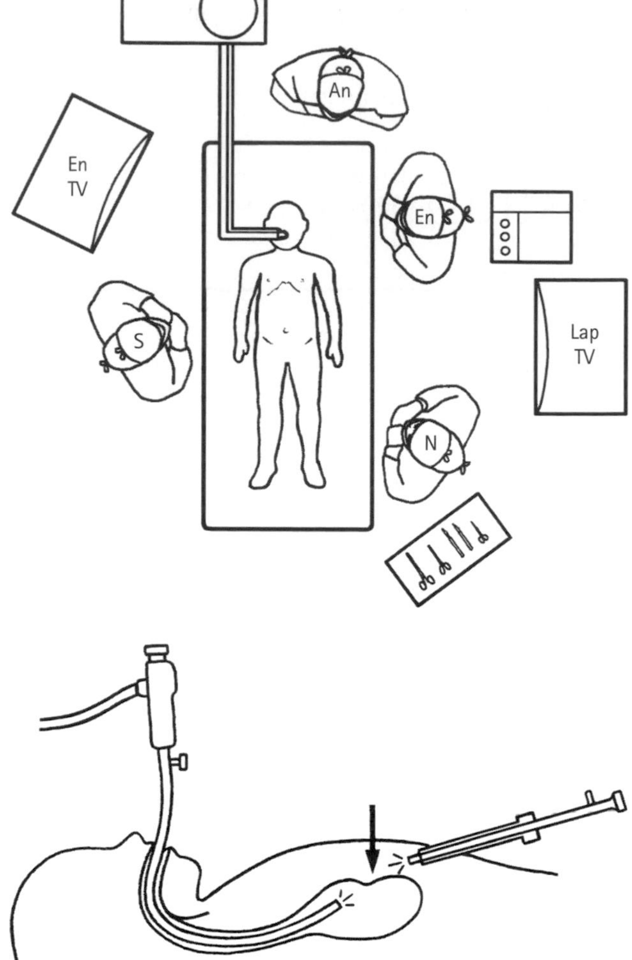

Figure 33.1

PREOPERATIVE PREPARATION

Investigations and preparation of the patient prior to laparoscopic gastrostomy are necessary, as for open or PEG procedures. Significant gastro-esophageal reflux and delayed gastric emptying are ruled out. Concomitant anti-reflux surgery may be considered if necessary. The patient (older children) and parents/carers (small children/infants) must be informed about the complications of gastrostomy, the advantages and disadvantages of the various types of gastrostomy devices available, and the possibility of the need to convert to either PEG or an open technique.

TECHNIQUE

Laparoscopic-assisted PEG

The patient is positioned supine as for insertion of PEG. The endoscopist stands on the top left hand of the patient, while the laparoscopist is on the right and the scrub nurse/assistant is opposite (to help both the laparoscopist and endoscopist). **(See Figure 33.1)**

An ideal gastrostomy site on the skin surface is marked before a pneumoperitoneum is established. A 3.5–5 mm cannula is inserted in the peri-umbilical region using the open technique. A pneumoperitoneum is created (4–6 mmHg). The peritoneal cavity is inspected for suitability of the PEG at both abdominal and gastric walls and a gastrostomy site is chosen. The endoscopist then passes a pediatric gastroscope into the stomach. It is important to keep both gastric and peritoneal insufflation to a minimum, and the balance between the two is changed as necessary throughout the procedure. A small skin and fascial incision to fit the size of the gastrostomy is made using a No. 11 blade. Under direct vision, a wide-bore needle is passed through this incision into the inflated stomach. The needle position is confirmed via the gastroscope and a guide-wire passed through the needle is snared gastroscopically and brought out through the mouth as for a standard PEG. A gastrostomy tube is then passed through the mouth and out of the abdominal wall. The position of the tube and the integrity of its track are then checked both gastroscopically and laparoscopically. If desired, the method allows fixation of the stomach to the abdominal wall by hitching sutures placed either percutaneously (see 'Laparoscopic gastrostomy' below) or intracorporeally by means of secondary laparoscopic cannulae and instruments.

The peritoneum is deflated and the umbilical wound is closed. The cannulae and gastrostomy sites are infiltrated with local anesthetic agents, at either the beginning or end of the procedure. Care must be taken not to damage the gastrostomy tube with the injecting needle.

PROBLEMS, PITFALLS AND SOLUTIONS

- Glare through the gastroscope as the result of disturbed light balance/intensity by the laparoscope. Withdraw the laparoscope into the cannula.
- In a scarred abdomen, laparoscopic adhesiolysis may be necessary. However, manipulation of the telescope around adhesions may allow adequate visualization of the stomach without adhesiolysis.
- Difficult view due to enlarged liver or spleen. Retraction through an additional cannula may prove helpful.

Laparoscopic gastrostomy (purse-string technique)

The patient is positioned supine with the surgeon standing on one or other side, at the end of the operating table (infants), or between the patient's abducted legs (older children). A nasogastric tube is inserted. The gastrostomy site is marked on the abdominal wall before a pneumoperitoneum is created. A peri-umbilical 3.5–5 mm primary cannula is inserted using an open technique. Under direct vision, two 3.5–5 mm working cannulae are placed, with the left being at or just above the umbilical level between the mid-clavicular and anterior axillary lines, and the right higher in the mid-clavicular line. **(See Figure 33.2)**

The liver is retracted anterio-superiorly by an atraumatic grasper through the right cannula and the exact site for the gastrostomy is marked on the stomach with a diathermy point or fine curved grasper through the left cannula. A 2-0 Vicryl® suture on a straightened-out taper-cut needle is introduced either percutaneously or through a 5 mm cannula into the peritoneal cavity. The stomach is then stabilized with an atraumatic grasping instrument and a single purse-string suture is placed on it (10–15 mm around the pre-marked site) using three long and deep bites and allowing 10 cm or more of the suture ends to remain free. A small incision to fit the size of the gastrostomy is made on the anterior abdominal wall using a No. 11 blade. The anesthetist is now asked to insufflate the stomach moderately through the nasogastric tube. The stomach is then stabilized gently and an appropriate incision to accommodate the gastrostomy is made in the gastric wall using a needle diathermy or scissors and a fine grasper through either the left cannula or the prepared site of the gastrostomy. Care is taken not to damage the suture. The gastrostomy is passed through the abdominal wall, guided carefully with an atraumatic grasper into the stomach, and the balloon is inflated. Care is taken not to damage the gastrostomy balloon. Alternatively, Seldinger technique and peel-away sheath (described below) are used to facilitate the insertion of the gastrostomy device. Flow through the gastrostomy and the absence of external leakage around the tube are checked by injecting saline through the gastrostomy before and after the purse-string suture is secured. **(See Figure 33.3)**

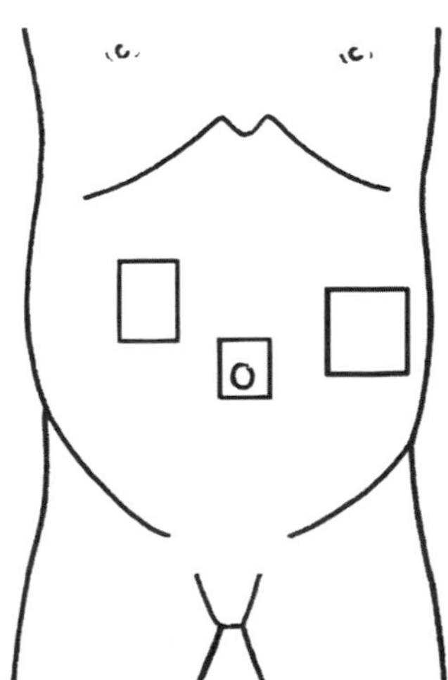

Figure 33.2

Using a pair of conventional fine, curved mosquito forceps through the abdominal wall entry site of the gastrostomy, the purse-string suture ends are pulled alongside the gastrostomy and tied externally, and hitched/secured around the tube or flange at or above the level of skin. The hitching configuration secures the stomach wall against the abdominal wall while the device is prevented from displacing outward. **(See Figure 33.4)**

When poor wound healing is expected or immediate postoperative peritoneal dialysis is necessary, absorbable suture material (PDS) or additional hitching intracorporeal or extracorporeal sutures may be used. Care must be taken to avoid damage to the device.

The pneumoperitoneum is evacuated and fascial incisions larger than 4 mm are closed. Local anesthetic agents may be used at the beginning or end of the procedure. Care is taken not to puncture the gastrostomy device with the injecting needle.

PROBLEMS, PITFALLS AND SOLUTIONS

Difficult access

- When the stomach is displaced as the result of a large hiatus hernia, kyphoscoliosis or large organomegaly, an additional cannula may be required for placing a retractor.
- Previous abdominal scarring may require adhesiolysis.

Difficult purse-string

Usually, less than 2 cm square or triangle formation purse-string through the stomach wall allows a secure inkwell formation (invagination) around the gastrostomy.

- A slightly inflated stomach may facilitate insertion of the purse-string.

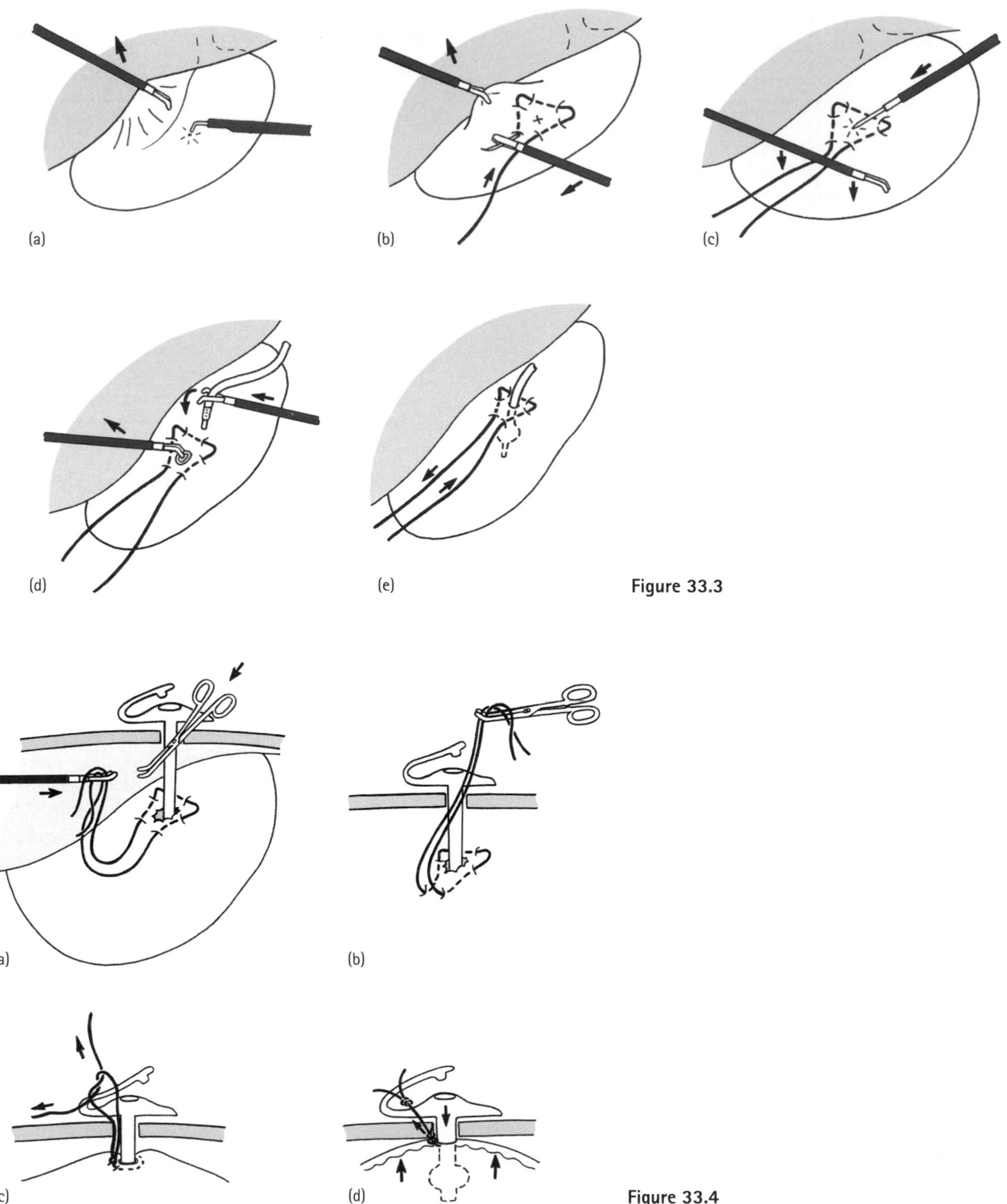

Figure 33.3

Figure 33.4

- Long and deep bites through the stomach wall prevent the suture from cutting through and provide a more secure purse-string. This is particularly so if the Seldinger technique and peel-away sheath is used to insert the gastrostomy.
- A wider placed purse-string may be necessary to prevent eversion of the gastrostomy site.
- Grasping the anterior gastric wall with an atraumatic grasper through the abdominal wall gastrostomy site may facilitate insertion of the purse-string. (**See Figure 33.5**)

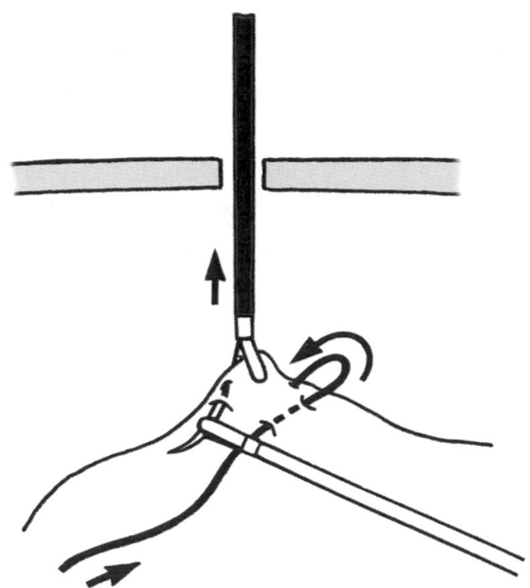

Figure 33.5

Tangling sutures

Long loops of intracorporeal suture may tangle around themselves, instruments and the gastrostomy device, which can be frustrating and difficult to untangle.

- Keep the suture ends well out of the operating field.
- In the case of a percutaneously placed suture, introduce and exit the needle at a site well away from the operating field and allow most of the suture to remain outside while the procedure is being continued.
- Keep the knot of purse-string in front of the gastrostomy.

Difficult incision/track formation on the anterior gastric wall through the purse-string

- The stomach should be inflated to create counter-traction against the penetrating force.
- The gastric incision is best made with a fine diathermy needle passed perpendicularly through the abdominal wall site of gastrostomy (without a cannula) into the stomach. Other fine scissors or straight graspers are less efficient. Minimal cutting/coagulation diathermy is used and care must be taken not to damage the purse-string suture.
- Seldinger technique and peel-away sheath are easier to use and more effective.

Suture snapping at the time of tying

- Use strong sutures such as 2-0 Vicryl®.
- Avoid weakening the material by direct handling of the suture intracorporeally or extracorporeally.
- Keep the purse-string formation simple, i.e. three bites only.
- Use multiple single (not double) throw of the suture for knotting.
- If necessary, place a new purse-string suture and/or additional hitching sutures.

Care must be taken not to perforate the gastrostomy device/balloon by advancing the balloon further into the stomach cavity.

Laparoscopic gastrostomy (hitching suture technique)

A nasogastric tube is inserted and the exact site of the gastrostomy is marked on the abdominal wall. A peri-umbilical 2.5–5 mm primary cannula and telescope allow adequate exposure and a pneumoperitoneum is created at a pressure of 10 mmHg. An appropriate incision to fit the size of the gastrostomy is made on the anterior abdominal wall. Atraumatic grasping forceps are then introduced through this incision (without a cannula) to retract the liver anterio-superiorly and mark and grasp the stomach at a desired site for the gastrostomy (usually high or mid-anterior stomach wall). Alternatively, a second cannula and atraumatic grasper are placed in the right upper quadrant region to retract the liver and manipulate and stabilize the stomach. Using a large needle on a strong monofilament suture (2-0-1 PDS, depending on the size of the patient), two U sutures are placed percutaneously through the abdominal wall, incorporating 1–2 cm of the anterior gastric wall, and out through the abdominal wall by a single maneuver while the peritoneal cavity is decompressed partially. Ideally, the sutures are placed along the long axis of the stomach, 2 cm apart. The sutures are then secured with mosquito forceps outside the abdominal wall. **(See Figure 33.6)**

The laparoscopic grasping forceps are now removed and the stomach is drawn slightly against the abdominal wall. The site of gastrostomy on the stomach wall is kept under vision by pulling the furthest stitch tight and leaving the nearer stitch slightly loose. The Seldinger needle is then positioned through the anterior abdominal wall gastrostomy site incision between the two U sutures. The anesthetist is then asked to insufflate the stomach while the needle is driven perpendicularly into the stomach between the sutures. Care must be taken not to drive the needle out through the opposite wall of the stomach or obliquely in between layers of the stomach wall. A guide-wire is passed through the needle into the stomach and the needle is withdrawn. Care must be taken not to displace the needle or guide-wire prematurely. Then the two hitching U sutures are pulled tight against the abdominal wall while a peel-away sheath over its graduated dilator(s) is passed over the guide-wire into the stomach. Gradually increasing the pressure with a gentle rotating maneuver facilitates safe and smooth entry of the dilator/peel-away sheath into the stomach. The dilators are withdrawn and the peel-away sheath is carefully maintained in position while a balloon button/tube gastrostomy is passed through it into the stomach. The sheath is partially peeled to accommodate the gastrostomy.

Once the balloon part of the gastrostomy has reached inside the stomach, the balloon is inflated to half its capacity

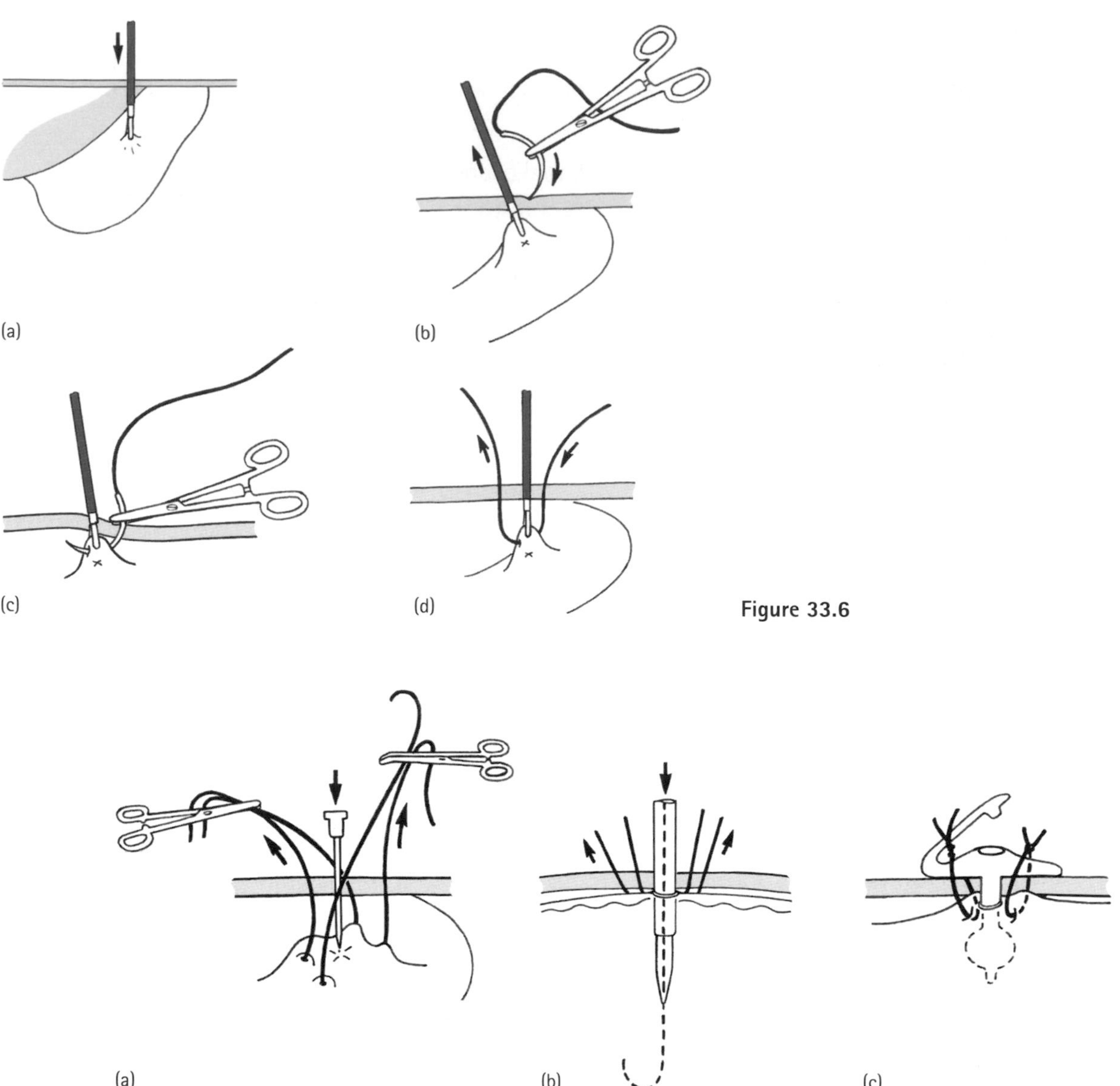

Figure 33.6

Figure 33.7

and the remaining part of the peel-away is removed. Check that the gastrostomy device is moving easily through the track by admitting 10–20 mL of sterile saline and aspirating some of the fluid back before inflating the balloon to its full 5 mL capacity. (**See Figure 33.7**)

Once the device is in place, the sutures are tied snug, but not too tight, over the button or flange of the tube gastrostomy. The pneumoperitoneum is evacuated and the umbilical wound is closed. Local anesthetic agents may be infiltrated into the wounds and around the gastrostomy at the beginning or end of the procedure. Care must be taken not to puncture the device with the injecting needle.

Alternatively, a diathermy point or fine scissors and graspers may be used to create a site for the gastrostomy through the stomach wall, as described for the previous technique.

PROBLEMS, PITFALLS AND SOLUTIONS

Difficult access

This can be dealt with in the same way as for the previous technique.

Difficult U sutures

- In older or obese children, placing a needle percutaneously in and out of the abdominal cavity may prove extremely difficult. In this situation either use an extremely large hand-held needle or consider other methods of insertion: purse-string technique or laparoscopic-assisted PEG, described earlier. Alternatively, a large straightened-out needle on a 2-0 PDS suture is passed percutaneously, close to the site of the gastrostomy, into the peritoneal cavity and placed through the stomach wall and back through the

abdominal wall approximately 1.5 cm or so distant from the site of entry using conventional and laparoscopic needle holders from outside and inside, respectively.
- A slightly inflated stomach may facilitate insertion of the suture.

Difficulty passing the dilator/peel-away sheath

- Effort must be made to introduce the Seldinger needle and dilators perpendicularly into the stomach.
- The hitching sutures must incorporate a good chunk of the stomach wall to avoid sutures cutting through the stomach while the dilator/peel-away sheath is being introduced.
- Graduated dilators, usually four sizes, penetrate through the stomach wall more easily than a single dilator.
- Often, the peel-away sheath catches the anterior abdominal wall fascia and the serosal surface of the stomach. Ensure that the abdominal wall incision is large enough and the dilator/peel-away system is passed perpendicularly into the stomach using gradually increased pressure and twisting maneuvers. A sudden and clear give is felt at the point of entry.
- Consider making a small nick on the surface of the stomach using either a diathermy point or scissors.

Difficulty passing the gastrostomy device

This occurs particularly when a short button gastrostomy is used.

- Split the peel-away sheath halfway down before passing the button gastrostomy; 14 Fr gastrostomy requires an 18 Fr peel-away.
- Consider not using the peel-away sheath and instead pass the gastrostomy device over the guide-wire. Here, care must be taken not to damage the valve mechanism of the button gastrostomy.
- Consider using a longer button gastrostomy or a temporary tube balloon device which may be changed in the clinic or on the ward several weeks postoperatively.

Suture snapping at the time of tying

Always use strong sutures (2-0 Vicryl® or PDS).

POSTOPERATIVE CARE

Postoperative analgesia in the form of an epidural infusion or intravenous morphine infusion is rarely necessarily. Local infiltration of the wound with an anesthetic agent provides adequate pain control and regular non-steroidal analgesia may be used for the first day or two postoperatively. The nasogastric tube is removed at the end of the procedure and the gastrostomy tube is aspirated 3-hourly with free drainage in between for the first 12–24 hours postoperatively. Usually, the gastrostomy tube/button is used for fluid and drugs at 12–24 hours and feeding at 24–48 hours. When poor wound healing or complications are expected or immediate postoperative peritoneal dialysis is necessary, as in renal patients, the use of gastrostomy is delayed for 3–7 days postoperatively.

COMPLICATIONS

In addition to the usual complications of access and pneumoperitoneum, which are exceedingly rare, especially when open technique laparoscopy is used, the following can also occur.

Technique-related complications

- Malposition of the gastrostomy. Examples include the balloon being inflated within the wall of the stomach and the tip of the gastrostomy being passed through the opposite wall of the stomach, with consequent peritonitis. This is more likely to happen when the Seldinger technique wire and dilators are used and therefore care must be taken to place the needle/wire carefully and ensure that the ends are within the lumen of the stomach before the dilators/peel-away sheath and the gastrostomy tube are placed. Inflate the balloon partially, check that the gastrostomy tube is moving freely within the track and the gastrostomy allows saline injection and aspiration freely before further inflating the balloon to its maximum capacity and tying the sutures. In difficult cases, consider placing a gastroscope to check the position within.
- In the U suture hitching technique, the size of the dilator/peel-away sheath is 4 Fr sizes larger than the gastrostomy device. Despite a minute visible leak, after the removal of the dilator/peel-away, this does not appear to cause problems when a balloon-tipped gastrostomy device is used.

Gastrostomy-related complications

Increased risks and frequency of gastro-esophageal reflux, inward or outward migration of gastrostomy, superficial leak infection and granulation tissue formation are known complications of gastrostomy whether placed laparoscopically or gastroscopically or through an open technique.

FURTHER READING

Croaker GDH, Najmaldin AS. Laparoscopically assisted percutaneous endoscopic gastrostomy. *Pediatric Surgery International* 1997; 12:2–3, 130–1.

Georgeson KE. Laparoscopic versus open procedures for long term enteral access. *Nutrition in Clinical Practice* [Suppl.] 1997; 12:S1–S2.

Humphrey G, Najmaldin A. Laparoscopic gastrostomy in children. *Pediatric Surgery International* 1997; 12:501–4.

34

Pyloromyotomy

TAKAO FUJIMOTO

INTRODUCTION

Infantile hypertrophic pyloric stenosis (IHPS) is a common surgical condition encountered in early infancy. The diagnosis is usually based on the clinical history, physical examination, 'palpable pyloric tumor' and ultrasonographic scanning of the abdomen. A contrast meal may be required in difficult and/or complicated presentations. Extramucosal pyloromyotomy is the standard treatment. Increasing numbers of pediatric surgeons use laparoscopy for pyloromyotomy. Compared with the open technique, laparoscopic pyloromyotomy produces less surgical trauma (forceful manipulation and bruising are avoided, significantly less peak value of stress marker – interleukin-6), earlier return to normal feed, and better cosmesis.

Although most surgeons use working cannulae for instruments, the author prefers direct insertion of the working instruments through the abdominal wall into the operating field.

Contraindications

ABSOLUTE

- Patients who are not fit for general anesthesia.

RELATIVE

- Hematologic disorders (abnormal coagulation profile).
- Suspected major abdominal scarring from previous abdominal surgery or peritonitis.

EQUIPMENT/INSTRUMENTS

Essential

- 3.0–5.0 mm access cannula for laparoscope and insufflation.
- 2.7–5.0 m 0–45° telescope.
- 3.0 mm atraumatic grasper for the duodenum.
- 2.0–3.0 mm retractable myotomy knife (arthrotomy knife or sheathed knife: endotome).
- 3.0 mm pyloromyotomy spreader.

Optional

- 3.0 mm monopolar and/or bipolar diathermy.
- Two cannulae for working instruments.

PREOPERATIVE PREPARATION

Hematological and biochemical analyses are necessary as for the conventional open procedure. Oral feeds are discontinued, intravenous fluid is commenced and a nasogastric tube is placed. Abnormal fluid, electrolytes and acid–base balance must be corrected prior to surgery.

TECHNIQUE

The procedure is carried out under general endotracheal anesthesia with complete muscle relaxation. A palpable

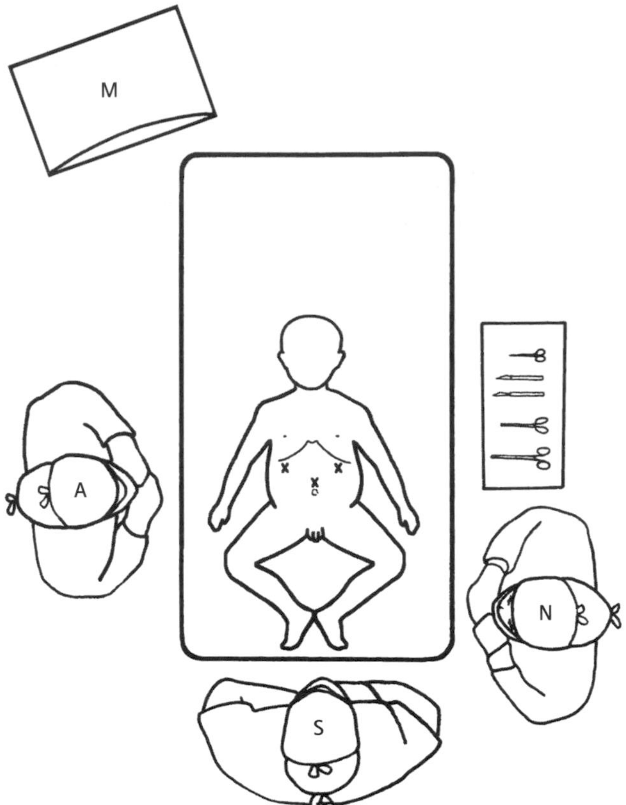

Figure 34.1

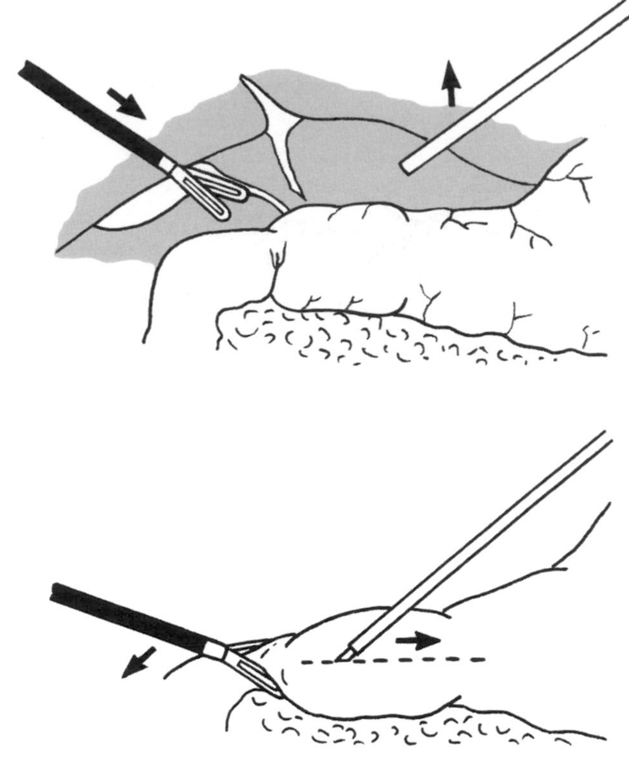

Figure 34.2

bladder may be emptied using the Crede maneuver. Placement of a nasogastric tube is ensured, a single dose of broad-spectrum antibiotics given, and the patient is placed in the supine position at the end of the operating table (or across the table). The video monitor is placed at the head of the table, and the surgeon stands at the end with the assistant to the patient's right and the scrub nurse on the left. The abdomen is scrubbed and draped in the usual fashion, and care is taken to clean the umbilicus meticulously.

The access sites are injected with local anesthesia (0.25 percent bupivacaine with epinephrine). While some surgeons routinely use a Veress needle technique for creating a pneumoperitoneum, the author prefers a peri-umbilical open procedure for insertion of the primary cannula. A pneumoperitoneum is created and maintained at a pressure of 8–10 mHg and insufflation flow of 0.5–1.0 L/min. In the right mid-clavicular line just below the costal margin (just above the liver edge), a No. 11 scalpel blade is used to make a 2–3 mm stab incision under direct vision. Similarly, a second stab incision is made just below the costal margin in the left mid-clavicular line. **(See Figure 34.1)**

Exposure

An atraumatic grasper is placed directly through the right upper quadrant incision and is used to retract the inferior border of the liver superiorly, and the hypertrophied pylorus is exposed. A retractable myotomy knife is inserted directly through the left incision. The working instruments (unarmed knife and grasper) are used to assess the extent of the hypertrophied pylorus by palpating the margins of the pylorus, as would be done with the thumb and forefinger in the open procedure.

The duodenum is then gently grasped just distal to the pyloric vein (pyloro-duodenal junction) and pulled anterio-inferiorly and the avascular surface of the pylorus is exposed. The proximal margin of hypertrophied pylorus (antro-pyloric junction) is usually seen as a deep fold in the wall of the stomach. Excessive and forceful manipulation can result in seromuscular laceration of the duodenum. **(See Figure 34.2)**

Pyloromyotomy

The knife is activated and a straight longitudinal seromuscular incision is made in the hypertrophied pylorus (preferably in a single stroke). The incision is started 1–2 mm proximal to the pyloro-duodenal junction (silver line) and extended into the gastric antrum 5 mm clear of the antro-pyloric junction. Most incomplete myotomies result from failure to extend the incision far enough proximally into the antrum. The incision has to be deep enough to allow the insertion of the pyloric spreader.

Once an adequate incision is made, the blade is retracted (deactivated) and the sheath of the arthrotomy knife is used to further split the hypertrophied muscle fibers (as the

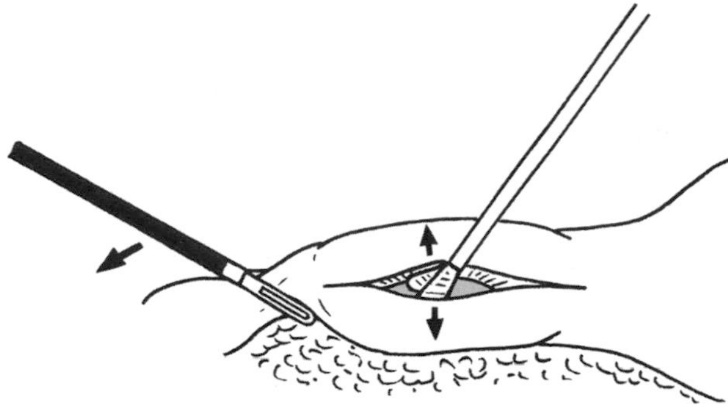

Figure 34.3

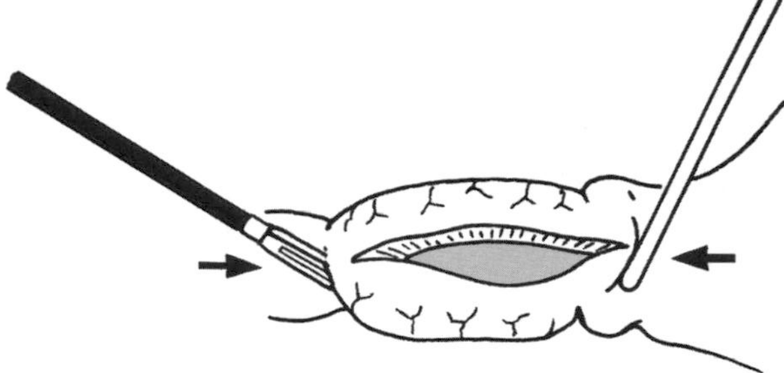

Figure 34.4

scalpel handle is used in the open procedure). Alternatively, one blade of the myotomy spreader is used to split muscle fibers further. The knife is then exchanged for a myotomy spreader, which is placed in the midpoint of the seromuscular incision, and the muscle is spread perpendicularly. Once the initial spread reaches the mucosa, several gentle distal and proximal spreads are usually required to complete the myotomy. Care must be taken to stop spreading 1–2 mm short of the pyloric vein. **(See Figure 34.3)**

An adequate myotomy is evidenced by a pale mucosa bulging through the muscle incision. An intact mucosa is tested by insufflating the stomach through the nasogastric tube with 100–150 mL of air. Greenish/yellow froth at the myotomy area is a sign of mucosal tear.

After a successful myotomy, the stomach is decompressed completely and the nasogastric tube is removed. The instruments are withdrawn under direct vision, the abdomen is decompressed and the peri-umbilical incision is closed using 3-0 absorbable sutures.

POSTOPERATIVE CARE

While some surgeons advocate an early full feed, the author prefers a gradual regimen starting at 4 hours postoperatively. The first feed is 5 mL/kg of an electrolytes solution, followed by 5 mL/kg of ordinary formula at 3-hourly intervals, with an increment of 5 mL/kg at every fourth feed and a full feed at 24 hours postoperatively. Feeding may be withheld for 3 hours if the infant vomits, and gastric lavage is considered in those who suffer significant postoperative vomiting. The infants are usually ready to leave hospital within 24–36 hours of surgery.

PROBLEMS, PITFALLS AND SOLUTIONS

Difficult access

- A supra-umbilical open incision for the primary cannula provides an ideal position for the telescope. Care must be taken not to allow more than 0.5–1.0 cm of the cannula to remain inside the peritoneal cavity.
- A low left instrument can be difficult to control and consequently myotomy will be difficult to perform. It is therefore important to keep the left upper quadrant stab incision just below the costal margin in the left mid-clavicular line.

Estimating the length of the pyloromyotomy incision required

- Start the incision 1–2 mm proximal to the pyloroduodenal junction and terminate at 3–5 mm proximal to the antro-pyloric junction.
- Avoid excessive manipulation and spreading at either end.
- Palpate (hold) the pyloric tumor between the non-activated knife or pyloric spreader and the duodenal grasper, and the myotomy incision should stretch from one to the other. **(See Figure 34.4)**

Difficulty engaging the pyloric spreader

- Cut the hypertrophied pylorus perpendicularly (not obliquely) and deepen the middle section of the incision.
- Further split the muscle fibers using the sheath of the arthotomy knife (non-activated blade) or one blade of the spreader. This maneuver may be enhanced by twisting the instrument inside the incision by 90°.
- Introduce the spreader perpendicularly into the middle section of the incision.

Bleeding

- Minor bleeding at the site of the myotomy is common and usually causes no problems.
- Hold the duodenum so that the avascular region of the pylorus is exposed for the incision.

COMPLICATIONS

Mucosal perforation

The risk of mucosal perforation is minimized by careful attention to the details described above. The risk is greater at the duodenal end of the incision. Mucosal perforation may be closed intracorporeally with or without an omental patch. Here, the nasogastric tube aspiration and intravenous fluid may be continued for 48 hours postoperatively. Some surgeons advocate closing the first myotomy (site of perforation) and starting a second myotomy. Conversion to open surgery should be considered.

Significant bleeding

Significant bleeding from the branches of the gastro-epiploic vessel can be controlled by low-voltage diathermy; minor bleeding requires no action.

Incomplete pyloromyotomy

The risk of incomplete myotomy is minimized by extending the incision well into the gastric antrum. A few intact fibers at the duodenal end usually cause no problem.

Incisional hernia at the site of ports

Oblique incisions, insertion of instruments and a formal suturing of incisions greater than 3 mm prevent omental hernia.

Wound infection

Appropriate cleaning of the umbilicus and a dose of perioperative antibiotics may prevent wound infection.

FURTHER READING

Bufo AJ, Merry C, Shah R et al. Laparoscopic pyloromyotomy: a safer technique. *Pediatric Surgery International* 1998; **13**:240–2.

Fujimoto T, Segawa O et al. Laparoscopic extramucosal pyloromyotomy versus open pyloromyotomy for infantile hypertrophic pyloric stenosis: which is better? *Journal of Pediatric Surgery* 1999; **34**:370–2.

Harris SE, Cywes R. How I do it: pyloromyotomy. *Pediatric Endosurgery & Innovative Techniques* 2001; **5**:405–10.

Tan HL, Najmaldin A. Laparoscopic pyloromyotomy for infantile hypertrophic pyloric stenosis. *Pediatric Surgery International* 1993; **8**:376–78.

35

Cholecystectomy

BEVERLY E. CHAIGNAUD AND GEORGE W. HOLCOMB III

INTRODUCTION

The birth of the laparoscopic revolution began in 1989 with the report by Reddick and Olsen of laparoscopic cholecystectomy in 25 patients. In that same year, Dubois et al. described the technique in 63 patients. The use of laparoscopy in children has had a more gradual acceptance; however, today, we see the technique being utilized by an ever-increasing number of pediatric surgeons. In just a few short years, laparoscopic cholecystectomy has become the preferred procedure for the removal of the gallbladder, not only in adults, but in children as well.

Indications

- Non-hemolytic cholelithiasis:
  - total parenteral nutrition
  - cholestasis
  - ileal resection
  - teenage pregnancy
  - oral contraceptives
  - obesity
  - biliary tract anomalies
  - idiopathic.
- Hemolytic cholelithiasis:
  - sickle-cell anemia
  - hereditary spherocytosis
  - thalassemia major.
- Biliary dyskinesia (uncommon).
- Acalculous cholecystitis (rare).

Contraindications

ABSOLUTE

- Uncorrectable coagulopathy.
- Inability to achieve an adequate pneumoperitoneum.

RELATIVE

- Common bile duct stones – need added experience with endoscopic sphincterotomy or laparoscopic choledochoscopy.
- Previous upper abdominal surgery.

In children the common bile duct can be very small and a second concern is misidentification of the common duct as the cystic duct, with resulting injury. Early in a surgeon's experience, routine cholangiography is suggested to identify these two structures accurately. After a number of cases, cholangiography can be utilized selectively, depending on the anatomy and concerns about common duct stones.

EQUIPMENT/INSTRUMENTS

The following instruments are considered the minimum number and types required for laparoscopic cholecystectomy.

Essential

- Telescope: 5 mm, 10 mm – 0° or 45°.
- Two video monitors.

- Two pairs of grasping forceps.
- Atraumatic dissecting instrument.
- Hook cautery or spatula.
- Cannulae: 5 mm or 10 mm.
- Cholangiocatheter.
- Laparoscopic clip applier: 5 mm or 10 mm.

Optional

- Specimen bag.
- Ultrasonic dissector.

PREOPERATIVE PREPARATION

The preoperative work-up includes liver function studies, especially total bilirubin, to evaluate for possible biliary obstruction, hepatic cell injury or inflammation. Ultrasound is the study of choice to document gallstones and evidence of bile duct dilatation/obstruction. In cases of presumed biliary dyskinesia a hepatobiliary nuclear medicine scan is helpful in evaluating liver function and excretion. A cholecystokinin-stimulated hepatobiliary nuclear medicine scan is the diagnostic test of choice for biliary dyskinesia. Poor excretion with reproduction of the patient's abdominal pain on injection of the cholecystokinin is generally thought to be diagnostic of biliary dyskinesia. If there is evidence of bile duct obstruction secondary to common bile duct stones, preoperative endoscopic retrograde cholangiopancreatography (ERCP) may be indicated in an attempt to remove the stones prior to laparoscopy. This depends on the expertise of the pediatric gastroenterologists and the condition of the patient. However, successful ERCP may decrease the need for laparoscopic or open common duct exploration.

For those non-sickle-cell children undergoing elective laparoscopic cholecystectomy without associated complications such as acute cholecystitis, jaundice or pancreatitis, preoperative admission is not required. The child arrives on the morning of surgery with the last solid food taken a minimum of 6 hours earlier.

With sickle-cell anemia, the hemoglobin S concentration must be lowered to at least 30 percent. These patients can be seen in the outpatient clinic 7–10 days prior to the operation for a transfusion of packed red blood cells to increase the hemoglobin level to 8–10 g/dL. The patient is often admitted to the hospital the night before surgery for intravenous hydration. Additional transfusions are given if necessary.

For patients with acute cholecystitis without common bile duct obstruction or pancreatitis, medical management is recommended initially. The patient is placed on bowel rest, nasogastric decompression, intravenous hydration, pain relief and antibiotics. Symptoms usually resolve and a cholecystectomy can be performed in 5–7 days. A second option is to discharge the patient until an elective operation is done 2–3 weeks later.

TECHNIQUE

The patient is positioned supine and general endotracheal anesthesia is administered. Cephalosporin is used in uncomplicated cases for preoperative antibiotic prophylaxis. An orogastric tube is inserted to decompress the stomach, as a distended stomach can impair visualization of the gallbladder, especially in young children. A Crede maneuver is utilized to empty the urinary bladder. Urinary catheterization is not routinely employed, especially in younger children, because of the potential complications of urethral instrumentation. However, it may be necessary in older children and teenagers or in patients with acute cholecystitis and an anticipated lengthy procedure. The patients are always prepped and draped widely.

Positioning

The operating surgeon stands on the patient's left and the assistant stands opposite the surgeon. A video monitor is positioned on either side of the patient, at the head of the table, which allows both the surgeon and assistant to view a monitor without having to turn around.

Trocar position

A four-incision (cannulae) technique is used in children, as in adults. The positions of the incisions are important, and placement of the cannulae should be modified according to the patient's age and body size.

INFANTS

A 5 mm incision is made in the umbilicus and extended through the umbilical fascia. A 5 mm blunt-tipped cannula is introduced into the abdominal cavity and insufflation with CO_2 is accomplished. The 5 mm telescope attached to the camera is inserted through the umbilical cannula. Three additional incisions are then created. A 3 mm instrument is inserted in the lateral aspect right upper quadrant (RUQ) through a stab incision with a No. 11 blade. A second 3 mm stab incision is made in the inguinal region and 3 mm grasping forceps introduced. This incision can be positioned here for cosmetic reasons as the instruments easily reach from the inguinal region to the gallbladder in small infants. A 5 mm port is placed in the left epigastrium (LUQ). This port should be placed as laterally as possible to allow adequate working distance between all instruments. The smaller the infant, the more important it is to position the instruments as widely as possible. If the epigastric port is situated in the midline, as in adults, it will be too close to the RUQ and umbilical cannulae and will not provide adequate working space in small children. If 3 mm instruments are not available. 5 mm instruments may be used in the RUQ and right lower quadrant (RLQ) positions. **(See Figure 35.1)**

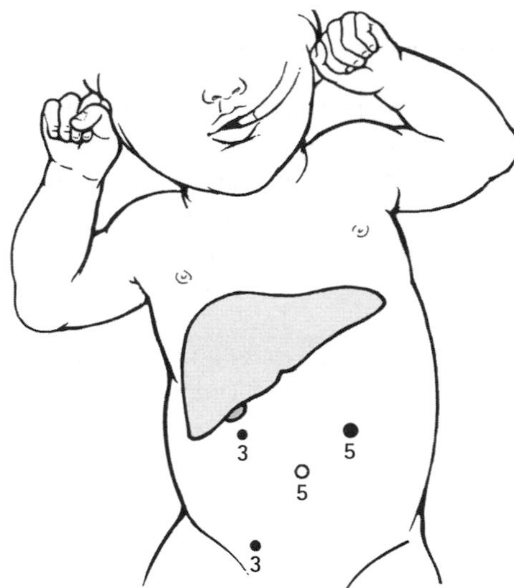

Figure 35.1

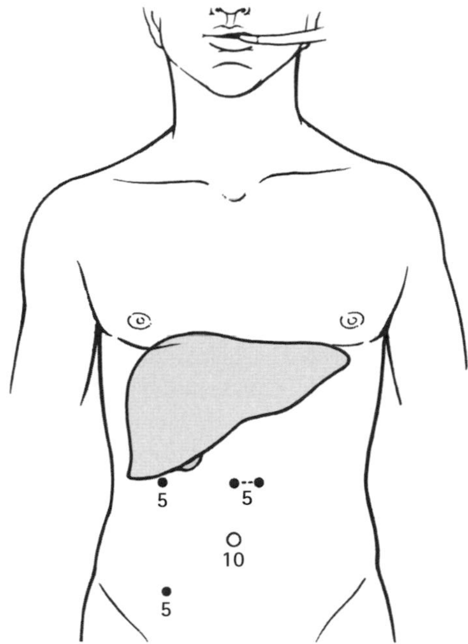

Figure 35.2

AGES 2 TO 18 YEARS

In this age group, optical visualization is usually sufficient with a 5 mm umbilical port. In the younger children, the umbilical cut-down technique is recommended. In the older children, the Veress needle may be used. The RUQ incision is positioned as in the infant. The (RLQ) incision is located at the level of the anterior superior iliac crest, a position slightly superior to that for infants. A 5 mm epigastric port is used. In younger children, this port is placed more laterally and, in the older child, it is moved medially toward the midline. The gallbladder can usually be exteriorized through the 5 mm umbilical incision if the cannula is removed. In some cases, it may be necessary to enlarge the umbilical incision or, if preferred, a 10 mm cannula and telescope may be used in older children. The gallbladder can usually be withdrawn through the 10 mm cannula. **(See Figure 35.2)**

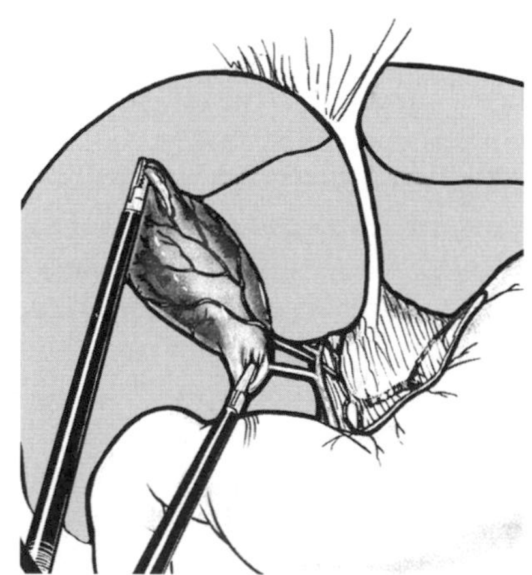

Figure 35.3

Operative dissection

After the insertion of all four instruments, either through cannulae or directly through the abdominal wall, the patient is placed in a slight reverse Trendelenburg position and the table is rotated to the left. This allows the colon and small bowel to fall away from the gallbladder. Dissection then follows a series of sequential steps.

- Through the right lower cannula, ratcheted atraumatic forceps are introduced and used to secure the fundus of the gallbladder, which is rotated superiorly and ventrally over the liver.
- A second pair of atraumatic forceps is inserted through the right upper port and is used to grasp the infundibulum of the gallbladder, which is retracted laterally, establishing a 90° angle between the cystic and common ducts. **(See Figure 35.3)**

The cystic artery, cystic duct and common duct in children can be quite small, and lateral retraction of the infundibulum is important to avoid misidentification of these structures. In cases of acute cholecystitis, there is often extensive edema and inflammation, making it difficult to grasp the gallbladder for retraction. In these cases, the gallbladder can be aspirated, resulting in decompression and making it easier to retract the gallbladder and expose the cystic and common ducts.

- After careful assessment of the cystic duct and common duct triangle, and once the correct anatomy is identified, two options exist.

The first option is to perform an intra-operative cholangiogram to confirm the correct anatomy and evaluate unsuspected cholelithiasis. The second option is to omit the cholangiogram and proceed with ligation and division of the cystic duct and artery. The decision depends on the surgeon's pediatric experience and confidence in the correct identification of the cystic and common ducts.

OPTIONS FOR CHOLANGIOGRAPHY

- One method involves placing a surgical clip across the cystic duct as close to the gallbladder as possible. A small lateral incision is made in the cystic duct just distal to the surgical clip. A cholangiocatheter or 4 Fr ureteral catheter is then passed through a purpose-made clamp (Olsen clamp) and directed into the cystic duct. The catheter is secured with the Olsen clamp and a cholangiogram is performed in the standard manner.
- In smaller children, the cystic duct can be very narrow, making it difficult to thread a catheter. An alternative method of performing a cholangiogram, which avoids making a lateral incision in the cystic duct, involves placing an atraumatic Kumar clamp across the infundibulum. This atraumatic clamp is introduced through one of the right abdominal cannulae and a 23 G sclerotherapy needle is passed through the side arm of the clamp and into the infundibulum just above the cystic duct junction. The cholangiogram is performed using fluoroscopy. Once the correct anatomy and the absence of choledocholithiasis have been confirmed, the sclerotherapy needle is removed and the Kumar clamp withdrawn. **(See Figure 35.4)**
- Another technique for cholangiography in children involves percutaneous puncture of the gallbladder. A small needle is inserted into the fundus of the gallbladder and the cholangiogram is performed through the gallbladder. A variation of this technique involves placing a clamp across the gallbladder at the cystic duct junction with direction of the needle into the dilated portion of the cystic duct.

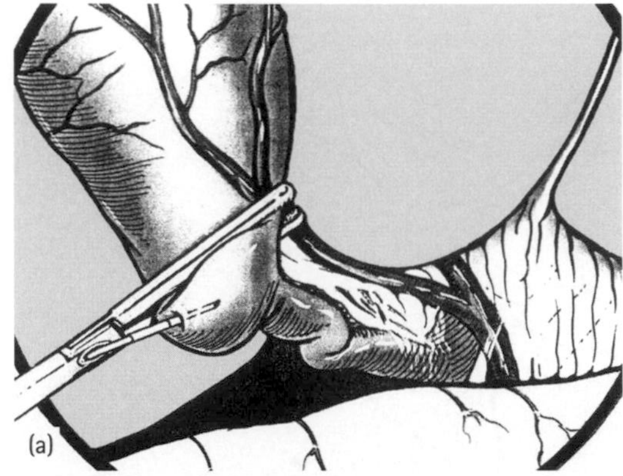

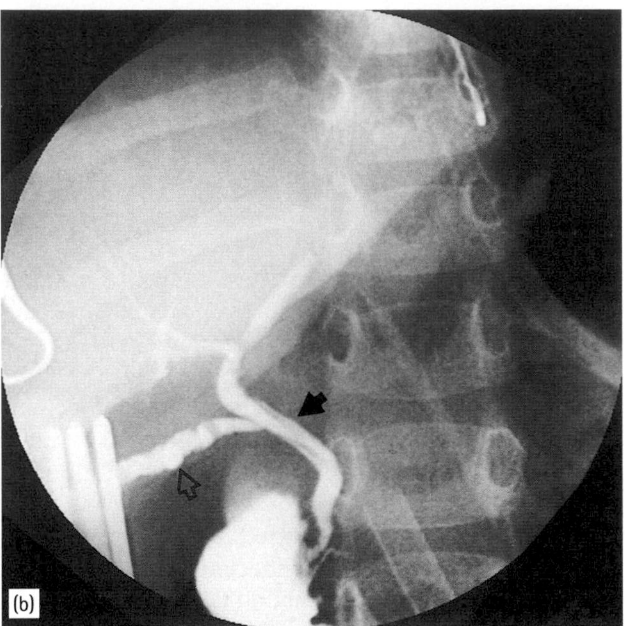

Figure 35.4

LIGATION AND DIVISION OF THE CYSTIC DUCT AND ARTERY

After cholangiography, a surgical clip is placed across the cystic duct adjacent to the infundibulum and the duct is then doubly clipped just distal to the first clip. The cystic duct is divided with scissors between the first and second clips. The cystic artery is carefully identified and then ligated and divided in a similar manner. **(See Figure 35.5)**

DISSECTION OF THE GALLBLADDER FROM THE LIVER BED

The gallbladder is then removed in a retrograde fashion using electrocautery. A variety of instruments may be used, including the hook cautery or the spatula. It is important to maintain hemostasis as mobilization of the gallbladder from the liver bed proceeds superiorly. Before the gallbladder is completely detached, the porta hepatis is carefully inspected for hemostasis and secure placement of the surgical clips. It is best to inspect the operative bed prior to removing the gallbladder completely, as it is easier to retract the liver superiorly with the gallbladder partially attached. Should entry into the gallbladder occur during dissection, it can be controlled with a pre-tied endoscopic loop. The perforation is grasped with forceps and the pre-tied loop is secured around the perforation and tightened. The suprahepatic and subhepatic spaces are irrigated with saline and the irrigant is inspected for blood and biliary contents. **(See Figure 35.6)**

EXTRACTION OF THE GALLBLADDER

Once the gallbladder is completely detached, it is extracted through the umbilical cannula. If it is large and inflamed or

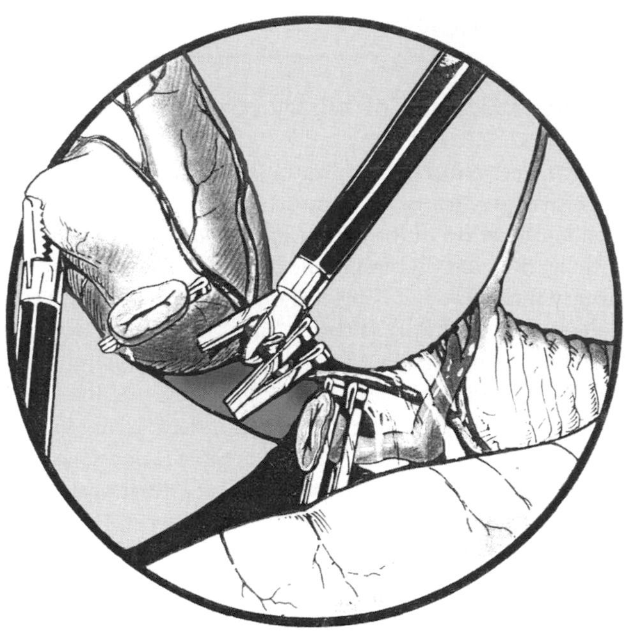

Figure 35.5

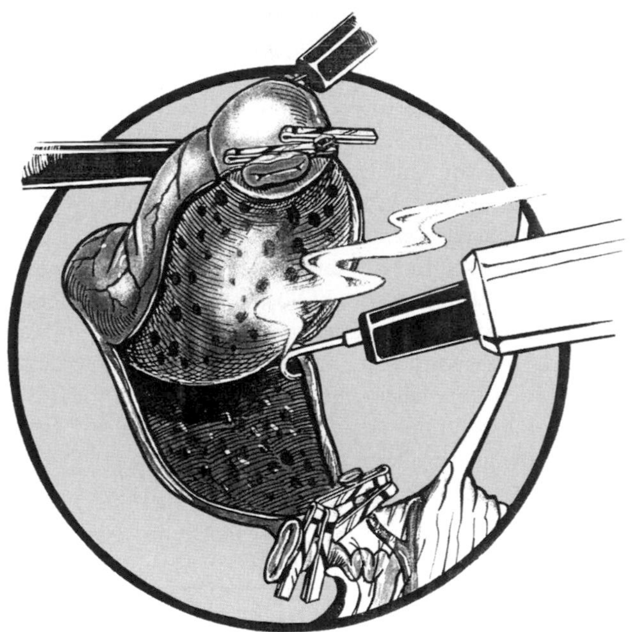

Figure 35.6

too distended with bile or stones to permit removal in this manner, the cannula is removed and the gallbladder is extracted through the umbilical incision. Should it still not be possible to remove the gallbladder, its neck is exteriorized and then grasped on each side with clamps and opened. The bile is aspirated and the stones removed, allowing the gallbladder to be advanced though the fascial opening. An alternative is to place the gallbladder in an endoscopic specimen bag to prevent spillage and contamination of the umbilical trocar site.

Once the gallbladder has been extracted, the telescope is re-introduced and the operative field again inspected for hemostasis. With hemostasis secured, the cannulae and instruments are withdrawn carefully, inspecting the peritoneal surface for hemostasis as each instrument is removed. Bupivacaine is instilled into the abdominal wall incisions for postoperative analgesia. The telescope is then removed and the abdomen is desufflated. The umbilical fascia is closed with 0 or 2-0 absorbable sutures. If possible, the fascia of the 5 mm incisions is approximated with 3-0 absorbable sutures and the skin incisions are closed in a subcuticular fashion. Sterile dressings are applied, the orogastric tube and urinary catheter, if inserted, are removed and anesthesia is terminated.

POSTOPERATIVE CARE

Postoperatively, the child is started on a clear liquid diet and is likely to be kept in hospital overnight for observation and analgesia. Pain is usually well controlled with acetaminophen with codeine. The child is advanced to a regular diet the following morning and most patients are ready for dismissal on the first postoperative day. All patients are seen 2 weeks postoperatively in the pediatric surgery clinic. Laboratory or radiographic evaluation is not routinely performed in the absence of symptoms.

PROBLEMS, PITFALLS AND SOLUTIONS

Preoperative ultrasound studies

As with all studies, the precision of the preoperative ultrasound study is operator dependent, and each surgeon must evaluate the expertise at his or her institution. If the common bile duct is of normal size, the only reason to perform a cholangiogram at the time of the laparoscopic cholecystectomy would be for delineation of the anatomy. Therefore, if the anatomy appears clear and there is no evidence of common duct involvement on the ultrasound, the cholangiogram can be omitted from the operative procedure.

Parental expectations with regard to chronic abdominal pain

The surgeon should be cautious about parental expectations regarding their child's symptoms. This is especially true in a child with chronic symptoms and only one or two small gallstones. It may be that the stones are not causing the patient's symptoms, and it is important to caution the parents that the symptoms may not resolve, especially if they are not related to the gallstones. This same is true for biliary dyskinesia, as there is certainly no guarantee that the symptoms of this disorder will resolve.

Adequate operative working space

Another potential pitfall is placing the instruments too close together to allow enough intra-abdominal working space. This is especially true in small children who require laparoscopic cholecystectomy. For this reason, the main working port, which is in the epigastrium, should be placed in the left subcostal region in small children and the most caudad port should be situated in the right inguinal crease region.

ERCP capabilities

It is important to understand the capabilities of ERCP and sphincterotomy in children in one's own institution in order to be able to plan the management of choledocholithiasis. This understanding is important in the preoperative evaluation of the patient with a suspected common duct stone, at operation in a patient with an unsuspected stone in the common duct found on cholangiography, and in the patient with persistent jaundice postoperatively in whom a stone is noted. The pediatric gastroenterologists in many children's hospitals are not trained or experienced in ERCP, which is therefore performed by their adult gastroenterology colleagues. If the adult colleagues are not comfortable dealing with this problem in children and the pediatric surgeon is not comfortable doing laparoscopic common duct exploration, it may be necessary to perform an open operation.

Exteriorization of the gallbladder

Extraction of the gallbladder poses another potential problem, especially in an overweight adolescent. Therefore, it is important that the fascial opening is large enough to extract the gallbladder so that there is no spillage of gallstones and biliary contents. If there is concern about the possibility of spillage, placement of the gallbladder in an endoscopic retrieval bag is prudent. In addition, enlargement of the fascial opening to an adequate size is important to remove some of these inflamed gallbladders.

Visualization

Two final pitfalls that are easily resolved are the lack of visualization of a distended stomach, which is easily solved with an orogastric tube for gastric decompression, and uncertainty about the correct anatomy. A basic principle of this operation is that if the anatomy does not look right, the surgeon should not hesitate to convert to an open operation.

COMPLICATIONS

Misidentification of biliary structures

Despite best efforts, complications can develop from the operative procedure. The most serious complication is misidentification of the common bile duct and cystic duct with ligation and division of the common bile duct. As previously mentioned, it is important to provide lateral traction on the cystic duct so that it forms a 90° angle of entry into the common bile duct. Even with lateral traction, misidentification of these two structures is possible, so a cholangiogram should be performed if there is any uncertainty about the anatomy in the triangle of Calot. Finally, if uncertainty persists, the surgeon should convert to an open procedure.

Injury to the right hepatic artery

Another complication is ischemia of the hepatic parenchyma in the distribution of the right hepatic artery. Occasionally, the right hepatic artery lies just inside the hepatic parenchyma in the gallbladder bed or in the plane of dissection between the gallbladder and the liver. In this situation, the right hepatic artery may be confused with the posterior branch of the cystic artery. It can be injured with cautery dissection of the gallbladder from the liver. When this occurs, the patient usually recovers uneventfully, but returns several days later with complaints of abdominal pain and leukocytosis. Usually, levels of the hepatic enzymes – alanine aminotransferase (ALT), aspartate aminotransferase (AST) and gamma-glutamyltranspeptidase (GGT) – are elevated. Ultrasound examination is usually unremarkable. These patients are best treated with conservative measures and their symptoms generally resolve after a few days, rarely with any long-term sequelae.

Bile leak

Biliary leak is rarely a problem in pediatric patients, but should be managed initially with percutaneous drainage followed by re-exploration if it persists. Routine drainage of the gallbladder bed is not indicated.

Postoperative bleeding

Postoperative bleeding is a rare problem in children, but the surgeon should use caution and inspect the area of dissection from the liver while the gallbladder remains attached to it, as this is the best way of visualizing the liver bed. Any areas of bleeding should be cauterized to prevent this postoperative complication.

Gallbladder perforation

Inadvertent entry into the gallbladder during dissection does not usually cause any postoperative sequelae, unless gallstones are spilled. This complication can be managed easily by grasping the perforation and securing a pre-tied endoscopic loop around it. Therefore, it is important to have endoscopic pre-tied ligatures in the operating room during the operation and not in a central storage area. If gallstones are spilled inadvertently, as many of them as possible should be removed and the area irrigated to remove any small stones and the biliary contents.

FURTHER READING

Holcomb GW III, Morgan WM III, Neblett WW III et al. Laparoscopic cholecystectomy in children: lessons learned from the first 100 patients. *Journal of Pediatric Surgery* 1999; **34**:1236–40.

Holcomb GW III, Naffis D. Laparoscopic cholecystectomy in infants. *Journal of Pediatric Surgery* 1994; **29**:86–7.

Holzman MD, Sharp K, Holcomb GW III et al. An alternative technique for laparoscopic cholangiography. *Surgical Endoscopy* 1994; **8**:927–30.

Newman KD, Powell DM, Holcomb GW III. The management of choledocholithiasis in children in the era of laparoscopic cholecystectomy. *Journal of Pediatric Surgery* 1997; **32**: 1116–19.

36

Splenectomy

AZAD NAJMALDIN

INTRODUCTION

Partial or total organ conservation is a major consideration in splenic surgery because of the long-term risks of post-splenectomy sepsis.

Indications

- Hematological disorders unresponsive to medical treatment.
- Traumatic injuries with life-threatening hemorrhage not amenable to repair or partial splenectomy.
- Benign cyst or abscess that is not amenable to conservative treatment, simple aspiration or partial resection.
- Painful splenomegaly.
- Primary or secondary splenic malignancy.

Laparoscopic splenectomy is an established technique, which offers a number of advantages over conventional open surgery. The minimally invasive technique is particularly attractive if cholecystectomy is also necessary. It offers an excellent view of the spleen and splenic hilum when the organ is small or moderately enlarged (to the umbilicus and iliac fossa). A laparoscopic-assisted (part laparoscopy, the remainder open surgery) or hand-assisted laparoscopy (one hand inside the peritoneal cavity through a special device to assist in an otherwise completely laparoscopic procedure) technique may be considered if the organ is massively enlarged.

Contraindications

ABSOLUTE

- Patients who are unstable hemodynamically.

RELATIVE

- Hemodynamically stable children with splenic and/or multiple injuries.
- Massive splenomegaly.
- Previous upper abdominal surgery and/or major scarring.

The role of laparoscopy in the management of cancer remains controversial. Portal hypertension and bleeding tendency are no longer regarded as absolute contraindications to laparoscopy because, in skilled hands, the risk of bleeding is less than with open surgery.

EQUIPMENT/INSTRUMENTS

Essential

- Four 3.5–12 mm cannulae, with an appropriate number of reducers if necessary (usually one 10–12 mm and three 5 mm cannulae).
- 5 mm or 10 mm preferably 30–45° angled telescope.
- 3.5–5 mm curved, double jaw action, preferably insulated, scissors with diathermy point.
- Two sets of 3.5–5 mm atraumatic, preferably curved and insulated, grasping forceps without ratchet.

- Fine 3.5–5 mm hook monopolar and bipolar diathermy.
- 3.5–5 mm atraumatic retractor.
- 3.5–5 mm suction/irrigation device.
- 5 mm clip applicator with appropriate 9 mm or larger clips (alternatively, a suture ligature may be used).
- Large (depending on the size of the spleen) strong, non-permeable retrieval bag.

Optional

- A fifth 3.5–5 mm cannula in case of difficult splenectomy.
- 3.5–5 mm atraumatic insulated grasping forceps with ratchet.
- 5 mm soft Babcock forceps or bowel clamp to hold the stomach, colon, omentum or splenic pedicle if necessary.
- 5 mm ultrasound shears (scissors and fine monopolar hook diathermy are still essential for fine dissection).
- 5–10 mm bipolar sealing device (LigaSure™ or equivalent) – a recently developed device, which offers advantages over conventional diathermy, ultrasound shears, clips and suture ligatures for small and large vessels including main splenic vessels.
- 5 mm pre-tied suture loops to add security to any large coagulated or clipped vessels/pedicle.
- A length of broad nylon tape or soft rubber tube to place around the spleen to manipulate the organ during dissection or to aid organ retrieval.

The size of cannulae used depends on the size of the instruments available. One large cannula should be placed at the site where the organ is eventually going to be retrieved. The size and length of the instruments are dictated by the size of the patient, the size of the spleen and the surgeon's preference. In general, the 5 mm instruments are less traumatic than 3.5 mm instruments, especially for manipulation and retraction of the body of the spleen.

PREOPERATIVE PREPARATION

Preparation of the patient prior to laparoscopic splenectomy is necessary, as for open surgery. Appropriate hematological and biochemical investigations should be undertaken and blood cross-matched. Liaison with the hematology and pathology services is particularly important. Steroid immunoglobulin and platelet cover should be arranged as necessary. Preoperative vaccination against pneumococcal, *Haemophilus influenzae* b and meningococcal infections should be performed. The advantage of preoperative CT or isotope imaging to localize or exclude the presence of accessory spleens is uncertain.

TECHNIQUE

General anesthesia with endotracheal intubation and muscle relaxation is essential. A nasogastric tube must be placed after the induction of anesthesia. A urinary catheter is only necessary if the bladder is palpable and cannot be emptied by expression. The abdomen should be palpated to assess the size of the spleen and determine the optimum positions of the cannulae.

The procedure may be performed with the patient positioned supine, completely lateral or anywhere in between. In general, the degree of lateral tilt depends on the size of the spleen, with the largest spleen being removed in a supine position. In a semi-lateral position (the patient is well padded, supported and strapped) access to the spleen can be improved further by rotating the table sideways and adding a slight head-up tilt. A lumbar support (either a break in the table or a soft towel placed under the dependent loin/lower chest) may improve access further. The surgeon and camera operator stand in front of the patient while the second assistant, if required, and scrub nurse stand opposite. The exact sites for the cannulae depend on a number of factors.

- Size and shape of the patient – closure to the costal margin in large patients and those with a narrow subcostal angle.
- Size of the spleen – further away from the costal margin in large spleens.
- Size of instruments available – close to the spleen for short instruments.
- Site of previous scars – avoid.
- Whether concomitant cholecystectomy is required.
- Surgeon's preference.

In the majority of cases (small and moderately large spleen) the primary cannula should be placed at or a few centimeters above and to the left of the umbilicus. A pneumoperitoneum is created using a flow rate of 0.5–1 L/min and pressure of 8–10 mmHg. After a preliminary exploratory laparoscopy, the site, size and number of working cannulae are finally decided. Under direct vision, the first working (secondary) cannula is placed in the epigastrium and the second to the left and sometimes below the primary cannula. These two cannulae are used for manipulation and dissection. The third working cannula is placed below and to the left of the last cannula for the retractor. Care must be taken not to place the cannulae too close to each other or the spleen, otherwise viewing and instrument function become difficult. Dissection may be facilitated by moving the telescope and/or instruments from one cannula to another. **(See Figure 36.1)**

Total splenectomy involves a number of sequential procedures.

- Division of the spleno-colic ligament, around the lower pole of the spleen to the lower margin of the spleno-renal ligament, is achieved using a combination

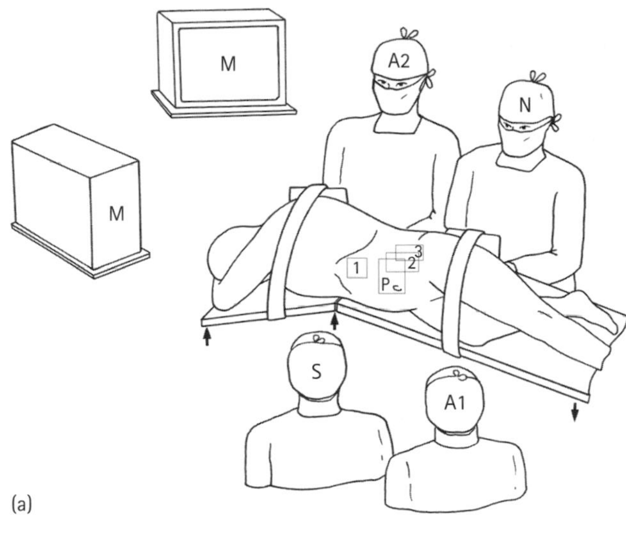

(a)

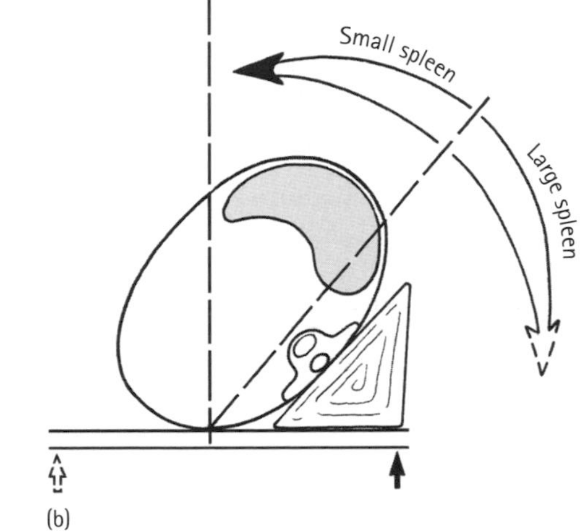

(b)

Figure 36.1

of bipolar diathermy and scissors, or monopolar diathermy with or without scissors, but ultrasound shears probably provide the most efficient method. Clips and ligatures are rarely required.

- Division of the gastro-splenic attachment (short gastric vessels) to the phrenico-splenic ligament. These dissections are facilitated by placing the ligament on a gentle stretch using atraumatic grasping forceps in the left hand while the spleen is retracted cephalad and/or laterally. Sometimes the spleen is very close to the fundus and lower esophagus, in which case division of the upper part of the gastro-splenic attachment may be accomplished using low-voltage fine monopolar hook diathermy or fine curved scissors with diathermy point. Care must be taken not to injure the splenic capsule or stomach wall. **(See Figure 36.2)**
- Once the colon and gastric attachments are released, a thorough search is made for accessory spleens.
- Dissection now proceeds towards the hilum of the spleen. The tail of pancreas is identified, and extreme care must be exercised to avoid injury to the pancreas, splenic capsule and splenic vessels. Traction and avulsion injury to small vessels in this region is a particular nuisance. The main splenic artery and vein are identified and mobilized individually over a distance of 1.5–2 cm. This is best achieved using a combination of sharp (fine, low-voltage hook monopolar or bipolar diathermy or scissors) and blunt (atraumatic pointed angled or curved dissecting forceps) dissection along and behind the upper border of pancreas a few centimeters away from the spleen. Extreme care must be taken at this stage to avoid injury to the vessels, with the predictable consequence of profuse bleeding. The splenic artery is divided first between ligatures or clips (double proximal clips and

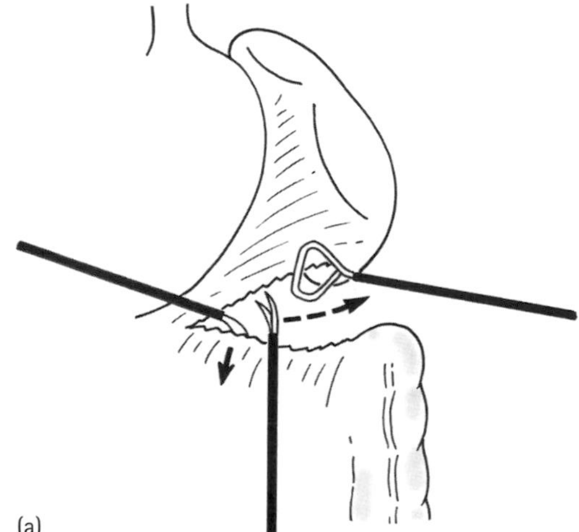

(a)

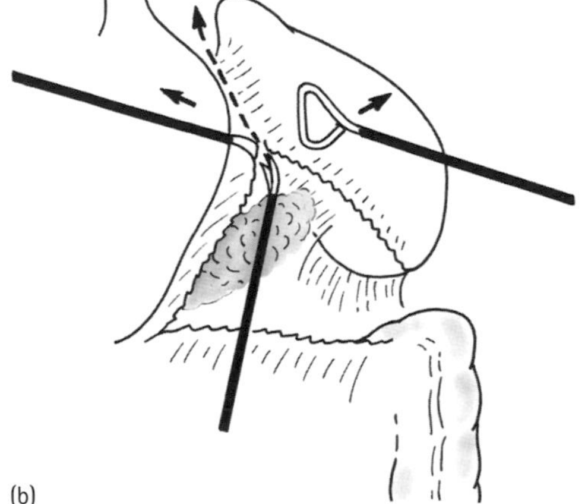

(b)

Figure 36.2

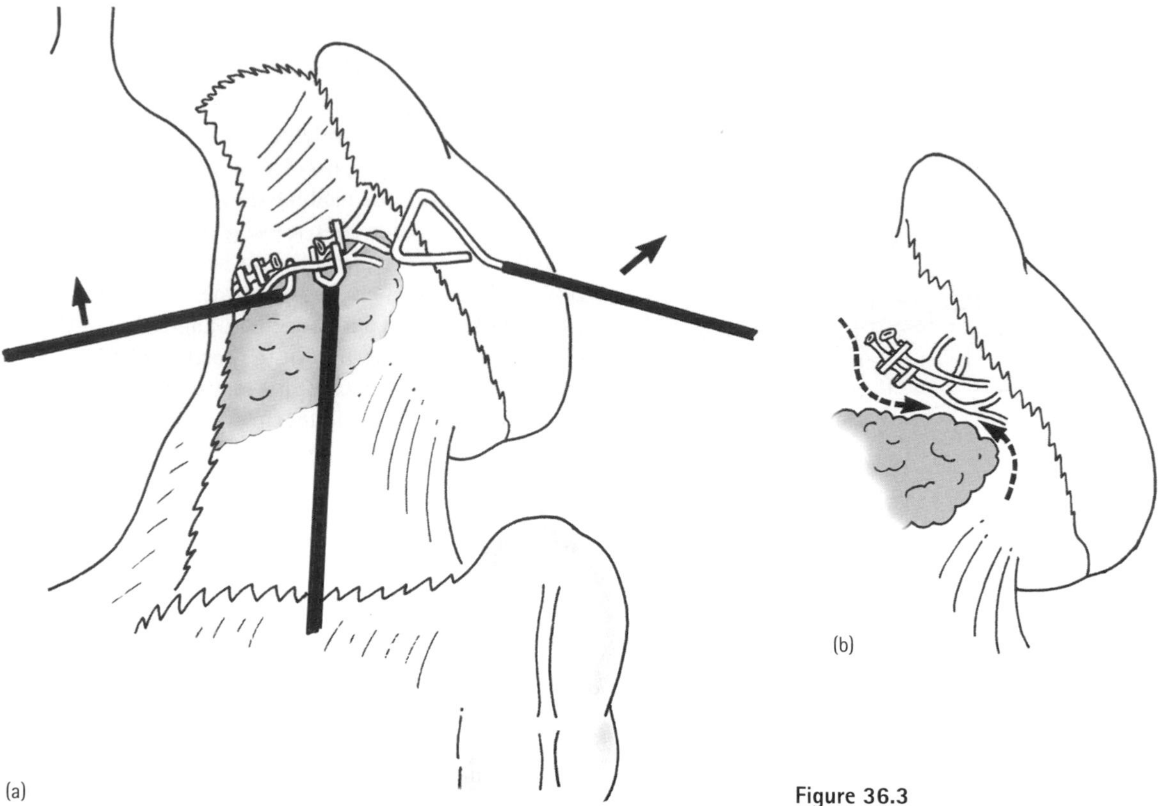

Figure 36.3

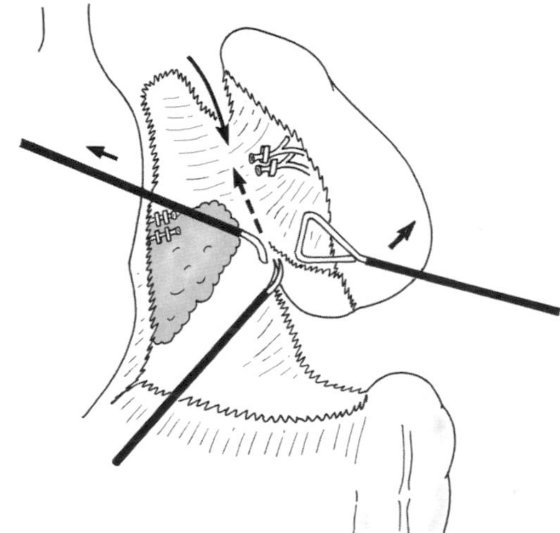

Figure 36.4

a single distal clip). The splenic vein is then divided in a similar fashion. This sequential maneuver interrupts the main blood supply to the spleen and thereby reduces the risk of subsequent major hemorrhage. Division of the artery prior to the vein significantly diminishes the size of the spleen through spontaneous venous drainage, which facilitates further manipulation and subsequent organ extraction. The recently developed LigaSure™ and plasma kineteic bipolar device provide a safe method of securing the main splenic vessels without the need for clips or ligatures. Any remaining vessels and hilar connective tissue are secured and divided using clips, diathermy, scissors or ultrasound shears. **(See Figure 36.3)**

- The body of the spleen is supported by the retractor in a cephalad or lateral direction. The spleno-renal and phrenico-splenic ligaments and any additional retroperitoneal attachments are divided using diathermy, scissors or ultrasound shears. It may be necessary to retract the spleen in a number of different directions to facilitate this move. **(See Figure 36.4)**
- The entire operative field is then inspected and complete hemostasis is ensured.
- Removal of spleen is accomplished using a retrieval bag placed into the peritoneal cavity via one of the larger cannulae (10–12 mm). Moving the telescope from one cannula to another may be necessary. The spleen, which is now completely free from intra-abdominal attachment, is then gently manipulated into the bag or, as this can be a slow and difficult process, the bag may be pulled over it. Care should be taken not to damage the splenic capsule at any time and this is best achieved by careful manipulation and avoiding grasping the spleen directly.

The neck of the bag is exteriorized through an extended cannula site or a strategically placed small abdominal incision, depending on the size of the

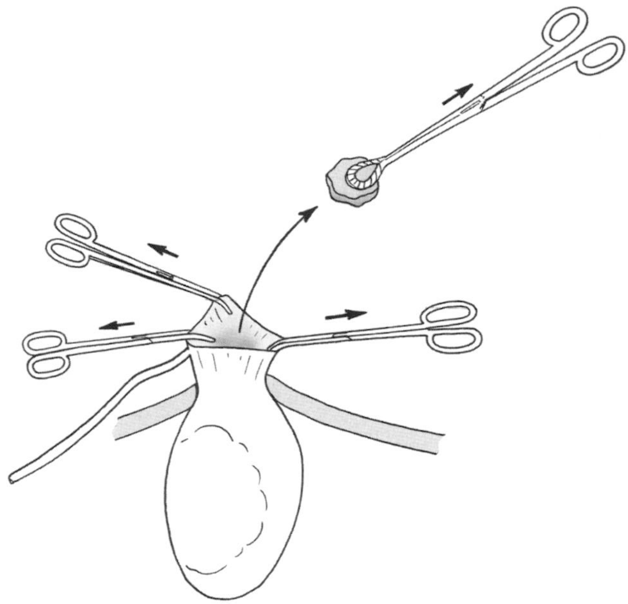

Figure 36.5

spleen and the patient's and surgeon's preference. The site of the chosen extended wound/incision should be discussed with the child and parents prior to surgery. The spleen can be fragmented in the bag using a pair of large artery forceps and extracted piecemeal using a sponge-holding forceps and suction. Extreme care must be taken not to damage the bag and spill the contents into the peritoneal cavity. **(See Figure 36.5)**

- The cannulae are removed and the pneumoperitoneum is evacuated. Cannulae sites larger than 4 mm in diameter and the site of spleen extraction are closed with absorbable sutures in the usual fashion. These incisions may be infiltrated with local anesthetic agents to provide postoperative analgesia.

POSTOPERATIVE CARE

Postoperative analgesia in the form of an epidural infusion or intravenous morphine infusion is rarely necessary beyond the first 12 hours. The nasogastric tube may be removed at this stage and the patient is fed at 24 hours. Regular oral non-steroidal analgesia may be used for the first day or two. The child is normally fit for discharge home at 36–48 hours postoperatively.

PROBLEMS, PITFALLS AND SOLUTIONS

As for all surgical procedures, conventional or laparoscopic, patient selection and meticulous attention to details are essential, particularly during the learning curve.

Difficult access and inadequate view

- The position of the patient is crucial. A semi-lateral position with a slight head-up tilt allows the stomach, greater omentum and intestine to fall medially under gravity. This position provides scope for moving the patient to a more lateral or supine position if necessary.
- Plan and position the cannulae carefully. Reposition one or more cannulae if required.
- Change telescope/instruments from one cannula to another.
- Use larger and/or angled telescope in difficult cases and when the operative field becomes blood-stained.
- An appropriate retractor is crucial, especially during the final parts of the procedure.
- Consider placement of an additional cannula/ instrument.
- Consider a hand-assisted technique or convert to open surgery if the spleen is very large or the operation difficult.

Bleeding

- Never grasp the spleen directly. Instead, use an atraumatic retractor or the side of instruments or tape around the spleen to manipulate.
- Use low-voltage diathermy to control blood vessels, in particular small, short or thin-walled veins.
- Double clip, suture ligate or seal (LigaSure™), or use additional pre-tied suture loops for major vessels.

Dissection at the hilum and around the tail of pancreas

- Small strands of connective tissue and small vessels in between larger vessels, spleen and pancreas must be handled carefully and secured individually. Some surgeons advocate the use of an EndoGIA® vascular stapler across the entire pedicle, which may or may not include the tail of pancreas (10–12 mm cannula required).

Accessory spleens

- A thorough search for splenunculi should be made as soon as the spleno-colic and gastro-splenic ligaments are divided. A blood-stained field or an untidy dissection increases the risk of missing splenunculi.

Organ retrieval

Placing the detached large spleen into a retrieval bag can be difficult. Extraction of the spleen from the bag piecemeal can be messy and potentially dangerous.

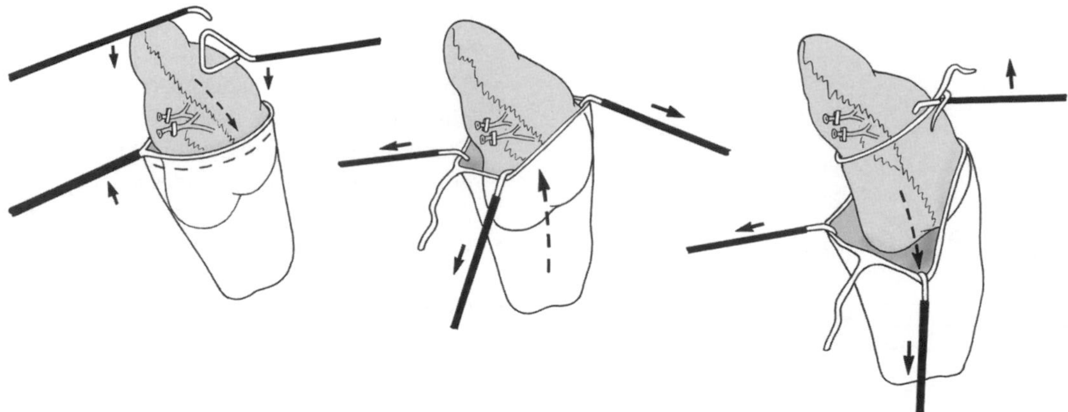

Figure 36.6

- Retrieval bags with a built-in drawstring and spring metal band on an introducer are available. It is relatively easy to use these devices as a fishing net to scoop up a small or medium-sized spleen.
- Large spleens are more difficult. An appropriately sized, tough and non-permeable bag is required. Graspers are used to triangulate the mouth of the bag by holding the posterior and side walls and moving the bag over the spleen from below or above.
- Wide tape or a long, soft, rubber tube/catheter can be placed around the spleen and the tape can then be grasped and used to manipulate the spleen into the bag.
- Avoid morcellator, as this can damage the retrieval bag.
- Retrieving an intact small/medium spleen requires a 2.5–5 cm long incision. **(See Figure 36.6)**

COMPLICATIONS

- Significant bleeding from an injured spleen prior to securing the hilar vessels or a major vessel usually mandates conversion to an open technique. However, provided the patient is hemodynamically stable, the experienced surgeon may attempt to place the spleen (small or medium) in a retrieval bag with a purse-string, which is tightened. This may allow isolation of the blood supply provided vision is not obscured.
- Bleeding from inadequately controlled blood vessels. Use appropriate retraction and suction/irrigation, swiftly identify the source and deal with it appropriately. Consider conversion to an open technique before losing too much blood.
- Thermal (diathermy, ultrasound) and mechanical (fine or traumatic instruments) injury to stomach, intestines and pancreas. Inspect and assess the injury, and consider laparoscopic repair at the end of the procedure.
- Recurrent symptoms from missed accessory spleen or auto-transplantation following capsular tear or spillage during organ retrieval. Consider a second laparoscopic procedure.

37

Pancreatectomy

THOM E. LOBE AND JAMES T. MOORE

INTRODUCTION

With modern pediatric instruments and experience, safe and effective laparoscopic pancreatic surgery becomes feasible as a logical extension of the laparoscopic procedures already performed every day. Careful consideration should be given to the indications for surgery of the pancreas. The procedure is essentially the same whether performed using an open or a laparoscopic technique. That being said, the laparoscopic approach has the potential to be less invasive and/or less traumatic than its open counterpart. In addition, the magnification inherent in the laparoscopic approach allows for better visualization and control of the pancreatic duct and small vessels supplying the pancreas (e.g. splenic vein tributaries).

Indications

- Pseudocysts.
- Vascular malformations.
- Trauma.
- Metabolically active focal lesions such as adenomas.
- Diffuse lesions such as persistent hyperinsulinemic hypoglycemia of the newborn (PHHN) and chronic pancreatitis.

Contraindications

ABSOLUTE

- Hemodynamically unstable patient.
- Severe respiratory compromise with inability to establish a pneumoperitoneum.
- Coagulopathy.

RELATIVE

- History of multiple upper abdominal procedures with significant adhesions.
- Prior pancreatic surgery.
- Portal hypertension.

EQUIPMENT/INSTRUMENTS

Essential

- 3 mm or 5 mm cannulae.
- 3 mm or 5 mm blunt and curved tip dissectors.
- 3 mm or 5 mm non-traumatic bowel graspers.
- Energy device for division of vascular structures:
  - LigaSure™ (bipolar sealant device)
  - Harmonic Scalpel®
  - monopolar hook or bipolar cautery.
- 3 mm or 5 mm laparoscopic scissors.

Optional

- Liver retractor.
- 5 mm clip applicator.
- Laparoscopic cholangiocatheter.
- 12 mm cannulae:
  - Endocatch device
  - laparoscopic stapling device
  - laparoscopic ultrasound probe.

PREOPERATIVE PREPARATION

Depending on the reason for the procedure, preoperative imaging can be extremely useful. In the case of an adenoma, computerized tomography (CT) scan or ultrasound can help in identifying the site of the lesion. This can be supplemented by the use of intra-abdominal ultrasound. Occasionally, preoperative angiography may also aid in localization. For pseudocysts, CT and/or ultrasound are used to evaluate the lesion and the need for drainage. In cases of metabolically active adenomas, the serum levels of relevant enzymes are measured, and other biochemical measurements are made to make the diagnosis. Surgery is only considered after a failure of suppressive therapy.

TECHNIQUE

Regardless of the indication, laparoscopic approaches to the pancreas are similar in most cases. Appropriate cannulae placement will maximize exposure and decrease the operative time and the risk of complications.

Patients are given a general anesthetic and positioned supine on a table that is suitable for fluoroscopy should a cholangiogram be necessary. They are placed at the end of the table (infant) or supine (older child) or in stirrups. The surgeon stands at the foot of the table and the assistant and scrub nurse on either side. Reverse Trendelenburg positioning helps to move abdominal viscera out of the operative field.

Cannulae positions

The authors prefer closed technique laparoscopy (Veress needle). However, in the setting of trauma, inflammatory disease, neoplasm or a large cyst, open technique laparoscopy is used. An umbilical or right upper quadrant (presence of umbilical scarring) primary cannula serves most purposes. Although a 5 mm cannula is often adequate, the size of the cannula is dictated by the procedure to be performed. A 12 mm cannula may be used if a linear stapler or intraoperative ultrasound probe is required. A 0° or 30° telescope provides an excellent view of the lesser sac and the entire pancreas.

After the initial inspection, two to three additional cannulae are inserted as needed. Cannulae size selection is a function of both patient size and the laparoscopic instruments to be used. We favor a 3 mm port in the right upper quadrant and a 5 mm port in the left upper quadrant. The larger port will accommodate a Harmonic Scalpel®, LigaSure™ or clip applier that can be used to divide vascular structures. For small babies, we use only 3 mm cannulae and divide small vessels with monopolar cautery. A third cannula may be necessary in the midline to provide additional retraction. (**See Figure 37.1**)

Access to the lesser sac

Since the pancreas is located in the lesser sac, the laparoscopic surgeon must know how to gain access to this region. For most cases this will be the first procedural step, but in certain circumstances (e.g. cystogastrostomy) the pancreas is approached via another route. The approach to the lesser sac is best undertaken with good gastric retraction.

In our experience, percutaneously placed sutures that pierce the abdominal wall, pass through the seromuscular wall of the greater curvature and then back through the abdominal wall are an excellent means of providing multipoint retraction of the stomach. The external ends of these sutures can be draped over or tied to a self-retaining retraction ring or bar to help lift the stomach out of the way.

The gastrocolic ligament is then divided using a LigaSure™, hook cautery or ultrasonic scalpel. In dividing this structure, the lesser sac is entered and the pancreas is visualized. (**See Figure 37.2**)

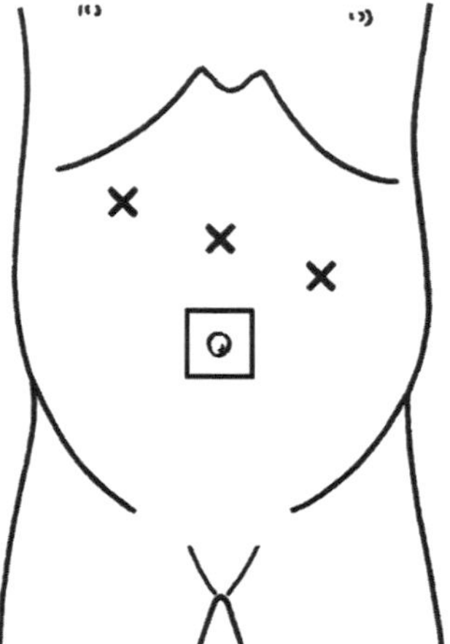

Figure 37.1

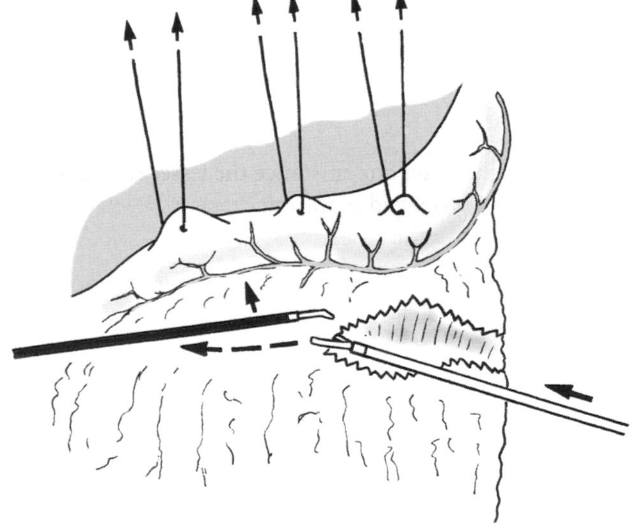

Figure 37.2

Special circumstances

- When a subtotal pancreatectomy is required, a Kocher maneuver is used so that the entire pancreas can be visualized. Also a cholangiogram is necessary to identify the biliary ducts and minimize the risk of duct injury.
- When suturing is necessary and anastomoses are required, the surgeon should be familiar with laparoscopic suturing and intracorporeal and extracorporeal knot tying. A laparoscopic linear stapler can be very useful for creating anastomoses and for securing and dividing the pancreas.
- The placement of drains is not routine and needs to be considered on an individual basis.

POSTOPERATIVE CARE

As in all laparoscopic procedures, postoperative pain is controlled with a combination of non-steroidal anti-inflammatory drugs and narcotics, and patients are encouraged to eat as soon as they are hungry and to return to normal activities as early as possible.

SPECIFIC PROCEDURES

Cystogastrostomy and cysto-enterostomy

Pancreatic pseudocysts can result from trauma or cholelithiasis-induced pancreatitis. In the absence of spontaneous resolution a cysto-enterostomy can be created relatively easily. The choice of what part of the gastrointestinal tract to use for drainage is a function of the cyst location. A preoperative CT scan is often helpful for planning the operative approach.

- In mature pseudocyst of the pancreas, open laparoscopy is the preferred technique. For lesions sitting directly behind the stomach and abutting the posterior wall, a cystogastrostomy is the procedure of choice. In the latter circumstance the lesser sac does not need to be opened as the approach to the pancreas is made through the stomach.
- A flexible pediatric gastroscope advanced into the stomach is used to localize the lesion by identifying the point of maximal anterior displacement of the posterior gastric wall. Alternatively, a laparoscopic ultrasound probe (12 mm umbilical cannula required) may be used to define the location and extent of the cyst.
- Once the location has been identified, two percutaneous retraction sutures are placed in the anterior gastric wall overlying the cyst. With elevation of the anterior gastric wall, a small gastrostomy is made with electrocautery. The gastrostomy must then be extended to visualize the posterior wall overlying the cyst. A laparoscopic linear stapling device is well suited to this purpose and provides excellent hemostasis. Alternatively, electrocautery may be used to enlarge the anterior gastrostomy. In this instance, intracorporeal suturing may be necessary to achieve complete hemostasis.
- A posterior gastrostomy overlying the previously defined cyst is created with electrocautery, thereby draining it into the stomach. Once again a linear stapler is used to extend the gastrostomy and provide hemostasis. In the event of persistent bleeding, a running, locking Vicryl® suture can be placed to achieve hemostasis. **(See Figure 37.3)**
- Finally, the anterior gastrostomy is closed with a stapler, laparoscopic suturing or a combination of the two. **(See Figure 37.4)**

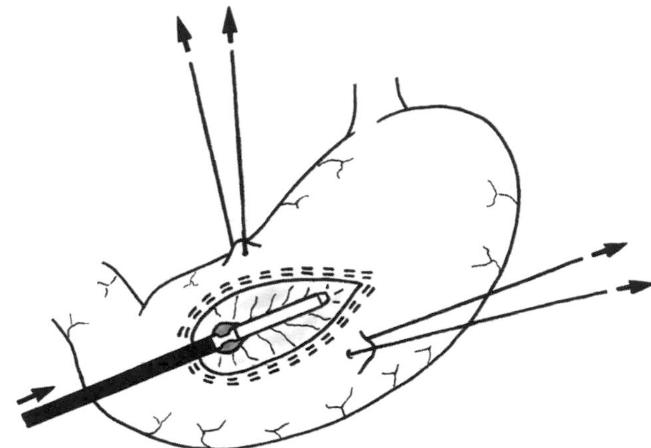

Figure 37.3

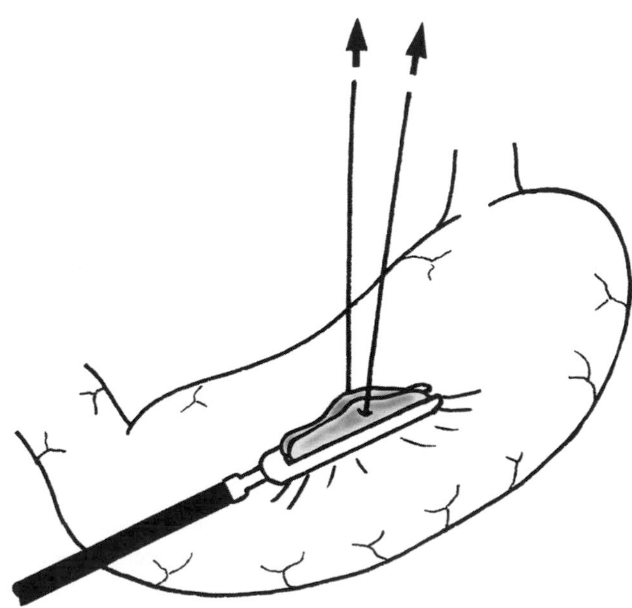

Figure 37.4

SPECIAL CONSIDERATIONS

If the location of the cyst precludes the formation of a cystogastrostomy, a cysto-enterostomy may have to be used for drainage. In this situation, it is often necessary to enter the lesser sac as described above. Once the cyst has been identified, a segment of jejunum is chosen for the anastomosis. This segment should be just distal to the ligament of Treitz but mobile enough to be brought up antecolic to the cyst without tension. After fixing the jejunum to the cyst with a single 3-0 silk, a small cystotomy and anti-mesenteric jejunotomy are made with electrocautery. Using a linear stapler with one blade in the cyst and one in the jejunum, a cystojejunostomy is then created by firing the stapler. The remaining cystotomy and jejunostomy can then be closed with staples or sutures.

When the cyst is abutting the duodenum, a cystoduodenostomy may be made. The procedure is similar to that described for a cystojejunostomy with two additional steps. The hepatic flexure is freed and the duodenum mobilized with a Kocher maneuver (see section below on subtotal pancreatectomy). Before attempting this procedure, the surgeon must be aware of the course of the biliary ducts and take measures to protect them from injury. The best way to do this is via a transcholecystic cholangiogram. The gallbladder is cannulated with an 18–22 G spinal needle (depending upon patient size) and contrast is injected under fluoroscopic control. Once the location of the ampulla has been established, a cystoduodenostomy is performed.

PROBLEMS, PITFALLS AND SOLUTIONS

Large cyst limits view and/or operative field

- A 30° scope allows versatility.
- Move the telescope from one cannula to the other, or consider placing an additional cannula.
- Consider percutaneous drainage of the cyst with a spinal needle; try to puncture the cyst at the planned site of the anastomosis.

Significant soft tissue edema at the anastomosis

- Use a hand-sewn anastomosis to accommodate a variety of tissue depths.
- If possible, use a different part of the cyst and/or bowel.
- Consider reinforcing the anastomosis with omentum.
- Consider leaving a closed suction drain near the anastomosis.

Proximity of bile duct difficult to assess

- Intra-operative cholangiogram with fluoroscopy and/or dye (e.g. methylene blue) helps to define the anatomy.
- Consider using a jejunal loop instead of the duodenum to drain the cyst.

Difficult antecolic approximation of the small intestine and cyst

- Pass bowel through transverse colon mesentery; mesenteric defect must be closed around bowel to prevent herniation.
- Consider a Roux-en-Y limb to drain cyst.

COMPLICATIONS

Bleeding from the anastomosis

- Avoid visible vessels when creating enterotomy/cystotomy.
- Cauterize smaller bleeding vessels.
- Control moderate bleeding with a running, locking suture or LigaSure™ device.

Anastomotic leak

- A small focal leak may be controlled with percutaneous drainage.
- A larger or expanding leak may require re-operation.

Pancreatitis

- Aggressive hydration and supportive care are mandatory.
- Antibiotics are rarely indicated.
- In cases of infected pancreatitis (culture proven), initiate antibiotics (imipenem) and consider open debridement.

Recurrent cyst

- Allow 6–8 weeks for original cysto-enterostomy to heal. In cases of recurrent or residual cysts, consider endoscopic versus laparoscopic approach for drainage.

Bile duct injury

- A small, clean injury to the bile duct may be repaired primarily with or without the use of a T-tube.
- Larger injuries necessitate ligation of the proximal duct with creation of a choledochojejunostomy.

Partial or subtotal pancreatectomy for PHHN

PREOPERATIVE PREPARATION

Infants or children with clinically significant persistent hypoglycemia should be evaluated for anatomic lesions or PHHN. In the former, surgical enucleation is a curative measure. Patients with PHHN remain the subject of some controversy. One school of thought recommends performing a 75 percent pancreatectomy to avoid the potential complications (diabetes and secretory insufficiency) while still allowing for a 50 percent chance of symptomatic relief. Others believe that, because there is such a high failure rate with the former approach, all patients should be subjected to a 95 percent pancreatectomy at the outset. Regardless of the approach, laparoscopy is an appropriate choice for surgery.

TECHNIQUE

Access is gained as described previously. A 12 mm port is used at the umbilicus if a stapler is to divide the pancreas. In small children the pancreas can often be mass ligated with a suture, in which case a 5 mm umbilical port is employed.

- Once the lesser sac is entered, the main splenic vessels are exposed by freeing the body and tail of pancreas posteriorly. The dissection is started at the midpoint along the lower border of pancreas and continued towards the tail.
- With the tail mobilized, the plane of dissection can be extended proximally to the chosen site of division. In larger children we use a 5 mm Harmonic Scalpel® for this dissection, but in babies a 3 mm hook cautery is sufficient. Once the splenic vein is visualized, a right-angled hook cautery or LigaSure™ is used to dissect and divide the numerous small veins that drain the pancreas posteriorly. When sufficient time is taken to do this, hemorrhage is rare. It is important to identify and avoid the course of the splenic artery at the superior edge of the pancreas. Using this technique, the pancreas can be mobilized from the tail to the junction of the splenic and portal veins. **(See Figure 37.5)**
- The pancreas is now freed from the splenic hilum laterally to the superior mesenteric artery medially.
- Attention is then turned to the duodenum, which must be freed laterally and rotated anteriorly and medially by a Kocher maneuver to expose the posterior and right sides of the pancreas. With downward traction on the transverse colon, the hepatocolic ligament is divided. This maneuver exposes the duodenum, which is then retracted medially and anteriorly while the lateral retroperitoneal attachments are divided with a hook cautery or Harmonic Scalpel®. **(See Figure 37.6)**
- After the pancreas has been mobilized, the surgeon should clearly identify the bile duct. The Kocher maneuver should facilitate this, but it may be necessary to perform a cholangiogram, as described earlier, to demonstrate the anatomy clearly.
- Once the bile duct has been identified, the pancreas can be freed to that point, leaving a 2–3 cm rim of pancreatic tissue medial to the duodenum. We find the

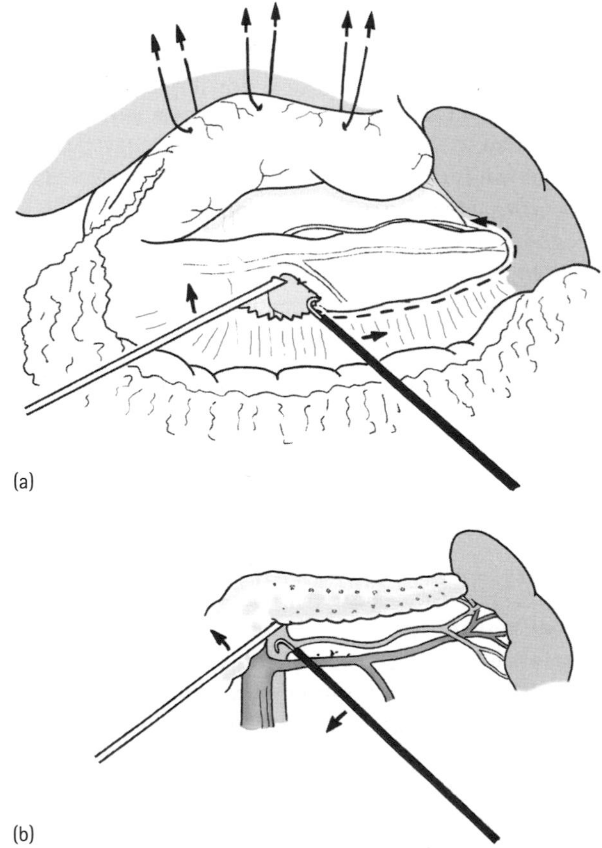

Figure 37.5

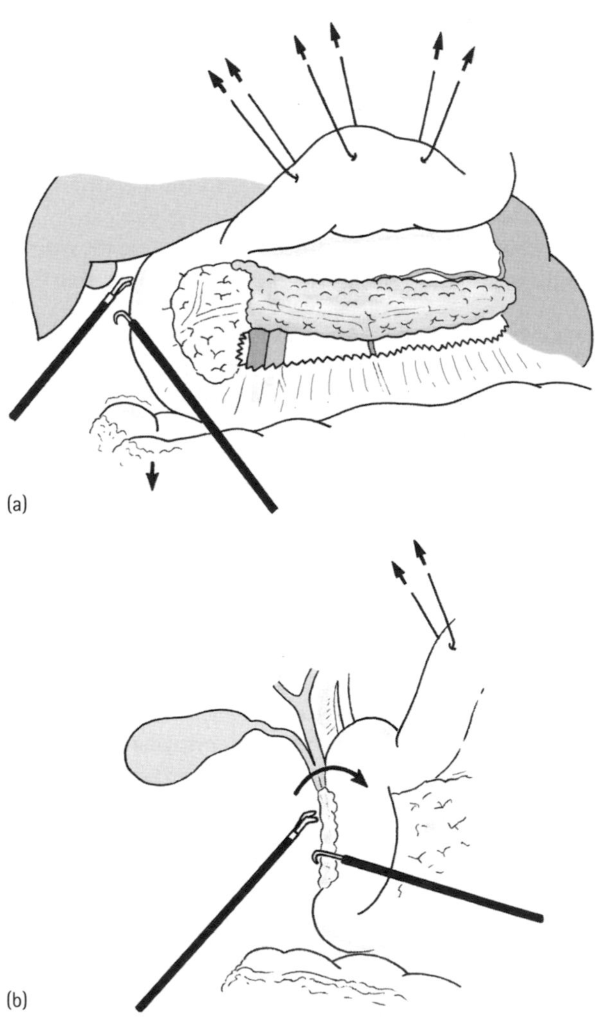

Figure 37.6

best tool for dividing the pancreas is the LigaSure™, which provides a seal sufficient to minimize or prevent leakage. We believe that the ultrasonic scalpel and the hook cautery deliver too much energy in the form of heat to be safe for this purpose when there are so many critically important structures in such a confined space. Alternatively, one can suture the cut surface of the pancreas or choose to reinforce the LigaSure™ seal by over-sewing it. In infants, it may be possible simply to ligate the body of the pancreas at the appropriate spot with a mass ligature or suture ligature. In larger patients, the endoscopic stapler may prove valuable to transect and seal the end of the pancreas.

- Once the pancreas has been divided, it is placed in a specimen bag. The end of the bag is then delivered through the umbilical port and the pancreas is morselated and aspirated and removed piecemeal with ring forceps.

PROBLEMS, PITFALLS AND SOLUTIONS

Poor visualization of the pancreas
- Ensure that the gastrocolic ligament is opened widely.
- Additional transcutaneous suture may improve gastric retraction.
- A 3 mm or 5 mm liver retractor may be used to elevate the stomach.
- An additional port may be required for downward traction on the colon.
- Reverse Trendelenburg positioning or table tilt will help move intervening bowel out of the operative field.

Proximity to the bile duct is difficult to assess
- Intra-operative cholangiogram with fluoroscopy and/or dye (e.g. methylene blue) helps to define the course of the bile duct.

Potential for significant bleeding during posterior dissection
- Extra-parenchymal dissection minimizes the risk of injury to branches of the pancreaticoduodenal artery and splenic artery, which tend to run within the substance of the pancreas.
- The approach to branches of the splenic vein must be systematic and meticulous.
- Small venous branches are easily controlled with cautery, whereas larger branches may require the LigaSure™.

Defining the margin of resection
- This decision is clearly experience-based, with the risk of persistent hypoglycemia weighed against the possibility of insulin dependence.
- We favor a more aggressive resection in neonates and infants, as their rates of persistent hypoglycemia are likely to be higher with less than a 95 percent resection.

COMPLICATIONS

Bile duct injury (see cystogastrostomy)
Bleeding
- In infants, mass ligature of the proximal margin prior to division of the pancreas minimizes the risk of bleeding.
- In larger children, two figure-of-eight silk sutures around the proximal inferior and proximal superior pancreatic edges help to control the marginal vessels.
- Use of a vascular load stapler or LigaSure™ device to divide the pancreas provides excellent hemostasis.

Pancreatic leak
- A visible pancreatic duct may be ligated using a figure-of-eight silk suture.
- Over-sewing the entire proximal resection margin with a running polypropylene suture will provide additional security against a leak.
- Consider the use of a closed suction drain in high-risk patients.

Pancreatitis (see cystogastrostomy)
Injury to the splenic vessels
- Unless the injury can be isolated and repaired, timely ligation of the vessels and splenectomy should be performed.

Resection of a functioning adenoma

- The lesser sac is entered and the pancreas sufficiently mobilized so that the entire area of pathology can be examined. It may not be necessary to free the splenic vein if an adenoma is clearly visible. Usually a single adenoma is found.
- Once the adenoma is visualized, it can usually be enucleated using the hook cautery, ultrasonic scalpel or LigaSure™. If the lesion is fairly large and involves the tail of the pancreas, a distal pancreatectomy (as described above) may prove easier than local enucleation.
- The specimen is then removed using a retrieval bag; a drain is usually not necessary.

PROBLEMS, PITFALLS AND SOLUTIONS

Difficult localization
- For small lesions, consider preoperative CT-guided localization with injection of dye.
- Intra-operative ultrasound may prove helpful.

Proximity to the bile duct is difficult to assess
- Intra-operative cholangiogram with fluoroscopy and/or dye (e.g. methylene blue) helps to define the course of the bile duct.

COMPLICATIONS

Bleeding

- The judicious use of cautery or the LigaSure™ device minimizes the risk of bleeding.
- Figure-of-eight suture ligatures may also be used to achieve hemostasis.

Pancreatic leak

- A small leak may be managed with percutaneous drainage.
- A larger or expanding leak may require re-operation.

Pancreatitis (see cystogastrostomy)

Vascular abnormality

Vascular malformations of the pancreas such as lymphangiomas or hemangiomas are variable and rare. A small hemangioma may be amenable to laser ablation or cryoablation. Larger lesions are best excised using the endoscopic stapler or LigaSure™. Both devices tend to prevent leakage at the suture line. A preoperative magnetic resonance angiogram (MRA) is usually helpful in localizing the lesion and planning the operation. If necessary, a formal pancreatectomy can be performed.

Trauma

While an unstable patient or one with evidence of trauma to multiple organ systems is not an appropriate candidate for laparoscopy, a stable patient with clinical or radiographic evidence of an isolated pancreatic injury may be explored with a laparoscope. The approach is the same as described for elective surgery. Once the pancreas is exposed, its anterior surface is inspected carefully.

Minor parenchymal injuries are best treated with external drainage and observation, whereas major parenchymal injuries or injuries to the pancreatic duct may require formal resection. If a distal pancreatectomy is performed, there is no need for drainage. The LigaSure™ device or laparoscopic stapler usually provides adequate closure of the stump.

38

Esophageal myotomy

CIRO ESPOSITO

INTRODUCTION

Esophageal achalasia is a functional disorder characterized by impaired motility of the distal esophagus and failure of the lower esophageal sphincter (LES) to relax in response to swallowing. The incidence is approximately 5 cases per million and only 5 percent of these are children. Conservative treatment with esophageal dilatations and/or botulinum toxin may give temporary relief of symptoms, but definitive therapy is surgical. The introduction of minimally invasive techniques has had a profound impact on the treatment of achalasia and has made surgical Heller's myotomy the treatment of choice.

Most pediatric surgeons prefer to perform an esophagocardiomyotomy as described by Heller using a laparoscopic approach, but some advocate a thoracoscopic myotomy. Some investigators have shown that the short-term and long-term outcomes after abdominal myotomy are superior to those obtained by the thoracic approach. The main disadvantages of the thoracic approach are assuring that the myotomy extends adequately below the gastroesophageal junction and the inability to perform a concurrent fundoplication. This can result in persistent or recurrent dysphagia, as well as significant gastro-esophageal reflux.

The principle of the procedure is to perform a myotomy 7–8 cm in length on the anterior wall of the lower esophagus. The myotomy should extend 1–2 cm onto the anterior wall of the stomach past the LES. The addition of an anti-reflux procedure is recommended to avoid secondary reflux, which is reported to occur in 10–30 percent of patients.

Indications

- Severe dysphagia.
- Malnutrition.
- Recurrent respiratory infections.
- Severe esophagitis.
- Mucosal metaplasia.

Contraindications

ABSOLUTE

- Hemodynamically unstable children.
- Esophageal perforation secondary to dilatations.

RELATIVE

- Previous upper abdominal surgery.
- Previous injections with botulinum toxin (increases the risk of perforation).

EQUIPMENT/INSTRUMENTS

Essential

- 5 mm or 10 mm Hasson trocar for the initial trocar insertion.
- Four 3 mm or 5 mm cannulae.
- 5 mm or 10 mm 30° telescope.
- 5 mm curved scissors with double-action jaw and diathermy.

- Three 3 mm or 5 mm atraumatic fenestrated grasping forceps.
- 5 mm monopolar hook.
- 3–5 mm atraumatic retractor.
- Two 5 mm needle holders.
- Umbilical tape.
- 5 mm laparoscopic scalpel.
- 5 mm suction/irrigation device.

Optional

- 5 mm clip applicator.
- 5 mm ultrasonic shears.
- 5 mm bipolar sealing device.
- Endoscopic peanuts.
- Suture assist devices.

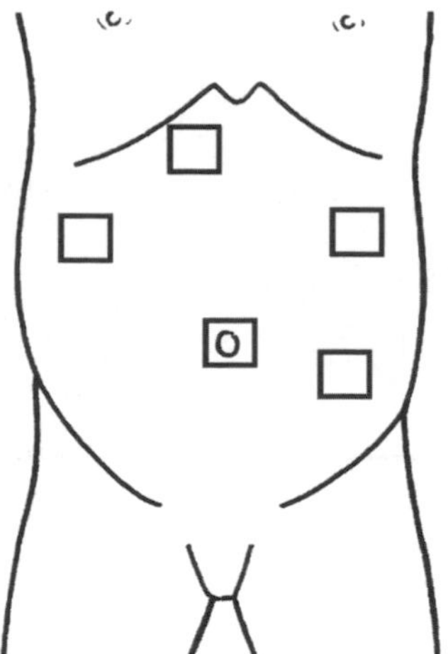

Figure 38.1

PREOPERATIVE PREPARATION

Three main investigations are performed in a child with a clinical suspicion of achalasia.

A plain chest X-ray may show a dilated esophagus or air/fluid level, or both. A contrast esophagram confirms dilatation and the absence of coordinated contraction of the esophagus. It also shows a failure of relaxation of the LES with the classic finding of the 'rat tail' of the esophagus. Upper endoscopy is also helpful in documenting a failure of relaxation of the LES and can be used to evaluate the status of the esophageal mucosa for evidence of esophagitis, mucosal metaplasia or other causes of stricture. Esophageal manometry is the most specific test, showing a failure of relaxation of the LES in response to swallowing with a high-pressure zone of the LES > 30 mmHg and the absence of peristaltic waves in the body of the esophagus.

TECHNIQUE

The operation is performed under general endotracheal anesthesia with orotracheal intubation. A nasogastric tube is placed and the bladder emptied if necessary using the Crede maneuver. The patient is placed supine or in the dorsal lithotomy position with the legs down. Smaller children may be placed near the end of the table with the legs crossed. Once the trocars have been inserted, the table is placed in reverse Trendelenburg of approximately 30°.

The theater and surgical team layout is the same as for anti-reflux surgery. A pneumoperitoneum is created (8–12 mmHg) and a five-cannulae technique is used. The first cannula (5–10 mm) is placed infra-umbilically for the telescope, and the other four cannulae (3–5 mm) are then placed under direct vision: one in the right upper quadrant, for a liver retractor; the second and third in the left upper quadrant and below the xyphoid process, respectively, for the working instruments; and the last lateral to the umbilicus to retract the stomach. (**See Figure 38.1**)

Esophagocardiomyotomy according to Heller's technique involves a number of sequential steps.

- Exposure of the abdominal esophagus and upper stomach is obtained by retracting the left lobe of the liver anterio-superiorly, and by placing traction on the stomach below the esophago-gastric junction with atraumatic grasping forceps.
- Dissection begins with the division of the esophago-hepatic ligament to expose the right crus. Exposure of the esophageal hiatus is completed, with the division of the phreno-esophageal membrane and the phreno-gastric ligament and blunt dissection on the surface of the left crus.
- A retro-esophageal window is then created. Care should be taken to dissect along the right crus, not the esophagus, in order to avoid injury to the posterior esophageal wall. The posterior vagus nerve is identified and is left undisturbed on the posterior esophageal wall.
- Umbilical tape is placed around the esophago-gastric junction and held with grasping forceps through the left lower cannula. This maneuver enables downward traction on the stomach and better visualization of the lower esophagus. Using blunt dissection, the lower few centimeters of esophagus are isolated. (**See Figure 38.2**)
- The myotomy is started anteriorly with a superficial incision through the muscle layer, 3 cm above the esophago-gastric junction. The incision is enlarged carefully with scissors. It is extremely important to keep the scissor blades parallel to the esophagus in the submucosal plain to avoid the risk of mucosal perforation. Alternatively, the myotomy can be carried out by stretching and tearing the circular muscle fibers with two laparoscopic graspers positioned in opposite directions. Once the submucosal plane is reached, the

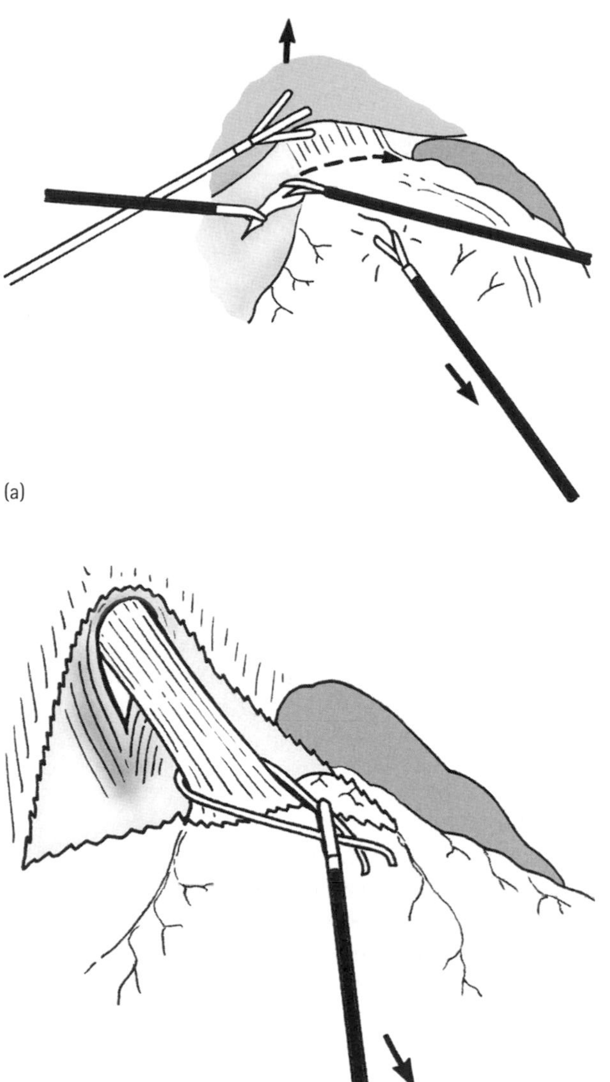

Figure 38.2

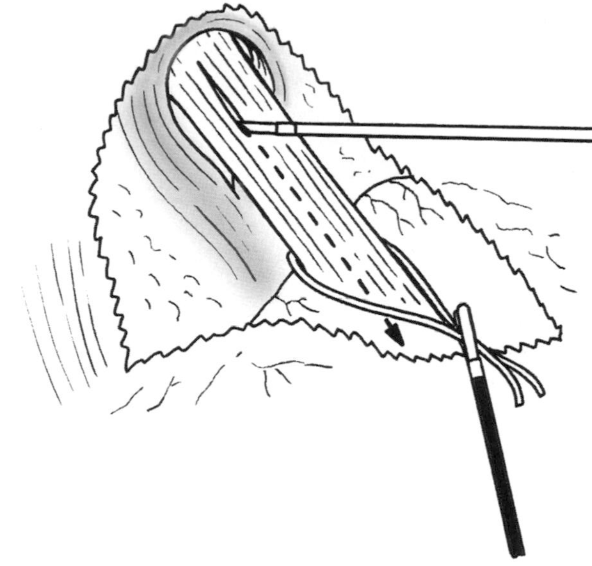
Figure 38.3

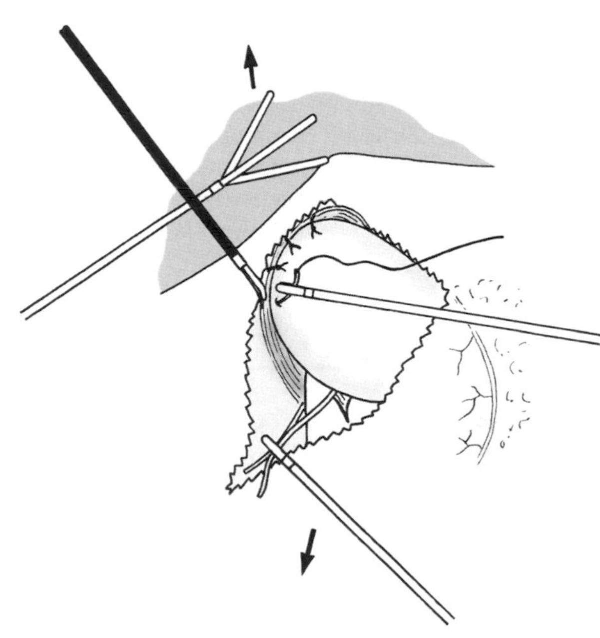
Figure 38.4

muscle layer is separated from the submucosa using blunt dissection and the myotomy is extended proximally for 5–6 cm and distally for 1–2 cm. Two muscular planes of the esophagus, the superficial longitudinal and the deeper circular, are clearly visible. The myotomy is stopped distally when the orientation of the gastric muscle fibers changes from circular to oblique and when the bridging vessels of the gastric submucosa appear. Bleeding from the divided muscle coat is minimal. Coagulation and division of the esophageal muscle fibers with monopolar diathermy may increase the risk of intra-operative or delayed mucosal perforation. **(See Figure 38.3)**

- Once the myotomy is completed, the esophagus and stomach are distended with air introduced through the nasogastric tube in order to check for signs of mucosal perforation. Alternatively, flexible esophagoscopy or methylene blue may be used. The former may prove helpful towards assessing the completeness of the myotomy.
- Because of the high incidence of significant post-myotomy gastro-esophageal reflux, an anti-reflux procedure is usually performed at the end of the procedure. The Dor anterior wrap, which also protects the exposed mucosal lining, is the procedure of choice in most cases. Other authors advocate Toupet or Nissen procedures. **(See Figure 38.4)**

- The cannulae are removed and the sites are closed with absorbable suture as necessary. Local anesthetic agents are used at all incision sites.

POSTOPERATIVE CARE

Regular non-steroidal injectable analgesia may be used for the first postoperative day. Epidural infusion is rarely necessary. The nasogastric tube is removed and gradual oral feeds resumed at 24 hours postoperatively (liquid diet for the first 24 hours, followed by semi-solid and finally solid over 15–30 days). Children are usually fit to leave hospital at 48–72 hours postoperatively.

Long-term follow-up is essential. The author advocates clinical assessment at 1, 6 and 12 months and yearly thereafter for the first 5 years. Residual symptoms of dysphagia and respiratory problems are encountered in less than 25 percent of cases. Contrast upper gastrointestinal and manometric studies at 12 months and 2 years should show a significant decrease in median esophageal diameter (from 50 to 25 mm) and steady esophageal pressure (from 30–40 to 12–17 mmHg) respectively. A 24-hour pH monitor helps in the detection of postoperative gastro-esophageal reflux. These examinations should be considered even when patients appear to be asymptomatic. Balloon dilatation may be considered for symptomatic residual stricture. Re-do laparoscopic surgery is reserved for those who suffer tight fundoplication or incomplete esophageal myotomy.

PROBLEMS, PITFALLS AND SOLUTIONS

As for all laparoscopic procedures, meticulous attention to details is essential to avoid problems or complications.

Inadequate view

- The importance of the position of the patient on the operating table and of the laparoscopic cannulae cannot be over-emphasized.
- A 30° telescope provides versatility and a 10 mm scope allows maximum light, which may prove helpful in difficult cases.
- Adequate liver retraction and mobilization of the distal esophagus are mandatory.

Bleeding

- In successful myotomy, minor bleeds are common but require no active treatment.
- The use of ultrasonic shears and monopolar diathermy may cause thermal injury to the mucosa.

COMPLICATIONS

Mucosal perforation

The gastro-esophageal junction is the commonest site. The thinness of the muscle layers in this region is regarded as a contributing factor. The risk is minimized by meticulous technique and the avoidance of thermal injury from diathermy and ultrasound energy. The risk is significantly higher in those patients who have undergone previous dilatation, botox injections or myotomy. A perforation that is identified per-operatively may be closed laparoscopically and the site protected by Dor anterior fundal wrap. Missed perforation or delayed perforation secondary to mucosal necrosis from thermal injury usually presents with symptoms and signs of peritonitis or mediastinitis 24–48 hours postoperatively. In these cases, a plain X-ray may confirm the diagnosis, and prompt medical and surgical therapy should be sought.

Dysphagia

Dysphagia can be secondary to an incomplete myotomy or a tight fundoplication. Residual dysphagia lasting more then a few weeks postoperatively should be investigated with barium swallow and manometry. A single pneumatic dilatation may solve the problem; however, re-do laparoscopic surgery may prove necessary.

Gastro-esophageal reflux

This complication may occur in 10–30 percent of children undergoing distal esophageal myotomy. The choice of concomitant anti-reflux procedure remains controversial. The patients are treated conservatively first, and anti-reflux surgery may be required in some.

Other complications

These may include pneumothorax, spleen injury, vagus nerve damage and visceral perforation.

FURTHER READING

Esposito C, Cucchiara S, Borrelli O, Roblot-Maigret B, Desruelle P, Montupet P. Laparoscopic esophagomyotomy for the treatment of achalasia in children: a preliminary report of eight cases. *Surgical Endoscopy* 2000; **14**(2):110–13.

Esposito C, Mendoza-Sagaon M, Roblot-Maigret B, Amici G, Desruelle P, Montupet P. Complications of laparoscopic treatment of esophageal achalasia in children. *Journal of Pediatric Surgery* 2000; **35**(5):680–3.

Holcomb GW, Richards WO, Riedel BD. Laparoscopic esophagomyotomy for achalasia in children. *Journal of Pediatric Surgery* 1996; **31**:716–18.

Mattioli G, Cagnazzo A, Barabino A, Caffarena PE, Ivani G, Jasonni V. The surgical approach to esophageal achalasia. *European Journal of Pediatric Surgery* 1997; **7**:323–7.

Tovar JA, Prieto G, Molina M, Arana J. Esophageal function in achalasia: preoperative and postoperative manometric studies. *Journal of Pediatric Surgery* 1998; **33**: 834–8.

39

Malrotation

STEVEN S. ROTHENBERG

INTRODUCTION

Malrotation is a common congenital anomaly, occurring in up to 2 percent of the population. The lesion may appear in a newborn with evidence of complete bowel obstruction, or individuals may remain asymptomatic throughout their entire lives. The direst consequence of malrotation is the development of intestinal volvulus, which can result in a life-threatening strangulation of the entire mid-gut. In this instance, failure to identify the etiology of the abdominal catastrophe and to operate immediately can result in severe short bowel syndrome or death.

However, malrotation may present with a myriad of other less dramatic symptoms, which can include evidence of partial proximal small bowel obstruction caused by intermittent volvulus, Ladd's bands, or a tortuous or kinked duodenum. It may also present as intermittent or chronic abdominal pain or, in younger infants, feeding intolerance. Some infants even present with what appears to be simple gastro-esophageal reflux. Because of the possible lethal implications of missing a possible malrotation and volvulus, it is incumbent on the pediatric surgeon to rule out this diagnosis in any child presenting with evidence of a small bowel obstruction not related to previous surgery. It is here that laparoscopy can play an extremely important role in both the diagnosis and therapy of this disease.

Indications

The indications for laparoscopy in the treatment of malrotation fall into two basic categories, diagnostic and therapeutic.

DIAGNOSTIC

Laparoscopy can be used to confirm malrotation in patients for whom radiographic confirmation is not possible. The gold standard for diagnosis is an upper gastrointestinal series and, to a lesser extent, ultrasound and barium enema, but at times these studies may be inconclusive and unable to differentiate between malrotation, which can volvulize, and partial fixation, which does not give rise to further risk.

THERAPEUTIC

Once malrotation has been confirmed, a laparoscopic approach can be used to perform the Ladd's procedure for surgical correction.

Contraindications

The only true contraindication is the child with apparent malrotation and volvulus who has signs of compromised bowel and hemodynamic instability. In these cases an emergency laparotomy should be performed.

Advantages and disadvantages

There are two true advantages of the laparoscopic approach: confirmation of the diagnosis in unclear cases, as discussed above, and the avoidance of major laparotomy with evisceration and extensive bowel manipulation, which can result in a prolonged ileus.

The major disadvantage is the difficulty in determining the bowel orientation and de-rotating the bowel through the limited access afforded by a laparoscopic approach.

EQUIPMENT/INSTRUMENTS

Essential

(3.0 or 5.0 mm, depending on the size of the patient.)

- Three or four 3.0–5.0 mm cannulae.
- 4 mm or 5 mm 30° wide-angle telescope. (A 3 mm lens can be used in smaller patients, but the wider view afforded by the 4 mm telescope greatly enhances the surgeon's ability to determine the orientation of the bowel.)
- Two atraumatic graspers (bowel clamps, De Bakey, Babcock) to manipulate and run the bowel.
- Curved scissors (insulated).
- Curved dissector (Maryland).
- Suction device.

Optional

- Hook cautery.
- Ultrasonic shears.
- 0 chromic Endoloops® (pre-tied suture ligatures) to perform the appendectomy.

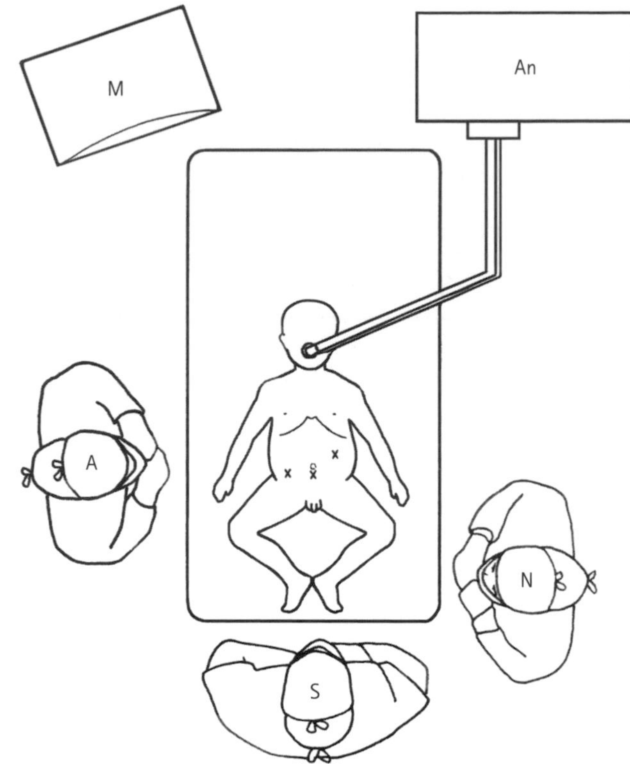

Figure 39.1

PREOPERATIVE PREPARATION

Little specific preoperative preparation is necessary. If the patient is asymptomatic with no obstructive symptoms, bowel preparation may be helpful to decompress the intestines to aid in the manipulation of the bowel.

TECHNIQUE

General endotracheal anesthesia should be administered and local anesthetic (0.25 percent marcaine) should be injected at each trocar site. A nasogastric tube should be placed, with plans to leave it in for at least 12–24 hours, depending on the difficulty of the dissection and the degree of bowel manipulation. The bladder should be emptied using the Crede maneuver, but a urinary catheter is not necessary.

The procedure is best performed with the patient supine and placed near the foot of the table. Larger children are placed in a dorsal lithotomy position (legs bent down) so that the surgeon can be between the patients' legs. The majority of the dissection occurs in the right upper quadrant and this position gives the surgeon the best access to this area.

If necessary, the surgeon can rotate to the patients' right or left in order to run the bowel. After the initial trocar has been placed, the patient should be put in reverse Trendelenburg position to give the best visualization of the duodenum. **(See Figure 39.1)**

Port placement

The procedure can usually be performed with three or four ports. The initial port is the camera port, which is placed at the umbilicus to allow optimal visualization of all quadrants of the abdomen. The positions of the right-hand and left-hand operating ports vary somewhat with the size of the patient. The majority of the dissection and bowel manipulation will occur around the duodenal sweep. Therefore the operating ports need to be placed to give good access to this area.

The surgeon's left-hand operating port needs to be in the right mid to lower quadrant, depending on the size of the child: the smaller the infant, the lower the port should be placed to allow adequate room for manipulation of the left-hand instrument. The surgeon's right-hand port should be placed in the patient's left mid to upper quadrant, slightly above the level of the camera port. This gives good access to the duodenum without causing 'dueling' with the telescope.

A fourth port is occasionally needed in the right upper quadrant. This is used to retract the liver in cases where it hinders visualization. This is accomplished by using the shaft of the instrument to elevate the falciform ligament and the left lobe of the liver.

The first step in the procedure is to confirm the diagnosis of malrotation. This is accomplished by examining the duodenal sweep, looking for the ligament of Treitz, and evaluating the fixation of the colon. With atraumatic graspers

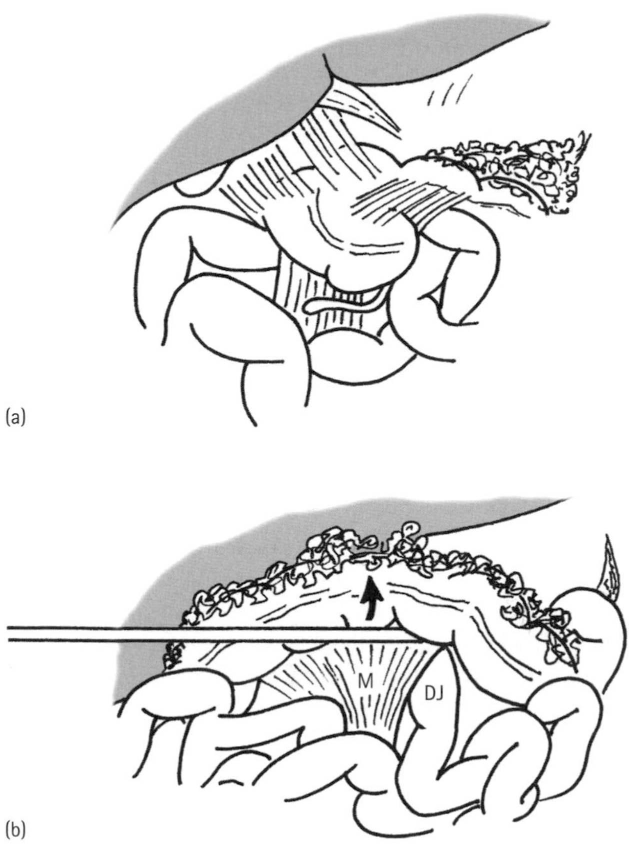

Figure 39.2

in the two operating ports, the C-loop is examined to check for proper orientation of the duodenum. If the duodenum clearly lies to the patient's right of the spine and is tortuous and covered by Ladd's bands, the diagnosis is confirmed. If it is not clear, the transverse colon should be elevated and the ligament of Treitz looked for. If there is fixation of the fourth part of the duodenum to the patient's left of the mesenteric vessels, there is at least a partial fixation and it is unlikely that volvulus will occur, even if the cecum is floating freely. At this point the procedure should be stopped. If no evidence of fixation is found, the surgeon should continue with the Ladd's procedure.

If the surgeon sees dilated ischemic loops of bowel (suggesting a volvulus with compromised circulation), an open procedure should be reverted to, to avoid any undue delay or bowel injury. **(See Figure 39.2)**

Mobilization of the duodenum

Because of the limited visual field afforded by the laparoscope, it can sometimes be difficult to determine the orientation of the bowel. Therefore it is important to work from known to unknown in order to prevent unnecessary or inappropriate manipulations. With an atraumatic grasper or curved dissector in the left hand port and scissors in the right port, the procedure starts with division of Ladd's bands and mobilization of the proximal duodenum. The duodenum is mobilized going from proximal to distal until it is free and can be placed along the right gutter, which often involves extensive mobilization of the duodenum and colon. Care must be taken not to cause bowel wall injury during the manipulation. Whenever possible, especially during mobilization of the C-loop, the adhesions to the bowel, rather than the bowel wall itself, should be used to manipulate the intestines. Often the duodenum is kinked up under the right lobe of the liver with the colon lying over it. The colon should be mobilized and displaced to the patient's left. It is then often necessary to place inferior traction on the duodenum and the proximal jejunum to expose the attachments under the liver. It may be necessary to use a fourth port to provide adequate retraction. Once the duodenum is free and can be laid out in the right gutter, the surgeon can proceed with de-rotation of the intestines. **(See Figure 39.3)**

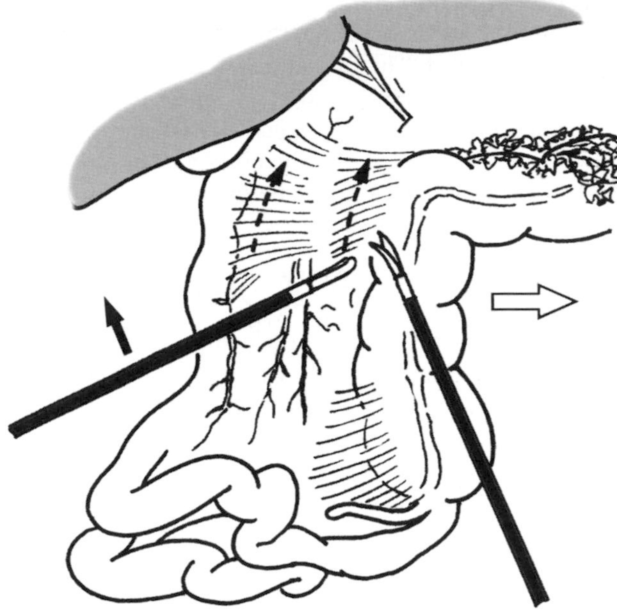

Figure 39.3

De-rotating the bowel

As already mentioned, it is often difficult to determine if the bowel is twisted or to what degree it is twisted. The best way to accomplish this with the limited field of view afforded by the laparoscope is to run the bowel from proximal to distal while limiting scope and instrument movement. This is accomplished with two atraumatic or bowel clamps. The surgeon passes the bowel from one clamp to the other in the right upper quadrant. The bowel is then placed over the stomach or in the right upper quadrant. This is facilitated by placing the patient in the Trendelenburg position. By maintaining visualization in the right upper quadrant and running the bowel in front of the lens, rather than tracking the bowel with the scope, it is easier to manipulate the bowel from clamp to clamp and to keep track of the appropriate orientation. If further bands are encountered, they can be divided as needed. This is continued until the cecum is reached. The large bowel is easily manipulated to the left and the small bowel placed in the epigastrium is allowed to fall back to the right gutter. During this portion of the procedure, if the bowel is twisted, it should be successfully de-rotated.

Broadening the mesentery

During mobilization of the duodenum, the base of the mesentery has already been significantly widened and denuded. This area should be checked after successful de-rotation of the bowel, but little further dissection should be necessary.

Appendectomy

The final step is to perform the appendectomy, which can be carried out either intracorporeally or extracorporeally. With the cecum already mobilized and lying to the left of the spine, the appendix is easily visualized. The appendiceal mesentery can then be stripped off the appendix using a curved dissector and monopolar cautery. Bipolar cautery, the ultrasonic dissector or any other vessel sealer can be used as well if already opened for the Ladd's procedure. The base of the appendix is then ligated with a series of three 0 chromic Endoloops®, two proximally and one 1 cm more distal. The appendix is then divided and taken out through the umbilical trocar site. A stapler can also be used, but this requires the placement of a 12 mm port and is significantly more expensive.

The alternative is to do this extracorporeally. With the cecum already mobilized, the appendix can easily be brought out through the umbilical port and ligation and division can be accomplished with standard cautery and suture.

Once the appendectomy is completed, the abdominal cavity is re-evaluated for hemostasis and then all trocars are removed. Fascial and skin closure is performed at all trocar sites.

POSTOPERATIVE CARE

In general, a nasogastric tube is left in place during the initial postoperative period. The length of time it is left in depends on how extensive the dissection has been, but it can usually be removed on the first postoperative day and a liquid diet started. However, if manipulation of the duodenum has been minimal, no nasogastric tube will be necessary.

Initial postoperative pain management is with intravenous morphine, which is usually required for only the first 24 hours postoperatively. Once patients are tolerating adequate liquids and are on oral pain medication, they can be discharged from the hospital. In most cases this is on the second or third postoperative day.

PROBLEMS, PITFALLS AND SOLUTIONS

Difficulty in evaluating the course of the duodenum

- Adequate visualization is the key to success. If the course of the duodenum cannot be adequately visualized, an extra port should be added to allow for better exposure. This may be used to elevate the left lobe of the liver if the duodenum seems to curl back up under the liver, or to retract the colon inferiorly to expose Ladd's bands better.
- Be sure that the intestines are truly malrotated. If the duodenum seems to be passing behind the transverse colon, make sure that the third or fourth portion of the duodenum is not fixed near the spine, even if it does not pass to the patient's left of the midline. A patient with incomplete rotation and adequate fixation may not be at risk for volvulus. An attempt to de-rotate the bowel of these patients and mobilize the duodenum to the right can be extremely difficult and result in injury to the duodenum, pancreas or bile ducts.

Loss of orientation

- This is the most difficult aspect of performing a Ladd's procedure laparoscopically. The relatively limited view afforded by the laparoscopic can make it difficult to tell how the bowel is twisted and in which direction it is being run. The key is to work from proximal to distal in a strictly stepwise fashion. This is facilitated by keeping the scope steady and running the bowel in front of it. If orientation is lost, the surgeon must restart from the duodenum – failure to do so may result in further torsion of the bowel and mesentery.

Injury to the bowel wall

- Because of the extensive nature of the bowel manipulation, it is very easy to injure the serosa or even perforate the bowel wall. This is especially true if there are extensive adhesions around the duodenum. Injury to the bowel wall is best avoided in this area by grasping the adhesions rather than the bowel wall itself. If using cautery or the ultrasonic shears to divide the attachments, care must be taken to avoid heat injury to the adjacent bowel.
- Injury to the bowel wall during de-rotation/running of the bowel is best avoided by using atraumatic bowel

clamps and grasping across the width of the bowel wall rather then grasping a small part and pinching the serosa.

COMPLICATIONS

Complications are most likely to arise from injury to the bowel wall or inadequate mobilization and de-rotation of the intestines. These problems are best avoided by performing meticulous dissection, avoiding thermal injury to the bowel wall, and maintaining proper orientation. A laparoscopic Ladd's procedure can be one of the most frustrating endoscopic procedures to perform because of the difficulty in visualizing all of the intestines at one time. Therefore the surgeon must be extremely patient and methodical in his or her approach or significant harm can be done. Great care must be taken to avoid injury to the superior mesenteric vessels, and if the surgeon cannot successfully de-rotate the bowel after two or three attempts, conversion to an open laparotomy should be considered.

Late peritonitis suggests an unrecognized bowel injury and should be investigated immediately. Whether to do this open or laparoscopically depends on the patient's overall condition and the experience of the surgeon. Postoperative obstruction could represent incomplete de-rotation or adhesion formation. An upper gastrointestinal series should be obtained to identify the site of the obstruction and determine whether re-exploration is indicated.

FURTHER READING

Bass C, Rothenberg SS. Laparoscopic Ladd's procedure in infants with malrotation without volvulus. *Journal of Pediatric Surgery* 1998; **33**:279–81.

Bax NM, Van der Zee DC. Laparoscopic treatment of intestinal malrotation in children. *Surgical Endoscopy* 1998; **12**: 1314–16.

Maziotti MV, Strasberg SM, Langer JC. Intestinal rotation abnormalities without volvulous: the role of laparoscopy. *Journal of the American College of Surgeons* 1997; **185**:172–6.

Yamashita H, Kato H, Uyama S et al. Laparoscopic repair of intestinal malrotation complicated by mid-gut volvulous. *Surgical Endoscopy* 1999; **13**:1160–2.

40

Intussusception

KIKI MAOATE

INTRODUCTION

Enema reduction remains the preferred treatment for intussusception, unless there is evidence of dead bowel or perforation. Laparoscopy provides a minimally invasive surgical option where attempts at enema reduction have failed to reduce the intussusception, or where enema reduction is contraindicated. It can be used also as a diagnostic tool where intussusception may be suspected clinically but ultrasonography and contrast enemas have proved inconclusive – this usually applies to intussusception confined to the small bowel.

Indications

- Failure to confirm the diagnosis by other means.
- Failure of enema reduction.
- Suspicion of a pathological lesion at the lead point.

Enema reduction remains the most effective and efficient non-operative method to reduce intussusception, and should be utilized as the first line of treatment unless there is evidence of peritonitis. However, enemas are not always successful, and surgery may be required.

Laparoscopic intussusception reduction is a relatively new technique. It is made easier when the small bowel is not excessively distended and there is no contamination from perforation or peritonitis.

Hand-assisted intussusception reduction laparoscopically in small children is technically possible but confers few advantages over an open procedure.

Contraindications

ABSOLUTE

- Hemodynamically unstable child.
- Small bowel obstruction with marked abdominal distension and distended bowel loops.

RELATIVE

- Perforation.
- Peritonitis.
- Previous surgery.

The principles of laparoscopic intussusception reduction are somewhat against historical teachings for open reduction. In contrast to the predominantly milking action used during open reduction (i.e. pushing the intussusception in retrograde direction to squeeze the intussusceptum proximally out of the intussuscipiens, rather than pulling it out), the technique involves a combination of pushing with assisted traction to the proximal bowel and eversion in the final component of reduction.

The working space during laparoscopic reduction is compromised when there is marked distension of small bowel. Laparoscopic-assisted intussusception reduction is an option if the laparoscopic approach alone is unsuccessful: the intussusception can be retrieved through a small wound, e.g. umbilical incision, extended to avoid the need for a major laparotomy wound or an incision directly over the intussusception.

Progression to a formal laparotomy should be undertaken if the laparoscopic approach is not feasible.

Advantages

- Laparoscopy may confirm complete reduction of the intussusception in children with a competent ileo-cecal valve that does not allow the small bowel to be outlined adequately.
- It can be used where attempts at enema reduction (including delayed repeat enemas) have reduced the intussusception only as far as the ileo-cecal valve, but the last part proves difficult to reduce. The region of the ileo-cecal valve is where an intussusception is most likely to become irreducible, and simple manipulation laparoscopically allows it to reduce without the need for laparotomy.
- Laparoscopy allows accurate assessment of suspected pathological lead points, such as a Meckel's diverticulum.

Disadvantages

- Vision is obscured by marked small bowel distension secondary to obstruction from the intussusception.

EQUIPMENT/INSTRUMENTS

- 3–5 mm 30° telescope.
- 3–5 mm (Hasson) trocars.
- Atraumatic bowel graspers (without ratchets).
- 3–5 mm Maryland dissector (without ratchets).
- 3–5 mm diathermy.
- 3–5 mm irrigation device.

PREOPERATIVE PREPARATION

Preoperative preparation is critical, as children often present acutely unwell over a 24-hour period or more: they may be dehydrated (from vomiting and third space loss), bacteremic or septicemic, and have an established small bowel obstruction. The hemodynamic condition of the child should be assessed. Appropriate fluid resuscitation is commenced and antibiotics given if the child appears septicemic. Intravenous fluid resuscitation should be commenced prior to gas enema reduction. A plain abdominal X-ray may be obtained before enema reduction is attempted to identify the intussusception, exclude free intraperitoneal air and document the degree of small bowel obstruction, but rarely does it alter subsequent management. Ultrasound of the abdomen is more reliable as a diagnostic tool. Alternatively, once the diagnosis has been confirmed, enema reduction can be commenced along standard intussusception reduction guidelines. Surgery is required where an enema has failed to reduce an intussusception, or where there is ongoing uncertainty about whether the intussusception has been fully reduced.

TECHNIQUE

The procedure is performed under general anesthesia with endotracheal intubation and muscle relaxation. A nasogastric tube should be inserted to deflate the upper gastrointestinal tract, especially where there is abdominal distension from the small bowel obstruction. The patient is positioned supine and towards the end of the bed. This allows the surgeon to move comfortably around the patient with the changing dynamics of the procedure. The primary port is placed through the umbilicus under direct vision (Hasson technique). Carbon dioxide is utilized to insufflate the abdominal cavity to 10 mmHg. The laparoscope is introduced through the umbilical port and initial intra-abdominal inspection includes:

- the feasibility of continuing the procedure, according to the amount of gut distension,
- identification of the intussusception,
- assessment of the amount of bowel ischemia and the likelihood of success with the laparoscopic approach,
- assessment of the degree of intra-abdominal contamination from peritonitis (if any).

After the exploratory laparoscopy, which may also need the assistance of other ports, two further ports are placed under direct vision. The preoperative enema may have already localized the intussusception, influencing the placement of the working ports. In the majority of cases, there will have been incomplete enema reduction of the intussusception as far as the ileo-cecal region or ascending colon. Two ports should be placed on the left side of the abdomen, either one above and one below the umbilicus or both below it. It is unusual to have to attempt reduction of an intussusception in the left upper quadrant. A third port can be inserted to assist with the reduction in the right side of the abdomen, if necessary: This may also be required as the reduction progresses to avoid overlap clashing of the instruments and telescope. **(See Figure 40.1)**

Milking the intussusception proximally is the 'ideal' method and historically, with open surgery, has been shown to be the safest technique. However, this may be difficult with the laparoscopic approach because of the limited working space available and poorer control with laparoscopic instruments (instead of the hand). Further, milking alone may not be sufficient; for this reason, proximal traction to the bowel is utilized to assist with reduction. **(See Figure 40.2)**

The most difficult part of the procedure is reduction at the ileo-cecal valve, which can usually be achieved by a combination of traction and eversion using the steady application of firm pressure. It may be necessary to introduce a grasper through a third working port to assist with the reduction. Once reduced, the bowel is assessed for viability and integrity (no perforation) and to exclude a pathological lead point. The abdominal cavity is irrigated with normal

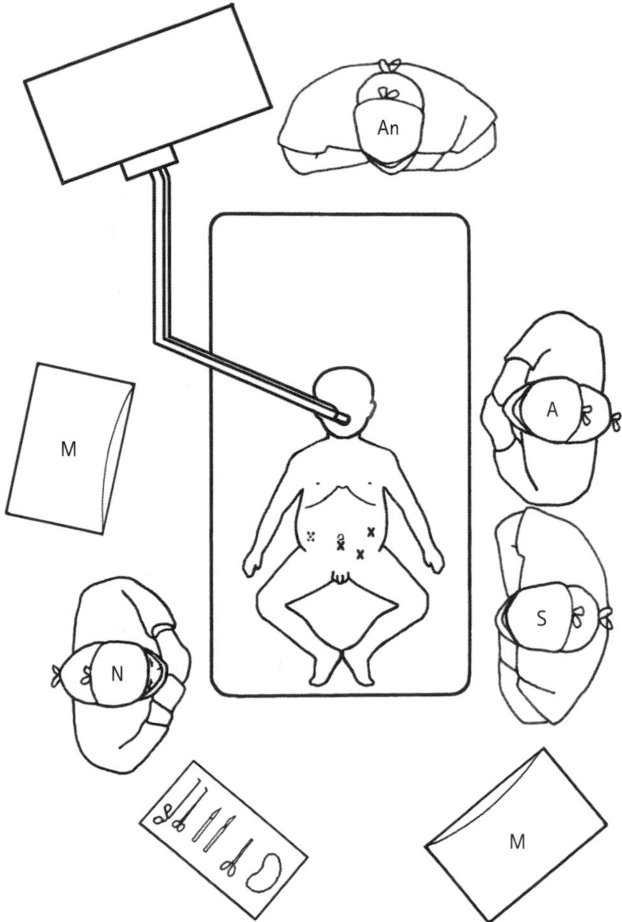

Figure 40.1

saline if there is contamination or turbid peritoneal fluid. The ports are removed and the abdominal wall and skin incisions closed with absorbable sutures. The wounds are infiltrated with additional local anesthetic.

If the intussusception cannot be reduced, the following options are available.

- Laparoscopic-assisted reduction with careful selection of the site of the wound to minimize its length and visualize reduction through the telescope.
- Conversion to an open procedure.

A urinary catheter is inserted only if there is a readily palpable bladder that cannot be expressed.

POSTOPERATIVE CARE

Morphine analgesia is required occasionally, but usually non-opiate analgesia is all that is necessary. Oral intake is started as soon as the child is no longer nauseated and is able to tolerate fluids; this may be delayed if there has been significant bowel obstruction. Children are usually discharged within 24 hours of a straightforward laparoscopic intussusception reduction.

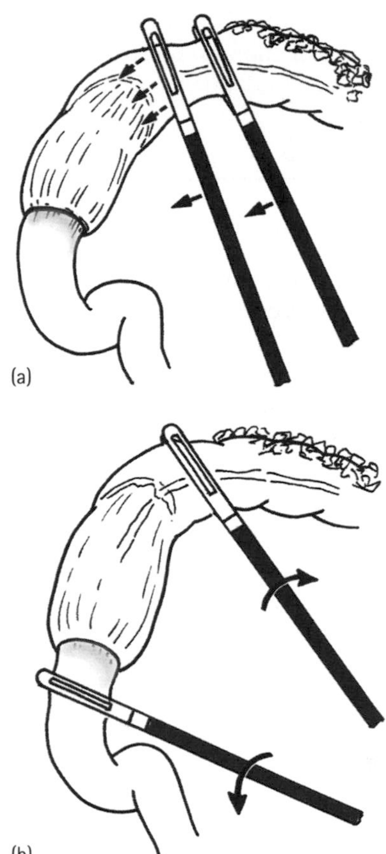

Figure 40.2 *(a) Milking maneuver; (b) traction maneuver.*

PROBLEMS, PITFALLS AND SOLUTIONS

- It is difficult to complete the procedure safely when the small bowel is grossly dilated. If visualization of the intussusception is compromised despite nasogastric suction and bowel retraction, conversion to an open procedure may be indicated.
- Anticipate the location of the pathology and place the ports to give maximum ergonomic advantage.
- Utilize the 30° angled camera to its full potential and rotate it through the ports as necessary for better vision and access.
- Introduce additional ports as needed.
- Be patient: do not rush the reduction, and apply firm and steady pressure.
- Conversion to an open procedure is not a complication and is better considered earlier than later in those cases with relative contraindications and moderately dilated bowel. An open approach should also be considered if the intussusception is likely to be due to a pathological lesion at the lead point, where there is difficulty with

initial gas reduction or where an attempt at laparoscopic reduction has failed.

COMPLICATIONS

Failure of laparoscopic reduction is not a complication.

- Inadvertent bowel perforation from the procedure or from ischemia preceding attempts at reduction of the intussusception. This may be evident from localized soiling of the peritoneal cavity. The bowel should be inspected carefully until the perforation is located. Simple suture repair with absorbable sutures to close the defect should be performed either laparoscopically or using an open procedure, depending on the expertise of the surgeon.
- Postoperative recurrence usually occurs within 24–48 hours. The initial symptoms recur, or the clinical features of a bowel obstruction continue. Ultrasonography may confirm the recurrence. Unless the bowel has been opened previously (e.g. resection required), a gas enema could be attempted initially, followed by a further surgical procedure if the enema is unsuccessful.
- A pathological lesion at the lead point may be difficult to recognize, but is more likely if the attempted enema reduction has been unsuccessful, or in association with some specific condition, e.g. Peutz–Jeghers syndrome. Pathological lesions are more likely to be irreducible, but if they are reduced, may not have the usual dimple appearance of Peyer's patch hypertrophy.

FURTHER READING

Cuckow PC, Slater RD, Najmaldin AS. Intussusception treated laparoscopically after failed air enema reduction. *Surgical Endoscopy* 1996; 10:671–2.

41

Meckel's diverticulum

STEPHEN R. POTTS

INTRODUCTION

Although present in only 2 percent of the population and generally asymptomatic in the majority of cases, the potential for Meckel's diverticulum to present in a variety of clinical, pathophysiological and symptomatic types must be fully considered in the management of this condition. Approximately 30 percent of these diverticuli contain heterotopic tissue, which is classically gastric or pancreatic but may be duodenal or colonic, and it is important that this is resected during the procedure to prevent recurrent problems.

Indications

- Acute inflammation, mimicking appendicitis.
- Acute or chronic bleeding from ulceration of the ectopic gastric mucosa.
- Intestinal perforation.
- Intestinal obstruction secondary to internal hernia or intussusception.
- Chronic abdominal pain.
- Asymptomatic but found at the time of abdominal exploration.

A diverticulum that is discovered inadvertently always provokes debate amongst surgeons as to whether it should be retained or removed. A reasonable policy is to remove the lesion if the general condition of the patient is satisfactory and there is no additional risk, as it has the potential to cause trouble in the future.

Contraindications

ABSOLUTE

- Hemodynamic instability secondary to massive bleeding, compromised bowel or sepsis.

RELATIVE

- Previous abdominal surgery.
- Perforation.
- Bowel obstruction with massively dilated proximal bowel.

EQUIPMENT/INSTRUMENTS

Essential

- Three cannulae for intracorporeal resection (usually 10–12 mm and 2–5 mm).
- 12 mm cannula for extracorporeal resection.
- 5–10 mm telescope, 0° or 30°, plus two 5 mm cannulae. These will be sited at the umbilicus, in the right aspect of the suprapubic area and the left iliac fossa, or in the anterior aspect of the right lumbar region and the left iliac fossa.
- Two atraumatic graspers.
- Monopolar or bipolar scissors.
- 5 mm clip applicator.
- Two 5 mm needle holders.

Optional

- Stapler/cutter, e.g. EndoGIA® (if used, this requires a 12 mm port).
- Endoloops®.
- Specimen bag.

PREOPERATIVE PREPARATION

As with any case of infection or bleeding, adequate preoperative resuscitation is the most important factor. In the case of acute presentation of a bleeding Meckel's diverticulum, the patient must be fully resuscitated with crystalloid and blood transfusion prior to surgery. Appropriate antibiotic cover must be given, as with any intestinal resection, generally with a second-generation cephalosporin.

If the patient presents with an acute abdomen and the diagnosis is unknown, a computerized tomography (CT) scan or ultrasound examination may aid in the diagnosis. In cases of rectal bleeding, a technetium scan should be performed if the presentation does not demand surgical intervention as an emergency. Technetium scan may be accurate in up to 85 percent of cases, but is likely to give a false-negative result in the case of active bleeding. Barium contrast studies may occasionally demonstrate a Meckel's diverticulum but are not routinely helpful.

TECHNIQUE

The procedure is carried out under general anesthetic with endotracheal intubation. Placement of a urinary catheter is generally not necessary. The patient is placed in the supine position. The table may be rotated with the left side down and head down as per appendicectomy to give a maximum unimpeded view to the right iliac fossa. The entire abdomen is prepared in case there is a need to place extra ports for intracorporeal resection. The operator stands on the patient's left, with a screen to the patient's right.

The primary cannula (10–12 mm) is placed at the umbilicus to allow for extracorporeal diverticulectomy if necessary and/or intestinal resection extracorporeally plus access for an endoscopic stapler if required. This may be done using a closed or open technique. The abdomen is inflated to 8–10 mmHg at a flow rate of 0.5–1 L/min with CO_2. Two 5 mm ports are then placed in the left iliac fossa and suprapubic area. While it is always best to remain within the principle of triangulation, i.e. camera position central with instruments lateral, many find it acceptable to use the umbilical port for the camera and the left iliac fossa and suprapubic ports as operating ports. However, it is always possible to shift the left iliac fossa instrument to the 10 mm camera port and use the 5 mm camera in the left iliac fossa port when desired.

The bowel is then examined in a thorough and sequential fashion.

- Locate the cecum and terminal ileum and run the bowel retrograde until the Meckel's diverticulum is encountered. (Remember that the diverticulum may be folded against the mesentery.) This is best accomplished by holding the telescope in a stable position and running the bowel in front of the scope using two atraumatic grasping forceps.
- Determine whether or not there is an omphalomesenteric or diverticulomesenteric band and, if present, divide/resect it. Assume the band has a blood supply. The band should therefore be diathermied and/or clipped.
- Display the diverticulum on the antimesenteric border of the ileum. Based on the configuration of the Meckel's diverticulum (i.e. the width of the base, suspicion of ectopic mucosa etc.), decide whether to resect in situ or extracorporeally.

Intracorporeal simple diverticulectomy

ENDOLOOP® TECHNIQUE

Introduce the Endoloop® through the left iliac fossa port, pass the suprapubic instrument through the loop and grasp the Meckel's diverticulum. Carry the loop over the Meckel's diverticulum to the base. Repeat the procedure with a second loop, and then again with a third loop, leaving a space for division between loops two and three. Divide the diverticulum leaving two Endoloops® on the retained bowel wall.

If this method is used, it is imperative that the surgeon is sure that the base of the Meckel's diverticulum is relatively narrow and that no ectopic mucosa or ulceration is left behind. **(See Figure 41.1)**

STAPLING TECHNIQUE

Make sure that the cutting/stapling device has an adequate jaw length to cover the entire base of the Meckel's diverticulum when closed. Remember that the tissue will extend when clamped and effectively expand. If the base extends past the length of the stapler, two applications may be required. It is important to not overly compromise the bowel lumen with the stapler, as this may cause a later obstruction. A hand-sewn closure may be required in these cases. It is therefore also essential that the operator has good suturing skills in this situation. **(See Figure 41.2)**

Intracorporeal resection and anastomosis

Additional working cannulae may be required to display the Meckel's diverticulum and adjacent bowel. Alternatively,

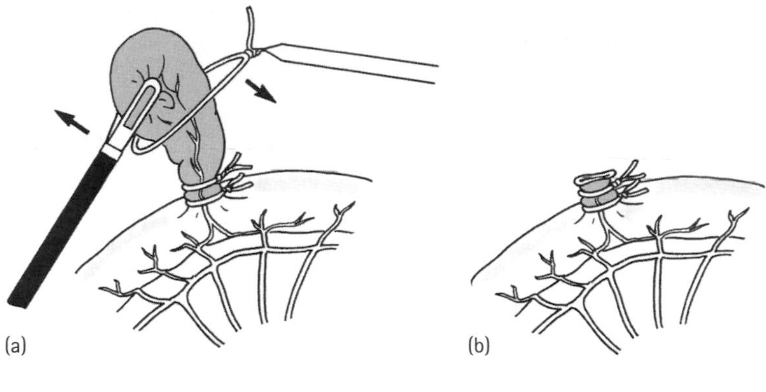

Figure 41.1

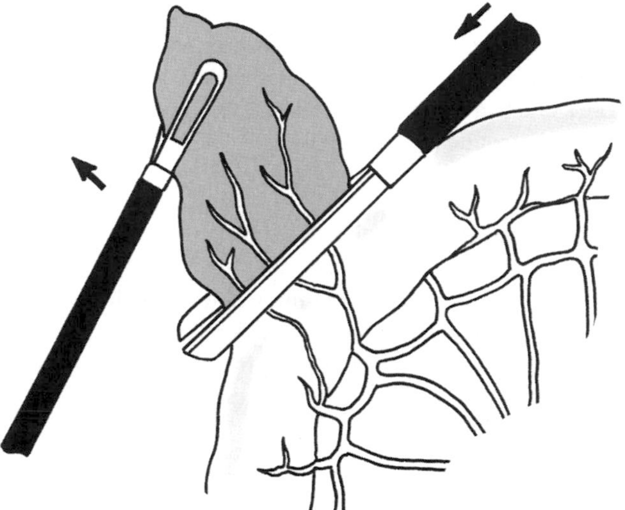

Figure 41.2

to reduce the number of ports required the bowel may be suspended by sutures placed through the abdominal wall. This technique produces better cosmesis and obviates the need for additional cannulae and instruments, which is an important consideration in small infants. Resection follows the standard principles of mesenteric division with bipolar instruments followed by anastomosis. **(See Figure 41.3)**

When locating the diverticulum in a patient whose preoperative diagnosis is uncertain, it is important that the surgical team inspects an adequate length of the bowel. Therefore the terminal ileum must be clearly identified: inspection carried out from distal to proximal commencing in the mid-small bowel runs the risk of the lesion being missed due to inaccurate location and the examination of an insufficient length of the bowel. Remember that the tendency is to overestimate the amount of intestine examined due to magnification on screen and the sometimes tedious nature of the inspection. If bowel should slip from the grasp of the instruments during inspection, start again from the ileo-cecal junction if there is any doubt about the position.

Potential stenosis must not be left in place, as this will lead to postoperative obstruction or recurrent abdominal pain. Remember that burying the Meckel's stump following resection by Endoloop® runs the theoretical risk of postoperative intussusception.

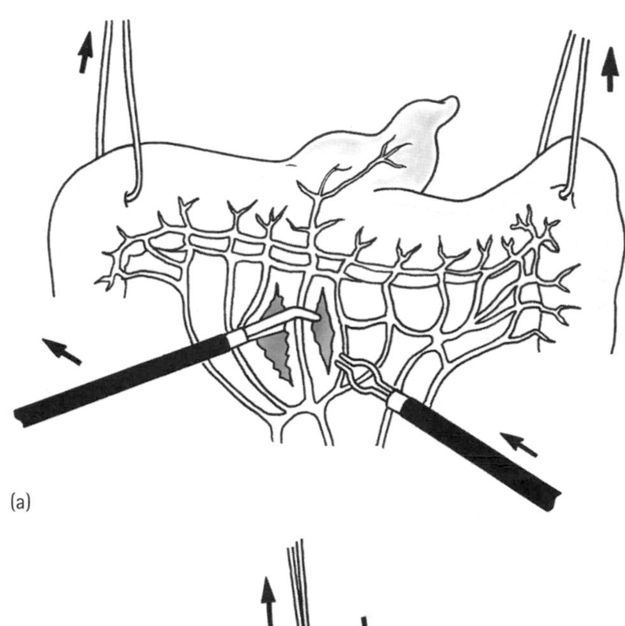

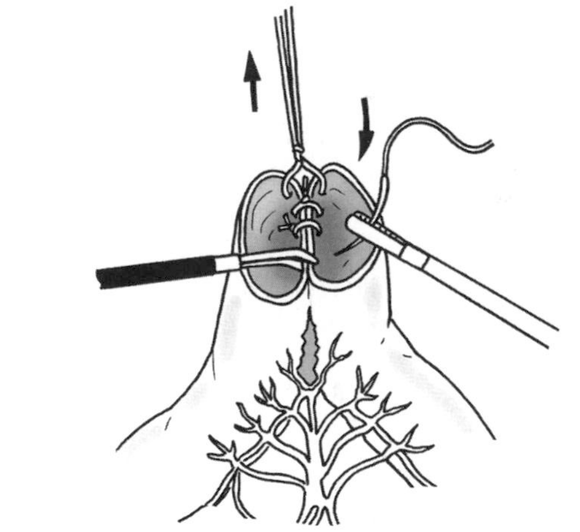

Figure 41.3

Extracorporeal resection

Extracorporeal resection of Meckel's diverticulum is carried out following standard surgical principles. A 10 mm

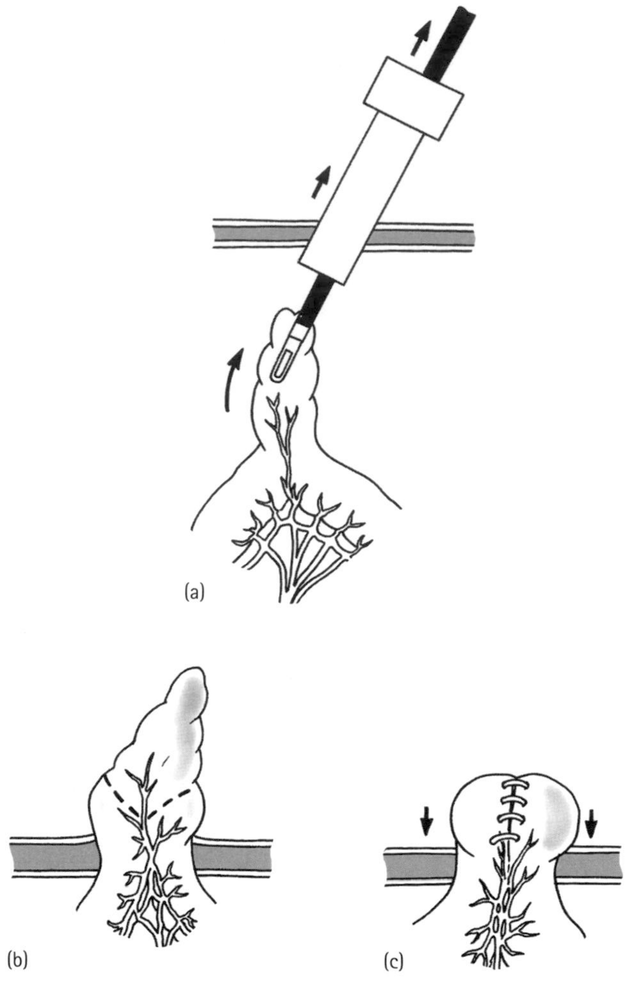

Figure 41.4

port should be used in this situation, to allow easy extraction of the diverticulum into the extracorporeal position and, most importantly, so that the anastomosis is not put under undue pressure where it is reduced into the abdomen following resection. Should replacing the bowel be problematical, splitting the rectus sheath or linea alba posteriorly in the midline above and below the wound will make reduction easier. **(See Figure 41.4)**

POSTOPERATIVE CARE

The management of postoperative pain should be based on local analgesia to the port sites (0.25 percent bupivacaine: the toxic dose is 2 mg/kg) and intravenous morphine infusion. The use of an epidural infusion is optional. Analgesia is seldom necessary beyond the first 24 hours, and can be replaced by the use of Voltarol and paracetamol used separately or in combination (these agents may be given orally or rectally, as dictated by the patient's condition).

It must be remembered that Meckel's diverticulum involves an intestinal resection and therefore requires a period of recovery beyond that of an appendicectomy, and care must be taken to ensure that the patient is fully established on oral intake before being discharged home – usually 36–48 hours postoperatively.

PROBLEMS, PITFALLS AND SOLUTIONS

Internal hernia

If this is encountered, the bowel may be compromised and it may be difficult to determine its correct orientation. If the bowel is ischemic or friable, the laparoscopic approach should be abandoned to avoid its inadvertent perforation. Otherwise, the bowel should be inspected from proximal to distal, looking for the site of the obstruction or band adhesion. If a volvulus is present, this maneuver should help to de-rotate the bowel.

Broad-based Meckel's diverticulum

As already mentioned, an attempt to amputate the Meckel's diverticulum with either Endoloops® or an endoscopic stapler may result in retained ectopic mucosa or compromise of the intestinal lumen. In these cases, a wedge or segmental resection is probably preferable.

Abscess

If the Meckel's diverticulum has perforated, treatment similar to that for a perforated appendix is carried out. The Meckel's diverticulum is resected as already described and then the peritoneal cavity is irrigated with antibiotic solution. If an abscess is present, a drain should be left in place. Also, a large, inflamed Meckel's diverticulum with perforation or exudates should be placed in an endoscopic specimen bag to avoid contaminating the wound on extraction.

COMPLICATIONS

- Incomplete resection of the diverticulum or ectopic mucosa with recurrence of symptoms.
- Stenosis from inappropriate placement of loops and staples.
- Leakage during intracorporeal resection with resulting postoperative sepsis and possible intra-abdominal abscess formation.
- Discharge from exposed mucosal surface after Endoloop® techniques, with complications as above.
- Dehiscence/herniation at port sites.

FURTHER READING

Brown RL, Azizkhan RG. Gastrointestinal bleeding in infants and children: Meckel's diverticulum and intestinal duplication. *Seminars in Pediatric Surgery* 1999; **8**(4):202–9.

Sarli L, Costi R. Laparoscopic resection of Meckel's diverticulum: report of 2 cases. *Surgery Today* 2001; **31**(9):823–5.

Schier F, Hoffmann K, Waldschmidt J. Laparoscopic removal of Meckel's diverticula in children. *European Journal of Pediatric Surgery* 1996; **6**(1):38–9.

42

Appendicectomy

FRANÇOIS BECMEUR AND FRANÇOIS VARLET

INTRODUCTION

Laparoscopic appendicectomy is one of the most common pediatric endoscopic procedures. It allows the novice pediatric surgeon to gain experience with laparoscopic techniques and instruments.

Indications

- Acute appendicitis.
- Appendicular mass and/or peritonitis.
- Suspected appendicitis in patients who present with abdominal pain.
- Chronic abdominal pain.
- As part of the surgical management of intussusception or malrotation or Hirschsprung's disease (biopsy or pull-through).
- Mucocele and suspected neoplasia.

Contraindications

ABSOLUTE

- Major cardiac or hemodynamic instability.

RELATIVE

- Pseudo-tumoral abscess in infants.
- Intestinal obstruction secondary to perforated appendicitis and peritonitis.
- Advanced peritonitis.
- Ventriculo-peritoneal shunts.

EQUIPMENT/INSTRUMENTS

Essential

- 5 mm or 10 mm 0° or 30° angled telescope.
- 5 mm or 10 mm trocar for the telescope.
- One to three cannulae – 3 mm or 5 mm, depending on the size of the instruments, the surgeon's preference and the complexity of the case.
- One or two pairs of atraumatic grasping forceps.
- Two to three Endoloops® and the introducer.
- Suction/irrigation device.
- Bipolar forceps.
- Scissors.

Optional

- 10 mm operative telescope.
- 50 cm long atraumatic grasping forceps.
- 12 mm cannula if an Endostapler is used.
- 10 mm cannula if an Endobag is used.
- Endostapler.
- 5 mm clip applicator.
- Monopolar hook.

- Endobag or a finger of a surgical glove to remove the specimen.
- Veress needle.

PREOPERATIVE PREPARATION

Preoperative evaluation may include abdominal ultrasound and/or computerized tomography (CT) scan to aid in the diagnosis, especially in adolescent females and chronically ill patients. Appropriate resuscitation with intravenous fluids is important prior to surgery, especially in patients with evidence of perforation. Preoperative antibiotics are routinely given: a single dose of cephalosporin is adequate in acute appendicitis; broad-spectrum coverage is necessary in perforated appendicitis. If the preoperative studies suggest a walled-off abscess, the surgeon may elect to drain it percutaneously under ultrasound/CT guidance and perform a delayed appendicectomy after 1–3 months.

TECHNIQUE

General anesthesia with endotracheal intubation and muscle relaxation is required. The use of nitrous oxide is prohibited, particularly in young children. The lower abdomen is carefully palpated to ensure that the bladder is empty; a palpable bladder can be emptied by expressing, and catheterization is rarely required. A nasogastric tube is usually necessary in cases of peritonitis and secondary intestinal obstruction.

The patient is placed in a supine position. Following insertion of the laparoscopic cannulae and visualization of the abdominal cavity and in order to facilitate exposure, the patient is placed in the Trendelenburg position with left lateral tilt. However, in cases of peritonitis, free pus should be aspirated under laparoscopic vision before the position of the operating table is changed. This will minimize the risk of spreading infective peritoneal fluid. A change of telescope from one cannula to another may also improve exposure.

Three-cannulae technique

TROCAR INSERTION

The sites of the cannulae may vary depending on:

- surgeon preference,
- the size of the patient,
- the site of the appendix (subhepatic, pelvic, retrocecal),
- the presence of mass or complications.

In general, an umbilical primary cannula and two working cannulae, one in the left iliac fossa and the other just to the right midline suprapubically, provide adequate exposure. After placing the first cannula, a look inside the peritoneal cavity helps the surgeon to decide the best sites for the cannulae to allow for an easy procedure. However, high working cannulae in the iliac fossa or both cannulae in the left iliac fossa may prove essential in pelvic appendicitis and large right-sided appendicular mass respectively. Suprapubic working cannulae produce the best cosmetic results. **(See Figure 42.1)**

After establishing a pneumoperitoneum to a pressure of between 8 and 12 mmHg, the procedure begins with an exploration of the abdominal cavity. The appendix is identified and the diagnosis of appendicitis confirmed. If there is no appendicitis, one must look for another cause of the abdominal pain. In the case of pus or abscess, the procedure begins with taking a sample of pus for a bacteriological analysis followed by aspiration of pus prior to any dissection.

MOBILIZATION OF APPENDIX

The appendix is gently and gradually released from its surrounding structures/organs (omentum, small bowel, cecum, bladder, female reproductive organs) using the tip or side of the grasping forceps. Avoid direct grasp if at all possible, because omentum easily bleeds and inflamed small intestine and cecum are easily perforated. The appendix may be grasped at a convenient, but healthy, site. An embedded appendix (behind the cecum or ileum) may be grasped at the base and a retrograde appendicectomy should be considered. In perforated appendicitis, a fecolith that is recognized on one operative X-ray or ultrasound scan should be localized and removed. **(See Figure 42.2)**

DIVISION OF MESENTERY

The mesoappendix is stretched and coagulated using a monopolar hook or monopolar scissors or a bipolar device. Care must be taken not to cause thermal injury to the base of the appendix, cecum or surrounding organs. If desired, clips may be used to secure the mesoappendix. Coagulation and division are then continued to near the base of the appendix,

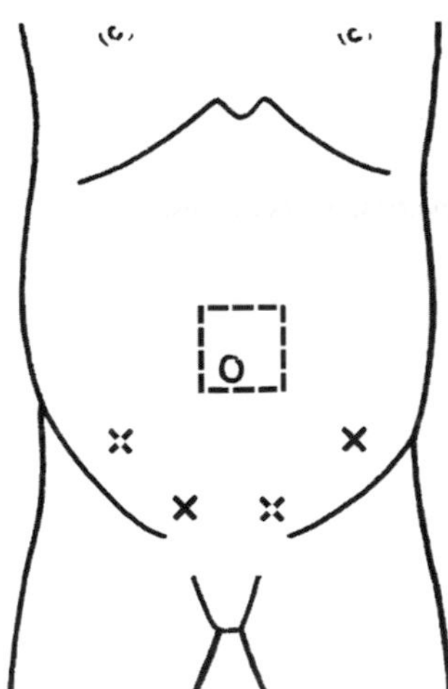

Figure 42.1

leaving the last few strands of tissue and blood vessels intact. This will minimize the risks of thermal injury and necrosis of the stump. In difficult cases (retro-cecal appendicitis, mass or advanced cases associated with peritonitis and intestinal dilatation), a fourth cannula for a retractor may prove necessary. In rare circumstances, mobilization of the right colon may be necessary in order to visualize and mobilize the appendix.

LIGATION AND DIVISION OF THE APPENDIX

Once released from its vascular attachments, the appendix is ligated and divided using either an intracorporeal or extracorporeal technique.

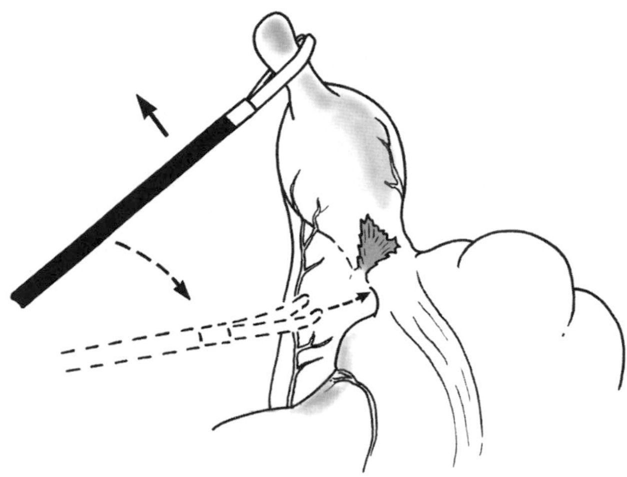

Figure 42.2

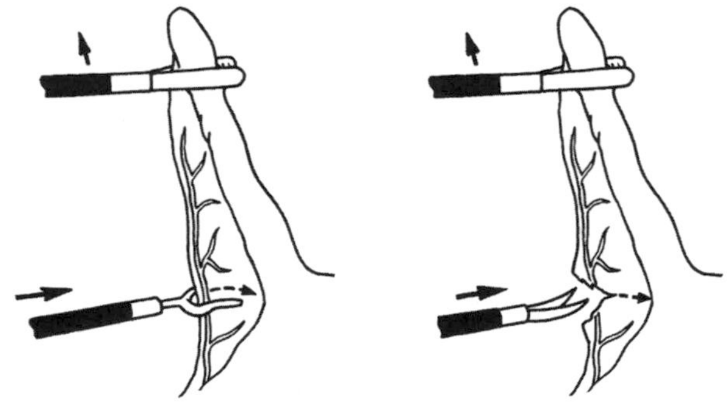

Figure 42.3 *Bipolar scissors to mesentery.*

Intracorporeal technique

The appendix is secured at it its base inside the abdominal cavity using absorbable suture ligature tied intracorporeally or extracorporeally. A pre-tied ligature (Endoloop®) provides an easier alternative. Usually the appendix is divided between two proximal and one distal ligature. A purse-string or figure-of-eight suture to bury the stump/base is only necessary if there is perforation at the base of the appendix. Alternatively, the entire mesoappendix and appendix (base) are secured and divided using an EndoGIA® stapler. **(See Figures 42.3–8)**

Specimen removal

Most appendices are retrievable through a large (10–12 mm) – usually the primary – umbilical cannula. The telescope has to be moved to one of the working cannulae. An Endobag or a finger of a surgical glove may be used to retrieve any large or swollen and friable appendix that will not pass through the lumen of the trocar. The site of extraction may or may not be extended. **(See Figure 42.9)**

Extracorporeal technique

The appendix is exteriorized through an extended laparoscopic cannula site (usually in or close to the right iliac fossa) and the procedure is completed using conventional instruments outside the abdominal cavity. This technique has the morbidity of wound contamination.

Two-cannulae technique

Two cannulae are inserted, a small one in the umbilicus under direct vision (for the telescope) and a large one (working cannula) in the midline above the pubic symphysis or right iliac fossa. Peritoneal fluid may be aspirated and the release of fibrinous adhesions may be achieved via the large working cannula. The appendix with its attached mesentery is then exteriorized through the site of the large cannula in a fashion similar to that described for the one-cannula technique, and the procedure is completed on the surface using conventional instruments.

One-cannula technique

A special 'operating' laparoscope with an operating channel is necessary. An appropriate sized (10–12 mm) cannula is

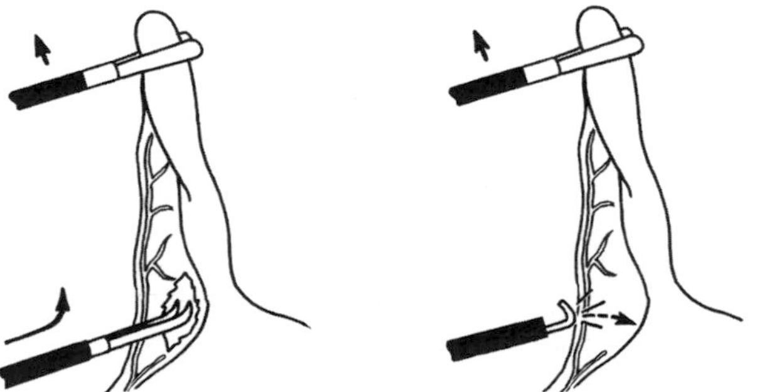

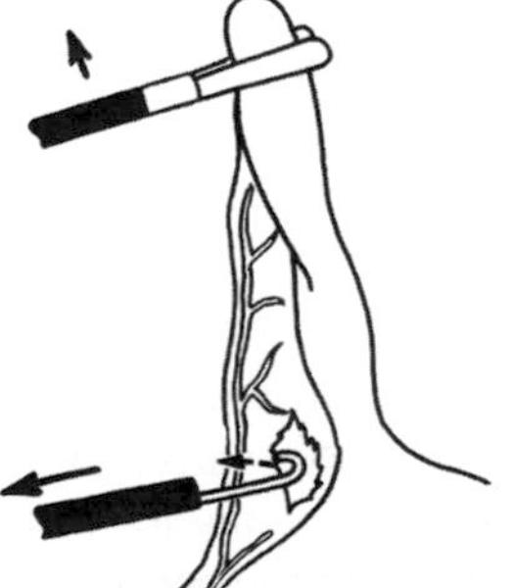

Figure 42.4 *Grasper and hook diathermy to mesentery.*

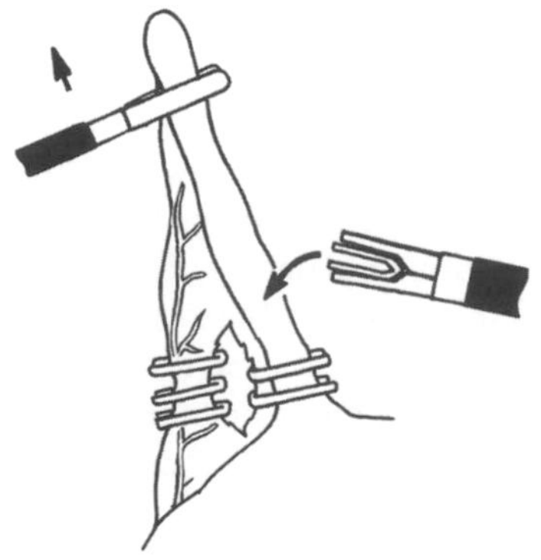

Figure 42.5 *Clips to both mesentery and appendix.*

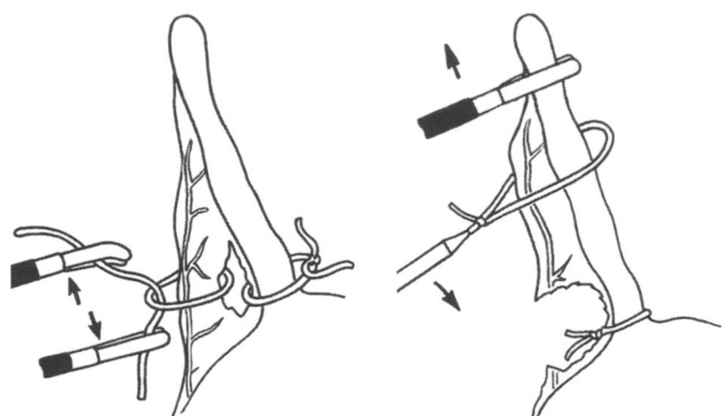

Figure 42.6 *Ligatures to both mesentery and appendix.*

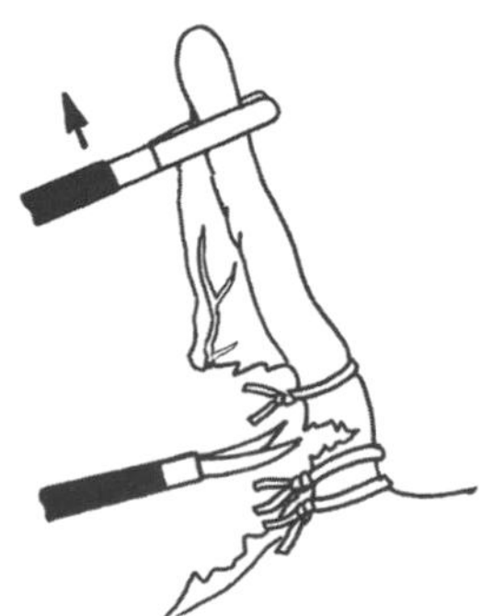

Figure 42.7 *Division of the appendix.*

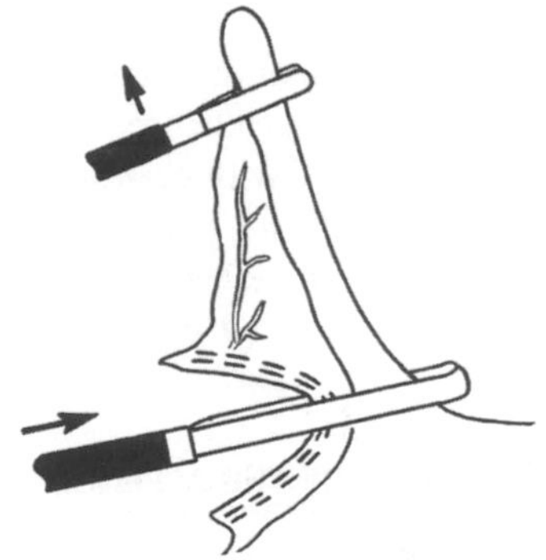

Figure 42.8 *Stapling mesentery and appendix.*

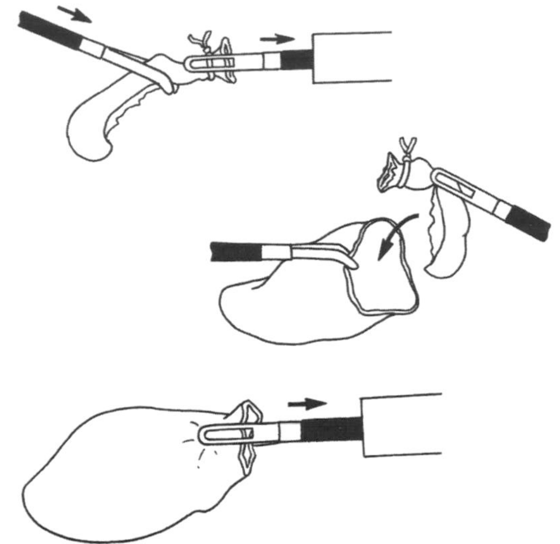

Figure 42.9

placed into the abdominal cavity (peri-umbilical or right iliac fossa) using either open or closed technique laparoscopy. A pneumoperitoneum is created (8–10 mmHg) and the appendix is localized. Peritoneal fluid/pus may be aspirated through the working channel and the appendix is grasped gently using a long atraumatic grasper. The appendix on its mesentery is then brought to the surface through the cannula site by pulling the appendix and the entire apparatus in one move. The technique is possible only if the appendix is freely mobile and minimally inflamed (less than 35 percent). An extended cannula site may allow exteriorization of a larger and more friable appendix. The technique may prove impossible in the presence of adhesions or appendix mass or when the appendix is embedded behind cecum or ileum, and has the disadvantage of significant wound contamination. **(See Figure 42.10)**

Peritonitis mass

Free fluid/pus is aspirated first and a sample is sent for microbiological examination. If necessary, the position of the operating table is then changed in order to improve exposure (as described earlier in this chapter). Appendicectomy is performed as described and the peritoneal cavity is then irrigated with saline. A small to medium sized palpable appendicular mass may be treated with laparoscopic appendicectomy. However, a large palpable mass, particularly one with a long-standing history, may be assessed under general anesthesia but treated with intravenous antibiotics and an interval appendicectomy at 6–12 weeks.

If a formal abscess cavity is encountered during the early stages of the procedure, a drain can be inserted under direct vision and brought out through the lowest trocar site. In this situation, interval appendicectomy is not always necessary.

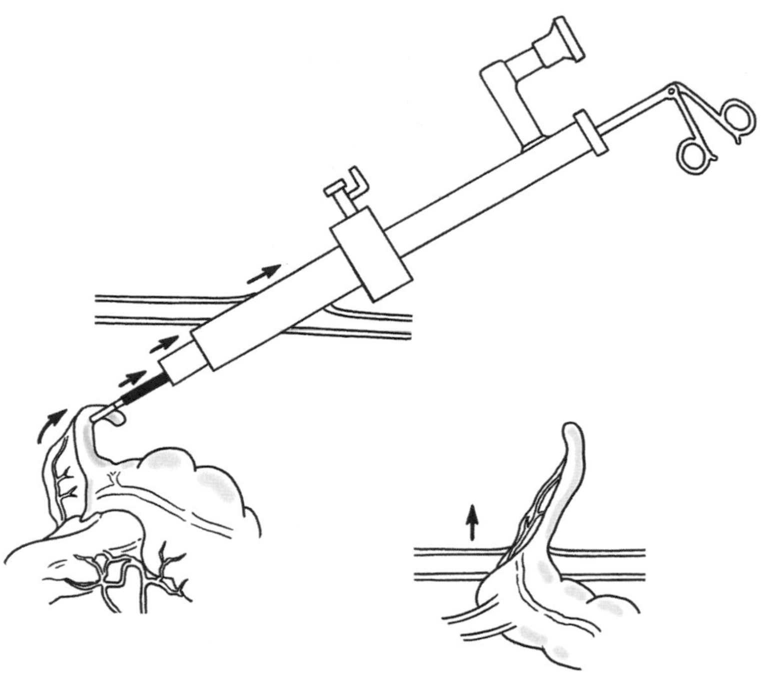

Figure 42.10

POSTOPERATIVE CARE

In cases of uncomplicated appendicitis, one to three doses of perioperative intravenous antibiotics provide adequate cover. Perforated appendicitis/peritonitis and appendicular mass require days of appropriate intravenous single-agent or triple-agent antibiotics. Although 12–24 hours of intravenous narcotic therapy provides adequate analgesia in non-complicated laparoscopic appendicectomy, a much longer duration (up to 2–3 days) is required in complicated cases because of ongoing irritation from peritonitis, ileus etc.

The nasogastric tube and/or urinary catheter are left in situ for as long as they are necessary, and oral fluid and feeds are resumed as tolerated. Patients are usually ready to be discharged from hospital by 1–3 days postoperatively following 'non-complicated' surgery, and by 4–7 days after treatment for 'complicated' appendicitis.

PROBLEMS, PITFALLS AND SOLUTIONS

Difficult access

A common cause of problems is misplaced working cannulae. It is therefore important to localize the appendix through the telescope before the working cannulae are placed. A one-port or two-port technique may be decided on in cases of simple acute appendicitis associated with minimal adhesions. In pelvic appendicitis, access and manipulation through low iliac fossae or suprapubic cannulae may prove difficult. Always consider changing the telescope and/or instruments from one cannula to another, changing cannulae position, or placing additional cannulae for retraction. In difficult cases, consider conversion to an open method.

Difficulties exposing the appendix and mesoappendix

This is not an uncommon problem in retro-cecal or advanced appendicitis. An extra cannula with an added instrument or retractor may allow better exposure. Consider retrograde appendicectomy or even mobilize the right colon as for open surgery. Rarely, the appendix mass may be found under the liver or even left iliac fossa (malrotation). In the case of a ruptured appendix, the main problem is the need to remove the entire organ.

Bleeding

Bleeding from the mesoappendix, omentum or the surface of adherent surrounding viscera can occur during the dissection, especially if the appendix is extremely inflamed and friable or in advanced appendicitis/appendicular mass. This is best avoided by maximizing exposure (position of patient/cannulae), gentle technique and cauterizing the appendicular vessels proximally and distally prior to dividing them. If bleeding is encountered, grasp the base of the appendiceal artery with an atraumatic grasper and apply low-power cautery. Care must be taken not to injure the cecum or the adjacent viscera or iliac vessels and ureter. If necessary, insert another cannula to allow a suction/irrigation device to be used.

Gangrenous/perforated appendix

If possible, avoid removing the appendix piecemeal. This risk is minimized by grasping the appendix at an intact/healthy point, gentle manipulation and the use of a retrieval bag. When the base of the appendix is sloughed or perforated, every effort must be made to prevent a leaking cecum by using a purse-string or figure-of-eight suture. Alternatively, and in difficult cases, a wide-bore drain may be placed close to the stump.

Advanced peritonitis/secondary intestinal obstruction

Adequate access may prove impossible due to adhesions and intestinal dilatation (inadequate pneumoperitoneum). If this is the case, convert to an open technique or consider conservative management and interval appendicectomy.

COMPLICATIONS

Bleeding

- Epigastric vessels – rare and avoidable. Keep the cannulae sites away from the vessels.
- Iliac vessels – extremely rare, but potentially dangerous. Meticulous technique (cannula insertion) and careful dissection and use of electrocautery (adhesions, mass) cannot be over-emphasized.
- Appendicular artery – rare and avoidable. Secure the vessels carefully using low-power coagulation or ligatures.

Intraperitoneal collection/abscess

This is a common complication following perforated appendicitis and/or peritonitis as in open technique appendicectomy. However, laparoscopy may reduce this risk though a wider exposure and suction and irrigation of the entire peritoneal cavity. Second-look laparoscopy and drainage under direct vision are an option, but require advanced laparoscopic skills.

Small bowel obstruction

As for open technique appendicectomy.

Wound infection

Stump leak

This may occur as the result of:

- weak and avascular base of the appendix,
- cheese-wire cut from tight ligature,
- diathermy burn: diathermy to an already tied-off appendix allows current to converge onto the narrowest part of the conducting organ. Use the diathermy sensibly before tying off the base.

FURTHER READING

Becmeur F, Bientz J. Surgical management of community-acquired peritonitis in children. *Journal de Chirurgie (Paris)* 2000; **137**:349–54.

D'Alessio A, Piro E, Tadini B, Beretta F. One-trocar transumbilical laparoscopic-assisted appendicectomy in children: our experience. *European Journal of Pediatric Surgery* 2002; **12**:24–7.

Rispoli G, Armellino MF, Esposito C. One-trocar appendicectomy. Sense and nonsense. *Surgical Endoscopy* 2002; **16**:833–5.

Valla JS, Steyaert H. Laparoscopic appendicectomy in children. In: *Endoscopic Surgery in Children.* Berlin: Springer-Verlag, 1999, 234–53.

Varlet F, Tardieu D, Limone B, Metafiot H, Chavrier Y. Laparoscopic versus open appendicectomy in children. Comparative study of 403 cases. *European Journal of Pediatric Surgery* 1994; **4**:333–7.

43

ACE procedure

SPENCER BEASLEY

INTRODUCTION

The laparoscopic antegrade continence enema (ACE) procedure is a refinement and simplification of the Malone procedure, which allows antegrade irrigation of the colon via a catheter tube passed through the appendicostomy stoma into the cecum. By regular emptying out of the entire colon and rectum, usually on an alternate-day basis, the child acquires a socially acceptable level of fecal continence.

Indications

- Spina bifida. Children with spina bifida who have fecal incontinence or require manual disimpaction of feces may benefit from a laparoscopic ACE procedure. Anorectal manometry is not required because virtually all spina bifida patients who have problems with the control of defecation are significantly improved following the procedure, irrespective of their initial manometric characteristics.
- Congenital anorectal anomalies in association with an abnormal sacrum or sacral agenesis, and in those who have poor anorectal sphincteric function following definitive surgery to correct the anomaly. Similarly, children who have poor anorectal control and ongoing fecal incontinence following surgery for Hirschsprung's disease have less soiling and empty their rectum more effectively after a laparoscopic ACE procedure.
- Some children with neuronal intestinal dysplasia or severe intractable constipation are improved after the procedure. The exact role of the ACE procedure in these patients is yet to be determined, but it is evident that the success rate is less than that achieved when it is performed for children with spina bifida. Minimum selection criteria for patients with neuronal intestinal dysplasia (NID) include:
  - evidence of decreased anorectal sensation as demonstrated on anorectal manometry;
  - previously proven ability to empty the rectum of fluid during rectal washouts.

Contraindications

- The standard laparoscopic ACE procedure as described here cannot be performed if an appendicectomy has already been performed, or where the appendix has or will be used for a Mitrofanoff procedure (urinary tract stoma) to manage the neurogenic bladder in spina bifida children. Consequently, the surgeon must always ensure that there is an appendix available prior to commencing the procedure. Check the history for previous appendicectomy, which may not always be obvious on clinical examination if the appendix was removed laparoscopically and scarring is minimal.
- Where access to the appendix is expected to be extremely difficult, such as in a child known to have extensive adhesions from previous abdominal operations. In this situation the threshold for proceeding is dependent upon the laparoscopic skills of the surgeon.
- Where the child has demonstrated an inability to empty the rectum of fluid adequately, as determined during attempts at rectal washouts.

The laparoscopic approach has a number of advantages over the conventional Malone procedure, including the following.

- A simpler operative procedure.
- A shorter operating time.
- No laparotomy wound.
- Less postoperative discomfort and a reduced requirement for analgesia.
- A stoma that can be used immediately for irrigations.
- A lower complication rate.

EQUIPMENT/INSTRUMENTS

Essential

- 5 mm 30° telescope.
- 5 mm Hasson blunt trocar and a 5 mm cannula (a cannula of a different caliber may be used).
- Two short 5 mm working cannulae and trocars.
- 5 mm laparoscopy instruments:
  - two atraumatic graspers
  - scissors
  - diathermy hook.
- Suture materials:
  - 2-0 absorbable suture on tapered needle for umbilical port (e.g. Dexon® or Vicryl®)
  - 4-0 absorbable suture for mucocutaneous anastomosis (e.g. Monocryl®).

PREOPERATIVE PREPARATION

The preferred site for the appendicostomy is marked on the skin preoperatively. In older, particularly non-ambulant, spina bifida children it is an advantage to situate the stoma where it is visible to the child, to make it easier for the child to insert the catheter. The eventual site of appendicostomy may not always coincide with this mark, because it depends also on the location and length of the appendix as determined at the time of laparoscopy.

TECHNIQUE

The child is anesthetized and placed in a supine position. Prophylactic intravenous antibiotics effective against bowel organisms (e.g. cephalosporin and metronidazole) are given at the induction of anesthesia. The whole anterior abdominal wall is painted with antiseptic solution, and the patient is draped.

Following local infiltration with 0.25 percent bupivacaine, a primary cannula (usually 5 mm) is inserted immediately inferior to the umbilicus using the open technique.

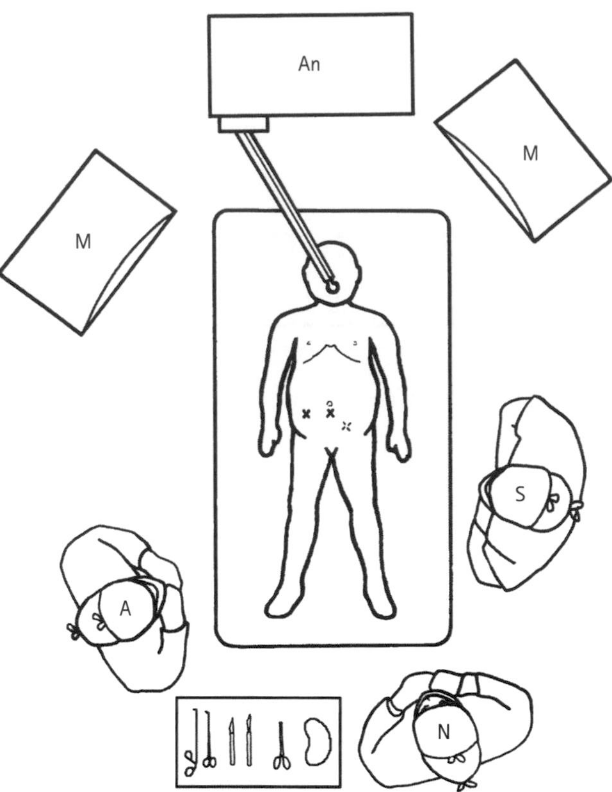

Figure 43.1

A pneumoperitoneum is created with CO_2 to a maximum intra-abdominal pressure of 10–12 mm Hg. The telescope is inserted through the cannula and a general exploration of the abdominal cavity is performed. **(See Figure 43.1)**

Location of the appendix

Often the appendix is clearly visible in the right iliac fossa. Spina bifida patients who have a ventriculo-peritoneal shunt in situ often have multiple filmy adhesions that prevent initial direct visualization of the appendix; these adhesions need to be divided using scissors or diathermy before the appendix can be found. Providing the appendix is visible in the right iliac fossa, is not retroperitoneal and access to it is not limited by peritoneal adhesions, a 7 mm transverse incision is made in the skin at the site previously marked on the skin. A 5 mm port is passed through the abdominal wall musculature directly into the peritoneal cavity.

Retrieval of the appendix

Laparoscopic grasping forceps are introduced through the 5 mm port to grab the tip of the appendix. They are then gently withdrawn, pulling the tip of the appendix into the end of the 5 mm port, which itself is slowly withdrawn through the abdominal wall. This maneuver also draws the appendix through the anterior abdominal wall to or beyond the level of the skin. The laparoscopic view will confirm that

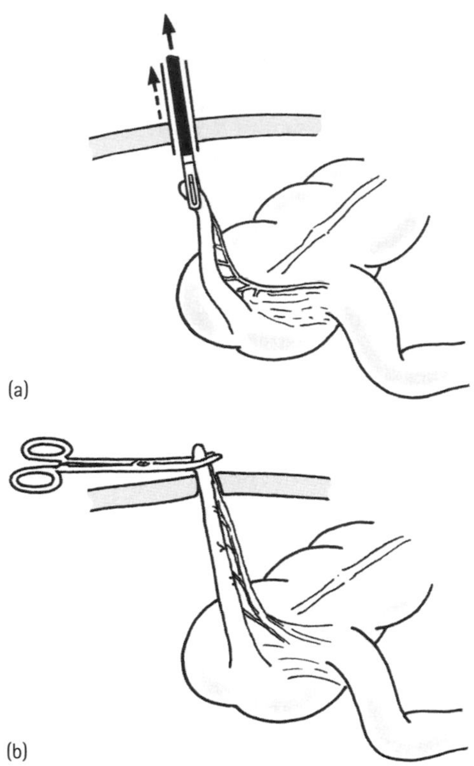

Figure 43.2

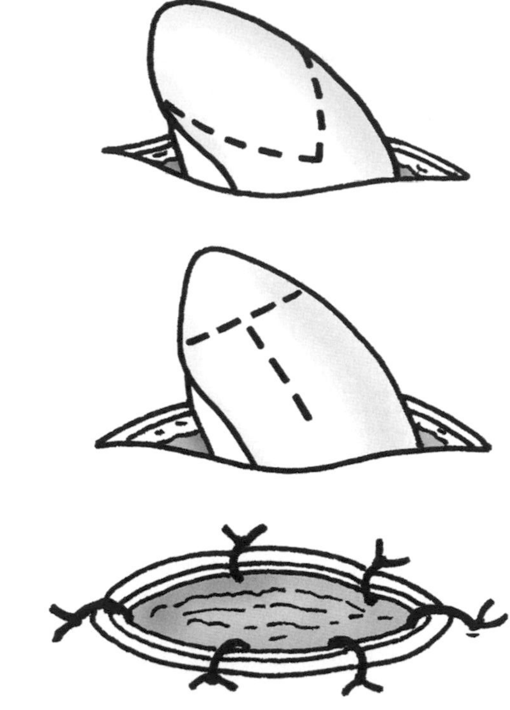

Figure 43.3

the appendix and its mesentery are not twisted or kinked. The distal-most edge of the mesoappendix is grasped with mosquito forceps as it is delivered into the wound, so that the appendix does not retract back through the abdominal wall. The laparoscopic grasping forceps can then be released. **(See Figure 43.2)**

Fashioning an opening on the tip of the appendix

The tip of the appendix can be opened obliquely, with the obliquity extending down the anti-mesenteric surface of the appendix for 10–12 mm. Alternatively, the tip of the appendix can be excised and an incision made down the anti-mesenteric border of the appendix for the same distance. This provides a good-sized opening in the appendix to facilitate subsequent catheterization and to reduce the likelihood of stenosis of the stoma.

Interrupted 4-0 absorbable sutures are placed between the dermis of the skin and the full thickness of the appendiceal wall around the perimeter of this opening. Usually six to eight sutures are required. **(See Figure 43.3)**

Catheterization of the stoma

A lubricated 8 Fr Foley catheter is introduced through the stoma into the cecum. Its unobstructed passage through the appendix into the right colon can be viewed through

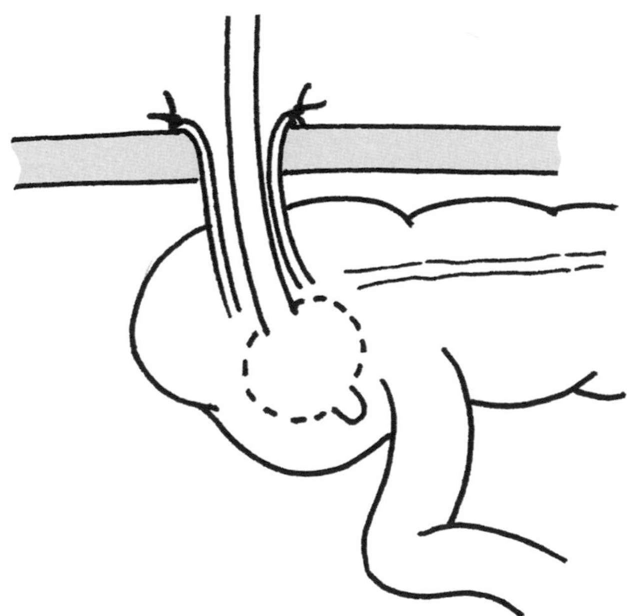

Figure 43.4

the laparoscope. Once in the cecum, the balloon of the catheter is inflated and the catheter is withdrawn gently until it becomes impacted at the internal orifice of the appendix. Insufflation of the peritoneal cavity is ceased, and the pneumoperitoneum is allowed to empty. The umbilical wound is closed in the normal fashion. Irrigation through the appendicostomy catheter can be commenced at any time. Most centers have a protocol for increasing the volume of irrigations over the first few days. **(See Figure 43.4, Table 43.1)**

Table 43.1 *Protocol for postoperative irrigation*

Day 0	Initial flush	20 mL	Saline
Day 1	First flush	350 mL	Saline
Day 2	Second flush	500 mL	Saline
	Additional flush (if no result from second flush)	500 mL	Saline Fleet enema via ACE

ACE, antegrade continence enema.

POSTOPERATIVE CARE

Saline irrigations can be commenced within hours of surgery. The usual practice is to put one teaspoonful of salt (5 g) into 500 mL of warm tap water. Tap water alone (i.e. without salt) may lead to hyponatremia, and phosphate enemas may cause hyperphosphatemia. One way that parents can check the concentration of salt in the irrigating solution is by measuring its specific gravity using an aquarium hygrometer.

The catheter is left in situ for 3–4 weeks, until the wound is fully healed and no longer tender. After the catheter has been removed, the stoma is only cannulated when a colonic irrigation is to be performed. The following equipment is needed.

- Size 8–12 Nelaton (short) catheter.
- Aqueous lubricating gel.
- Spigot.
- Syringe 60 mL – 'catheter tip'.

The volume and frequency of irrigations are determined according to response.

PROBLEMS, PITFALLS AND SOLUTIONS

Unable to locate the appendix

The appendix is retroperitoneal or cannot be readily located, or is not sufficiently mobile to be brought directly through the abdominal wall. In this situation a 5 mm working port is placed in the left iliac fossa. Grasping forceps introduced through this port can be used in conjunction with grasping forceps introduced through the now second working port in the right iliac fossa at the likely site of appendicostomy to manipulate the bowel and expose the appendix. Once the appendix has been located, it can be mobilized more fully by dividing its peritoneal attachments or mobilizing the cecum. Care must be taken to preserve the mesoappendix. Once mobilized, forceps passed through the right-sided port can pick up the tip of the appendix and the procedure continues as described earlier.

Multiple adhesions that obscure the appendix or limit its mobility

As already mentioned, multiple filmy adhesions are common in children with a ventriculo-peritoneal shunt in situ, as in many patients with spina bifida. Adhesions in the right lower quadrant are best divided to allow safe access to the appendix. These maneuvers are achieved by introducing two working ports, one 5 mm port in the left iliac fossa and a second 5 mm port at the site of anticipated appendicostomy in the right iliac fossa. The adhesions can be broken down by a combination of gentle retraction and disruption, and with diathermy dissection. Care must be taken to avoid damage to the ventriculo-peritoneal shunt, which should be relocated elsewhere in the abdomen if it is encountered in the operative field.

Appendix short or scarred, with obliteration of its lumen

The child may have had previous (often unrecognized) appendicitis, resulting in the appendix becoming scarred or fibrotic, and its lumen may be obliterated. If the lumen of only the distal half of the appendix is obliterated, it can be sacrificed, and the appendix retained from the point at which it has a lumen sufficient to enable cannulation. If the whole appendix is fibrotic, either a Chait cecostomy tube can be inserted directly into the cecum through a purse-string suture that is also used to anchor the cecum to the ventral abdominal wall, or a non-refluxing vascularized conduit can be constructed using the cecum or ascending colon.

No appendix

Sometimes a child has had a prior appendicectomy for acute appendicitis, or the appendix has been used for urinary diversion (e.g. in spina bifida). Where there is no appendix available, a non-refluxing vascularized conduit can be constructed from the ascending colon or cecum, or a laparoscopic-guided button cecostomy tube can be inserted.

COMPLICATIONS

Closed loop obstruction

Theoretically, the foramen between the appendix and the lateral abdominal wall may cause a closed loop bowel obstruction if small bowel herniates through it and becomes trapped. In practice, however, this seems to be a very rare event and does not occur often enough to justify routine closure of the space.

Stomal stenosis

This is by far the most common complication of the ACE procedure, whether performed as an open procedure (reported incidence 10–33 percent) or laparoscopically (27 percent). It is more likely to be related to:

- the size of the opening in the distal end of the appendix;
- whether there is ischemia of the distal appendix as a result of compression of the mesoappendix as it passes through the abdominal wall musculature;
- from excessive tension, such as when the appendix is short or the abdominal wall thick (as in obesity);
- skin growing over the stoma between catheterizations.

Stenosis is less likely to occur if the appendix is sitting comfortably without undue tension, and if the appendix is opened obliquely to produce at least 10 mm length at the mucocutaneous junction. In some children, a thin layer of skin grows across and may obscure the stoma in the time between catheterizations, particularly when they are performed every second or third day. This can be dealt with by re-introducing a Foley catheter and leaving it in situ for several weeks, or by increasing the frequency of irrigations (thus shortening the interval between catheterizations). Alternatively, a long-stemmed Chait cecostomy tube can be inserted.

Pseudo-polyp

This is a rare complication, and is secondary to trauma during repeated cannulation of the appendix. It presents as difficulty introducing the irrigation catheter in the absence of evidence of stenosis at skin level, or as stomal bleeding after catheterization. It is more likely to occur where there is a long history of resistance during the introduction of cannulae, and usually occurs at the level of the external oblique muscle.

Leakage

About 5 percent of ACE procedures cause troublesome leakage between irrigations. The amount of leakage may be reduced by a variety of maneuvers, including the following.

- Leaving in an indwelling Foley catheter with its balloon inflated and on slight traction.
- Placement of a specially designed soft Silastic® plug into the appendicostomy stoma.
- Application of a Tegaderm™ occlusive dressing.

FURTHER READING

Lynch AC, Beasley SW, Robertson RW, Morreau PN. Comparison of results of laparoscopic and open antegrade continence enema procedures. *Pediatric Surgery International* 1999; **15**:343–6.

Malone PS, Ransley PG, Kiely EM. Preliminary report: the antegrade continence enema. *Lancet* 1990; **336**:1217–18.

Singh SJ, Cummins G, Manglick P et al. How to test the safety of a homemade antegrade colonic washout fluid. *Pediatric Surgery International* 2002; **18**:81–2.

Webb HW, Barraza MA, Crump JM. Laparoscopic appendicectomy for management of faecal incontinence. *Journal of Pediatric Surgery* 1997; **32**:457–8.

Wing NA, Findlay FJ, Beasley SW, Dobbs BR, Robertson RW. Does anorectal manometry predict clinical outcome after laparoscopic ACE procedures in children with spina bifida? *Colorectal Disease* 2001; **3**:185–8.

44A

Laparoscopic pull-through for Hirschsprung's disease

MUNTHER J. HADDAD

INTRODUCTION

Surgery has been the accepted treatment for Hirschsprung's disease since Swenson's description of the first successful pull-through operation in 1948. A variety of procedures have been developed over the years, including the Soave and Duhamel operations. As originally described, these were all three-stage procedures with an initial colostomy, subsequent pull-through and then closure of the stoma. Subsequently many surgeons have performed successful two-stage procedures and, more recently, single-stage pull-throughs without a covering colostomy.

The choice of technique will depend, in part, on the age and weight of the child, but also, importantly, on the help of an expert histopathologist. Before contemplating a single-stage procedure, facilities must be available for rapid examination of biopsy specimens by frozen section to confirm the presence of ganglion cells at the site of the pull-through.

The Soave procedure is ideally suited to the laparoscopic approach. The view is excellent and biopsies can be taken from any part of the colon to look for ganglion cells. The colon is easy to mobilize laparoscopically and the blood supply is easy to control. The aganglionic colon is removed transanally and the anastomosis then completed by hand at the anus before reduction of the bowel into the pelvis. Although the laparoscopic Soave operation can be performed as a three-stage or two-stage procedure, the potential benefits of a single-stage procedure are greatest.

Indications

- Infants and children with short-segment Hirschsprung's disease.

Contraindications

ABSOLUTE

- An indeterminate transition zone.
- Lack of histopathology expertise for rapid frozen section analysis.
- Major associated life-threatening congenital malformations.

RELATIVE

- Failure to achieve adequate preoperative decompression.
- Recurrent severe enterocolitis.
- Long segment disease with a transition zone in the ascending colon.
- Total colonic aganglionosis.

EQUIPMENT/INSTRUMENTS

Essential

- 5 mm telescope, preferably with a 30–45° viewing angle.
- Four 3–5 mm trocars.

- Fine L-hook monopolar forceps.
- 3–5 mm bipolar diathermy forceps.
- Two 3–5 mm atraumatic grasping forceps.
- 3–5 mm curved scissors.
- 3–5 mm curved needle holder.

Desirable

- 5 mm ultrasonic knife or shears.
- 3–5 mm retractor.
- 5 mm clip applicator.

PREOPERATIVE PREPARATION

The diagnosis of Hirschsprung's disease should be confirmed by rectal suction biopsy before considering a pull-through operation. A lower gastrointestinal contrast study may help define the extent of the aganglionic segment if a single-stage procedure is contemplated.

Standard bowel preparation should commence 24 hours prior to surgery. A rectal washout should be performed on the evening prior to surgery. Routine hematology and biochemistry investigations should be requested and blood sent for typing. Diaper cream should be applied to the perineum. Arrangements should be made for frozen section analysis of biopsy specimens.

TECHNIQUE

This procedure is performed under general anesthesia with endotracheal intubation and muscle relaxation. Intravenous cannulae should be sited on the upper limbs as necessary, leaving the lower limbs free because they will lie within the operative field. A nasogastric tube should be sited. Prophylactic broad-spectrum intravenous antibiotics are administered. The Bovie return electrode plate should be attached to the back of the chest. The bladder may be catheterized or simply emptied by the Crede maneuver.

Small infants are placed transversely across the operating table in a supine position. An arm board may be affixed to the side of the table to widen it for longer infants. Older children can be placed either obliquely on the table or along the table in a conventional manner. The surgeon stands near the head of the child and the main video monitor is placed in a gaze-down position at the foot of the patient, directly in line with the pelvic dissection. Stirrups are positioned to support the legs and a towel or jelly bag is placed behind the pelvis. The trunk, pelvis and lower limbs of the child are prepared front and back with aqueous Betadine antiseptic. The lower limbs and pelvis are raised by the assistant while a large sterile drape is placed behind the patient covering most of the operating table, jelly pad

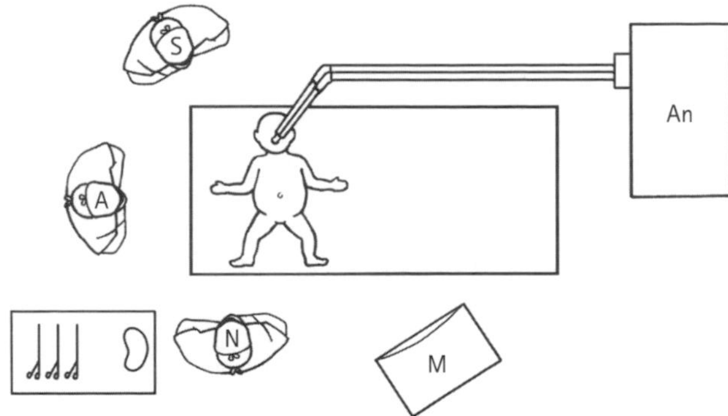

Figure 44A.1

and stirrups. In this way the legs can be moved freely to allow free access to the perineum without re-draping. **(See Figure 44A.1)**

Abdominal procedure

A pneumoperitoneum of 8–12 mmHg CO_2 is established using a standard open or Veress needle technique. A 0° telescope is inserted high in the right iliac fossa and used to site working ports as follows.

1. Right upper quadrant: 5 mm port, 2–3 cm to the right of the midline, approximately 2 cm below the liver edge.
2. Left lateral quadrant: 5 mm port, sited just below or above the level of the umbilicus in the anterior axillary line.
3. Suprapubic or low left iliac fossa (optional): 3 mm port, placed in the suprapubic skin crease to the left or right of the midline, taking care to avoid the bladder or female pelvic organs. **(See Figure 44A.2)**

Ports 1 and 2 are the main working ports. The third port is optional but useful for retracting the colon during the pelvic dissection. A moderate Trendelenburg tilt on the operating table encourages the small intestine to slide out of the pelvis.

Before the pelvic dissection can begin, the transition zone must be established. A change in caliber of the colon may be obvious as the bowel is examined laparoscopically. The transition zone may be visible on the contrast enema. However, a biopsy must be taken from the colon distal to the transition zone to confirm normal innervation by frozen section before starting the endorectal dissection. Multiple biopsies can be taken from the colon if necessary and this is a straightforward laparoscopic procedure: the colon is steadied with atraumatic grasping forceps and a small wedge of seromuscular tissue is removed with curved endoscopic scissors. Each biopsy site is closed with a suture to mark the position. If there is any doubt about the innervation of the bowel, the procedure should be terminated and a stoma opened. The pull-through can be completed once a definitive pathology result becomes available.

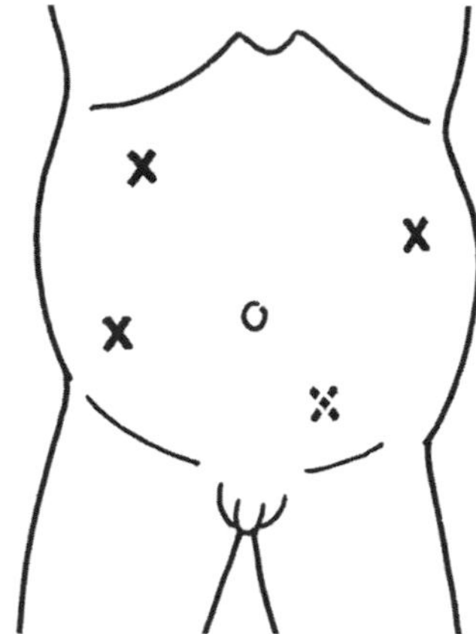

Figure 44A.2

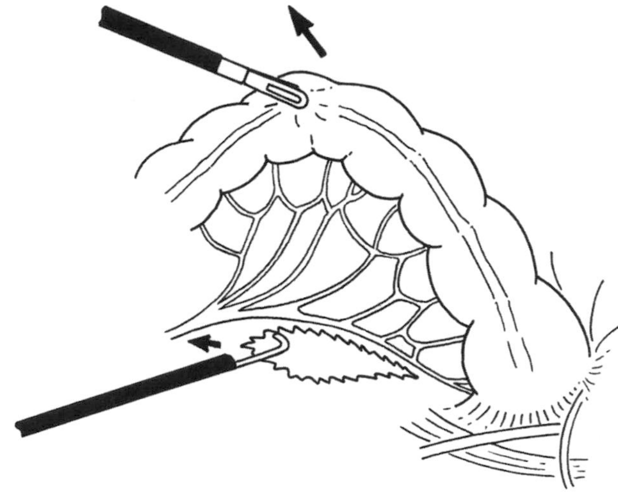

Figure 44A.3

Mobilization of the colon and rectum

The recto-sigmoid is grasped with atraumatic forceps through the left lateral port and lifted upwards. This displays the mesocolon and the vessels. A window is opened in the sigmoid mesentery behind the superior rectal vessels using scissors, an L-shaped cautery hook or a Harmonic Scalpel® through the right upper quadrant port. The superior rectal vessels are then cauterized or clipped and divided. **(See Figure 44A.3)**

The rectum is mobilized, staying close to the bowel wall to avoid injury to the autonomic nerves in the pelvis. Both ureters should be identified and preserved. The rectum is held with grasping forceps through the left lateral port and pulled over to the left to place tension on the mesentery. L-hook cautery, a Harmonic Scalpel® or endoscopic bipolar diathermy scissors through the right upper port is used to divide vessels running on the rectum as close to the bowel wall as possible. The instruments are then switched over and the rectum retracted over to the right so that the vessels on the left side of the rectum can be divided. In this way a circumferential close rectal dissection can be performed. Mobilization should continue down into the pelvis anteriorly until the level of the prostate or cervix is reached. Great care should be taken to avoid the ureters at this point and the vas in males. Posteriorly, dissection is continued down to the level of the fifth sacral vertebra. This dissection will divide the middle rectal vessels. **(See Figure 44A.4)**

After the pelvic dissection has been completed, the proximal colon must be mobilized for the pull-through. If the transition zone is in the distal sigmoid colon, minimal mobilization is necessary, but if the transition zone lies in the proximal sigmoid, the left colon must be mobilized up to the splenic flexure. This dissection is accomplished by holding the descending colon under tension with grasping forceps through the right upper quadrant port and dividing the lateral peritoneal reflection with scissors, L-cautery diathermy hook or ultrasonic scalpel through the left lateral port. The colon is then lifted forwards and dissection is continued medially behind the bowel, taking care to avoid damage to the inferior mesenteric pedicle and the marginal arcade.

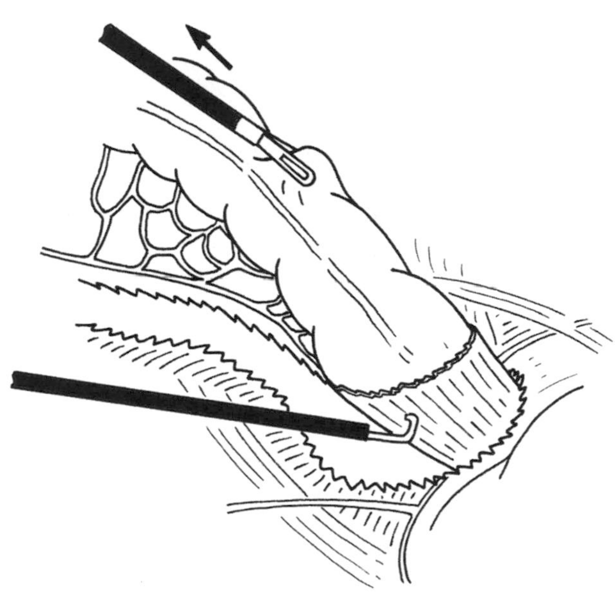

Figure 44A.4

After the abdominal phase of the dissection has been completed, the pneumoperitoneum is released, but the ports are left in place to allow a final inspection at the end of the operation.

Perineal procedure

The surgeon and assistant move to the end of the operating table. The child's lower limbs are placed in the stirrups to expose the perineum. Six O-silk traction sutures are placed

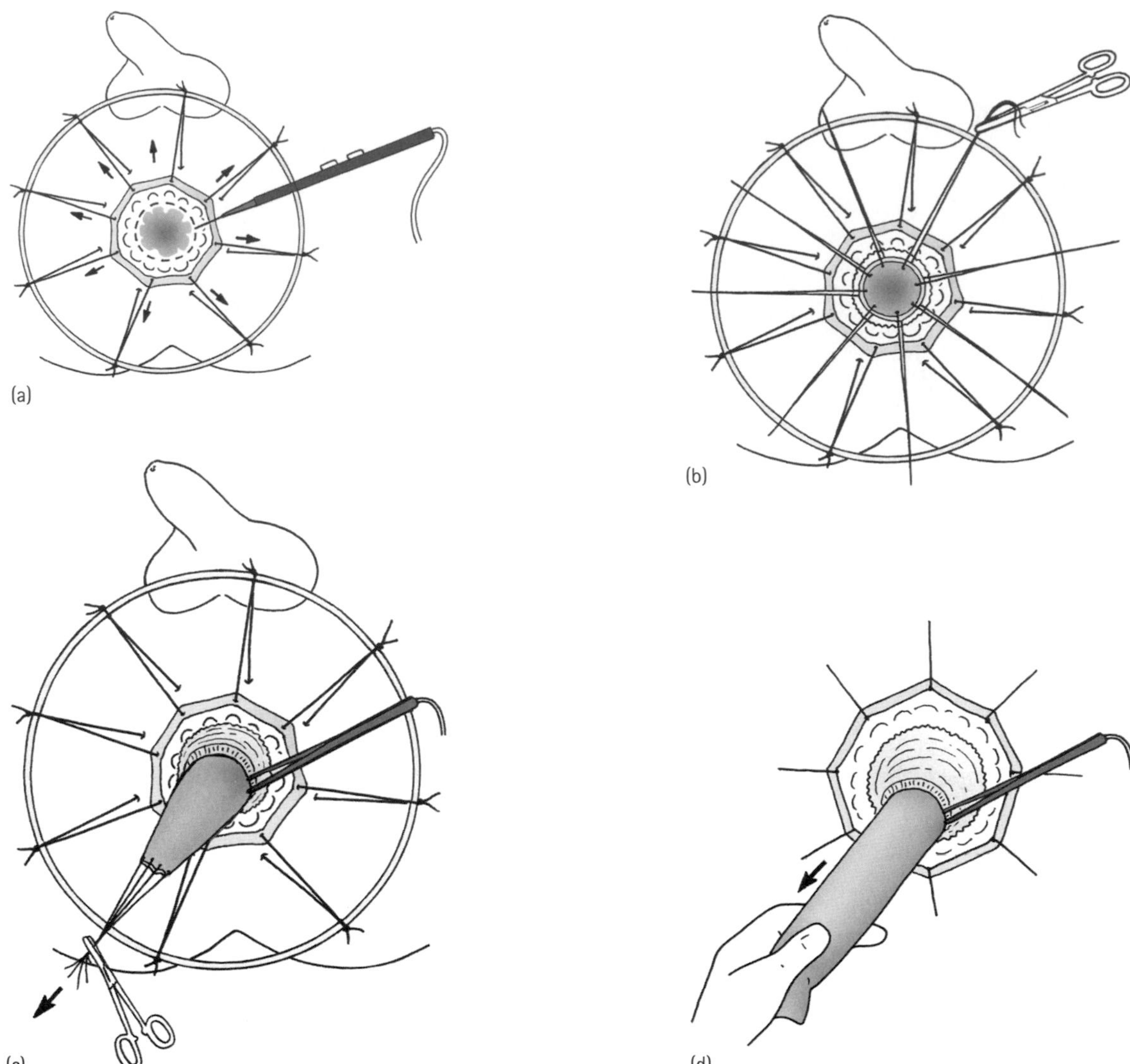

Figure 44A.5 *Radial traction sutures at the anal verge and a circumferential incision above the dentate line; (b) traction sutures to the mucosa; (c) developing a plane; (d) traction on the mucosal cuff and continuous dissection between the mucosa and muscle layers.*

around the anal verge, taking generous bites of the peri-anal skin, and tied around a ring retractor. This exposes the ano-rectal mucosa for the endorectal dissection. Great care must be taken to avoid damage to the anal sphincter by excessive stretching during the subsequent dissection.

A circumferential incision is made through the mucosa of the rectum 5–8 mm above the dentate line, depending on the size of the infant, using monopolar diathermy with a conventional handset and fine needle. It is important to stay superficial to the internal sphincter.

A plane is developed between the mucosa and the internal sphincter by sharp dissection. Once the edge of the mucosa is elevated, a series of 4-0 sutures can be inserted for traction. Meticulous technique is necessary at this stage to stay in the correct plane between the mucosa and the white fibers of the internal anal sphincter. A combination of blunt and sharp dissection is necessary, using bipolar diathermy for hemostasis. Once the submucosal plane has been established, the dissection becomes much easier.

As the dissection proceeds, the relative absence of bleeding is noted because the bowel has already been mobilized and separated from its mesentery during the preliminary laparoscopic phase. As the dissection progresses proximally, the rectal cuff will turn inside out and prolapse through the anus so that the site of the most distal biopsy can be seen. (**See Figure 44A.5**)

The muscular cuff of the rectum can be divided circumferentially at this point and trimmed to leave a 5–6 cm sleeve around the neorectum. The muscular cuff is divided posteriorly down to within 1–2 cm of the sphincter using monopolar diathermy and then allowed to retract back into the pelvis. Dividing the rectal cuff increases the capacity of the neorectum. (**See Figure 44A.6**)

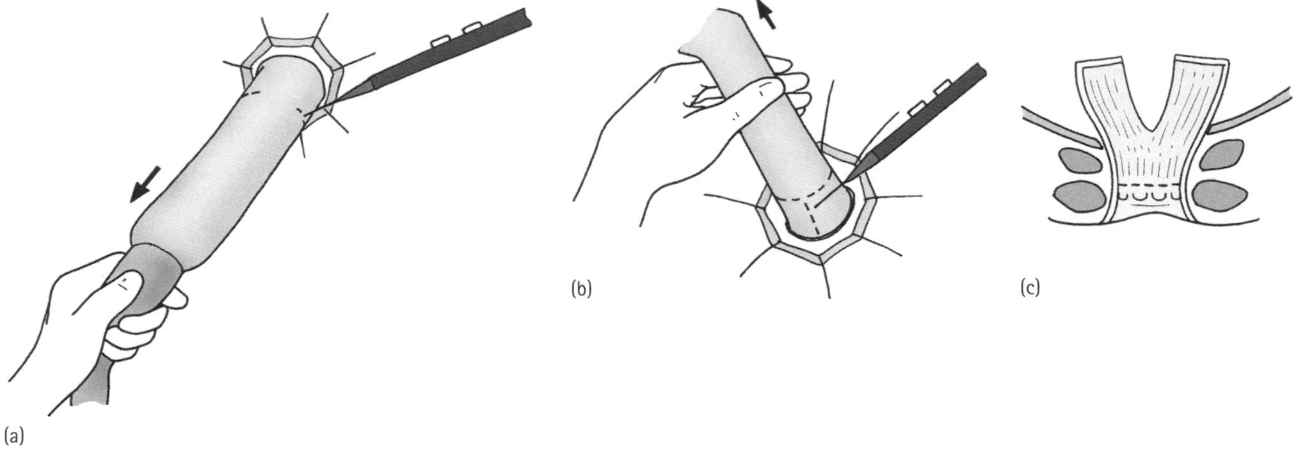

Figure 44A.6

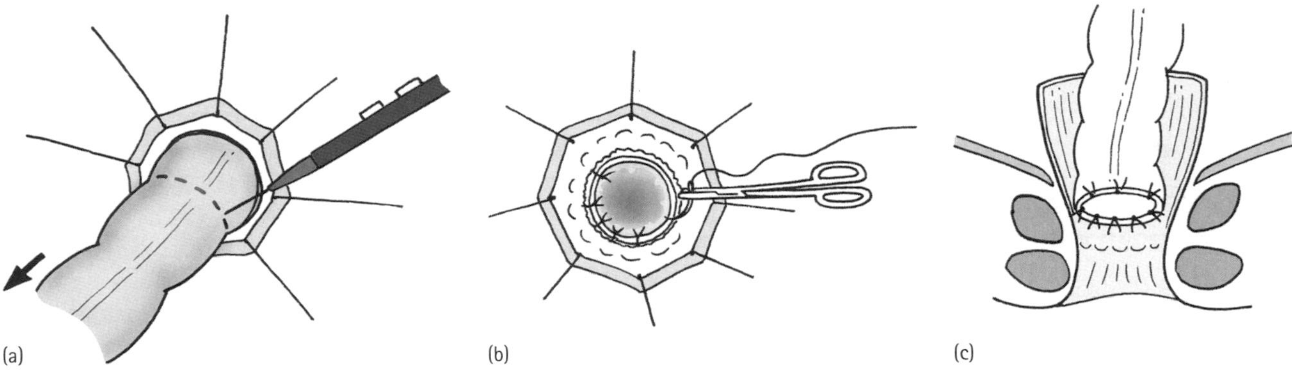

Figure 44A.7

The colon is pulled down through the rectal cuff and transected at a level with normal innervation. Usually this will be 5–6 cm above the transition zone. If there is any doubt about the innervation at this level, a full circumference 'donut' specimen of colon should be sent for frozen section to confirm the presence of ganglion cells in all quadrants of the bowel wall. After the bowel has been divided, the aganglionic colon/rectum should be submitted for histological analysis with the proximal end tagged with a suture.

The orientation of the colon should be checked in case the mesentery has twisted. The colon is then anastomosed to the distal mucosa of the rectal cuff. The anastomosis is completed with 20–24 full-thickness sutures of 4-0 Vicryl®. The ends of these sutures should be left long to aid inspection of the entire circumference of the anastomosis. Additional sutures may be required. When the anastomosis is satisfactory, the sutures are trimmed. (**See Figure 44A.7**)

The anal retraction sutures are removed and the anus returns to a normal position. A gentle rectal examination can be performed as a final examination of the anastomosis, and a loose roll of Vaseline gauze is left in the anus.

Completion of the operation

The surgeon and assistant change their gowns and gloves before returning to the abdomen. The pneumoperitoneum is re-established and a laparoscope inserted for final confirmation of hemostasis. The colon can be seen to lie comfortably along the posterior abdominal wall and an assessment must be made of the risk of small bowel herniation behind the colon. If necessary, the colon should be tethered to the posterior abdominal wall with a series of fine Vicryl® sutures. The pneumoperitoneum is finally evacuated and the port sites closed with 4-0 Vicryl® sutures to the deep fascia and Steristrips® to the skin.

Modifications for children with an existing colostomy

A similar procedure can be performed in children with a colostomy. The colostomy is taken down and the proximal and distal colons are divided using transverse linear staplers. No attempt is made to anastomose the two ends. The closed stapled ends of the proximal and distal colon are approximated by three or four 3-0 Vicryl® sutures and dropped back into the peritoneal cavity. The wound is closed and the laparoscopic abdominal procedure proceeds as described above. During the perineal phase, the rectum everts and is divided in the normal fashion. Traction will then deliver the two closed ends of the colon sutured together. The proximal colon is divided at a convenient point and the colo-anal anastomosis completed, as previously described.

Formation of a stoma

If total colonic aganglionosis is identified during the preliminary laparoscopic phase of the operation, or if there are problems determining the innervation of the colon, it is wise to abandon the procedure in favor of a stoma. A 3 cm incision is made in the skin of the abdominal wall at the proposed site for the stoma. The colon is exteriorized at this point and opened to fashion a stoma. Prolapse of the stoma can be prevented by fixing the bowel to the anterior abdominal wall with a few non-absorbable sutures placed laparoscopically.

POSTOPERATIVE CARE

- Intravenous antibiotics are continued for 48 hours.
- Fluids are allowed by mouth on postoperative day 1 and normal diet can be resumed by day 2.
- Most children can be discharged from hospital on the third postoperative day.
- Diaper cream must be applied liberally three to four times a day for at least 6 weeks to minimize perineal excoriation.
- Patients are reviewed at 6 weeks postoperatively. A gentle rectal examination is performed to check the anastomosis, and the anus is calibrated with Hegar dilators.
- Anal dilatation is not necessary unless the anastomosis is very tight, which is unusual.

PROBLEMS, PITFALLS AND SOLUTIONS

Poor view of the colon

This is caused either by inadequate decompression of the colon or poor positioning of the port sites. It is essential to achieve effective decompression of the bowel if a single-stage pull-through is planned. This will require daily or twice-daily rectal washouts. If the child remains subacutely obstructed despite regular washouts, the aganglionic segment is, in all probability, long and a stoma should be opened with a view to a staged pull-through.

No obvious transition zone

If the rectal washouts have been very effective, or the colon is defunctioned by a stoma, there may be no visible change in the caliber of the colon at the transition zone. Evidence from a previous contrast enema may help determine the site of the transition zone. If the site of the transition zone is unknown, the first biopsy should be taken from the distal sigmoid colon and sent for rapid frozen section analysis. Whilst this specimen is being processed, further biopsies should be taken from the ascending, transverse and descending colons. The appendix should be removed and sent for analysis. The importance of ensuring normal innervation of the colon at the site chosen for the pull-through cannot be stressed highly enough. The onus of responsibility is on the histopathologist, because the consequences of a pull-through in transition zone bowel can be disastrous. If there is any doubt, the procedure should be abandoned and a stoma raised.

Long segment disease

Mobilization of the descending, transverse or even ascending colon may be required. This will add considerably to the duration of the operation. Additional working ports may be necessary. Whilst a laparoscopically assisted ileo-anal pull-through is technically feasible, judgment is necessary as to whether the child would do better with an ileostomy and a staged pull-through. This is usually the case with neonates.

Difficult hemostasis

Bipolar diathermy, the ultrasonic scalpel and clips should be used as required. Preservation of the marginal arcade of the colon is essential to ensure a good blood supply to the distal bowel. This becomes particularly important as dissection proceeds to the splenic flexure and transverse colon.

Ischemic pull-through

The most common explanation is inadequate mobilization of the colon during the preliminary abdominal phase of the operation. If the descending colon is used, the splenic flexure must be taken down. The orientation of the colon should be verified to ensure that the blood supply has not been twisted. The pneumoperitoneum should be re-established and the colon examined as it runs down into the pelvis.

COMPLICATIONS

- Bleeding. Major bleeding is uncommon provided care is taken with the blood supply to the colon.

- Injury to the bowel. Inadvertent injury to the bowel is usually caused by unnoticed Bovie contact, which can be avoided by ensuring it is only operated on under direct vision.
- Injury to the ureters, vas, bladder and pelvic autonomic nerves. This risk is minimized by a close rectal dissection in the pelvis, as with the open Soave procedure.
- Anastomotic stenosis. Stenosis may occur at the site of the anastomosis itself, which is usually caused by ischemia or an anastomotic leak. Stenosis at the level of the rectal stump may be prevented by division of the muscle cuff in the posterior midline. More proximal stenosis in the neorectum is invariably ischemic in origin.
- Anastomotic leak. This is uncommon but usually caused by a combination of ischemia and tension at the anastomosis. Conservative treatment is rarely successful and inevitably leads to anastomotic stenosis. Once the diagnosis is confirmed, an ileostomy should be opened. This will defunction the colon and allow the anastomosis to heal. An ileostomy will not jeopardize the blood supply of the colon and is preferable to a colostomy for this reason.
- Preliminary outcome data following laparoscopically assisted pull-through appear comparable to those for conventional open surgery.

FURTHER READING

Carcassonne M, Guys JM, Morrison-Lacombe G, Kreitmann B. Management of Hirschsprung's disease: curative surgery before 3 months of age. *Journal of Pediatric Surgery* 1989; **24**:1032–4.

Cilley RE, Statter MB, Hirschl RB, Coran AG. Definitive treatment of Hirschsprung's disease in the newborn with a one-stage procedure. *Surgery* 1994; **115**:551–6.

Georgeson KE, Cohen RD, Hebra A et al. Primary laparoscopic-assisted endorectal colon pull-through for Hirschsprung's disease: a new gold standard. *Annals of Surgery* 1999; **229**:678–82; discussion 682–3.

44B

Duhamel pull-through for Hirschsprung's disease

BENNO M. URE, NATALIE K. JESCH AND RAINER NUSTEDE

INTRODUCTION

In children with Hirschsprung's disease the ideal method for large bowel resection is still under debate. For many years the Swenson, Soave, Rehbein and Duhamel techniques have been used as standard methods. The introduction of minimally invasive surgery has made it possible to perform the abdominal part of the operation via laparoscope. Compared with Swenson and Soave, the laparoscopic Duhamel pull-through procedure is more challenging due to the lack of space in the pelvis, especially in newborns.

Indications

- All levels of Hirschsprung's disease including total colonic Hirschsprung's disease.
- Other intestinal neuronal malformations that require pull-through surgery.
- Re-do surgery.

Contraindications

ABSOLUTE

- Enterocolitis with diarrhea, fever, leucocytosis.

RELATIVE

- Previous abdominal surgery/major scarring.

An enterostomy is not a contraindication for the procedure.

EQUIPMENT/INSTRUMENTS

In most patients, 3 mm instruments are used. However, in older patients with a large rectum, 5 mm instruments are more appropriate. We prefer to use a 5 mm telescope for all patients, as this provides adequate visualization.

Essential

- 5 mm telescope (30° angled).
- Two 6 mm cannulae with appropriate reducer.
- Three 3.5 mm cannulae.
- Standard set of 3 mm instruments:
  - monopolar hook,
  - hook scissors,
  - curved scissors,
  - two atraumatic curved graspers without ratchet (Kelly clamps),
  - two atraumatic straight graspers with ratchet,
  - suction/irrigation device.
- 5–3 mm reducer.
- A standard set of surgical instruments for rectal anastomosis (scissors, pincets, Langenbeck hooks for anal exposition, mosquito clamps, large curved clamp, monopolar cautery device).
- Set of Hegar bougies (numbers 5–12).
- Stapler devices for anal anastomosis (55–75 mm).
- Absorbable sutures:
  - 2-0: fascia around the umbilical cannula, ligation of the rectum,
  - 3-0: holding sutures at the rectal stump,

- 4-0: closure of the biopsy sites, closure of the rectal stump, closure of the abdominal wall fascia,
- 5-0: anal anastomosis according to Duhamel.

Optional

- Bipolar coagulation forceps and/or ultrasound shears.

PREOPERATIVE PREPARATION

The preparation includes the standard preoperative work-up for Hirschsprung's disease, which is described in Chapter 44A. The diagnosis is established by rectal suction biopsy. A contrast enema may give information about the extent of the disease. If possible, a colostomy should be avoided and the bowel should initially be treated by daily enemas and washouts. The procedure seems to be easier at 2–6 months of age compared to in older children.

The patient is admitted the day before surgery and the bowels are prepared with colonic enemas and antegrade washout.

TECHNIQUE

General anesthesia with endotracheal intubation and muscle relaxation is mandatory. A central venous line may be placed for safe intra-operative and postoperative venous access and parenteral nutrition. Intravenous antibiotic prophylaxis (e.g. a second-generation cephalosporin) is commenced after the introduction of anesthesia. The bowels are further decompressed using on-table irrigation and suction. The patient is placed in the supine position at the lower end of the operating table.

The abdomen, genital region, buttocks and upper legs are disinfected. After sterile draping, the bladder is catheterized and emptied and the catheter is spigotted.

The surgeon stands on the right of the patient, the camera assistant further down on the right, and the second assistant and scrub nurse on the left. Two monitors are used, one on each side of the table.

Five cannulae are used, two 6 mm and three 3.5 mm. The first cannula (6 mm) is introduced via an open infra-umbilical approach. The fascia around the cannula is closed with a 2-0 purse-string suture. A pneumoperitoneum is created at a maximum pressure of 8 mmHg. All the other cannulae are positioned under visual control. The second 6 mm cannula in the right upper abdomen is used for the scope, the cannula in the right lower abdomen for the cautery hook, forceps or scissors, and the cannula in the left upper abdomen for a second working instrument. Other grasping forceps can be introduced via the infra-umbilical and left lower abdominal cannulae, as needed for exposition,

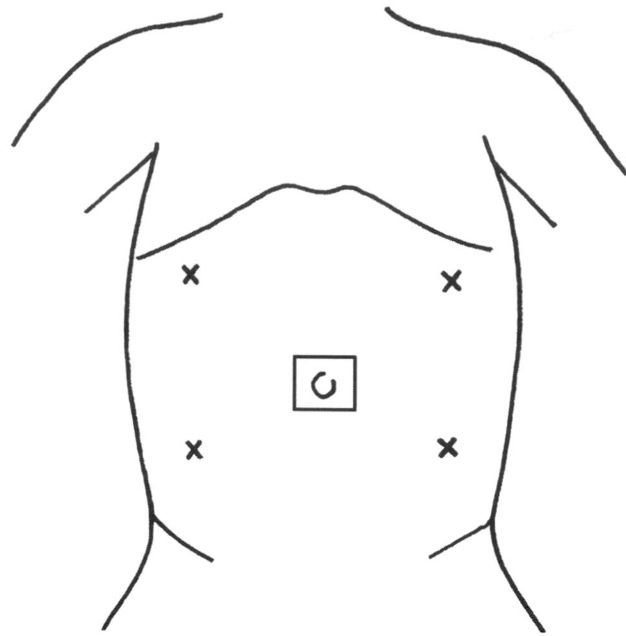

Figure 44B.1

and held by an assistant. A 5–3 mm reducer is needed when 3 mm instruments are introduced via the infra-umbilical cannula (6 mm). **(See Figure 44B.1)**

As in all pull-through surgical procedures, the laparoscopic Duhamel involves a number of sequential steps.

Multiple colon biopsy

Two or more extra-mucosal biopsies are taken using scissors and a grasping forceps for immediate examination by a pathologist. The first sample is taken from the recto-sigmoid junction and the next from the sigmoid colon, followed by others higher up as needed. The biopsy sites are closed using intracorporeal absorbable sutures. **(See Figure 44B.2)**

Colorectal mobilization

Mobilization of the rectum and sigmoid colon is performed using a monopolar dissecting hook, which is introduced via the cannula in the right lower abdomen, and grasping forceps, introduced via the cannula in the left upper abdomen. The preparation starts at the recto-sigmoid junction and is continued as close to the bowel wall as possible, taking down multiple small vessels. Individual large vessel ligations are not usually necessary.

The ureters and vas deferens in boys are identified and preserved. Initially, the dissection is performed in the direction of the rectum. The lateral and anterior peritoneal fold is opened and the rectum is mobilized circumferentially down to approximately 3 cm above the anus. The length of

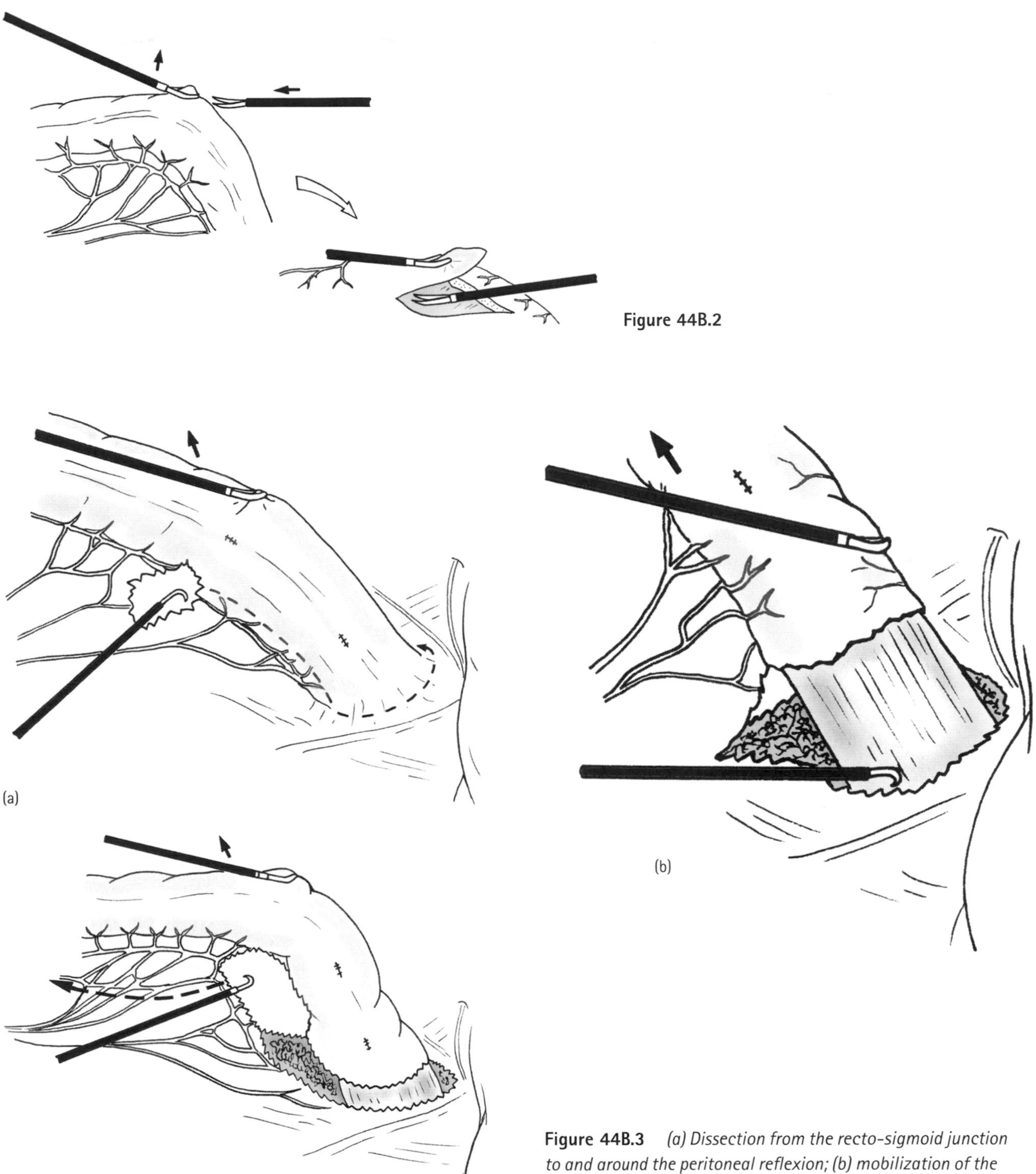

Figure 44B.2

Figure 44B.3 *(a) Dissection from the recto-sigmoid junction to and around the peritoneal reflexion; (b) mobilization of the rectum; (c) dissection extending proximally.*

the rectal stump can be determined using a Hegar bougie through the anus which is monitored via the laparoscope. Care must be taken not to damage the iliac vessels, the bladder, the vagina in females, and the urethra and prostate in males. (**See Figure 44B.3**)

Once the results of the biopsies are known, the mobilization is extended proximally as far as indicated. The marginal colonic blood supply must be preserved for the pull-through colon (above the transection line). The assistant on the left side of the table may use one or two pairs of atraumatic forceps through the umbilical and/or left lower abdominal cannulae in order to improve exposure. Moving the colon from one side to the other and placing forceps to retract the bladder improve viewing.

When higher mobilization (splenic or hepatic flexure) is required, the scope is moved into the infra-umbilical cannula and the surgeon stands to the lower right or left side of the patient, as needed. The right upper or lower and the left lower abdominal cannulae are used for mobilization of the descending, transverse or right colon. Mobilization of the splenic and hepatic flexures usually necessitates division of the middle and right colic vessels in between clips or ligatures. Care must be taken not to damage the spleen, pancreas and duodenum.

In patients with total colonic aganglionosis, complete laparoscopic mobilization of the colorectum to and including the terminal ileum may prove time-consuming. A transverse mini-laparotomy in the right lower abdomen may allow an open technique resection and fashioning of a protecting double-loop ileostomy.

Transection and closure of the rectal stump

The rectum is transfixed just below the intended transection line using 2-0 percutaneously introduced holding stitches medial to the inferior epigastric vessels. These sutures facilitate:

- pelvic exposure,
- rectal transection,
- closing of the stump,
- colon pull-through.

The rectum is transected using monopolar hook scissors, and fecal soiling is minimized using a suction device. Closure of the stump is achieved in two layers – the first continuous and the second interrupted using absorbable 4-0 sutures. The integrity of the suture line may be checked by trans-anal insertion of water into the stump.

The retrorectal space is created using blunt dissection. Grasping forceps are introduced through the infra-umbilical cannula with their tip pointing anteriorly as low as possible within the retrorectal space. The tip of the forceps may now be palpated posteriorly through the anus just above the dentate line. This will represent the site for the pull-through. The abdomen is desufflated and the cannulae are left in place. **(See Figure 44B.4)**

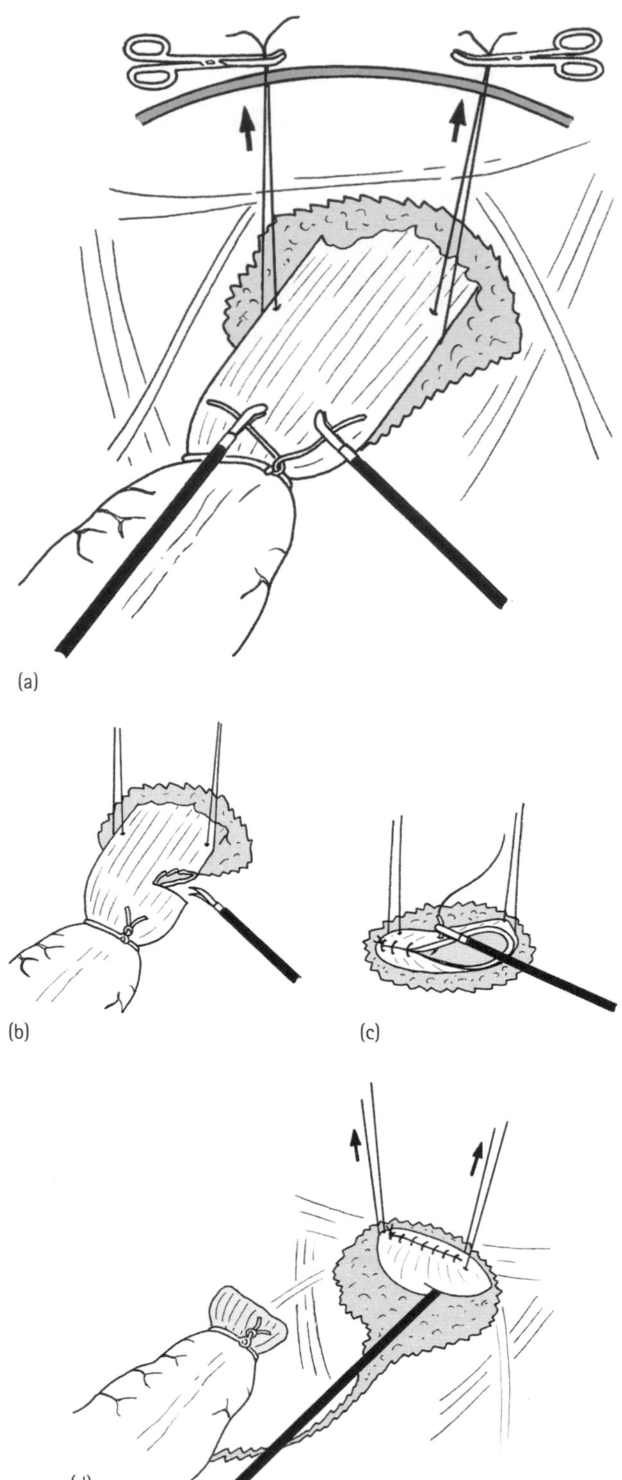

Figure 44B.4

Perineal dissection

The hips are flexed and abducted, the anus is gently dilated and the anal canal is kept open using two small retractors. A posterior semicircular incision is made approximately 0.5 cm above the dentate line and the previously inserted intra-abdominal grasping forceps are pushed through. Four 4-0 stay sutures are introduced at the lateral, anterior and dorsal margins of the semicircular rectal opening. **(See Figure 44B.5)**

A second, but larger, pair of curved grasping forceps is rail-roaded from below into the peritoneal cavity (following the previously introduced grasping forceps from above). A pneumoperitoneum is recreated and the transected colon is grasped and carefully pulled through. Orientation of the colon is ensured laparoscopically. The pulled-through colon is transected a few centimeters proximal to the aganglionic distal colon and the anastomosis is done using 5-0 absorbable sutures.

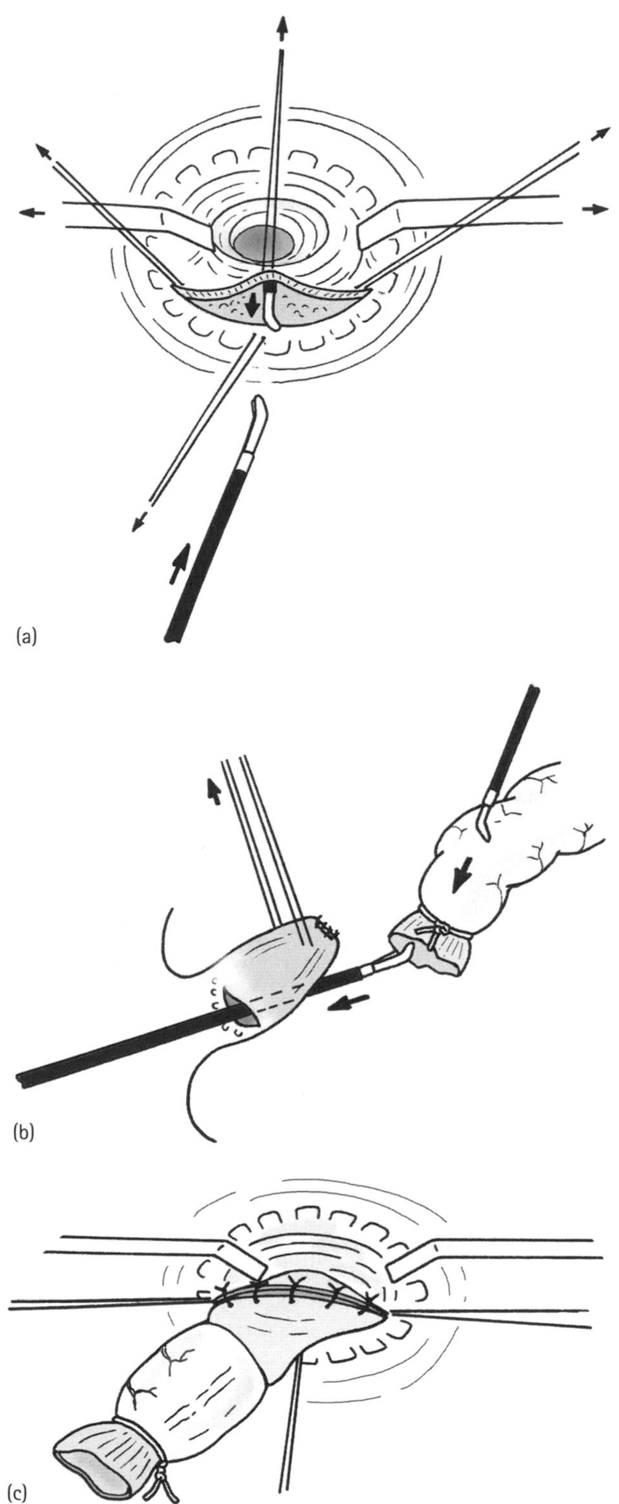

Figure 44B.5 *(a) Posterior semicircular incision with a grasping forceps through from above; (b) pull-through; (c) anterior aspect of the anastomosis.*

Once the circular anastomosis has been completed, a side-to-side anastomosis is carried out using a 55–75 mm stapler introduced through the anus. The introduction of the stapler is facilitated by the previously placed stay sutures. It is absolutely critical that safe positioning of the stapler is ensured before it is activated. An ideal anastomosis leaves less than 1 cm of blind rectal stump above the staple line. Finally, a silicon rectal tube may be inserted into the pull-through colon and fixed with tape. (**See Figure 44B.6**)

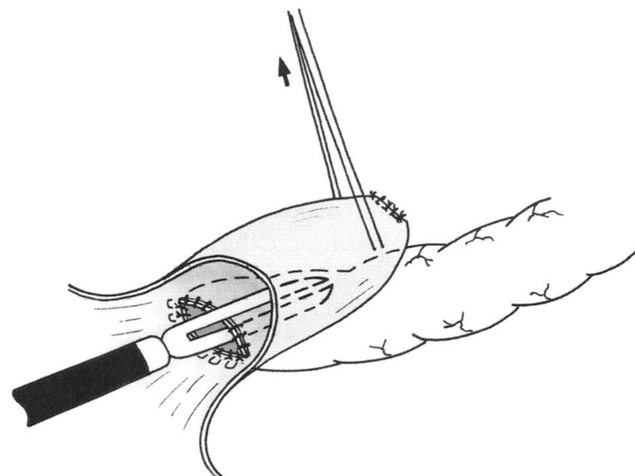

Figure 44B.6 *Stapler in position.*

The cannulae are removed under visual control and the fascia is closed by 4-0 absorbable sutures. Adhesive strips are used for skin closure.

POSTOPERATIVE CARE

The urinary catheter is removed 24–48 hours postoperatively. The rectal tube is gently irrigated with saline solution daily and removed after the first stool. Intravenous morphine infusion or epidural analgesia might be required for a day or two. Prophylactic antibiotics may be used for 24–48 hours. Oral feeds may be started at 48 hours postoperatively.

PROBLEMS, PITFALLS AND SOLUTIONS

There is a considerable learning curve for laparoscopic Duhamel technique, and experience with suturing and intracorporeal knotting is essential.

Difficult exposure

The following steps improve exposure.

- Appropriate positioning of the patient, surgeon and cannulae.
- Additional cannulae and instruments to retract and manipulate.
- Preoperative and on-table bowel preparation/ decompression.

- A urinary catheter.
- Moving telescope/instruments from one cannula to another.
- Changing the positions of the surgeon/assistants.
- Retracting bladder/uterus anterio-superiorly using instruments or percutaneous sutures.
- Percutaneously placed transfixation sutures to maintain/retract the position of the rectum.
- Meticulous technique and the avoidance of bleeding.

Bleeding

Bleeding from mesenteric or pararectal vessels is usually avoidable. Keep the dissector line close to the rectal/colon wall. Ultrasound shear, LigaSure™, or a sealing bipolar device greatly facilitates dissection and minimizes the risk of bleeding.

Problems with biopsies

The risks of inadequate or crushed specimens as well as of mucosal perforation are minimized using appropriate techniques and delicate 3 mm instruments.

High/total colonic aganglionosis

In this category of patients, the procedure may become time-consuming. Therefore consideration should be given to the following.

- Additional cannulae and instruments.
- Change of telescope/instruments from one cannula to another.
- Change of surgeon's position.
- The use of ultrasound shears/LigaSure™ or bipolar sealing device for dissection.
- A mini-laparotomy to supplement the initial laparoscopic approach.

Colostomy

A pre-existing colostomy does not preclude the laparoscopic approach. Minor modification to the position of the cannulae may be required. A stoma may be mobilized, re-fashioned or closed during the pull-through procedure.

COMPLICATIONS

Minor and/or serious complications during and after laparoscopic Duhamel pull-through are rare. As for the open technique, in the Duhamel pull-through operation the risks are reduced by appropriate technique and attention to details. Conversion to an open method must be considered in all difficult procedures.

- Bleeding.
- Leak from the suture/staple lines.
- Ischemia of the distal part of the pull-through colon.
- Rotation of the pull-through colon.
- Stenosis/rectal spur.
- Incontinence.
- Constipation.
- Residual aganglionosis.

FURTHER READING

Bax NMA, van der Zee DC. Laparoscopic removal of the aganglionic bowel according to Duhamel–Martin. In: Bax NMA, Georgeson KE, Najmaldin A, Valla JS (eds), *Endoscopic Surgery in Children.* Berlin: Springer, 1999.

de Lagausie P, Berrebi D, Geib G, Sebag G, Aigrain Y. Laparoscopic Duhamel procedure. Management of 30 cases. *Surgical Endoscopy* 1999; **13**:972–4.

Moog R, Becmeur F, Kauffmann-Chevalier I, Sauvage P. Minimally invasive surgery in the treatment of Hirschsprung disease. *Annales de Chirurgie* 2001; **126**:756–61.

Ure BM, Bax NM, van der Zee DC. Laparoscopy in infants and children: a prospective study on feasibility and the impact on routine surgery. *Journal of Pediatric Surgery* 2000; **35**:1170–3.

45

Intestinal resection and stoma formation

THOMAS H. INGE

INTRODUCTION

Although minimally invasive colorectal techniques have been incorporated into the practice of adult general surgery since the mid-twentieth century, it was not until the early 1990s that advanced laparoscopic colorectal surgery was routinely performed. Over the last decade, pediatric surgeons have also minimized access for intestinal surgery, and currently laparoscopically assisted total colectomy and partial intestinal resections are being performed routinely in children.

While the techniques described here can be adapted for many conditions, this chapter focuses specifically on laparoscopically assisted total colectomy with jejunal pouch reconstruction for ulcerative colitis, ileocolectomy for Crohn's stricture, and minimally invasive enterostomy. Further information may be obtained by referring to Chapters 44A and 44B.

EQUIPMENT/INSTRUMENTS

For children weighing more than 20–30 kg, 5 mm instrumentation is commonly used. For infants and toddlers weighing <20 kg, 3.5 mm instruments are most appropriate. The following lists include instruments that are essential and those that are optional for these advanced procedures in children.

Essential

- Telescope, 30°.
- Babcock grasper.
- Two atraumatic (Debakey-type) tissue graspers.
- Tissue scissors.
- Curved dissector.
- 'L'-hook dissector with electrocautery (diathermy).
- Suction/irrigator system.
- Needle driver.
- Ultrasonic (Harmonic®) scalpel.
- Endoscopic linear stapler.
- Bipolar electrocautery.

Optional

- LigaSure™ device with laparoscopic hand pieces.
- Radially expandable 5 mm short trocars.
- Endoscopic clip applicator.

LAPAROSCOPICALLY ASSISTED COLECTOMY

Indications for total colectomy

- Chronic ulcerative colitis.
- Total colonic aganglionosis.
- Familial adenomatous polyposis.

Contraindications for laparoscopic colectomy

ABSOLUTE

- Toxic megacolon (the patient is usually critically ill with dilated intestine increasing the chance for perforation with manipulation and impairing visualization).

- Severe, chronic dilatation of the colon (difficult to manipulate bowel and impaired visualization).
- Fulminant ulcerative colitis with hemodynamically significant intestinal hemorrhage.

RELATIVE

- Peritonitis.

If any of these conditions exist, conventional open subtotal colectomy with terminal ileostomy should be considered.

Preoperative preparation

When considering colectomy and continent reconstruction for ulcerative colitis, it is imperative that the surgeon be as certain as possible that the diagnosis of ulcerative colitis is correct, since 20 percent of patients with inflammatory bowel disease cannot be accurately classified and are given a diagnosis of indeterminate colitis. Patients with Crohn's disease (regional enteritis) generally do poorly after operations designed for the definitive treatment of ulcerative colitis. Routine testing prior to operation includes colonoscopy with biopsy to exclude skip lesions and ileal involvement that would be consistent with Crohn's disease. Esophago-gastro-duodenoscopy must also be performed to exclude granulomatous inflammation of the foregut, which would again be suspicious for Crohn's disease. Upper gastrointestinal contrast study with small bowel follow-through can demonstrate subtle signs of small bowel obstruction, strictures, fistulas and mucosal inflammation, which would also cast doubt on the diagnosis of ulcerative colitis. Finally, serologic testing to characterize the relative levels and isotypes of antineutrophil cytoplasmic antibody and anti-*Saccharomyces cerevisiae* antibody can be helpful in classifying patients with inflammatory bowel disease.

One of the most common indications for total colectomy in children is medically refractory ulcerative colitis. Bleeding, complications of immunosuppression (growth retardation, delayed puberty) and risk of subsequent carcinoma are also indications for operation. The operative techniques for the abdominal colectomy for ulcerative colitis are similar to those used for patients with total colonic Hirschsprung's disease, although reconstruction options differ and are covered elsewhere in this volume. Patients with total colonic Hirschsprung's disease also require downsizing of instrumentation, and 3 mm working ports are routine.

Laparoscopic total colectomy is considered an advanced procedure and can be technically demanding. For ulcerative colitis patients who are not undergoing operation on an urgent basis, elective total proctocolectomy with pouch reconstruction is often performed. When acute symptoms necessitate more urgent surgical treatment, total colectomy with temporary ileostomy can be done. When advanced laparoscopic procedures are carried out, families are always advised that conversion to open surgery is a possibility. As with open surgery, both mechanical and antibiotic preparations of the colon are needed prior to elective laparoscopic total colectomy. Polyethylene glycol solution (40 mL/kg over 6 hours, by mouth or nasogastric tube) is given on the day prior to surgery. Oral neomycin (20 mg/kg) and erythromycin base (20 mg/kg) are also administered on the day prior to operation at 1 p.m., 2 p.m. and 11 p.m. Finally, parenteral antibiotics and stress dose steroids are given immediately prior to operation.

Technique

GENERAL

The child with ulcerative colitis is positioned in the lithotomy position on the operating table, with the hips slightly flexed to avoid interference with the arc of the laparoscope. Special care is taken to ensure that the lateral aspect of the lower leg is well padded and that weight is distributed to the heel to prevent a peroneal nerve injury and calf muscle ischemia, respectively. Rigid sigmoidoscopy is performed to exclude active rectal mucosal ulceration. If active disease is seen in the rectum, this should be considered an indication for a staged approach. For total colectomy, the monitors are placed on opposite sides of the table. The monitors can be moved up towards the patient's shoulders or down towards the feet as the resection proceeds cranially or caudally, respectively. After induction of general anesthesia, a nasogastric tube is placed. A urinary catheter is inserted after the patient is draped. The presence of a prior diverting stoma is not a contraindication to laparoscopy; however, additional care will be needed for safe abdominal entry because of the risk of adhesions to the anterior abdominal wall.

COLONIC MOBILIZATION AND RESECTION

A 12 mm vertical midline incision is made into the depth of the umbilicus and the abdominal cavity is insufflated using either a Veress needle or open technique, according to the surgeon's preference. An intra-abdominal pressure of 15 mmHg is optimal for exposure in teenagers, while 10–12 mmHg is usually sufficient for younger children. A 12 mm radially expanding trocar is then placed in the umbilicus. Although conventional trocars provide adequate access, radially expandable trocars are most useful because they penetrate the abdominal wall as a low-profile sheathed needle that is subsequently dilated, decreasing abdominal wall trauma. In addition, because these trocars *expand within* the thin abdominal wall of children, they are held securely in the tissue and do not tend to move with instrument insertion and removal.

Four 5 mm trocars are placed into the abdomen in the right and left upper and right and left lower quadrants at the edge of the rectus muscle. The right lower quadrant trocar should be properly positioned between the umbilicus and the anterior superior iliac spine in case this trocar

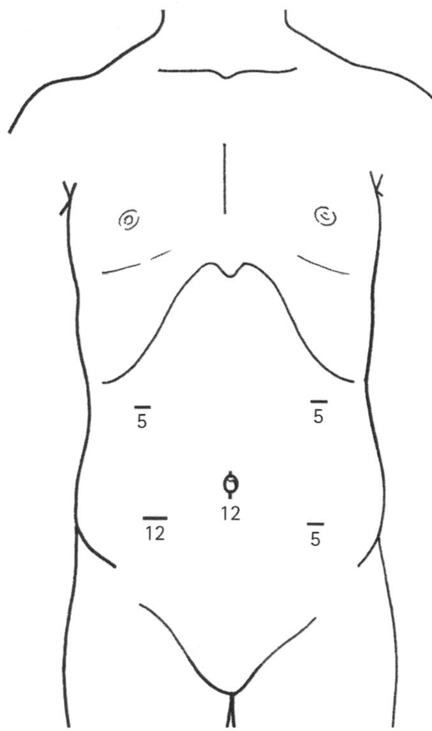

Figure 45.1

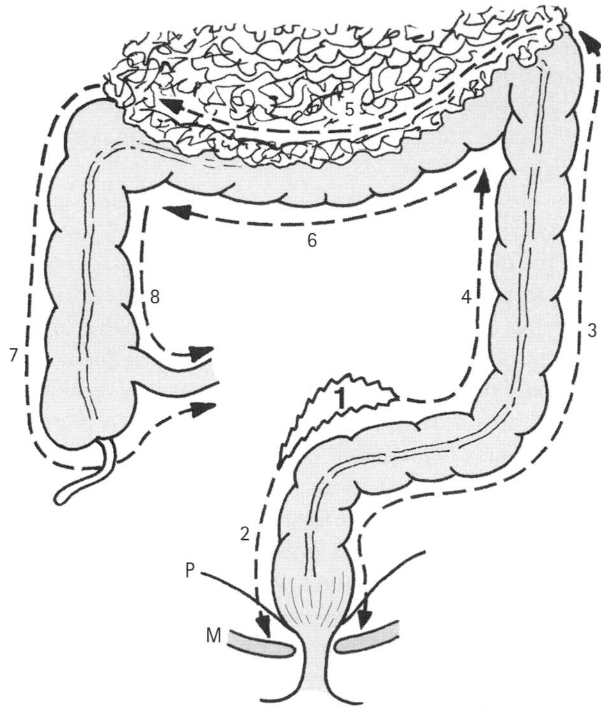

Figure 45.2

needs to be enlarged for the creation of a diverting ileostomy. **(See Figure 45.1)**

The operation begins with a careful general exploration of the abdominal cavity, with particular emphasis on excluding ileal inflammation which would be indicative of Crohn's disease. The colectomy commences in the pelvis with an entry into the mesentery near the recto-sigmoid junction. Hook electrocautery or the ultrasonic scalpel is used. This dissection is primarily postero-lateral to the bowel and can be carried distally almost to the level of the levators. The further one proceeds with this dissection, the easier and faster the subsequent dissection from the perineum. This is usually an avascular plane that can be exploited with ease. The plane is deliberately kept close to the bowel wall, as it is preferable to risk injury to the bowel (which will be removed as specimen) rather than to surrounding pelvic structures. The surrounding structures that it is most important to avoid are the pelvic autonomic nerve supply, vas deferens, posterior urethra and prostate in males, vagina and adnexal structures in females, ureters and iliac vessels. For benign pediatric conditions, the general principle of staying close to the bowel should be followed throughout the procedure. The establishment of good exposure posterior and lateral to the rectum also makes it much safer to perform the more hazardous anterior portion of the dissection. The endpoint of the dissection anteriorly is the prostate in the male and the cervix in the female. An additional disposable instrument, the bipolar coagulating shears, is sometimes useful for this pelvic dissection. The bipolar shears further reduce the risk of cautery injury to adjacent structures.

Next, the mesenteric dissection continues proximally, with the surgeon reducing the risk of bleeding by staying near the sigmoid colon where vessels are of smaller caliber. In addition, this technique maximizes the distance between the dissection plane and the left ureter below. 'Gravitational retraction' of small bowel is accomplished by rotating the operating table rightward during dissection of the left colon, and later leftward during dissection of the right colon. The fusion fascia (white line of Toldt) of the left colon is opened up to the splenic flexure. This maneuver frees the left colon from the lateral abdominal wall, allowing inspection of the mesentery. Next, the mesentery is readily divided. The LigaSure™ device allows for rapid progress in the mesentery with satisfactory hemostasis. Occasionally, larger vessels may require surgical clips prior to division. If difficulty is encountered dissecting the splenic flexure, it may be helpful to proceed more proximally to mobilize the transverse colon; the mesenteric dissection can then proceed from both directions towards the splenic flexure. **(See Figure 45.2)**

The patient is placed into the reverse Trendelenburg position and the omentum is reflected cephalad to expose the transverse colon. This position gives maximal exposure of the transverse colon by gravitational retraction of the small bowel into the pelvis. The omentum is usually preserved with its gastric blood supply intact by elevating the omental apron and dividing the colonic attachments. To perform this maneuver, the assistant retracts superio-anteriorly on the omentum while the surgeon retracts infero-posteriorly on the colon. The gastrocolic ligament is thus exposed and divided from left to right. During the course of this dissection, the camera is rotated to the port site that most conveniently places the telescope between the surgeon's left-hand and right-hand ports.

The dissection continues around the hepatic flexure, taking care to remain near the colon wall at all times to avoid the duodenum below. The white fusion fascia of the right colon is opened next and the colon is rotated medially to free the mesentery from the underlying retroperitoneal structures. This is usually an avascular plane. The mesenteric division continues towards the ileo-cecal junction. At this point, if immediate pull-through is planned, the ileal pouch is prepared.

If a staged reconstruction is planned, an endoscopic linear stapler is used to divide the rectum distally in the pelvis. The endoscopic stapler is introduced through the right lower quadrant port (12 mm). The small size of the pediatric pelvis and the relatively large stapler dictate a necessarily oblique line of transection of the rectum. The colectomy specimen can then be delivered intact by enlarging the right lower quadrant port site. The bowel is transected at the ileum and a final inspection is made to ensure that the mesentery is not rotated. Standard techniques for Brook ileostomy are used.

PREPARATION OF THE TERMINAL ILEUM

The terminal ileum can be brought down to the anus as a straight-pipe ileo-anal reconstruction, or folded upon itself into a J-pouch configuration, depending on the surgeon's preference. The J-pouch serves to arrest small bowel peristalsis and, secondarily, functions as a small fecal reservoir to limit the number of evacuations per day. The ileal J-pouch can be constructed using an extracorporeal mini-laparotomy technique or by using an intracorporeal, transanal stapled technique. Many surgeons consider the extracorporeal technique to be the most straightforward method. After completion of the laparoscopic colectomy, a 5–7 cm suprapubic transverse mini-laparotomy is performed. Ideally, this incision is positioned so low that care must be taken to avoid injury to the bladder, which can be easily accomplished using laparoscopic guidance. Through this mini-laparotomy, the terminal ileum is further mobilized by dividing the posterior peritoneal attachments that tether the ileum down in the right lower quadrant. The terminal ileum is exteriorized through the mini-laparotomy and divided just proximal to the ileo-cecal valve using a linear stapler. Folding the terminal ileum on itself and tacking it into place using anti-mesenteric approximation stitches then creates the 8–10 cm J-loop. An enterotomy is made in the loop and a 45 mm or 60 mm endoscopic stapler is inserted from proximal to distal and fired. An alternative technique is to perform an enterotomy into the apex of the loop at this point, and insert the stapling device distally to proximally to divide the opposing bowel walls. A common cavity, or pouch, is thus created. The endoscopic device is preferred for pouch creation because it has a smaller external profile and thus can easily be manipulated into the lumen of a child's small bowel. In addition, the endoscopic stapler approximates tissue using three rows of staples on either side of the cutting blade rather than the two rows that are seen with standard staplers used for open surgery. As usual, care is taken to resect any blind end of terminal ileum beyond the pouch cavity to avoid a potential area of fecal stasis. (**See Figure 45.3**)

It is critical that the ileal mesentery be adequately mobile to allow the pouch to reach the pelvis without tension. Through the suprapubic mini-laparotomy, proximal mesenteric dissection must be performed as proximal as possible under direct vision. Traction sutures placed in the apex of the loop can provide tension on the mesentery during this mobilization, and can later be used for positioning the pouch for ileo-anal anastomosis. The mesenteric mobilization can be difficult because of the limited exposure provided by the suprapubic laparotomy. However, further *laparoscopic* mobilization of the ileal mesentery can be achieved after mini-laparotomy. The extracorporeal ileal pouch can actually be used to 'plug' the mini-laparotomy defect to prevent gas leakage during re-insufflation. After re-establishment of pneumoperitoneum, the anterior abdominal wall is raised, effectively stretching out and thinning

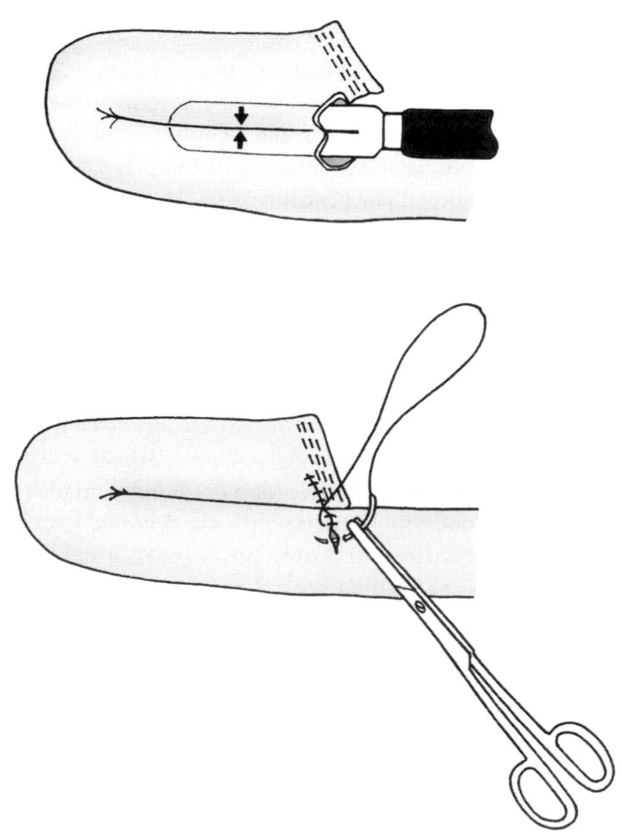

Figure 45.3

the ileal mesentery within. This additional retraction and exposure aids the surgeon by allowing a more precise laparoscopic dissection of the mesentery cephalad towards the duodenum and origin of the superior mesenteric artery, thereby gaining length to permit a tension-free transfer of the J-pouch to the pelvic floor.

PERINEAL DISSECTION AND ILEO-ANAL ANASTOMOSIS

Whether the pouch construction is performed extracorporeally or intracorporeally, definitive reconstruction after total colectomy requires that the ileal pouch be brought through the pelvic floor and anal sphincter complex. This is accomplished using an endorectal mucosectomy from the perineum, which allows removal of the entire colon specimen transanally. The ileum is brought through the rectal muscle sleeve and the ileo-anal anastomosis is fashioned. This technique is a safe option since the genitourinary structures and pelvic autonomic nerves are not directly in jeopardy with this plane of dissection. The technique can be applied in infants as well as in adolescents.

The legs are raised to expose the perineum. For optimal exposure, circumferential traction sutures are placed to evert the mucocutaneous junction of the anus. Alternatively, the Lone Star retractor can be used for this purpose. Fine-needle-tipped cautery is used to develop a submucosal plane, beginning 0.5–1 cm above the dentate line. This plane is carefully followed proximally until the plane of the laparoscopic rectal dissection is reached, at which point prolapse of the devascularized, pale rectal wall occurs. The muscle sleeve is then divided circumferentially, leaving the mucosal lining in continuity with the colectomy specimen above. **(See Figure 45.4)**

The colectomy specimen is pulled through the pelvis and out of the body. The pouch is brought down into the pelvis and the surgeon ensures that no twisting of the mesentery has occurred. The ano-rectal anastomosis is fashioned using circumferential 3-0 absorbable sutures. If the pouch was completely created extracorporeally, the procedure is completed by closure of the mini-laparotomy. If there remains any common wall within the center of the pouch at this point, transanal application of a linear stapler is used to complete the pouch. A decision about whether to perform a temporary protective loop ileostomy is made by assessing the blood supply to the pouch, the degree of tension and proctitis, corticosteroid use, and the patient's general medical and nutritional condition. Many surgeons routinely perform a diversion to protect the pouch and anastomosis from leakage. **(See Figure 45.5)**

Postoperatively, a nasogastric tube is left in place until there is evidence of gas and stool in the ileostomy bag. Stress dose steroids are maintained for 48 hours and tapered rapidly thereafter. A contrast study of the pouch is done through the distal loop of the ileostomy after 6 weeks to exclude leak or stricture and ensure adequate pouch emptying prior to ileostomy reversal.

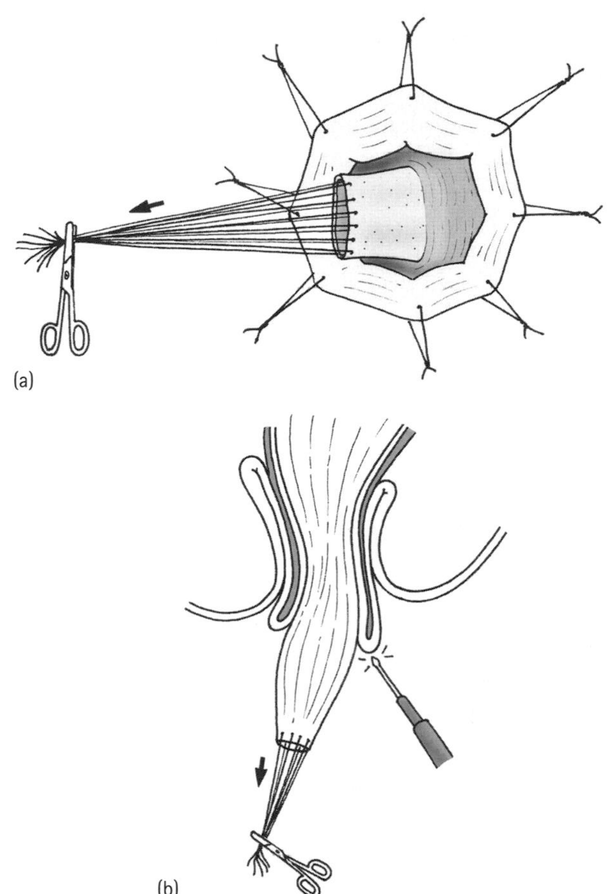

Figure 45.4 *(a) Traction on the mucosal sleeve and a submucosal plane is developing; (b) the rectal muscle sleeve is divided (see also Chapter 44A).*

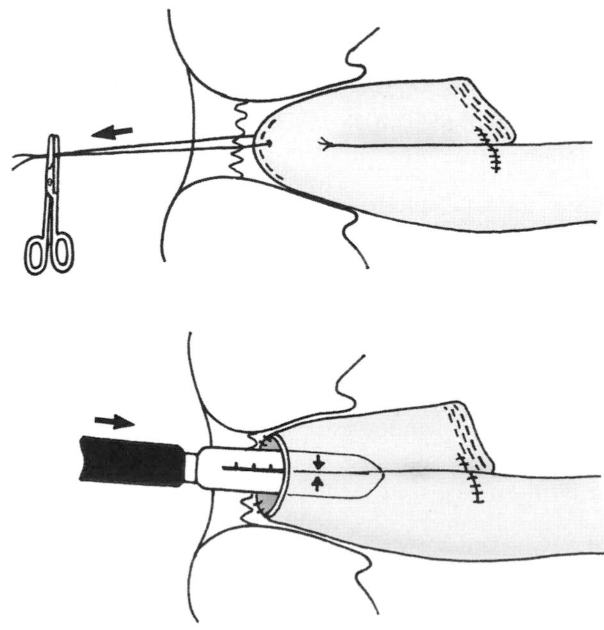

Figure 45.5

ILEOSTOMY FORMATION

Loop ileostomy to protect an ileo-anal reconstruction can be performed at the conclusion of the procedure. Provided the right lower quadrant trocar site was placed a suitable distance from the iliac crest, the site can be enlarged somewhat and a proximal ileal loop readily exteriorized for stoma formation. For other patients who need ileal diversion (e.g. perineal septic complications of Crohn's disease or trauma), an appropriate ileostomy site can be marked preoperatively. A laparoscope is placed into an umbilical trocar site and a right lower quadrant Babcock grasper can be used to grasp an ileal loop. This grasper, trocar and bowel are exteriorized together, and the wound is enlarged as needed for ileostomy.

Problems, pitfalls and solutions

VISUALIZATION

Adequate visualization is the key to safe and efficient laparoscopic surgery. Significant improvements in visualization can often be afforded simply by changing the position of the table to take best advantage of gravity to expose the area of surgical interest. In addition, when difficulties arise with visualization or interference between instruments, additional port placement should always be considered before tolerating suboptimal conditions. For the pelvic dissection, the bladder and uterus may need to be manipulated for proper exposure. Even though the bladder has been evacuated, it may be necessary to retract it up and out of the way for the pelvic dissection. This is readily accomplished by placing a suture on a large curved needle through the abdominal wall at the suprapubic position. A portion of bladder wall is then incorporated and the needle is passed out of abdominal wall, where the suture is tied. The uterus can be similarly retracted if necessary.

MESENTERIC DISSECTION

The mesenteric dissection is certainly the most tedious portion of the total colectomy and numerous challenges can emerge. Mesenteric hemorrhage can be a significant problem. In addition to LigaSure™ use, traditional bipolar electrocautery can be helpful to control point bleeding. Surgical clips may be used for large vessels as well. If there is difficulty with visualization of the colonic mesentery, colonic mobilization or ileal mesenteric mobilization, another adjunctive technique is hand-assisted laparoscopy. This procedure is especially well suited for a hand-assisted technique since the port can be placed in the suprapubic mini-laparotomy that will subsequently be used for J-pouch construction.

PELVIC CONSIDERATIONS

Distal mobilization of the rectum can be tedious and there is considerable risk of injury to surrounding structures in the tight space of the pelvis. The key to safe dissection is to remember that posterior to the bowel there is far less risk of injury since the important structures are largely anterior to the rectum. If the plane is first developed posteriorly and then laterally, using blunt and careful cautery dissection, the procedure will be successful. In the male, increased vascularity will be encountered near the prostate anteriorly, and dissection should cease as the prostate is approached. In small children, the pelvic cavity is too small to accommodate the 12 mm endoscopic stapler and therefore rectal transection may take place as low as possible.

Once the ileo-anal anastomosis has been fashioned, the mesentery should again be inspected from above to ensure that there is no twist that may compromise the blood supply. Also, if undue tension is apparent, the mesentery can again be released as needed before closure of the abdomen.

PARTIAL INTESTINAL RESECTION

Indications

- Ileal stricture in Crohn's disease.
- Meckel's diverticulum.
- Intussusception.
- Intestinal duplications.
- Colonic or small bowel stricture after enterocolitis.
- Severe chronic constipation.
- Mesenteric cysts.
- Intestinal lymphangioma.
- Intestinal web.
- Congenital stricture.

Contraindications

- Lack of peritoneal cavity (prior peritonitis and adhesion formation).
- Significant abdominal distension due to bowel obstruction (obscures visualization).
- Inability adequately to mobilize the bowel and mesentery.

Preoperative preparation

There are far more pediatric indications for partial intestinal resection than for total colectomy. When planning a minimally invasive operative procedure, it is important to have a complete understanding of the extent and severity of the intra-abdominal pathology so that errors can be avoided during surgery. There are several relative contraindications to minimally invasive bowel resection, most of which require initial laparoscopic exploration for complete assessment. Open conversion should be considered if there is lack of an adequate peritoneal cavity (prior massive peritonitis with adhesion formation and obliteration of the cavity), inability to visualize the pathology adequately due to the dilated intestinal loops in patients with bowel obstruction, and inability to mobilize the intestine or mesentery safely (avoiding peritoneal contamination and injury to adjacent structures). It is also important to consider how the anastomosis will be fashioned (intracorporeal or extracorporeal). This decision requires consideration of patient factors as well as skill on behalf of the surgeon. Since resectional procedures usually require enlargement of a port site for specimen removal, an extracorporeal anastomosis may well be the most efficient technique to use, especially in the smaller patient with a thin abdominal wall. In older patients with thicker abdominal walls, extracorporeal anastomosis might require a larger laparotomy, and therefore intracorporeal anastomosis may be the best choice.

Ileal stricture associated with Crohn's disease is an ideal indication for laparoscopic partial bowel resection. Indeed, Milsom and colleagues demonstrated more rapid improvement in pulmonary function and shorter recovery times for patients who underwent laparoscopic compared to open ileo-colic surgery. The preoperative work-up includes contrast study of the gastrointestinal tract to exclude other pathology before isolated resection is undertaken. In addition, contrast-enhanced computerized tomography (CT) scan of the abdomen and pelvis can be very useful for determining the relationship between the ileal stricture and the right ureter. A large inflammatory mass from prior ileal perforation impinging on the ureter would lower the threshold for performing an open laparotomy. Preoperative percutaneous drainage of a right lower quadrant abscess may also be of benefit. To reduce the risk of infectious complications, preoperative mechanical and antibiotic bowel preparation is indicated, as described above. If stricture is so severe that bowel preparation cannot be adequately performed, or unexpected purulence is encountered during the dissection, or the patient is on high doses of corticosteroids at the time of operation, diversion with a loop ileostomy at the conclusion of the procedure should be considered. Parenteral antibiotics are administered immediately prior to operation. For patients who are taking long-term corticosteroids, stress dose corticosteroids are also administered parenterally prior to operation.

Technique

The stomach and urinary bladder are decompressed. The patient is positioned supine and secured to the table. The video monitor is placed to the patient's right, and the surgeon stands to the left of the patient's abdomen, while the assistant stands to the left of the patient's chest. Port placement is similar to that used for appendectomy: umbilical 12 mm (surgeon's right hand), left lower quadrant 5 mm (scope), suprapubic 5 mm (surgeon's left hand), and a fourth

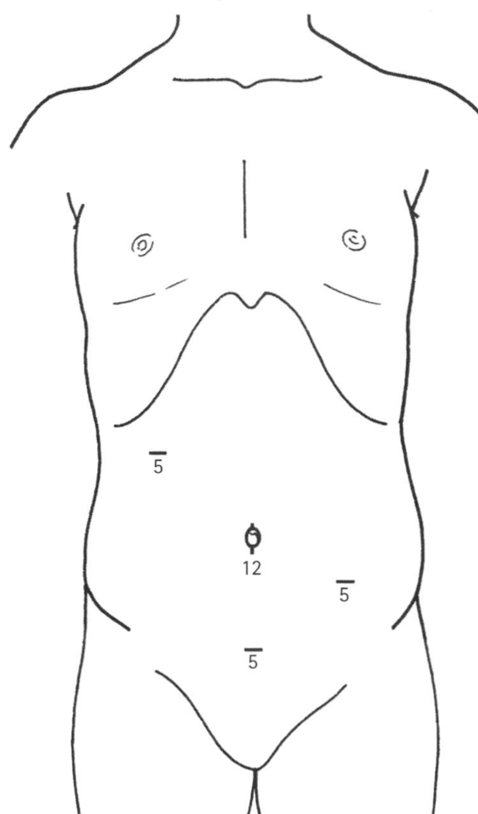

Figure 45.6

5 mm site in the upper abdomen (assistant's grasper). **(See Figure 45.6)**

Any adhesions in the right lower quadrant are divided using hook cautery or ultrasonic scalpel dissection. The omentum is manipulated away from the ileo-cecal region and placed into the epigastrium. The small intestine is examined from ileum to duodeno-jejunal flexure to exclude other sites of active disease. Terminal ileal strictures and the associated fibrosis usually require ileo-cecal resection to remove the grossly diseased bowel. To mobilize the right colon, the cecum is retracted medially with an atraumatic grasper and the white fusion fascia is divided using the ultrasonic scalpel (or scissors/hook cautery). The entire right colon is mobilized up to the hepatic flexure, taking care to avoid injury to the underlying duodenum. Next, the ileum is mobilized enough to identify the ileal mesentery accurately. A soft, relatively normal-appearing area of ileum is identified proximal to the fibrotic, strictured bowel and a 45 mm or 60 mm endoscopic stapler is applied to the ileum in a soft area of bowel just proximal to the stricture. The stapler is clamped for a 10-second count prior to dividing the bowel to ensure maximal hemostasis. Next, a suitable area for division of the right colon distal to the stricture is identified, and the mesentery is divided toward this target region. The ileo-colic mesentery can be foreshortened due to prior inflammation, thus a slow, deliberate dissection is needed to avoid bleeding. In addition, care is taken to stay adjacent to the bowel wall, which reduces the risk of injury to the right ureter. For this dissection, often the ultrasonic scalpel will suffice, but the LigaSure™ can also be used. Although an endoscopic stapler can also be used, it may be a more costly option.

INTRACORPOREAL ANASTOMOSIS

Once the colon is transected, the specimen is placed to the side and the anastomosis is performed. The ileum is juxtaposed to the right colon with two 3-0 absorbable sutures. These tacking sutures approximate the transected ends and the anti-mesenteric borders 3 cm from each end to facilitate introduction of the stapler. Opposing enterotomies are made near the staple lines using an ultrasonic scalpel (or scissors with cautery), and the opening is enlarged by gentle spreading with a grasper. A 45 mm endoscopic stapler is used for the anastomosis. The enterotomy is closed using a single-layer running absorbable suture. The mesenteric defect is closed with permanent suture to prevent internal herniation. The specimen is removed by enlarging the umbilical port site to 3–4 cm. Fascia and skin are then closed at the umbilical site, and skin alone is closed at the other 5 mm sites. **(See Figure 45.7)**

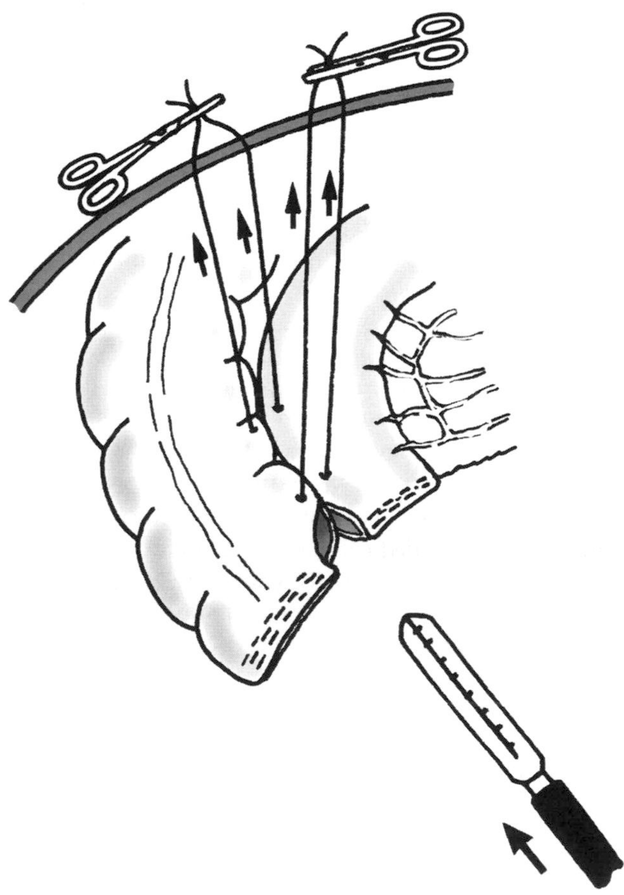

Figure 45.7

EXTRACORPOREAL TECHNIQUE

The procedure outlined above is an advanced laparoscopic technique. Many of the benefits of laparoscopy can also be realized using the laparoscopically assisted method, provided the bowel and mesentery are not particularly edematous or thickened. Once the right colon and terminal ileum are mobilized, the ileum is delivered through a 4–5 cm mini-laparotomy at the umbilical trocar site. The stricture and more distal bowel can be manipulated up and exteriorized until a loop containing the stricture is free. The remainder of the operation, including mesenteric and bowel transection and ileo-colic anastomosis, can be performed using traditional open techniques. Once the fascia is closed, the umbilicus is easily reconstructed.

UMBILICAL CLOSURE

Some surgeons deliberately avoid making an incision through the umbilicus because of concern for cosmesis and/or wound complication. In reality, there is a cosmetic *advantage* if a midline skin incision centered in the umbilicus is used, and complications can be avoided by meticulous skin closure. Umbilical port site infections are rare due to a paucity of fat in the midline cicatrix between the skin and fascia at the umbilicus. For closure, no attempt is made to perform more difficult subcuticular techniques that can result in umbilical granuloma formation. Rather, the skin incision is closed using simple, interrupted, fast-absorbing suture material (e.g. 4-0 Vicryl Rapide® or plain gut).

In most patients, the nasogastric tube can be removed on the morning after the operation, and oral intake can commence once gastrointestinal function has returned.

Problems, pitfalls and solutions

CONTAMINATION

If intracorporeal anastomosis has been selected, there is a risk of intra-abdominal contamination due to the enterotomies that are made. This contamination can be minimized by setting up the anastomosis with stay sutures such that the assistant's port can be utilized for suction rather than presenting or manipulating bowel.

BLEEDING

The stapled anastomosis is always at risk of *intraluminal* staple line hemorrhage, which can go unnoticed intraoperatively. To reduce the risk of staple line bleeding, the endoscopic staplers should be clamped down on the tissue for a full 10-second count prior to activating the cutting blade. If bleeding is noted within the bowel lumen at the staple line, this can often be controlled with either bipolar cautery or a surgical clip.

PROBLEMS OF SPECIMEN DELIVERY

Specimen delivery can represent a challenge at the conclusion of the procedure. Due to the visual complexity of the umbilicus, a reasonably significant incision can be obscured in this region. A size discrepancy between the specimen and the umbilical defect can easily be corrected by placement of a probe and groove into this port site after removal of the trocar. With a No. 11 blade, the fascia and skin are opened simultaneously superiorly and inferiorly until the specimen can be delivered. Since the blade follows the groove, there is no risk of injury to bowel below.

Some patients undergoing partial intestinal resections may be too small for application of the linear stapler. In these patients, the surgeon will either need to exteriorize the bowel ends for extracorporeal anastomosis or will need to be able to perform intracorporeal hand-sewn anastomosis to restore intestinal continuity.

COLOSTOMY FORMATION

Indications

- High imperforate anus.
- Hirschsprung's disease.
- Peri-anal complications of Crohn's disease.
- Fecal diversion for severe peri-anal sepsis or peri-anal/rectal trauma.

Contraindications

- Tense abdominal distension.
- Systemic toxicity.
- Severely dilated colon that obscures laparoscopic visualization and bowel manipulation.

Conventional open sigmoid colostomy is usually performed through a small left lower quadrant exploratory laparotomy through which the bowel is subsequently exteriorized. Occasionally, difficulties can be encountered with accurate identification of the appropriate segment of colon for stoma formation. This problem is commonly solved by further enlarging the incision. The major advantage of laparoscopic colostomy is that it affords visualization of the entire hindgut superior to that of the open technique without the abdominal wall wounds having to be any larger than is necessary for the stoma itself. Confirmation of the proximal/distal orientation of the colon is simplified, and there is a reduced risk of wound complications (dehiscence and infection) since the wounds are smaller. Finally, leveling biopsies and colostomy can also be performed for patients with Hirschsprung's disease who are not candidates for a one-stage operation. **(See Figure 45.8)**

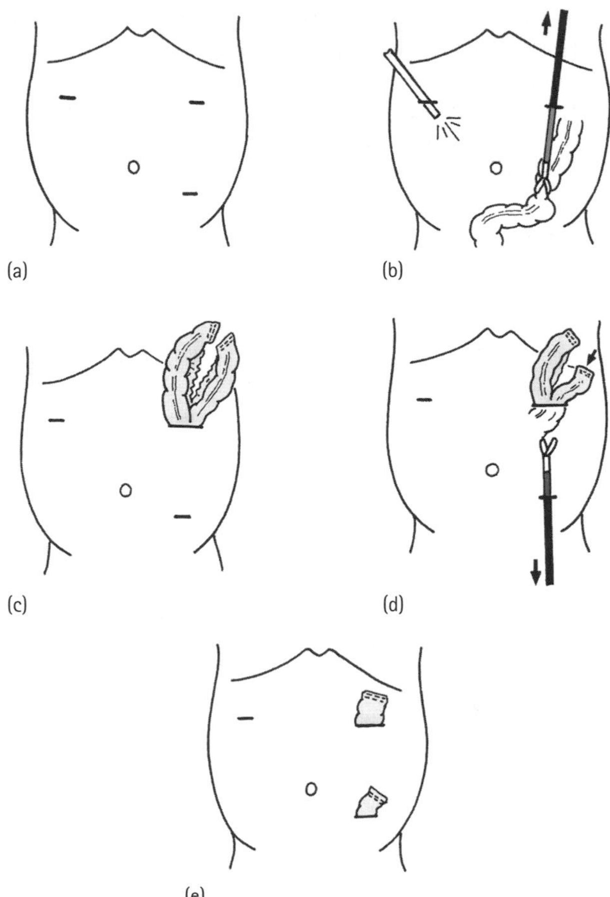

Figure 45.8

Technique

A technique for completely diverting colostomy for high imperforate anus is described to illustrate the principles of this procedure. Preoperatively, sites for the active stoma in the left upper quadrant and mucus fistula in the left lower quadrant are marked. A 4 mm or 5 mm trocar is placed in the right upper quadrant site, a 10 mm trocar at the left upper quadrant site, and a 5 mm trocar is used in the left lower quadrant site. After laparoscopic exploration is performed through the right upper quadrant telescope, bowel segments for a divided colostomy are chosen. The proximal sigmoid colon is engaged with an atraumatic bowel grasper inserted through the left upper quadrant site. The instrument, trocar and 4–5 cm loop of sigmoid colon are exteriorized as a unit. Next, a mesenteric defect is created externally and a 30 mm endoscopic stapler is used to divide the bowel extracorporeally. Using cautery, the mesenteric defect is enlarged appropriately and the distal end is gently replaced into the peritoneal cavity.

The abdomen is re-insufflated and a grasper is inserted into the left lower quadrant trocar site to grasp the stapled end of the Hartmann's pouch. This end is then partially exteriorized through the left lower quadrant trocar site.

If a 5 mm trocar was used at this site, only a corner of the staple line will exteriorize, due to size discrepancy. The pneumoperitoneum is next evacuated and the right upper quadrant trocar is removed. The bowel at each site is secured by circumferentially approximating fascia to the seromuscular intestinal wall using fine absorbable suture. The staple line is then opened and the stomas are matured in the usual fashion. If a loop sigmoid colostomy is desired, the 10 mm trocar can be placed in the left lower quadrant site, which can then be enlarged as needed for convenient exteriorization of the sigmoid loop.

Problems, pitfalls and solutions

Distended loops of bowel may obscure adequate visualization. In this case, the right upper quadrant trocar site may need to be positioned (or repositioned) closer to the midline. In addition, for patients with a patent anus, rectal irrigation can be considered if abdominal distension is noted.

Thickened or distended bowel may be difficult to externalize through the trocar sites. In this event, the port sites may need to be enlarged using a spreading force from an external hemostat or using external cautery.

Complications

HEMORRHAGE

To perform advanced laparoscopic procedures safely, the surgeon must be familiar with numerous hemostatic techniques, including the use of the energy devices described throughout this chapter. In addition, there are other important considerations and techniques. Knowledge of the major vascular supply of the bowel allows the surgeon to prevent major bleeding by preparing for major vessel control prior to transection. However, if rapid hemorrhage is encountered, it is rare that it cannot be controlled by the quick application of a curved dissector (clamp) to occlude the vessel while a definitive control strategy is contemplated and enacted. That definitive strategy may be the introduction of another well-placed trocar if needed for additional exposure or suction. Bipolar cautery can then be used effectively. Surgical clips and Endoloops® can also be helpful to control bleeding, depending on the length of exposed vessel that is available. For bleeding that is difficult to pinpoint, a valuable technique is to introduce a gauze sponge into the abdomen (10 mm trocar site) to localize bleeding as in an open procedure. A sponge can also be used to pack-off an area of oozing temporarily. Finally, if hemorrhage cannot be controlled laparoscopically, the sponge can be grasped and used to apply pressure to an area of bleeding to limit blood loss as the surgeon converts to open laparotomy.

ANASTOMOTIC LEAK

To prevent delayed recognition of an anastomotic leak, it is helpful to 'test' the anastomosis before completion of the procedure. This can easily be done by placing the anastomosis under saline and compressing the bowel proximally and distally to rule out an air leak. Any bubbles from the anastomosis can be identified and the leak controlled directly with interrupted sutures placed laparoscopically.

INJURY TO INTRA-ABOMINAL AND PELVIC STRUCTURES

During laparoscopic intestinal surgery, the risk of injury to the duodenum, ureters, iliac vessels, vas deferens, prostate, nervi ergentes, vagina, urethra and small bowel is clearly a concern. Recognition of the usual anatomic relationships between the specimen bowel and these structures is crucial. Adequate visualization and meticulous dissection close to the bowel wall are needed to avoid inadvertent injury.

COLOSTOMY PROLAPSE

A major problem after colostomy formation is stoma prolapse. To prevent this, the portion of the sigmoid chosen for exteriorization is proximal, near the descending/sigmoid junction. In this way, the fixation of the descending colon to the abdominal wall reduces the ability of the bowel to prolapse through the fascia, and laparoscopic suture fixation to the inner abdominal wall is not usually required.

FURTHER READING

Beals DA, Georgeson KE. Laparoscopic total colectomy. In: Bax NMA, Georgeson KE, Najmaldin A, Valla J-S (eds), *Endoscopic Surgery in Children.* Berlin: Springer, 1999, 254–60.

Diamond IR, Langer JC. Laparoscopic-assisted versus open ileocolic resection for adolescent Crohn disease. *Journal of Pediatric Gastroenterology and Nutrition* 2001; **33**:543–7.

Georgeson KE. Laparoscopic-assisted total colectomy with pouch reconstruction. *Seminars in Pediatric Surgery* 2002; **11**:233–6.

Milsom JW, Hammerhofer KA, Bohm B, Marcello P, Elson P, Fazio VW. Prospective, randomized trial comparing laparoscopic vs. conventional surgery for refractory ileocolic Crohn's disease. *Diseases of the Colon and Rectum* 2001; **44**:1–8.

Rothenberg SS. Laparoscopic segmental intestinal resection. *Seminars in Pediatric Surgery* 2002; **11**:211–16.

46

Inguinal hernia

FELIX SCHIER

INTRODUCTION

The basic step of inguinal hernia surgery in children is ligation of the hernia sac at the internal inguinal ring. In a conventional open inguinal herniotomy the sac is identified in the inguinal canal through an incision on the abdominal wall. With the laparoscopic approach, the neck of the sac is identified from within the peritoneal cavity at the internal ring. The laparoscopic approach is a logical procedure that allows precise definition of the anatomy and precise suture placement to close the internal inguinal ring.

Indications

- Unilateral or bilateral indirect inguinal hernias.
- Doubt about the contralateral side.
- Doubt about the type of hernia (indirect, direct, femoral).
- Recurrence following previous open or laparoscopic surgery.
- Suspected other intra-abdominal pathology.

Contraindications

- Massive bowel dilatation.
- Children weighing <1500 g with short anatomical distance between the umbilicus and inner inguinal ring or otherwise limited abdominal cavity space which makes access and instrument manipulation difficult.
- Anesthesiologic concerns relating to CO_2 insufflation.

Advantages

- Leaves the cord structures untouched. This eliminates the risk of iatrogenic testicular ascent.
- Reduced risk of testicular atrophy and vas injury, particularly in recurrent hernias.
- Technically simple in experienced hands.
- The risk of missing an uncommon direct or femoral hernia is reduced because the type of hernia is clearly defined with the laparoscopic view.
- Inspection of the internal genitalia in girls to exclude testicular feminization syndrome.
- Incarcerated hernias can be reduced under direct vision with simultaneous inspection of bowel for signs of ischemia. Immediate repair of the hernia is then possible.
- Reduced risk of bladder injury.

Disadvantages

- Cannot be performed under regional anesthesia.
- Trocar placement in small children requires practice.
- Requires skill in laparoscopic suturing and instrument manipulation within a confined space.
- Slightly higher recurrence rate (3.5 percent compared to 1–2 percent), especially for direct and femoral hernias.

EQUIPMENT/INSTRUMENTS

- 5 mm trocar and 5 mm 0° laparoscope (to be inserted at the umbilicus).
- Two 2 mm working trocars (to be inserted at the left and right middle abdomen).

- Two 2 mm needle drivers.
- 2 mm scissors.
- 4-0 non-absorbable monofilament suture (cut to a length of 7 cm), for closure of the inner inguinal ring. A cutting needle is preferred because this is less likely to slip in the needle driver during intracorporeal suturing.
- 4-0 absorbable suture to repair the site of the primary port at the umbilicus.
- Steristrips® for the skin.

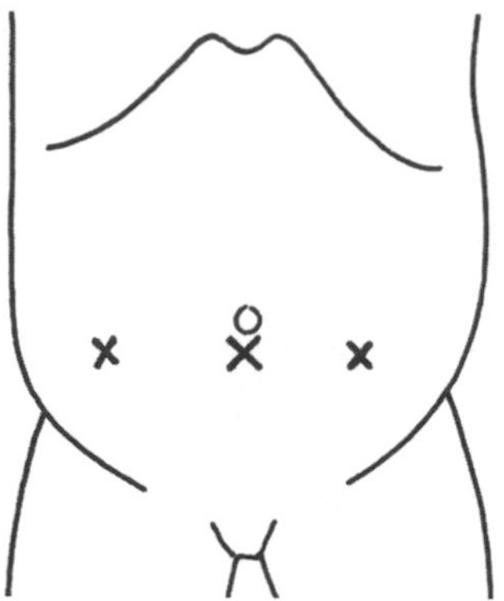

Figure 46.1

PREOPERATIVE PREPARATION

Older children should be instructed to empty their bladder prior to surgery. If this is not possible, the bladder should be expressed prior to insertion of the ports. A urinary catheter is rarely required.

Monitors and equipment should be located in the operating room in such a way that the surgeon has unimpeded access to both sides of the patient if necessary.

TECHNIQUE

General anesthesia with endotracheal intubation is essential. A nasogastric tube may be inserted. A urinary catheter is rarely required.

An infra-umbilical skin incision is the preferred entry site for the Veress needle and the primary cannula because this is simple to close at the end of surgery. A pneumoperitoneum is created with CO_2 at a flow rate of 0.4 L/min and a maximum pressure of 12 mmHg. Two additional 2 mm trocars are placed, one on either side of the primary cannula. The surgeon stands on the opposite side of the patient from the hernia (and changes side during surgery for bilateral herniotomies). **(See Figure 46.1)**

The needle of the suture is inserted directly through the skin near the deep inguinal ring and grasped from inside. We use a 4-0 monofilament non-absorbable suture attached to a cutting needle, because the cutting needle is less likely to slip in the jaws of the needle driver. The suture is cut to 7 cm in length, which facilitates closure of the internal ring and intracorporeal knot tying. Closure of the internal ring is simplified if two needle drivers are used. A needle driver with a ratcheted handle is held in the dominant hand and one without a ratchet in the non-dominant hand.

A single N-shaped suture is used to ligate the hernia sac at its neck. The suture bites should include peritoneum and some underlying connective tissue at the deep ring (transversalis fascia). Care must be taken not to injure vas or vessels. Incising the peritoneum is probably unnecessary. **(See Figure 46.2)**

There are no technical differences between girls and boys, although absence of the vas and vessels simplifies the procedure. In older children (>10 years) closure of the deep inguinal ring can be difficult. Lowering the intra-abdominal pressure by partial evacuation of the pneumoperitoneum and applying external pressure over the deep ring with a finger will both aid suture tightening.

In bilateral hernias after completion of the first side repair, the suture is left uncut with the needle attached inside the peritoneal cavity. The second side is then repaired with a second suture. Following repair of both sides, both sutures are grasped in a needle driver and trimmed. Finally the suture ends and both needles are removed together with one of the 2 mm trocars. Alternatively, a single suture 12 cm in length may be used to repair both sides.

After evacuation of the pneumoperitoneum, the remaining cannulae are removed. A 4-0 absorbable suture is used to close the umbilical port site. The port-site incisions are infiltrated with local anesthetic and then closed with Steristrips®.

In teenage children, simple closure of the internal ring may be associated with an increased risk of hernia recurrence. Some surgeons advocate a formal 'repair' of the posterior wall of the inguinal canal for these children. Suture closure of the neck of the sac carries a risk of recurrence for direct inguinal and femoral hernias. Peritoneal incision and formal anatomical repair are required for these hernias.

POSTOPERATIVE CARE

Children may be fed after recovery from anesthesia and discharged home later the same day. Oral or rectal acetaminophen may be required for analgesia during the first 24 hours postoperatively.

PROBLEMS, PITFALLS AND SOLUTIONS

- Massively dilated bowel makes the manipulation of instruments and needles difficult, particularly in small infants. Decompression of the stomach with a nasogastric tube may help.

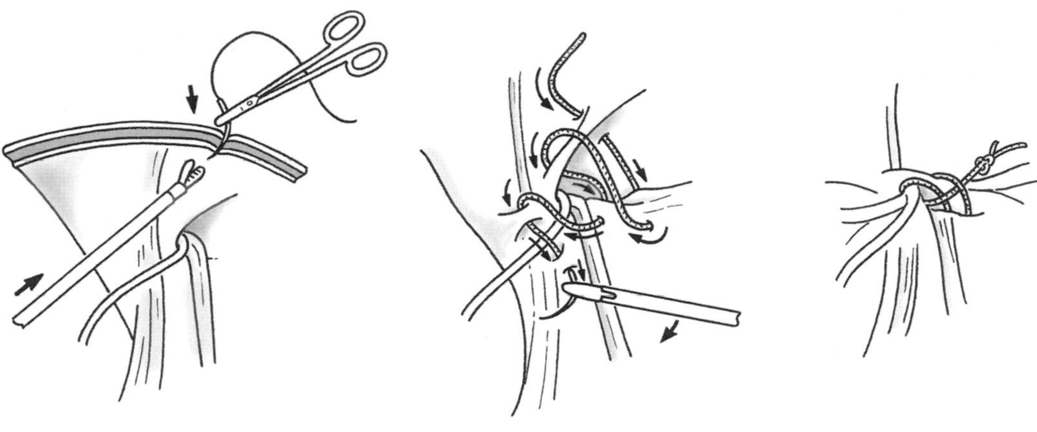

Figure 46.2 *Repair of indirect hernia.*

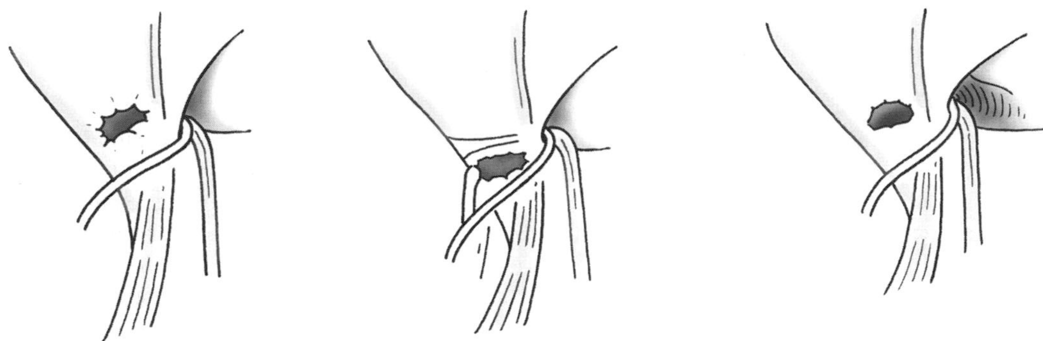

Figure 46.3 *(a) Direct; (b) femoral; (c) combined direct and indirect.*

- If the most medial stitch is placed too far lateral to the epigastric vessels, there is an increased risk of recurrence. The misplacement of this stitch usually occurs because of concern about damaging the epigastric vessels or the vas. Practically all recurrences occur medially, never laterally. The risk of recurrence can be minimized by including some of the deeper connective tissue at the margin of the internal inguinal ring with the peritoneum.
- Direct inguinal and femoral hernias, and combinations thereof, are identified more frequently during laparoscopic repair than during open surgery. This is particularly so in recurrent cases. **(See Figure 46.3)**

In a personal series of 358 cases, there were 3 percent direct hernias, 1 percent femoral hernias and 1 percent hernias-en-pantaloon. Unusual hernias require formal anatomical repair and not simple ligation of the sac.

- Occasionally, irritating minor bleeding from a small vessel in the lateral abdominal wall adjacent to the deep ring is encountered. This will stop once the deep ring is ligated.
- In boys with a patent processus vaginalis, a pneumoscrotum will develop as the peritoneal cavity is insufflated. This may be expressed through the ligated hernia opening or, preferably, allowed to resorb spontaneously.
- A contralateral patent processus vaginalis will be found in 15–30 percent of cases. This should be closed in the manner described above.

COMPLICATIONS

- There is a potential for intestinal or vascular injury in any laparoscopic procedure. In newborns the 4-0 suture needle appears large and must be manipulated carefully within the peritoneal cavity. Turning large needles within small cavities may result in inadvertent laceration of the epigastric or testicular vessels. Although an extensive subperitoneal hematoma may develop, the bleeding will invariably cease spontaneously. Although careless, puncturing bowel wall with the needle tip is of no consequence.
- If the Veress needle is not inserted sufficiently deeply into the abdominal cavity, an extraperitoneal insufflation will ensue. The peritoneum is lifted

off and vision is restricted. The extraperitoneal CO_2 will be absorbed within 10 minutes and a further attempt can then be made to establish a pneumoperitoneum. This is no reason to convert to the open approach.
- The recurrence rate following laparoscopic hernia repair in children is presently 3–5 percent. This will decrease further in the future with improved suturing and knot-tying techniques. Placing sutures as medially as possibly and as close as possible to the epigastric vessels minimizes this risk.

FURTHER READING

Schier F. Direct inguinal hernias in children, the laparoscopic aspect. *Pediatric Surgery International* 2000; **16**:562–4.

Schier F, Danzer E, Bondartschuk M. Incidence of contralateral patent processus vaginalis in children with inguinal hernia. *Journal of Pediatric Surgery* 2001; **36**:1561–3.

Schier F, Montupet Ph, Esposito C. Laparoscopic inguinal herniorrhaphy in children: a three-center experience with 933 repairs. *Journal of Pediatric Surgery* 2002; **37**:395–7.

Section D: Urology

47

Cystourethroscopy – basic technique

UWE FRIEDRICH AND R. VETTER

INTRODUCTION

Most morphological anomalies of the lower urinary tract can be demonstrated reliably during childhood using diagnostic imaging. However, systematic pathological classification of abnormalities of this part of the efferent urinary system often requires endoscopic urological investigation as well. The more sophisticated instruments currently available make endoscopy a safe examination procedure, and its use may avoid complications, for example those attributable to concomitant pathology unrecognized until the time of major reconstructive surgery. Advances in pediatric anesthesia, moreover, make the decision to subject a child to endourological diagnostic procedures easier. Our own experience of more than 5000 cystourethroscopic procedures in children has shown them to be characterized by precise timing, stringent criteria for patient selection, and strict adherence to a post-procedural observation period. All pediatric urologists should have a sound understanding of the basic technique of cystourethroscopy. Its therapeutic value is a reflection of the expertise of the endo-urological surgeon. In fact, the results of the examination are an important part of overall case management and should be recognized as such.

Indications

DIAGNOSTIC

- Persistent recurrent urinary tract infections.
- Hematuria.
- Diagnostic work-up and when tumor is suspected.
- Bladder-emptying disorders in patients with pathomorphogical anomalies detected on ultrasound, other imaging modalities and urodynamic (e.g. thickening of the urinary bladder wall, residual urine, or suspected urinary calculi).
- Localization of the ureteric orifices in patients with duplex or ectopic ureters, radiographically silent kidneys, single kidneys and renal ectopia.
- Evaluation of the position and configuration of the ureteric orifice – and the length of the submucosal ureteric course – prior to anti-reflux surgery.
- Investigation of urogenital anomalies – if necessary in combination with vaginoscopy – in patients with a urogenital sinus or ambiguous genitalia.
- Urethral duplication.
- Diverticula of the urethra or bladder.
- Proximal and midshaft hypospadias.
- Symptomatic or asymptomatic supravesical urinary retention (Grade II–IV).
- Suspected recto-vesical, recto-urethral and urethro-vaginal or vesico-vaginal fistulas.

THERAPEUTIC (WITH OR WITHOUT RESECTOSCOPY)

- Meatal stricture with calibration.
- Urethral valve, urethral stricture and syringocele.
- Urethral polyps.
- Sub-orifice anti-reflux injection therapy.
- Insertion or removal of ureteral stents (Friedrich and Vetter 1998, Friedrich et al. 1997).
- Stretching of microbladder.
- Foreign body removal.
- Treatment of urinary calculi.
- Ureterocele.
- Bladder neck injections as a treatment for incontinence.
- Lavage of the urinary bladder.

Contraindications

- Decompensated urinary retention concomitant with urosepsis.
- Acute urinary tract infection (to minimize the risk of ascending infection).
- Impassable stricture of the urethra and bladder neck, especially during the first 6 months of life (alternative treatment: temporary vesicostomy or antegrade intervention).
- Small infant (i.e. premature baby) – because of the danger of urethral injury.
- Anesthesia intolerance.
- Lack of suitable instruments and equipment.

Where there has been previous surgical reconstruction of the lower urinary tract, the pros and cons of subsequent endoscopic exploration need to be considered carefully (Gillenwater et al. 1996). For example, in patients with previous bladder reconstruction for bladder exstrophy, hypospadias or epispadias repair, and previous bladder neck injections, care must be taken to avoid complications such as mechanical injury of the bladder or rupture of the bladder neck during endoscopy. The risk of injury can be minimized by choosing the right endoscopic instruments – from the wide spectrum of both flexible and rigid cystoscopes available – for the lower urinary tract constellation presented by the individual case.

EQUIPMENT/INSTRUMENTS

Essential

To investigate the entire spectrum of pathomorphological anomalies found in pediatric patients up to the age of 14 via cystourethroscopy, a pediatric urologist needs access to a broad assortment of equipment.

COMPLETE ENDO-UROLOGICAL WORKSTATION IN THE OPERATING ROOM

- Operating table with adaptors for positioning and X-rays, including loops for infants and anatomically shaped cups for older children.
- High-intensity light source (halogen or xenon).
- Power source with diathermy – laser and wide adaptation range, in particular for resectoscopy.
- Flushing guidance system including a drainage catheter – ready-mixed bag (3 L) containing a mixture of sorbitol, mannitol (Purisole) and saline.
- Local disinfection (penis, introitus vaginae and surrounding area).
- Instrument gel with local anesthetic agent.
- Instrument tray for scopes, gauze, sponge holder and containers.

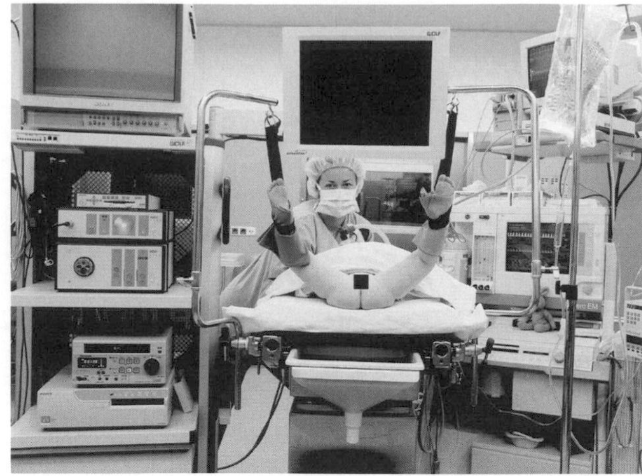

Figure 47.1

- Cystoscope and accessories.
  - Premature infant–term infant:
    - 7.5–9.5 Fr
    - cystourethroscope with straight and angled optics.
  - Term infant–adolescent:
    - 9.5–17.5 Fr
    - cystourethroscope with replaceable straight and angled optics
    - flexible cystourethroscope 9.5 Fr with a 3 Fr instrument channel.
- Resectoscope and accessories.
  - Premature infant:
    - 7.5 Fr cystoscope with a 3 Fr instrument channel for an electric cable with a small scalpel.
  - Term infant–adolescent:
    - 9.5–19.5 Fr resectoscope with an electric hook, button or loop electrode as well as a scalpel (for further information, see Chapters 6 and 50).
- Biopsy forceps and clamps.
- X-ray unit for performing radiological examination during the intervention (image intensity). **(See Figure 47.1)**

9.5 FR CYSTOURETHROSCOPE WITH A COMPLETE RANGE OF ACCESSORIES

All endoscopes have an instrument channel with a diameter of at least 3 Fr as well as a flushing and draining channel; cystoscopes with this configuration can perform the most important diagnostic and therapeutic functions. In addition, flexible ureteral catheters with a mandrin of 3–5 Fr are necessary. For ureteral submucosal and bladder neck insertion, the urologist should have a 10.5–14.5 Fr cystoscope with permanently installed angled optics and an O'Donnell needle or flexible injection cannula. The hypodermics are supplied by the major manufacturers pre-filled with the required substances. **(See Figure 47.2)**

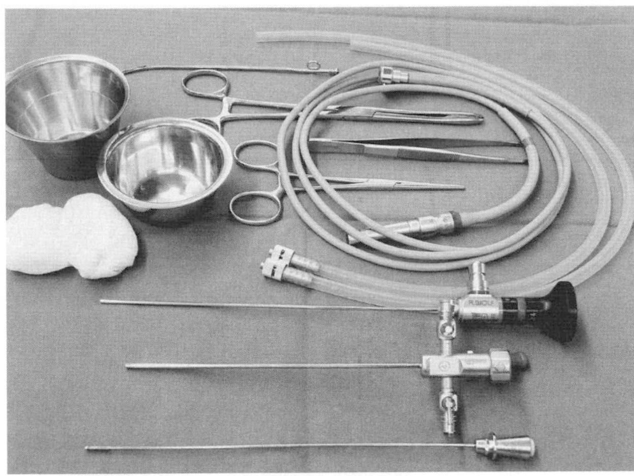

Figure 47.2

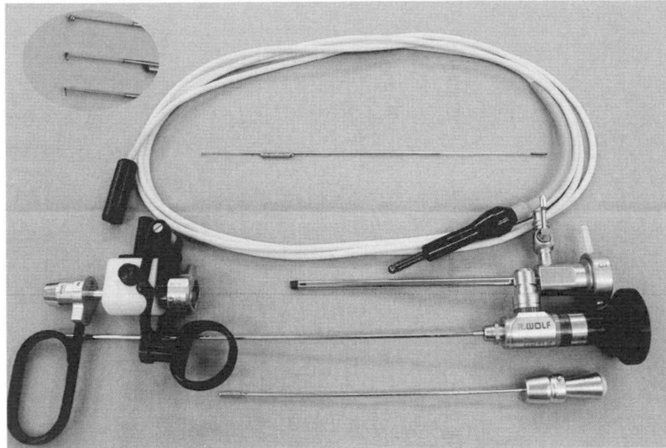

Figure 47.3

9.5 FR RESECTOSCOPE FOR TERM INFANT WITH HOOK ELECTRODE

- High-intensity light source (halogen).
- Power source with wide adaptation range, in particular for resectoscopy.
- Flushing guidance system including a drainage catheter – ready-mixed bag (3L) containing a mixture of sorbitol and mannitol (Purisole).
- Local disinfection (penis, introitus vaginae and surrounding area) with antiseptic.
- Lignocaine gel.
- Complete array of instruments for the administration of anesthesia (including intubation) and for patient surveillance (including electrocardiogram monitoring). **(See Figure 47.3)**

Optional

- Imaging equipment (including endoscopic tower camera, television screen and video recorder/printer).
- Sonography equipment (e.g. for checking stents or locating urinary calculi).
- Evans' blue dye, e.g. for the localization of ectopic orifices.
- Stent cystoscope (12 Fr) with angled optics for the insertion of the valve-DD-ureteral stent with an oval instrument channel for the passage of the vulnerable anti-reflux valve.

TECHNIQUE

Objectives and capabilities

As a rule, examinations of this kind are performed on pediatric patients under general anesthesia after the potential benefits and risks have been explained to the parents fully and written informed consent has been obtained. Pediatric patients present for the examination in a fasting state. During the first 6 months of life such examinations always require admission to hospital; for toddlers and older infants, the procedure may be performed on an outpatient basis, depending on their initial status. Soon after the induction of anesthesia and prior to the instrumentation, appropriate intravenous antibiotics should be given to all patients. Postoperatively, antibiotics are continued in the presence of infected urine. In all cases the urethrovesical tract is subjected to a comprehensive evaluation including the following:

- Assessment of genitalia and urinary meatus.
- Assessment of urethra.
- Evaluation of the pars diaphragmatica urethrae and the colliculus seminalis.
- Diagnosis of urethral valves or urethral stricture.
- Precise assessment of the sphincter region and bladder neck.
- The size of the urinary bladder.
- The urothelial and wall configuration of the bladder.
- Assessment of the vesical trigone.
- Evaluation of the ureteric orifices: location, form and function, sometimes with the aid of terminal probing if there is no supravesical retention. In patients with significant structural anomalies of the urethra (e.g. in conjunction with neurogenic disorders or peg-shaped bladder), the injection of Evans' blue dye during chromocystoscopy can be an extremely useful aid for locating the ectopic orifice.
- Checking of stents, including testing of valve functions.

Every examination begins with an inspection of the external genitalia and evaluation of the external urinary meatus in order to avoid the injuries frequently associated with the sequelae of strictures. In addition to the age of the child, the configuration of the external meatus represents an important criterion for selecting the correct instrument size. The examination of male children is more difficult than that of girls. Preputial tear – a common injury during urological examinations in male children – should be avoided.

The child is placed in the lithotomy position in preparation for the examination, with the buttocks approximately flush with the front edge of the operating table. The legs are spread apart with the knees up; in toddlers, the legs may be suspended in loops, and in older children, immobilized in anatomically shaped cups. Damage caused by excessive pressure, especially at nerve exit points, should be prevented by cushioning the affected regions. It is important to adhere to the position described above: only by good access to the urethra will the examiner be able to follow its course exactly during instrumentation. This constellation plays an especially important role during intra-operative cystourethroscopy planned within the limits of surgical supravesical reconstruction of the urinary tract. The surgeon sits at the end of table, between the child's legs, with the assistant, scrub nurse and instrument table on the right.

Two examination techniques are widely used.

1 Sliding insertion of the instrument with the obturator by touch and replacement of the latter with the optics after placement of the cystourethro-resectoscope in the urinary bladder.
2 Insertion of the cystoscope under visual guidance – either directly or indirectly using the imaging equipment and screen (the latter technique is used in cases in which a problematical urethra is expected – especially in male children).

The second insertion technique described above is safer and should, for this reason, be used routinely. The instruments are inserted into the meatus. This can be achieved in the male after very gently stretching the prepuce – only to expose the external urinary meatus – by first inserting the device vertically and then lowering the optics into the proximal third of the urethra, causing the tip of the device to slide atraumatically into the urinary bladder. The urinary bladder of female children can be reached immediately after overcoming the short urethra. Labial adhesions may have to be separated first. **(See Figure 47.4)**

The instrument should never be inserted forcefully or shoved into the bladder; instead, it should always be advanced by touch with extreme sensitivity; otherwise there is a substantial risk of injury. Should the examiner encounter mechanical resistance due to inappropriate instrument diameter or a mechanical obstacle, the examination should be terminated immediately. Once the cystoscope is in the urinary bladder it is routine to submit the urine for analysis and culture.

When the bladder has been filled to medium capacity with the Purisole solution, the examiner initially performs a general overview before doing a more detailed examination. The view of the bladder interior may be impaired by cloudy urine or bloody secretions; in such cases, repeated flushing is required to provide an unimpeded view. Both

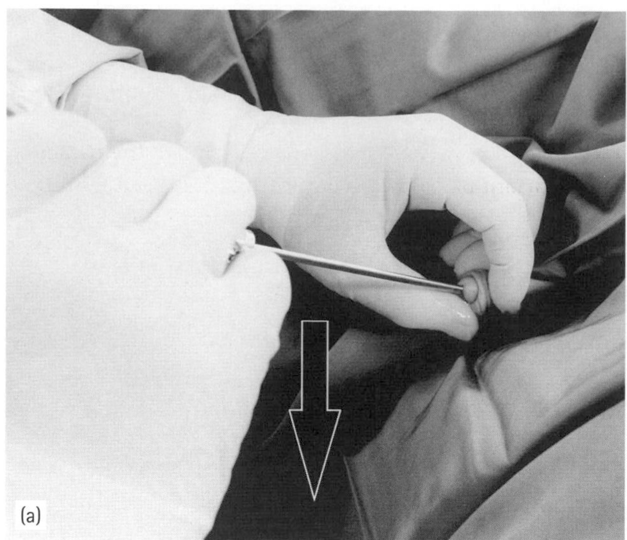

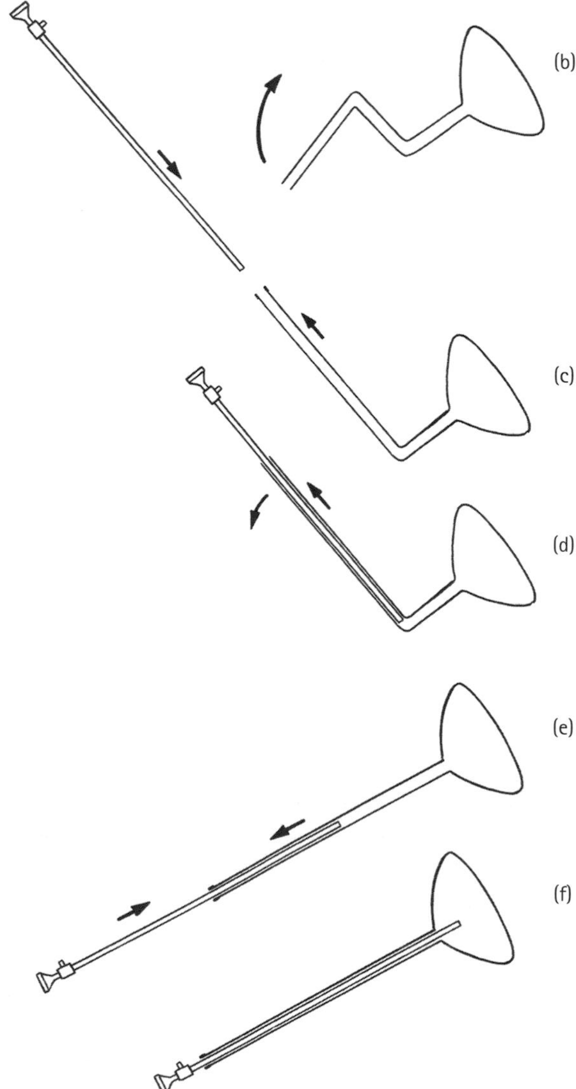

Figure 47.4 *Cystourethroscopy. Note how the penis and telescope are maneuvred.*

straight and angled optics are used for this procedure. By turning or lowering the optical device, the examiner can view first the infundibulum and then the remaining regions of the urinary bladder.

The evaluation of the vesical trigone and the orifices is an important part of the examination. It is useful to evaluate the urinary bladder at various stages of filling in order to assess its shape, the intravesical ureteric course and possible parostial (para-ureteric) diverticula. Terminal probing of the ureter and intravenous injection of dye are two feasible methods for evaluating difficult pathology of the ureteric orifices.

Following complete emptying of the bladder, insertion of the straight optics and adjustment of retrograde flow, the examiner can evaluate the urethra while carefully withdrawing the instrument. This applies, in particular, to the evaluation of the male urethra to exclude a wide range of pathological structures. It is especially important to evaluate the bladder outlet, bladder neck and pars diaphragmatica of the urethra while the bladder is empty; otherwise the automatic sphincter-opening reflex will impede – or even preclude – the gathering of diagnostic information about this section of the lower urinary tract. Furthermore, the sphincter structures, ectopic ureters, valves, syringoceles or collicus anomalies are easy to recognize and evaluate. In many cases, survey cystoscopy is followed by resectoscopy; the former procedure constitutes an important preparatory step for carrying out the latter procedure safely. After viewing the remainder of the urethral course, the examiner brings the examination to a close by emptying the bladder and carefully removing the instrument.

POSTOPERATIVE CARE

Because of the tremendous advances that have been made in the development of instruments for cystourethroscopy in recent years, this technique is now a safe diagnostic procedure in the hands of a skilled examiner. The obligation to keep the child under observation after the examination results more from the necessity of surveillance after the administration of general anesthesia and less from possible sequelae of the examination method itself. Usually cystourethroscopy takes place within the framework of an overall diagnostic work-up in a pediatric patient with severe anomaly; in such cases there is often an objective requirement to follow up the patient in hospital. This follow-up may include general surveillance of the child, observation of micturition and measurement of body temperature. Depending on the child's overall status, ambulatory examinations are possible for children 6 months of age and older; the pros and cons should be weighed carefully in cooperation with the parents. When this approach is used, the examiner should wait for the child's first micturition after cystoscopy before allowing discharge from hospital. In contrast, resectoscopy should always be followed by observation in hospital.

PROBLEMS, PITFALLS AND SOLUTIONS

The surgeon must be familiar with the instruments and test all components prior to surgery.

- Incompatibility of various parts and components of instruments and equipment.
- A small, but otherwise normal, urethra may require calibration and gentle serial dilatation, which facilitates insertion of the cystoscope. Such dilatation should cause no bleeding, and forceful calibration must be avoided.
- Poor visibility, which occasionally occurs in the urinary bladder or urethra as a result of cloudy sediment-containing urine or hemorrhage from an inflamed or traumatized urothelium. In this situation, it is advisable to perform the examination with the urinary bladder partially filled and irrigate continuously with Purisole or saline. Cleaning the tip of the instrument may also be helpful. It is usually not necessary to change instruments. Should significant bleeding become apparent towards the end of the examination, a bladder catheter should be inserted upon completion of the procedure. In more severe cases, the child may require intravenous infusion.
- Missed diagnosis may result from inadequate view or examination. To identify some lesions, e.g. just behind the bladder neck, the examination must be carried out in an empty bladder: use one hand to press the bladder suprapubically and turn the angled 30–45° cystoscope in an upward direction.
- A small or medium-sized ureterocele may be missed if the bladder is over-distended.
- Heavy bleeding is usually caused by deeper epithelial tears, particularly in the more vascular bladder neck. Such bleeding may require careful electrocoagulation. Urethral bleeding in boys usually stops with manual compression of the penis or perineum. Bladder catheterization and in-hospital observation are mandatory for 24–48 hours postoperatively.

Minor bleeding usually results from rough handling or from rapid distension and decompression of the bladder.

- The presence of a Mullerian or recto-urethral fistula may allow the cystoscope to enter the wrong track. Keep the scope in contact with the roof (dorsal aspect) of the urethra.
- Even if the cystourethroscopy is preceded by a diagnostic micturition cystourethrogram, surprise findings, e.g. syringocele, ureterocele or diverticulum, can occur.
- An impassable urethra may be due to congenital abnormalities, such as atresia, diverticulum or stenosis

from previous surgery and scarring: the initial introduction of a guide-wire or the use of a smaller caliber scope may allow safe instrumentation. In difficult cases, consider termination of the procedure, other imaging or diagnostic modalities and a vesicostomy.

COMPLICATIONS

There are few data available on the rate of complications following endo-urological examinations in children. In our experience, the incidence of serious complications following cystourethroscopy – including cystourethroscopy followed by resectoscopy – has been 0.7 percent. This low complication rate shows that diagnostic and therapeutic endo-urological procedures are safe. Not surprisingly, this technique has become firmly established at all institutions with departments of pediatric urology.

- Significant hemorrhage (see 'Problems, pitfalls and solutions' above).
- Injury to urethra and bladder which may or may not be recognizable at the time of surgery.
  - Never use force, especially in small infants or where there are suspected anomalies or pathology.
  - When a significant false passage (via falsa) is created, terminate the procedure and drain the bladder suprapubically.
  - Minor bladder injury may be treated with an indwelling bladder catheter, whereas major injury requires surgical repair.
  - Antibiotics are usually required.
  - Significant extravasation may require formal surgical drainage.
  - Look out for signs of urethral stricture by following the patient up.
- Sepsis following straightforward instrumentation is usually prevented by peri-operative and postoperative antibiotics and appropriate follow-up.
- Symptomatic micturition (pain and frequency) is treated expectantly, but follow-up and re-investigation may be required in persistent cases.

FURTHER READING

Friedrich U, Vetter R. Use of pyeloureteral DD stents in children. In: Yachia D (ed.), *Stenting the Urinary System.* Oxford: Isis Medical Media, 1998, 141–9.

Friedrich U, Vetter R, Jorgensen TM, Muhr M. Experimental and clinical experience with new pyeloureteral stents in paediatric urology. *Journal of Endourology* 1997; 11(6): 431–9.

Gillenwater JY, Grayhack JT, Howards SS, Duckett JW. *Pediatric Urology.* St Louis, MI: Mosby-Year Book, 1996.

48

Submucosal injection of ureter – vesico-ureteric reflux

PREM PURI

INTRODUCTION

Primary vesico-ureteric reflux (VUR) is the most common urological anomaly in children and has been reported in 30–50 percent of those who present with urinary tract infection (UTI). The association of VUR, UTI and renal parenchymal damage is well established. Reflux nephropathy is present in 3–25 percent of children and in 10–15 percent of adults with end-stage renal failure. There has been no consensus regarding when medical or surgical therapy should be used. A number of prospective studies have shown low rates of spontaneous resolution of high-grade reflux. Moreover, observation alone carries a risk of renal scarring. Ureteric re-implantation by open surgery on the bladder is effective in curing reflux, but the operation is not free of complications, and its indications are disputed.

Since its introduction, endoscopic correction of VUR has become an established alternative to long-term antibiotic prophylaxis and open surgical treatment. The long-term effectiveness of endoscopic STING (subureteral injection of polytetrafluoroethylene) for VUR in a series of 258 patients involving a 17-year follow-up period has been confirmed. Injection of polytetrafluoroethylene appears to be safe for the treatment of VUR.

Recently, a number of other tissue-augmenting substances have been used endoscopically for subureteric injection. Dextranomer microspheres in sodium hyaluronic acid solution (Deflux) is a recently developed organic substance comprising 80–250 μm microspheres. It has been reported that dextranomer/hyaluronic acid copolymer is biodegradable, has no immunogenic properties and has no potential for malignant transformation. Dextranomer microspheres in sodium hyaluronic acid solution consists of microspheres of dextranomers mixed in a 1 percent high-molecular-weight sodium hyaluronan solution. Each milliliter of the system contains 0.5 mL sodium hyaluronan and 0.5 mL of microspheres.

Indications

- High-grade primary VUR (grade III–V).
- VUR in duplex renal systems.
- VUR secondary to neuropathic bladder and posterior urethral valves.
- VUR in failed re-implanted ureters.
- VUR into ureteric stumps.

EQUIPMENT/INSTRUMENTS

- Disposable Puri catheter for injection – a 4 Fr nylon catheter onto which is swaged a 21 G needle with 1 cm of the needle protruding from the end of the catheter. **(See Figure 48.1)** Alternatively, a rigid needle can be used.
- 1 mL syringe.
- Deflux paste.
- All cystoscopes available for infants and children can be used for this procedure. **(See Figure 48.2)**

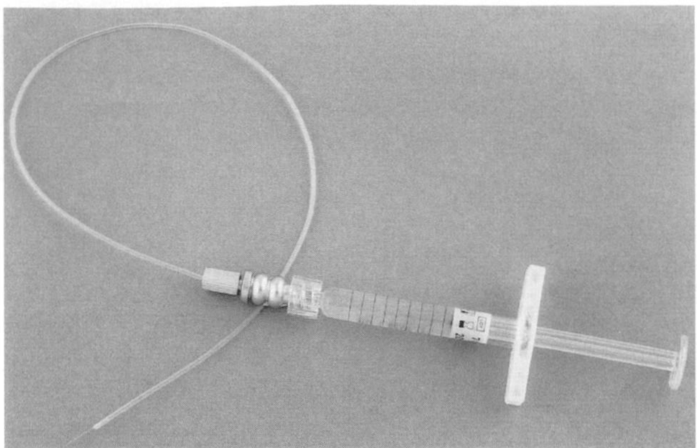

Figure 48.1

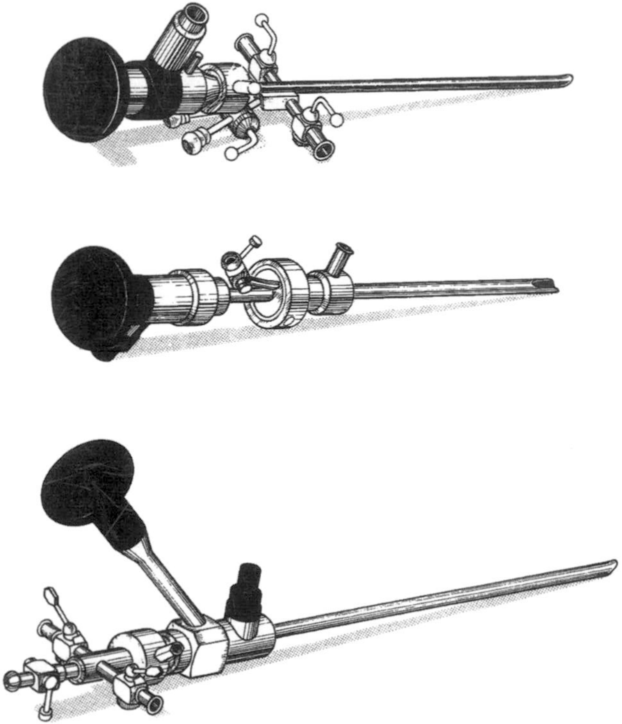

Figure 48.2

TECHNIQUE

The procedure is performed under general anesthesia with the patient in the lithotomy position. The cystoscope is passed and the bladder wall, trigone, bladder neck and both ureteric orifices inspected. The bladder should be almost empty before proceeding with injection, since this helps to keep the ureteric orifice flat rather than away in a lateral part of the field.

The injection of Deflux paste should not begin until the operator has a clear view all around the ureteric orifice. The purpose is to create a mound or 'hillock' by injecting the paste into the submucosal layer; this effectively prevents retrograde flow of urine through the ureteric orifice. Under direct vision through the cystoscope, the needle is introduced under the bladder mucosa 2–3 mm below the ureteric orifice at the 6 o'clock position. In children with grades IV and V reflux with wide ureteric orifices, the needle should be introduced not below but directly into the entrance of the ureteric orifice. It is important to introduce the needle with pinpoint accuracy. Perforation of the mucosa or the ureter may allow the paste to escape and result in failure.

The needle is advanced about 4–5 mm into the lamina propria in the submucosal portion of the ureter and the injection is started slowly. As the paste is injected, a bulge appears in the floor of the submucosal ureter. During injection the needle is slowly withdrawn until a 'volcanic' bulge of paste is seen. The needle should be kept in position for 30–60 seconds after injection to avoid extrusion. Most refluxing ureters require 0.3–0.6 mL Deflux for correction.

A correctly placed injection creates the appearance of a nipple on the top of which is a slit-like or inverted crescent-shaped orifice. The non-injected ureteric roof retains its compliance while preventing reflux. (**See Figure 48.3**)

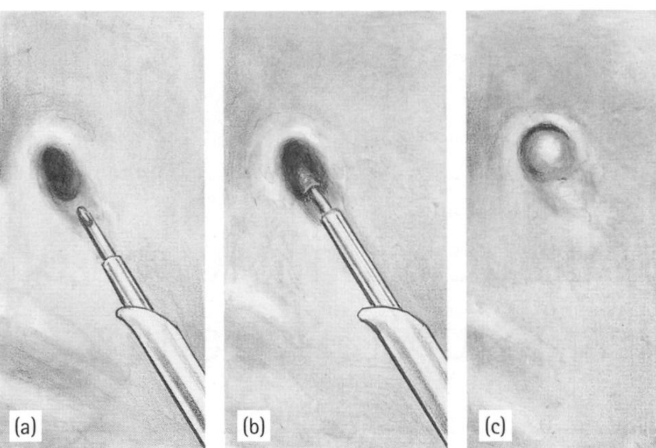

Figure 48.3

POSTOPERATIVE CARE

Postoperative urethral catheterization is not necessary. The majority of patients are treated as day cases. Co-trimoxazole is prescribed in prophylactic doses for 3 months after the procedure. Micturition cystography and renal ultrasonography are performed 3 months after discharge. A follow-up micturating cystogram and renal and bladder ultrasonographic scan are obtained 12 months after endoscopic correction of reflux.

PROBLEMS, PITFALLS AND SOLUTIONS

Problems related to the procedure are rare.

Paste extrudes from the needle hole immediately after injection

This is most likely to occur if the needle is removed too quickly. Extrusion is minimized if the needle remains in situ for 30–60 seconds after completion of the injection. Despite this, a small amount of paste extrusion is common; it will stop spontaneously and, provided the 'hillock' produced by the paste is correctly located, cure of the reflux can be anticipated.

Bulge appears in the wrong place

If the bulge appears in an incorrect place, e.g. at the side of the ureter or proximal to it, the needle should not be withdrawn. Instead, it should be moved so that the point is in a more favorable position.

No mound or hillock appears

This may indicate that the tip of the needle has been introduced too far and the injection is peri-ureteric and not submucosal. Stop further injection and remove the needle. Depending on how much material has been injected already, the needle may be introduced into the correct position and injection recommenced.

COMPLICATIONS

Persistent or recurrent reflux

Sometimes the reflux is not abolished by the initial injection. In other patients there is recurrence after the initial correction has been confirmed on micturating cystography. About 15–20 percent of refluxing ureters require more than one endoscopic injection of paste for correction.

Vesico-ureteric junction obstruction

Vesico-ureteric junction obstruction is an occasional complication following STING. A recent multi-center survey of STING procedures in 12 251 ureters in 8332 patients revealed vesico-ureteric junction obstruction in 41 (0.33 percent) ureters that was sufficiently severe to require re-implantation.

FURTHER READING

Chertin B, DeCaluwe D, Puri P. Endoscopic treatment of primary grades IV and V vesicoureteral reflux in children with subureteral injection of polytetrafluoroethylene. *Journal of Urology* 2003; **169**:1847–9.

Puri P. Endoscopic correction of vesicoureteric reflux. *Current Opinion in Urology* 2000; **10**:593–7.

Puri P. Endoscopic treatment of vesicoureteral reflux. In: Gearhart JP, Rink RC, Mouriquand PDE (eds), *Pediatric Urology*. Philadelphia: WB Saunders, 2001, 411–22.

Puri P, Chertin B, Velayudham M et al. Treatment of vesicoureteral reflux by endoscopic injection of Dextranomer/Hyaluronic acid copolymer: Preliminary results. *Journal of Urology* 2003; **170**:1541–4.

49

Endoscopic insertion of ureteric stent

A.K. TAGHIZADEH AND DUNCAN T. WILCOX

INTRODUCTION

Retrograde insertion of a stent into the ureter is commonly performed by the pediatric urologist. It is a simple procedure but occasionally and unexpectedly can be difficult. This chapter describes the retrograde technique. Antegrade stenting is an alternative to the retrograde method, but requires puncture of the collecting system, and is usually in the realm of the interventional radiologist.

Indications

Insertion of a ureteric stent is a temporary measure to improve the drainage of the kidney in situations such as the following.

- Urinary extravasation not responding to conservative measures.
- Upper urinary tract obstruction associated with pain, infection or decline in renal function.
- As an adjunct to other endoscopic urinary procedures.

Contraindications

ABSOLUTE

- Patient unfit for general anesthesia.
- Complete ureteric stricture, identified by retrograde fluoroscopy.

RELATIVE

There are circumstances in which stenting may be expected to be difficult and alternative treatment is considered.

- The presence of active urinary infection should be treated with caution. If stent insertion is an elective procedure, it should be postponed until the infection has been controlled. However, if pyonephrosis is considered, relieving the obstruction is urgent. In this situation percutaneous nephrostomy may be considered more appropriate.
- In idiopathic vesico-ureteric junction obstruction associated with a mega-ureter, the obstruction will often be too tight to allow retrograde or antegrade stenting. It may be easier to place the stent into the mega-ureter at open operation.
- A very dilated and tortuous ureter may be difficult to stent, as the guide-wire tends to coil in the capacious ureter.
- Previous reconstructive surgery to the urethra, bladder neck, trigone or ureter may make retrograde stenting very difficult.

PREOPERATIVE PREPARATION

Before the operation, the appropriate imaging should be reviewed and must be in theater. Microbiology results must be checked so that antibiotic prophylaxis can be adjusted accordingly. Retrograde stenting can be unexpectedly difficult and so parents and patients should be aware of the potential difficulties and be prepared for the insertion of an antegrade stent if required. On rare occasions it is necessary to undergo an open exploration if there is urinary perforation with extravasation during the procedure.

EQUIPMENT/INSTRUMENTS

Essential

The choice of cystoscope will be determined by the size of the patient and the caliber of the urethra. The cystoscope should have a working channel and ideally this should be large enough to accommodate the stent. However, this is sometimes not possible in children. A 10 Fr cystoscope with a 4 Fr working channel is most commonly used. In an infant, a 7.5 Fr integrated cystoscope with a 3 Fr working channel is more suitable.

- Telescope, preferably a 30°.
- Light source and light lead.
- Irrigation fluid – may be water, saline or glycine solution if no additional procedures are being performed.
- Guide-wire, e.g. a 0.035 guide-wire with a straight tip, although a smaller 0.025 guide-wire may be necessary in smaller children.
- Facilities for screening must be available.
- Water-soluble X-ray contrast.
- The type of stent used is a matter of personal preference. Silicone stents are softer and have good biocompatibility. Polyurethane stents are the commonly used alternative. Polyurethane stents are easier to place because they have a lower friction coefficient, and they are more rigid and therefore better at resisting bucking as they are pushed in. The diameter of the stent chosen can vary between 3.5 Fr and 6 Fr. The length of the stent can be estimated from a plain abdominal X-ray. 'Multilength' stents have several curls to their tails, which unwind to a varying degree to adapt to a wider range of length of ureters.
- Cystoscopic forceps.

An assistant should be scrubbed and available. Ureteric stenting cannot be performed alone.

Optional

- Video camera, monitor and stack.
- Hydrophilic coated guide-wire (e.g. Terumo Glidewire®) may be useful under certain circumstances (see below).
- Catheterizing bridge for the cystoscope and a 70° telescope.
- Availability of an ultrasound machine, when antegrade stent insertion becomes necessary.

TECHNIQUE

The patient is given a single dose of prophylactic antibiotic at induction.

Position the patient supine on the operating table. The table should allow screening with the image intensifier, allowing the screening arm to move under the table and X-rays to be taken through the table. If a camera and monitor are being used, the TV stack should be placed on the same side of the patient as the fluoroscopy monitor. This will make it easier for the surgeon to change his or her line of vision from one to the other.

The patient's buttocks should be well supported and close to the end of the table. The legs need to be supported so that the hips are abducted and flexed to about 45°. For an infant this may be achieved by placing silicone pads under the knees. The knees and calves of an older child may be placed in crutch supports. Good alternatives are the pneumatic supports in which the calves and feet are placed in boots. These allow easy positioning without placing a strain on the knees. Placing the feet in pole stirrups is not satisfactory, as it tends to over-flex the hips and knees whilst applying undue pressure to the inner thighs, ankles and around the leg straps. **(See Figure 49.1)**

The cystoscope is connected to the light source, video and irrigating fluid, lubricated with an aqueous gel and passed into the bladder. The bladder is drained of urine and inspected and the ureteric orifice on the side to be stented is identified.

The following steps then depend on whether the size of the working channel of the cystoscope is wide enough to accept a ureteric catheter or stent.

If the cystoscope has a wide enough working channel, the following steps should be performed. It is helpful to begin by mapping out the ureter and pelvi-calyceal system by performing a retrograde ureterogram. An open-ended ureteric catheter, e.g. size 6 Fr, is passed down the cystoscope. The ureteric catheter should have been flushed, so that injection does not result in the introduction of air bubbles, which may give the appearance of filling defects. The tip of the catheter is passed about 0.5 cm into the ureter. If it cannot be maneuvered into the ureter, it may be easier first to pass the guide-wire into the ureteric orifice, sliding the catheter over it and then removing the guide-wire. **(See Figure 49.2)**

The contrast for the retrograde study should be diluted to half strength with saline. Full-strength contrast will tend to make it difficult to visualize the guide-wire, stent or stones on X-ray screening. A retrograde ureterogram is taken by gently injecting contrast; it is seldom necessary to inject more than 10 mL into a normal collecting system. A dilated ureter and pelvis may require a significantly larger volume. Performing the retrograde ureterogram will give information not only about pathology, but also about the anatomy of the pelvi-calyceal system. Contrast in the collecting system will therefore allow the surgeon accurately to place the

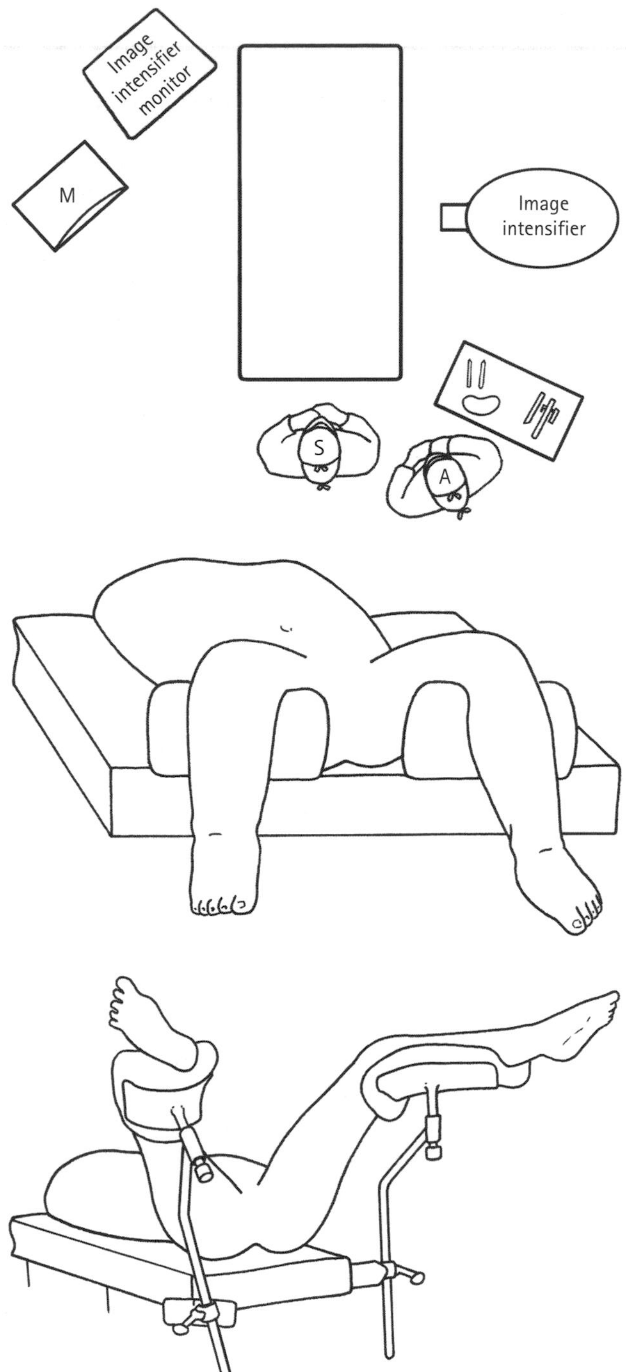

Figure 49.1

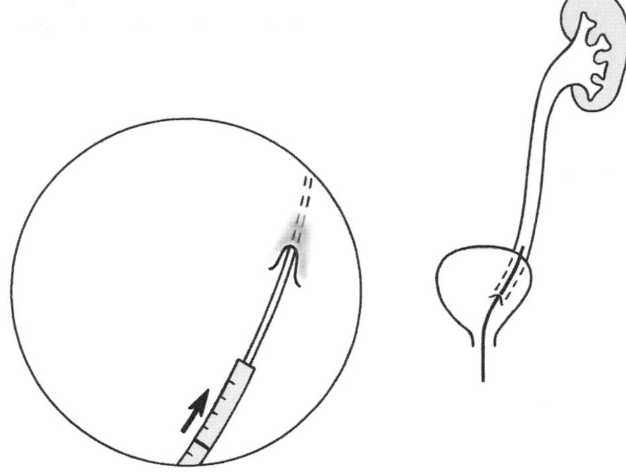

Figure 49.2

guide-wire and then the stent into the renal pelvis, and will identify complications such as the guide-wire or stent leaving the ureter.

Once a ureterogram has been performed, the next step is to place the tip of a guide-wire into the renal pelvis.

The role of an assistant becomes very important from the time the guide-wire starts being used. His or her crucial task is to support and secure the positions of the guide-wire, stent and pusher as they leave the cystoscope. As devices are loaded onto and moved along the guide-wire, it should be held as still and straight as possible. The surgeon must be able to attend to the camera and fluoroscopy monitors, checking and maintaining the position of the instruments within the urinary tract. If the cystoscope drifts out of position, there is a danger that it will drag the guide-wire out of the ureter. At the same time, the assistant must make sure that the position of the guide-wire is not lost either by being pushed in inadvertently by the surgeon or slipping out under its own weight. A guide-wire that has come out of the ureter may be very difficult and sometimes impossible to replace once the ureteric orifice has become a little edematous following instrumentation.

The next stage requires a guide-wire to be passed through the cystoscope up the ureter and into the renal pelvis. This is straightforward if a ureteric catheter is still in place in the distal ureter. Whilst the end of the ureteric catheter is being held steady, the guide-wire is fed up into it. The end of the guide-wire is fed up into it – flexible end first. The guide-wire is passed into the ureter until X-ray screening confirms the position of its tip in the renal pelvis. The ureteric catheter is then carefully removed without altering the position of the guide-wire. There is a danger at this point that, as the catheter is removed, it will drag the guide-wire out with it. One way of avoiding this is for the surgeon to hold and control the guide-wire whilst the assistant removes the catheter, or visa versa. The guide-wire is held by the surgeon about 5 cm from the distal end of the ureteric catheter, and the assistant then pulls the catheter out until it stops against the surgeon's fingers. While the assistant holds the catheter without pulling, the surgeon then moves his or her grip another 5 cm down the wire. The process is repeated until the proximal end of the catheter leaves the cystoscope and the surgeon takes hold of the guide-wire proximal to it. The position of the guide-wire should then be checked again with screening at this stage and adjusted as appropriate. **(See Figure 49.3)**

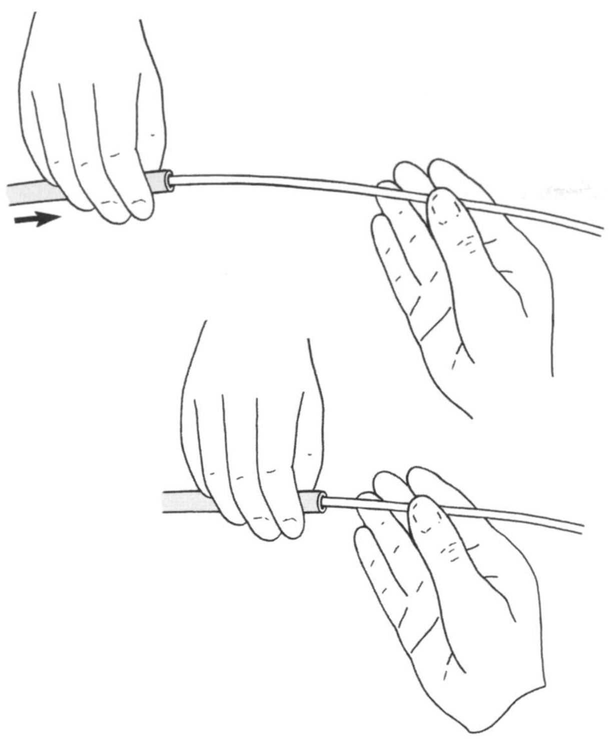

Figure 49.3

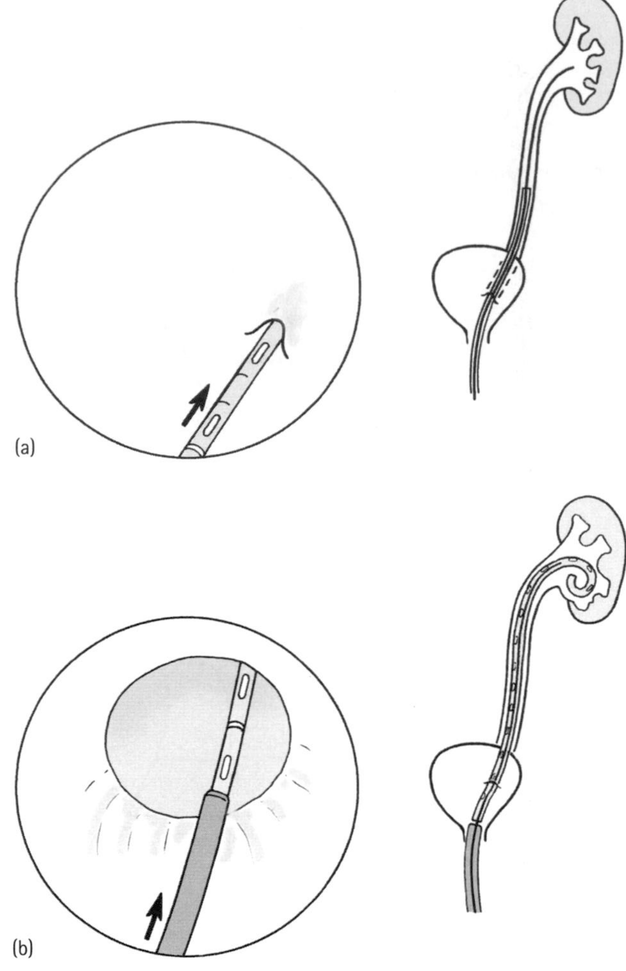

Figure 49.4 *(a) Stent through left ureteric orifice; (b) pusher at the bladder neck.*

Once it has been confirmed that the tip of the guide-wire is in the renal pelvis, the stent is fed onto it. There is usually a slight bevel on the end of the stent to be inserted first. It is worthwhile inspecting the stent in order to be familiar with its distance markings.

The stent is passed over the guide-wire, through the cystoscope and into the bladder. This is done by holding the cystoscope in the left hand and moving the stent over the guide-wire with the right hand. It helps if the assistant keeps tension on the guide-wire, ensuring that it is not removed inadvertently. A 'pusher' that is supplied with the stent is also fed onto the guide-wire and used to advance the stent when it is within the cystoscope. During these maneuvers the assistant should take particular care that the guide-wire does not move. The surgeon, meanwhile, keeps the stent and ureteric orifice in view. As the stent is gradually pushed in, the cystoscope is moved back towards the bladder neck so that there is more stent in view, and therefore more warning before the end of the stent reaches the ureteric orifice. **(See Figure 49.4)**

There are two ways of checking that the stent has been pushed far enough in. One involves using fluoroscopy to check that the proximal end of the stent is in the renal pelvis. The other involves watching the cystoscopy views of the lower end of the stent and observing the markings on the stent that indicate its remaining length. Once a good position is achieved, the guide-wire is removed. Brief use of continuous X-ray screening as the wire is slowly pulled will show the upper end of the stent curl up as it leaves the guide-wire. The cystoscopy view will also demonstrate a similar curling of the lower end in the bladder as it comes off the guide-wire. Care is taken to make sure that the distal end of the stent does not rest on the trigone. **(See Figure 49.5)**

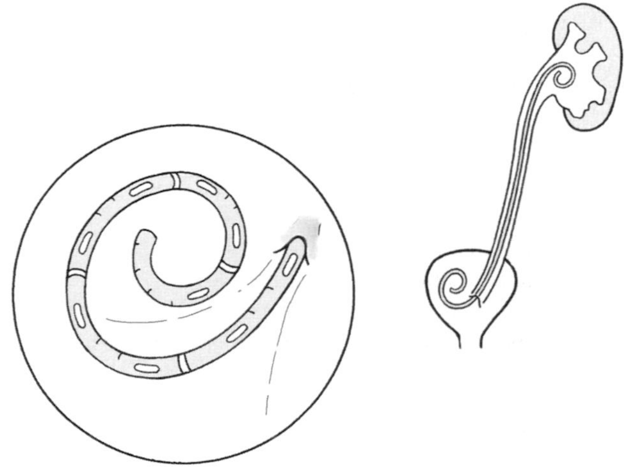

Figure 49.5

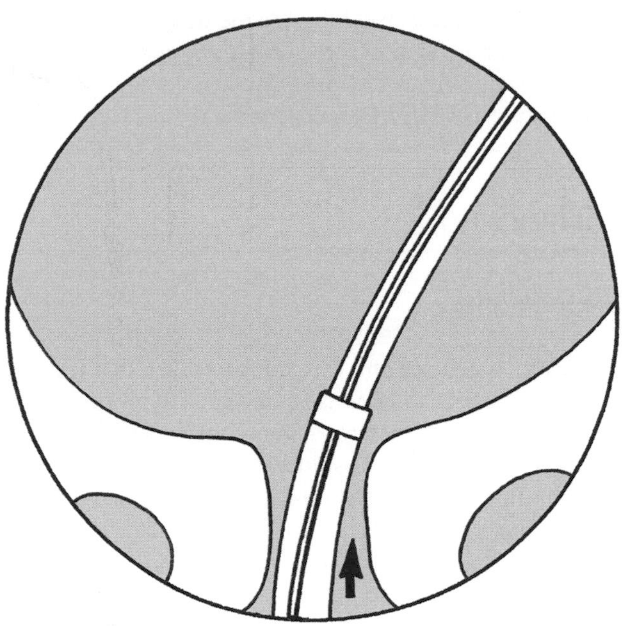

Figure 49.6

The position of the stent can be adjusted after the guide-wire has been removed by using cystoscopy forceps.

If the working channel of the cystoscope is too narrow for a ureteric catheter and stent, a different technique has to be used to place the stent. A guide-wire alone is simply passed via a cystoscope, through the ureteric orifice, up the ureter until its tip is at the level of the L1–L2 transverse process. The cystoscope is then removed from the urinary tract, leaving the guide-wire in place, and the stent is inserted without using a cystoscope. The stent is then passed onto the guide-wire and slid up, again using the pusher. The differences with this technique are the absence of a view of the lower ureter, and the absolute dependence on X-ray screening. The stent should be advanced more slowly so that its position can be checked more frequently with screening. It is important that the pusher is used so that the radio-opaque marker is on the end closest to the stent. This will help identify the position of the lower end of the stent on screening. Identifying that the lower end of the stent has reached a satisfactory position has to be inferred from the X-ray position of the marker on the pusher. This position is reached when, on anterio-posterior screening, the marker starts to move laterally from the midline position of the urethra, which coincides with it reaching the level of the superior border of the symphysis pubis. **(See Figure 49.6)**

The pusher is held in position while the guide-wire is gradually removed under screening. The upper and lower ends of the stent will be seen to curl if they are correctly positioned in the renal pelvis and bladder. This should be checked by cystoscopy.

POSTOPERATIVE CARE

Unless there are other reasons, such as obstructive pyelonephritis, it is not necessary to continue with antibiotics once the stent is in place. It is not uncommon for patients to report troublesome symptoms with the stent. Irritation of the trigone will cause urinary frequency, which tends to improve if the bladder is allowed to fill, lifting the stent off the trigone. Hematuria or discomfort may occur with physical activity. Loin pain during voiding is the result of intravesical pressures being transmitted to the renal pelvis. Occasionally, if too much of the stent has been left in the bladder, it can enter the urethra, and may even be visible in females – this requires replacement of the stent.

PROBLEMS, PITFALLS AND SOLUTIONS

Cannot identify the ureteric orifice

- Avoid indwelling urethral catheters preoperatively, as these will cause mucosal edema.
- Empty the bladder of urine: clear irrigation fluid will give a better view.
- Over-distending the bladder, especially if done repeatedly, will make the bladder mucosa bleed and should be avoided. Turn off the irrigating fluid if the bladder is adequately filled and there is a good view.
- A clue to the location of the ureteric orifice can be found by looking for the contralateral orifice, noting its position in the bladder, and then following the inter-trigonal bar to the corresponding position on the other side of the bladder.
- Consider the likelihood of an ectopic ureter.

Cannot feed the guide-wire into the ureteric orifice

The angle of entry of the wire allowed by the scope may be too oblique for the position of a particular ureteric orifice, so that the catheter or guide-wire skims across it. The angle of entry can be controlled independently of the cystoscope by using a catheterizing bridge if the cystoscope is large enough. This is fitted to the cystoscope and provides a deflecting arm at its tip that can angle the guide-wire in a more downward direction. It will not fit all cystoscopes. It is best used with a 70° telescope, which will allow a view of the tip of the wire as it is deflected downwards.

Cannot maneuver the tip of the guide-wire past the level of obstruction

Care should be taken not to perforate the wall of the ureter with the guide-wire by using excessive force.

- If possible, a ureteric catheter should be passed over the guide-wire to a point just below the level of the obstruction. This creates a shorter fulcrum, allowing the guide-wire to be more effectively pushed beyond the obstruction.
- The guide-wire should be substituted for one with a hydrophilic coating. These are soft and extremely slippery, and will often pass an obstruction where a standard guide-wire has failed. They need to be made wet before they are inserted in order to activate their hydrophilic coating. They are not the first choice of guide-wire as their coating makes them difficult to handle.
- A ureteroscope may be used to guide the wire through the obstruction under vision.

The lower end of the stent has been pushed all the way into the ureter

This is a difficult situation to correct. Removal may require ureteroscopy, percutaneous puncture and removal by an interventional radiologist, or removal at open operation.

Cannot maneuver the stent over the guide-wire into the ureter

Without a cystoscope, placing a relatively rigid stent over a soft guide-wire may allow both the wire and stent to coil inside the bladder. In this situation, consider:

- using a softer stent,
- using a rigid guide-wire,
- placing a small scope alongside the wire/stent so that the procedure is monitored under vision as well as by image intensifier. Care must be taken not to injure the urethra, especially in small patients.

COMPLICATIONS

Ureteric injury

The ureter is delicate and care must be taken that it is not injured. Excessive force must be avoided at all times. If a guide-wire or stent does not advance through a stricture or around a stone, forcing should not be tried.

If the guide-wire, catheter or stent perforates the ureter or collecting system, special care should be taken. If a stent can be correctly placed at the end of the procedure, little further needs to be done, other than a course of antibiotics. However, the situation will often have arisen because of a difficulty such as an impassable obstruction. In this situation, it is unlikely that a stent will be successfully placed. Antibiotics are required, and drainage of the injured urinary system should be established with the placement of a percutaneous nephrostomy.

The forgotten stent

The patient must not be lost from follow-up with a stent in situ. The patient and parents should be aware that the stent will need to be removed at a future date. A stent register will help avoid this problem.

50

Endoscopic treatment of posterior urethral valves, ureteroceles and urethral strictures

RANJIV MATHEWS

INTRODUCTION

The endo-urological management of lower urinary tract abnormalities in infants and children has become possible with the development of smaller fiberoptic endoscopes and therapeutic instrumentation. Endo-urological techniques are now used in the initial management of posterior urethral valves, ureteroceles and urethral strictures in children.

General principles

- It is typically performed using retrograde techniques.
- The diagnosis is confirmed and intervention performed at the same operative procedure.
- The lithotomy approach is utilized – older children are placed in stirrups, infants and younger children have their legs elevated on bolsters.
- The surgeon works from between the patient's legs.
- The instruments are placed behind or to the right of the surgeon. An assistant, when required, typically stands to the right of the surgeon to facilitate the passage of wires and catheters.
- Cautery with a foot-switch is required.
- Fine cystoscopes minimize urethral trauma.
- Offset cystoscopes allow instruments and catheters to be introduced easily.
- Warmed irrigation fluid reduces heat loss.
- Peri-operative antibiotics are utilized.
- A video system with the ability to obtain photographs is used to document the operative findings.

POSTERIOR URETHRAL VALVES

Posterior urethral valves (PUVs) are congenital obstructing lesions that occur in boys. They may be suspected on antenatal ultrasonography by the presence of bilateral hydro-uretero-nephrosis, dilatation of the bladder and prostatic urethra, and bladder neck hypertrophy. Oligohydramnios or anhydramnios may be noted during prenatal evaluation. Fetal morbidity is considerably greater in the presence of decreased amniotic fluid. Fetal intervention has been attempted to improve renal function in the presence of normal urinary parameters, although the risk to the mother and fetus remains high, and renal function may remain poor. Antenatal diagnosis permits prenatal counseling and planning for immediate postnatal management.

In some boys, PUVs may not be identified in infancy, but may present later in childhood with voiding problems, incontinence, recurrent infections or early signs of renal deterioration. Antenatal ultrasonography has decreased the number of patients presenting in later life.

Posterior urethral valves were first described in 1919 by H.H. Young. He described three types of valves. Type I valves (95 percent of patients) are made up of leaflets that extend distally from the verumontanum. During voiding, the leaflets billow outwards and cause obstruction. Type II valves are hypertrophied mucosal folds proximal to the verumontanum and are not considered obstructive. Type III valves (5 percent of patients) comprise a near-complete membrane distal to the verumontanum. Recently, it has been suggested that all patients have Type III valves that, with initial postnatal manipulation, are converted to the appearance of Type I valves.

Immediate postnatal management involves stabilization of the infant and antibiotic therapy. Urethral catheterization to provide urinary tract drainage is a critical first step. Postnatal radiographic evaluation includes ultrasonography and micturating cystourethrogram (MCU). It is important to ensure that the catheter is removed during the voiding phase and fluoroscopic evaluation undertaken. Hypertrophy of the bladder neck and dilatation of the posterior urethra with faintly visible valve leaflets confirm the diagnosis.

Initial management in the infant and older child involves endoscopic incision of the valves. An initial vesicostomy may be required in the premature infant and in those whose urethra is too small to accept a cystoscope.

Equipment

ESSENTIAL

- 6.5 Fr, 8 Fr and 10 Fr pediatric cystoscopes. **(See Figure 50.1)**
- Resectoscope with hook or loop electrode.
- Blunt-tipped electrode and electrocautery machine with foot pedal.
- Video camera.
- Light source.
- Warmed irrigation fluid.

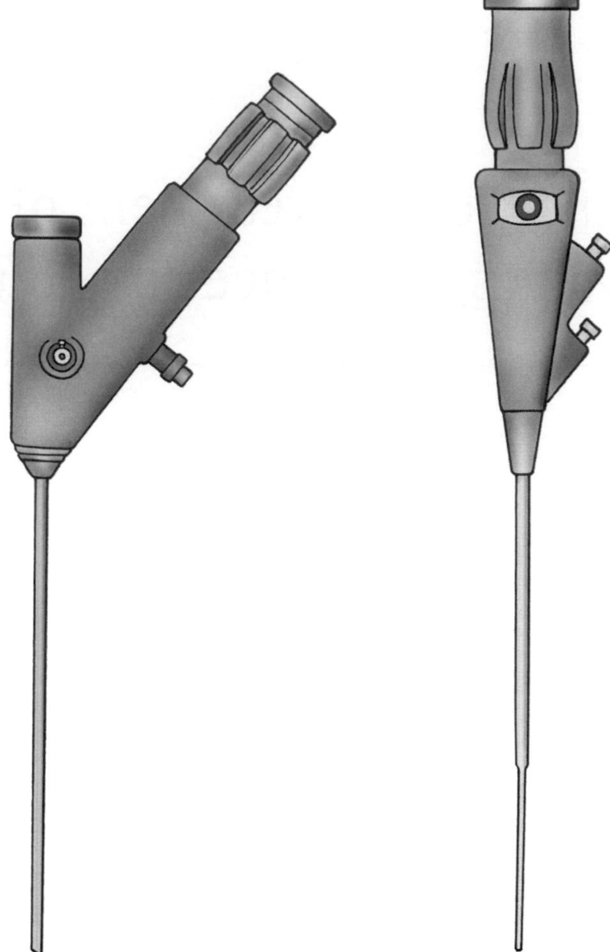

Figure 50.1

Technique

Infants are placed with their legs on bolsters; older children are placed in stirrups in the standard lithotomy position. Hyperextension of the extremities should be avoided during positioning. Antibiotic prophylaxis is administered. The lower abdomen is included in the field of skin preparation so that vesicostomy may be performed if necessary. **(See Figure 50.2)**

The cystoscope should be introduced as atraumatically as possible. If the external urethral meatus appears tight, gentle dilatation or meatotomy will prevent it from tearing. Most infant urethras should accept a 6 Fr cystoscope without much difficulty. The penis is held between the thumb and forefinger of the left hand. Holding the penis with the fingers on its lateral aspect and gently stretching it will permit insertion of the cystoscope into the anterior urethra. The barrel of the urethra should be clearly seen prior to advancement of the cystoscope to prevent undermining of the urethra and the creation of false passages. As the posterior urethra is approached, the water inflow is discontinued and gentle pressure on the partially filled bladder will demonstrate the valve leaflets. The valve leaflets may be incised with a laser fiber or blunt cautery probe through the smallest cystoscopes. Alternatively, a pediatric resectoscope with a cutting electrode can be used. Cold knife incision leads to bleeding and rapid obscuring of visualization. Incision of valve leaflets is also preferred to ablation, as the latter can lead to later stricture. Incisions are made at the 5 and 7 o'clock positions. An additional incision in the midline 12 o'clock position is performed in those who have a complete membrane (Type III). After the valves have been incised, the full bladder can be gently pressed to demonstrate the good urinary stream achieved. **(See Figure 50.3)**

Postoperative care

A catheter may be left in place for 24 hours and most patients can be discharged home as soon as they are medically stable. A postoperative ultrasound examination will confirm bladder emptying. Close follow-up of renal function and ultrasonography will detect renal deterioration

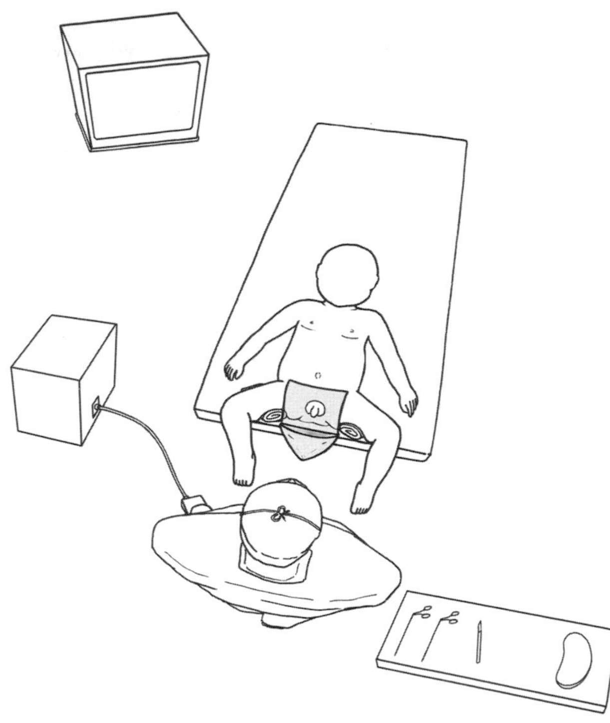

Figure 50.2

early. Referral to a pediatric nephrologist is recommended, particularly in those who develop renal deterioration or may need renal replacement. All patients are maintained on postoperative antibiotics.

Problems, pitfalls and solutions

Bleeding is encountered rarely when incision is undertaken with a cautery or laser. A cold knife is more likely to cause bleeding, which rapidly obscures visualization of the valves and urethra. When bleeding occurs and obliterates the view of the valves, the procedure should be stopped and a urethral catheter inserted.

Complications

- Inadequate incision of valves may be noted on postoperative evaluation. This may be managed with repeat incision. Inadequate bladder drainage despite adequate valve incision may require vesicostomy or upper tract diversion using proximal cutaneous ureterostomies.
- Excessively aggressive electrocautery ablation of valves can lead to later development of urethral strictures.
- Ongoing urethral obstruction from incomplete ablation of the valves: a further endoscopic resection is performed.
- Urethral stricture at the level of the valves: this may be related to cautery damage at the time of the initial valve ablation. Measures required to correct the stricture range from radial balloon dilatation under continuous fluoroscopic control to cold knife incision to open resection of the stricture, according to its length and response to previous manipulations.

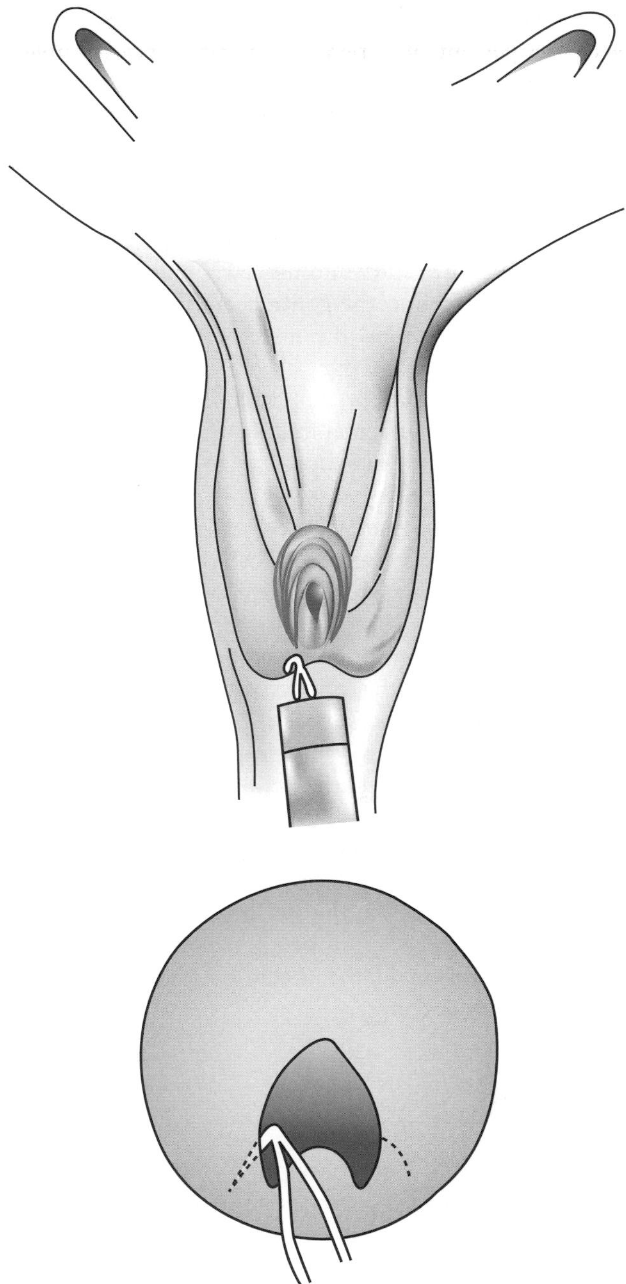

Figure 50.3

URETEROCELES

Ureteroceles are a dilated segment of the distal ureter. Most have a stenotic orifice located in the bladder. Ureteroceles are most common in girls and are associated with a duplex system. They tend to be in an ectopic location (in the bladder neck or extending into the urethra) and can prolapse into the urethra and lead to bladder outlet obstruction. Single-system ureteroceles are more common in boys and are usually in an orthotopic location (within the bladder).

Antenatal diagnosis of a duplex system and its associated ureterocele can be made with a significant degree of certainty. Postnatal ultrasonography confirms the diagnosis. MCU will identify reflux into the lower pole ureter of the duplex system or into the contralateral ureter. Typically, the bladder wall behind the ureterocele may evert with bladder filling.

Some patients may present later in childhood or in adult life with an incidental finding of a non-obstructing ureterocele, or with discomfort due to the presence of a stone in the ureterocele.

The need for intervention is determined by the size of the ureterocele and the presence of obstruction. Ureteroceles identified in childhood are typically associated with duplex systems and reduced function of the upper pole moiety. Secondary obstruction of the lower pole moiety may also occur. Evaluation of the kidneys with renal scintigraphy clarifies the relative function of the renal moieties.

Incision of the ureterocele to improve drainage can be performed in infancy. Early drainage may allow some recovery of upper pole function or permit functioning units to continue to grow. Endoscopic incision of the ureterocele may unmask reflux into the ipsilateral lower pole ureter or the contralateral ureter as the attachment of the ureters in the trigone may be compromised in the presence of a large ureterocele. Incision of the ureterocele can also lead to reflux into the same ureter.

Equipment

ESSENTIAL

- 6.5 Fr, 8 Fr and 10 Fr pediatric cystoscopes.
- Resectoscope with hook or loop electrode.
- Blunt-tipped electrode and electrocautery machine with foot pedal.
- Video camera.
- Light source.
- Warmed irrigation fluid.

Technique

Patients are positioned in the same way as for the endoscopic management of PUV. Antibiotic prophylaxis is used. Initial endoscopic evaluation identifies the location and extent of the ureterocele. The locations of the ureteral orifices are noted. Identification of the ipsilateral lower pole ureteric orifice is important to avoid its injury. Additionally, distal extension of the ureterocele through the bladder neck into the proximal urethra should also be noted.

Overfilling of the bladder during initial evaluation should be avoided to prevent collapse or eversion of the ureterocele. Although the ureterocele appears as a distended entity, incision can be difficult if the wall collapses away from the electrode being used. A hot electrode is used for incision, and entry into the ureterocele can be confirmed by direct visualization. When a ureterocele extends into the urethra, the distal extension should be incised to prevent a residual 'windsock' that may cause persistent obstruction. **(See Figure 50.4)**

Once the ureterocele has been incised, the inner wall will collapse and allow the ureter to drain freely, usually without causing postoperative reflux. Incision should be made in the most dependent part of the ureterocele. Patients that present with a stone in the ureterocele may be managed by incision, enabling the stone to be manipulated into the bladder and then fragmented.

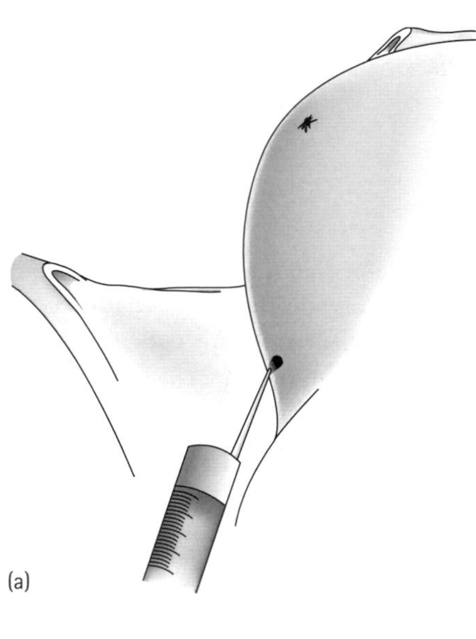

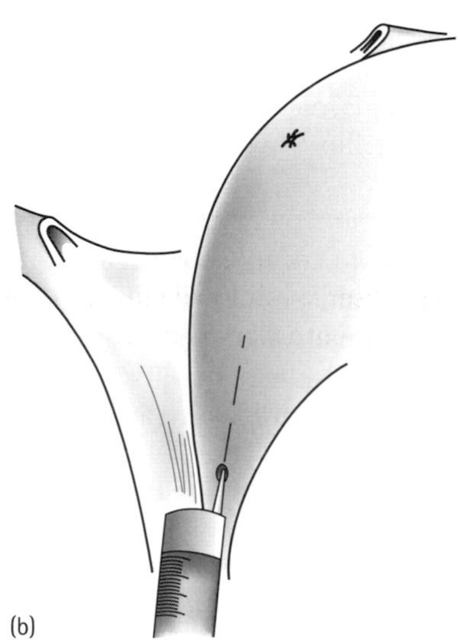

Figure 50.4 *(a) Incision of a left intravesical ureterocele; (b) incision of a left ureterocele extending into the urethra.*

Postoperative care

Most patients can have incision of the ureterocele as a day procedure. Antibiotic prophylaxis is continued postoperatively until the presence of reflux has been excluded. Follow-up ultrasonography is used to check the status of the segment drained by the ureterocele. MCU is used to establish whether there is vesico-ureteric reflux post-incision. Additionally, diuretic renal scintigraphy is used to confirm adequate drainage and functional improvement of the upper pole segment following the procedure. If the ureterocele subserves a duplex system and good drainage is achieved, this may be the only treatment required. Ureteroceles that do not cause obstruction may not require intervention.

Problems, pitfalls and solutions

Bleeding is noted rarely following incision of a ureterocele. Use of a cold knife may increase the frequency of this complication. Placement of a catheter and bladder irrigation should allow this to be managed effectively.

Complications

- Inadequate incision of the ureterocele will lead to ongoing obstruction. This may be noted on postoperative ultrasonography as a persistently dilated ureterocele in the bladder. Repeat incision may be performed. This problem is more likely to arise if the initial incision in the ureterocele has been too small.
- Injury of the ipsilateral or contralateral ureteric orifice should be managed with ureteric stenting if identified at the time of surgery. If noted in the postoperative period, ureteric stenting (e.g. double J ureteric stent placement) may be attempted or, if significant injury is present, percutaneous nephrostomy followed by primary repair may be required.
- Persistence of reflux or recurrent infections in the upper pole moiety may require later ureteric re-implantation and possible upper pole partial nephrectomy if it functions poorly. Since many ectopic ureteroceles subserve minimally functioning upper pole segments, eventual hemi-nephro-uretectomy may be required.
- Ongoing obstruction from ureterocele: further endoscopic incision or deroofing of ureterocele may be required.
- Deterioration of subserved upper pole moiety may require hemi-nephro-ureterectomy.
- Ongoing vesico-ureteric reflux: when associated with reasonable function of related renal moieties, this may require common channel ureteric re-implant (in the case of a duplex system).

URETHRAL STRICTURES

Rarely, urethral strictures in children may be congenital. More often, they are seen following valve ablation or secondary to trauma (including urethral instrumentation). The management of strictures is based on their etiology and length. Congenital strictures are typically managed in infancy with initial vesicostomy and secondary open reconstruction or serial radial dilatation. The immediate management of strictures may be with urethral dilatation or placement of a suprapubic tube. Short strictures may be managed with retrograde incision using a cold knife. Longer ones may be managed with combined antegrade and retrograde endoscopy. Evaluation of the length of the stricture is performed using retrograde urethrography, which may be combined with voiding cystography with contrast instilled through a suprapubic tube.

Equipment

ESSENTIAL

- 6.5 Fr, 8 Fr and 10 Fr pediatric cystoscopes.
- Resectoscope with cold knife.
- Urethral dilators.
- Video camera.
- Light source.
- Warmed irrigation fluid.

DESIRABLE

- Holmium/YAG laser.

Technique

The patient is positioned in the same way as described for PUV. If a suprapubic tube has been placed, both it and the abdomen are prepped into the field. Endoscopy is performed to the level of the stricture. The area of stricture is initially passed (if possible) with a guide-wire that is advanced into the bladder. The resectoscope with a cold knife is used to incise the stricture at the 12 o'clock position. In strictures that are not passable but appear short on radiographic evaluation, a combined approach is used. A cystoscope is inserted via the suprapubic tube site and antegrade endoscopy is performed to the level of the stricture. A resectoscope is inserted into the urethra to the level of the stricture. The light on the resectoscope is turned off and the light on the suprapubic cystoscope is used for visualization. Incision is performed towards this light.

Steroids may be instilled for patients who have recurrent strictures. The holmium laser may also be used for incision, allowing the use of smaller scopes.

Postoperative care

After incision of the stricture, a Silastic® urethral catheter is placed and left to drain for at least 3–5 days. Retrograde urethrography will show whether incision has been adequate. Long-term follow-up is indicated to check for recurrence. Rapid recurrence despite multiple incisions may require definitive management with open urethroplasty.

Problems, pitfalls and solutions

Bleeding following endoscopic management is possible but rare. Utilization of a Foley catheter for 24–48 hours will stop most bleeding problems following the incision of strictures.

Complications

- Undermining of the urethra during endoscopy is also possible. This may be successfully managed with urethral catheterization.
- Recurrence of the stricture following incision may be managed with repeat incision or dilatation. Further recurrence or worsening of the stricture despite this may be an indication for open surgical resection of the stricture and reconstruction of the urethra.

FURTHER READING

Gearhart JP, Rink R, Mouriquand P (eds). *Pediatric Urology.* Philadelphia: WB Saunders, 2001.

Walsh PC, Retik, AB, Vaughan, D, Wein A (eds). *Campbell's Urology,* 8th edn, Vol. 2. Philadelphia: WB Saunders, 2002.

51

Endopyelotomy

JOHN-PAUL CAPOLICCHIO

INTRODUCTION

The principle of endopyelotomy is derived from the Davis intubated ureterotomy. Endopyelotomy may be considered the treatment of choice in children with uretero-pelvic junction obstruction (UPJO) *secondary* to failed open pyeloplasty. The difficulty and morbidity of open re-operative pyeloplasty make percutaneous endopyelotomy (PCEP) an attractive consideration, with further advantages of reduced convalescence. The high success rate of pediatric open pyeloplasty makes this an uncommon indication, and therefore endo-urological experience is a prerequisite. The majority of the literature related to children deals with the percutaneous or antegrade approach, but the development of smaller ureteroscopes will contribute to greater applicability of the retrograde approach in the future. The poor results of endopyelotomy in children with *primary* UPJO combined with the promising evolution of laparoscopic pyeloplasty in children suggests that endopyelotomy should not be contemplated in this situation. Finally, endopyelotomy with the cutting balloon is another retrograde option, but is presently not practical in the pre-pubertal child because of the size of the balloon (10 Fr). Simple balloon dilatation of the UPJ without incision should be avoided in view of the poor results. **(See Table 51.1)**

Indications

- UPJO secondary to failed open pyeloplasty.
- UPJO and concomitant renal lithiasis.
- UPJO in an adolescent in the absence of aberrant crossing vessels (relative).

Contraindications

ABSOLUTE

- Severe kyphoscoliosis or restrictive lung disease impeding prone positioning.
- Stricture longer than 2 cm or complete obliteration of the ureteral lumen (inability to pass a guide-wire).
- Ectopic kidney (pelvic, malrotated, horseshoe).

RELATIVE

- Primary UPJO.
- UPJO secondary to aberrant crossing vessels.
- Poor differential renal function.
- Massive hydronephrosis.

EQUIPMENT/INSTRUMENTS

Essential

- Bolsters for prone positioning.
- C-arm for fluoroscopy.
- Operating table that accepts fluoroscopy, with stirrups and arm rests.
- Betadine prep. solution (non-alcohol-based iodine).
- Syringes and contrast medium.
- Two pediatric cystoscopes (10–14 Fr: 5 Fr working port preferable, the first for cystoscopy and the second for nephroscopy). If necessary, one can proceed with only one cystoscope by re-sterilizing it whilst the patient is being repositioned.

Table 51.1 *Advantages and disadvantages of different endo-urologic options for the surgical management of uretero-pelvic junction obstruction*

Approach	Pro	Con
Open pyeloplasty	*Highest success* Single procedure	Pain, convalescence, cosmesis (less with dorsal lumbotomy)
Laparoscopic pyeloplasty	Reproduces the principles of open surgery Improved cosmesis and convalescence	*Steep learning curve*
Percutaneous endopyelotomy	Tiny incision, less pain, convalescence, cosmesis *Proven results in properly selected patients* Available instrumentation, i.e. cystoscope	Higher morbidity from percutaneous access compared to retrograde techniques Lower success rate than open surgery
Retrograde endoscopic endopyelotomy	No skin incision, outpatient procedure	Lowest success rate, *few outcome data in children* Expense of mini-ureteroscope Potential poor visualization Potential ureteral trauma Second procedure for removal of stent
Retrograde balloon endopyelotomy	No skin incision, outpatient procedure	Lowest success rate, *few outcome data in children* No direct visualization Cost of catheter Ureteral trauma from 10 Fr balloon catheter Second procedure for removal of stent

- Endoscopic alligator forceps.
- 5 Fr end-flushing ureteral catheter.
- 0.035 Teflon-coated guide-wire.
- Foley catheter, skin stapler, craniotomy drape with suction drainage.
- 18 G Chiba needle.
- Fascial incising needle and Amplatz dilator set, heavy scissors.
- Warm irrigation fluid (normal saline and non-electrolyte water solution, e.g. glycine).
- Angled, fine-tip Greenwald electrosurgical probe.
- 5 Fr ureteral balloon dilator; 5 mm diameter, 4 cm long balloon with 0.035 guide-wire channel (can substitute with balloon angioplasty catheters).
- Leveen inflation syringe with pressure gauge.
- Malekot nephrostomy tube (12 Fr).
- 4.7–6 Fr double pigtail stents with 0.035 guide-wire channel (multiple lengths, measuring tape).

Optional

- Operating table that permits prone perineal access.
- Flexible pediatric cystoscope (for prone cystoscopy).
- Fascial balloon dilator (for adolescents, instead of Amplatz dilators).
- 13 Fr peel-away sheath with introducer (instead of Amplatz dilators).
- 10 Fr dual lumen access sheath (for quicker insertion of second safety wire).
- Pediatric resectoscope or nephroscope or 200 μ holmium laser (instead of Greenwald probe).
- 10/5 Fr endopyelotomy stent or 5 Fr Salle stent (instead of double J stent).
- 3 Fr, 4 Fr and 6 Fr end-flushing ureteral catheters, Kumpe angiography catheter (for difficult guide-wire access across the UPJ).
- Multiple guide-wires 0.018, 0.025, 0.035; Teflon-coated, straight-tip and J-tip hydrophilic guide-wires (for difficult guide-wire access across the UPJ).
- Superstiff guide-wire (for tract dilatation through fibrotic tissue).

Additional equipment for retrograde endoscopic endopyelotomy

- 4.6 Fr semi-rigid mini-ureteroscope.
- Three-way stopcock, intravenous extension tubing, 60 mL syringe.
- 7.5 Fr flexible ureteroscope and 10 Fr ureteral access sheath (optional, for adolescents).
- 20 W holmium laser with 200 μ fiber (optional).

Additional equipment for retrograde cutting balloon endopyelotomy

- Acucise™ balloon catheter.

PREOPERATIVE PREPARATION

Anesthetic and surgical considerations are similar to those of open surgery, with the caveat that the patient should be able to tolerate prone positioning. Blood count and serum creatinine are obtained and blood cross-matched. The majority of patients will already have an indwelling percutaneous nephrostomy, which should be cultured preoperatively and prophylactic antibiotics administered. If the surgeon is unfamiliar with percutaneous renal access, an interventional radiologist should be present. Renal access can be obtained through an upper or preferably middle calyx, a consideration that should be remembered when an acute decompression becomes necessary after failed pyeloplasty. Never perform an endopyelotomy after failed infant pyeloplasty without waiting at least 2 months for transient edema to resolve; a temporary nephrostomy is indicated instead. It is also imperative to obtain a copy of the operative report in referred cases of failed pyeloplasty in order to ascertain if crossing vessels were found and properly dealt with. The issue of crossing vessels and endopyelotomy outcomes is considered controversial, but this author believes that patients with crossing vessels are poor candidates for endopyelotomy. Preoperative spiral computerized tomography (CT) scan may be needed for clarification.

TECHNIQUE

The technique consists of four basic steps: guide-wire access across the UPJ, establishment of a percutaneous tract, incision of the UPJ, and stenting of the UPJ. **(See Figure 51.1)**

Percutaneous endopyelotomy

The operation is performed with general anesthesia and endotracheal intubation with antibiotic cover. The procedure can be performed entirely in the prone position if a flexible pediatric cystoscope and an operating table that allows prone access to the perineum are available. Commonly, the

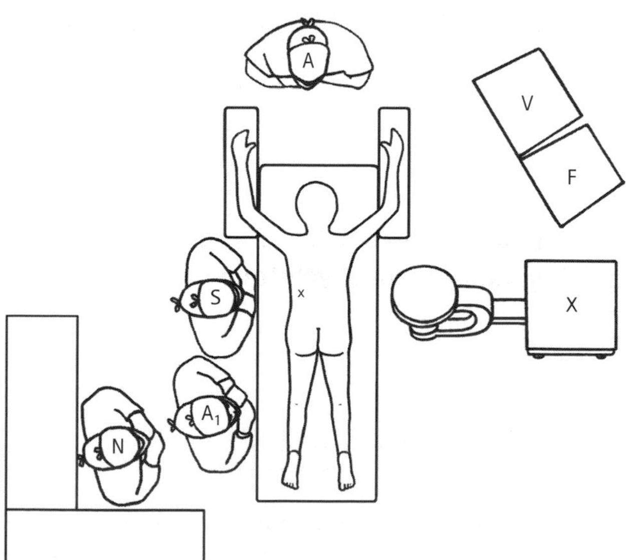

Figure 51.1

retrograde guide-wire insertion is performed in the supine lithotomy position, with time spent repositioning prior to percutaneous access. One may be tempted to forego repositioning patients with indwelling nephrostomy tubes in the hope of establishing antegrade guide-wire access through the UPJ. This usually fails and results in more time lost repositioning the patient twice.

Cystoscopy is performed with a cystoscope of age-appropriate size, preferably with a 5 Fr working channel which permits an end-flushing catheter. In the absence of a working channel of this size, a guide-wire can be passed up the ureter through a smaller working channel. The cystoscope is then removed, a 5 Fr end-flushing ureteral catheter is passed over the guide-wire and the wire is removed. It is important to place the catheter tip within the intravesical ureter such that the entire ureter can be opacified during uretero-pyelography. This allows one to assess for concomitant ureteral pathology, especially in infants who may have had the ureter instrumented during a failed pyeloplasty.

It may take time to visualize the length of UPJ stenosis, especially with the combination of a very narrow UPJ and a large pyelo-calyceal system. In such cases, an already indwelling nephrostomy tube, if present, can be utilized for simultaneous antegrade pyelography.

After assessment and confirmation of UPJ stricture length less than 2 cm, the retrograde 5 Fr ureteral catheter is advanced across the UPJ and into the renal pelvis. This is accomplished by first passing a 0.035 Teflon-coated guide-wire into the renal pelvis through the ureteral catheter. The gradation on the catheter at the level of the ureteric orifice within the bladder is noted for later reference. Difficult passage of the guide-wire should be dealt with by the usual tricks; hydrophilic guide-wires are especially helpful. One should be gentle with attempted guide-wire passage so as to avoid mucosal trauma, which can impair nephroscopy. It is best to exhaust all options from below since antegrade cannulation is usually more difficult. Though it is not mandatory to have the ureteric catheter across the UPJ, establishing guide-wire access across the UPJ is an absolute requirement. **(See Figure 51.2)**

A Foley bladder catheter is then inserted, the balloon inflated and the ureteral catheter secured on the Foley. The patient is repositioned prone and access to the retrograde catheter established by directing the ends of the Foley and ureteral catheters between the legs and to the surface. Proper padding is required for the head, chest, knees and feet. The Foley catheter position is verified to avoid pressure on the legs or genitalia.

Percutaneous access to the kidney is obtained if a nephrostomy tube is not already indwelling. Access through a middle pole posterior calyx is preferred. An upper pole approach may be used for concomitant removal of a lower pole or upper pole renal stone. It is helpful to avoid placing the access through the scar from a prior pyeloplasty. Access is achieved by an interventional radiologist at the author's institution. Briefly, an 18 G Chiba needle is passed under

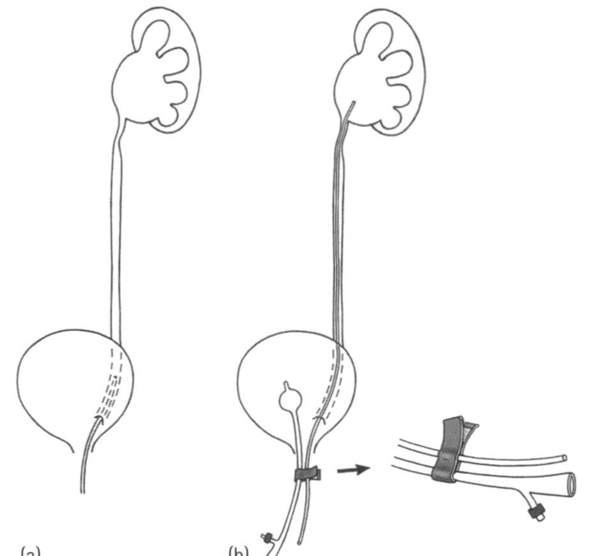

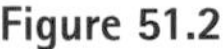

Figure 51.2

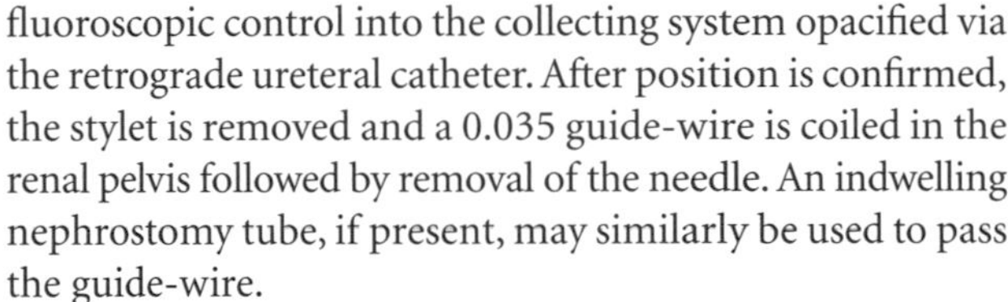

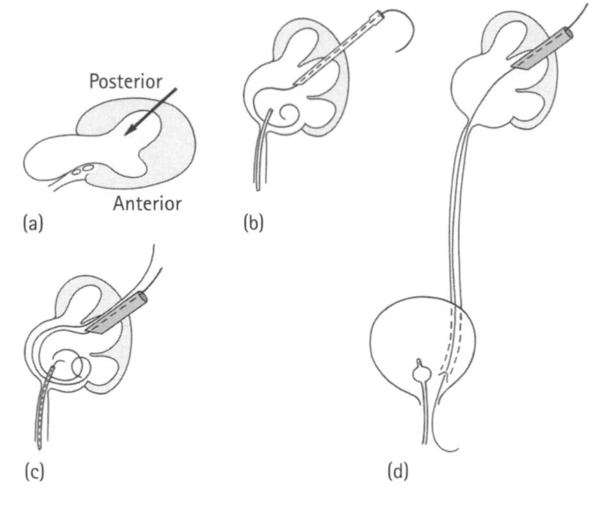

Figure 51.3

fluoroscopic control into the collecting system opacified via the retrograde ureteral catheter. After position is confirmed, the stylet is removed and a 0.035 guide-wire is coiled in the renal pelvis followed by removal of the needle. An indwelling nephrostomy tube, if present, may similarly be used to pass the guide-wire.

A 6 mm incision is made in the skin adjacent to the guide-wire and the fascial incising needle is then passed. The combined 8/10 Fr Amplatz dilator and sheath is lubricated and used to dilate the tract with a corkscrew motion. Dilatation occurs over the guide-wire, care being taken to avoid kinking it. Contrast or air is injected retrogradely to outline the renal collecting system, ensuring that dilatation does not occur past the calyx. Once the 10 Fr outer sheath is fluoroscopically confirmed in the collecting system, the 8 Fr inner dilator is removed and a second guide-wire coiled in the renal pelvis (safety wire). The 10 Fr sheath is removed and the 8 Fr dilator re-inserted over the working wire, while the safety wire is secured to the paper drapes with a skin stapler.

The tract is incrementally dilated with lubricated Amplatz dilators over the 8 Fr dilator, taking care under fluoroscopic control to avoid kinking the guide-wire and not to dilate too medially. Once dilation up to 20 Fr is performed, an 18 Fr working sheath is placed. This 18 Fr working sheath is trimmed with heavy scissors to a length that can accommodate the cystoscope/nephroscope. The size of the patient will determine the length of nephroscope required, which in turn dictates the caliber of the access tract. The working sheath should be large enough to allow easy return of irrigation fluid around the endoscope and guide-wire. In adolescents, the 30 Fr fascial dilating balloon can be used to dilate the tract more quickly and with less trauma.

Having established the working tract, nephroscopy is performed with an 11 Fr cystoscope or 14 Fr pediatric nephroscope. The retrograde ureteral catheter is identified, through which a 0.035 guide-wire is passed retrogradely. This wire is grasped through the nephroscope with alligator forceps and then pulled out through the working tract, providing through-and-through control. Once the working wire is controlled externally at both ends, the percutaneous guide-wires coiled in the renal pelvis and the retrograde ureteral catheter are removed. The previously noted gradation of the ureteral catheter is now used as a reference to determine the length of the ureter precisely, which in turn determines the length of double pigtail stent used later. Precise measurement of the length of double pigtail stent is helpful to avoid accidental placement of the distal pigtail within the urethra, which can easily happen with a through-and-through guide-wire. **(See Figure 51.3)**

Nephroscopy continues, confirming adequate access and visualization of the UPJ. One also assesses for any arterial pulsations in the site of planned incision. The Greenwald electrode is inserted for planning of the incision site. Alternative methods of incision include the smaller caliber holmium laser fiber, bearing in mind that the guide-wire can be damaged by laser energy. Cold knife incision can also be performed with a urethrotome or sickle-shaped knife. The cold knife methods allow for more precise cutting, but there is a potential for bleeding and obstructed vision.

If the UPJ stenosis is too narrow and impedes access for electrode positioning alongside the indwelling guide-wire, the stenotic segment can be gently balloon dilated to slightly enlarge the lumen. The 5 Fr/5 mm balloon ureteral dilator is slipped antegradely over the working wire until the balloon straddles the UPJ. The balloon is filled with dilute contrast and inflated slowly at the lowest pressure needed mildly to expand the waist under fluoroscopy. The Leveen syringe attached to a pressure gauge is needed for controlled dilatation. If the 4 cm long balloon does not waist, one should suspect that the length of stricture has been underestimated.

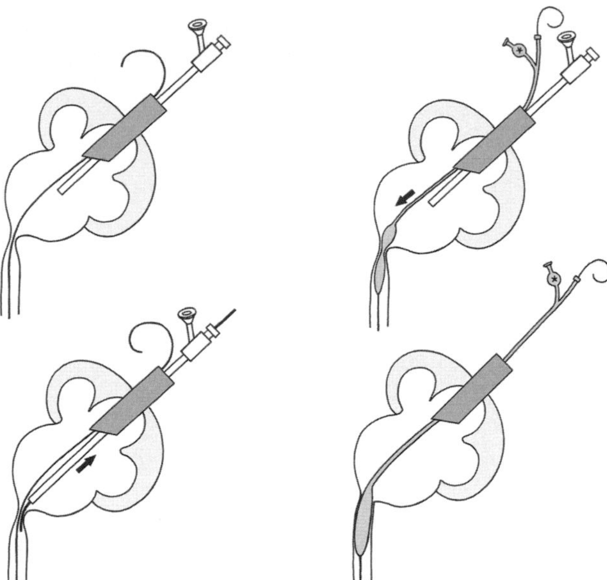

Figure 51.4

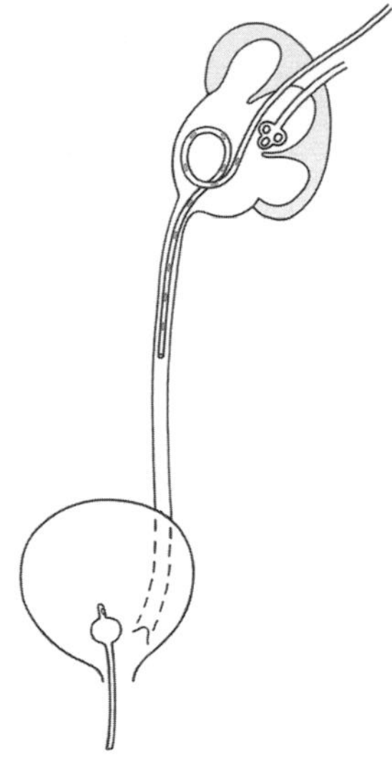

Figure 51.5

At this point the warm irrigation fluid should be temporarily switched to a non-electrolyte solution. Incision is performed by pushing the cold electrode to the distal limit of the stricture, activating the electrode with 50–75 W of pure cutting current, and dragging the entire nephroscope back, while swinging laterally. One should avoid cutting in an antegrade fashion, as a ureteral perforation will quickly occur and prevent access to the remainder of the more proximally located stricture. The full thickness of the ureter is incised – sighting of peri-ureteral fat indicates its depth.

Having completed the incision, the balloon dilator is re-inserted to verify that waisting has resolved, thus confirming the success of the incision. Resolution of waisting is demonstrated by the appearance of the full balloon profile at low-pressure inflation (less than 1 atm). This step is mandatory in cases with abundant peri-ureteral fibrosis and if bleeding after incision obscures vision. This step is omitted at some centers because of the added cost of the balloon catheter and pressure syringe. At a minimum, a nephrostogram should be performed to document antegrade passage of dye and extravasation at the incision site. **(See Figure 51.4)**

The final step is stenting of the incision with drainage of the kidney, for which three options exist. The classic approach is the tapered Smith endopyelotomy stent, which is a percutaneous nephro-ureteral stent that is 10 Fr at the level of the skin, kidney and UPJ and 5 Fr within the bladder. The external component can be quite cumbersome. A common approach is to use a 5–6 Fr double pigtail ureteral stent and a separate percutaneous 12 Fr nephrostomy tube. Though effective, this requires a second anesthetic to remove the pigtail stent. This author's approach consists of the combination of a 12 Fr percutaneous nephrostomy and a 5 Fr percutaneous nephro-ureteral Salle stent. The Salle stent is trimmed such that the distal limb ends within the distal ureter, avoiding bladder spasms and misplacement of the distal pigtail within the urethra.

The guide-wire is removed, the percutaneous drains secured to the skin and all catheters left to gravity drainage. **(See Figure 51.5)**

Retrograde endoscopic endopyelotomy

The entire procedure is performed in the supine lithotomy position. The first step, similar to PCEP, consists of cystoscopy, retrograde pyelography and guide-wire access into the renal pelvis.

Ureteroscopy is accomplished with the mini-ureteroscope, thus usually avoiding the need for dilatation of the distal ureter. A large syringe attached to the irrigation port of the endoscope via extension tubing and a three-way stopcock is helpful for pressure irrigation to distend the ureteral orifice.

The anatomy of the incision site is inspected in a similar way to that for the PCEP. A very narrow lumen is handled in the same fashion as PCEP, except that the endoscope must be removed in order to pass the 5 Fr balloon dilator.

Incision is carried out with the same principles as PCEP. A 2 Fr Greenwald electrode or 200 μ laser fiber is the only option. Again it is important to pull the endoscope and the probe back while swinging laterally, going from a proximal to distal direction along the ureter. The flow of irrigation fluid and consequently vision are improved with the use of the smaller caliber laser fiber. The adjacent guide-wire can be exchanged for a 4–5 Fr ureteral catheter, thus providing an outlet for drainage and some improvement in the flow of irrigation fluid. Ureteral access sheaths should be used with caution in children younger than 10 years of age.

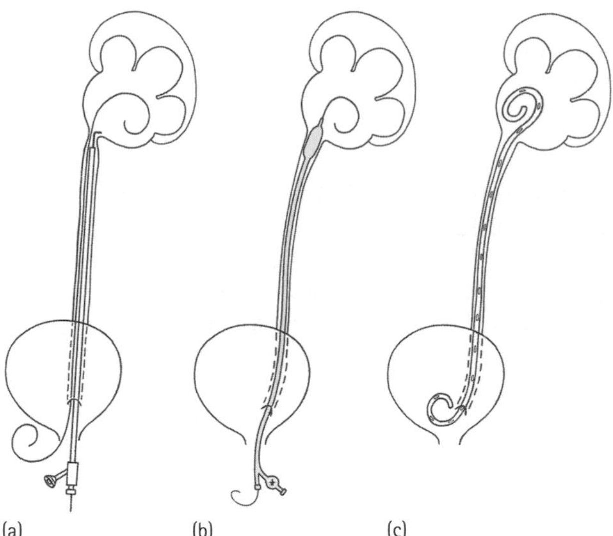

Figure 51.6

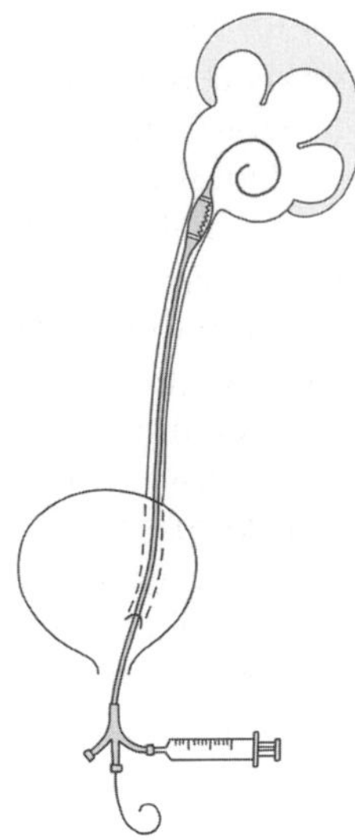

Figure 51.7

Similar to PCEP, the balloon dilator is inflated to assess the caliber of the incision. The guide-wire is exchanged for a double pigtail ureteral stent or internal, tapered endopyelotomy stent. A Foley catheter is inserted and the child admitted for overnight observation. **(See Figure 51.6)**

Retrograde cutting balloon endopyelotomy

The entire procedure is performed in the supine lithotomy position. The ureter should be large enough to accommodate the 10 Fr diameter of the deflated balloon, essentially limiting the applicability of this technique to full-grown adolescents.

The first step, similar to PCEP, consists of cystoscopy, retrograde pyelography and guide-wire access into the renal pelvis. The Acucise catheter is introduced with the cutting wire aligned in the lateral orientation. The balloon is positioned across the UPJ under fluoroscopy. Then it is partially inflated to verify waisting and to confirm lateral orientation of the cutting wire. Simultaneously, the balloon is inflated to 2.2 mL while applying 75 W of pure cutting current for 5 seconds. The waist should disappear. The balloon is left inflated for 10 minutes in order to tamponade any bleeding. **(See Figure 51.7)**

The balloon is deflated and the catheter is withdrawn and exchanged for a double pigtail ureteral stent or internal, tapered endopyelotomy stent.

POSTOPERATIVE CARE

The Foley catheter is removed the following morning. On postoperative day two, a nephrostogram is performed to verify antegrade passage of dye and resolution of extravasation. The nephrostomy tube is removed under fluoroscopic control and the Salle stent is then capped and curled beneath a dressing. The absence of leakage, pain and fever permits discharge of the patient the following morning, with prophylactic antibiotics. The Salle stent is pulled out percutaneously during an outpatient appointment 6 weeks later. Similarly, any internal stents placed during retrograde endopyelotomy are removed 6 weeks later under a second (general) anesthetic.

Follow-up renal ultrasound is obtained 1 month after stent removal and a diuretic renogram 2 months thereafter. Late failures have been reported, especially in younger children, and consequently postoperative follow-up into adolescence is recommended. Options for late failures include repeat endopyelotomy, laparoscopic redo pyeloplasty, open redo pyeloplasty with or without renal pelvic flap extension or ureterocalycostomy.

PROBLEMS, PITFALLS AND SOLUTIONS

The UPJ cannot be traversed with the 0.035 guide-wire

This can be due to a very narrow stricture, an eccentric lumen or ureteral tortuosity. The patient is lowered into the Trendelenburg position to straighten the ureter. Short bursts of pressure inflation with the contrast syringe attached to the ureteral catheter can also be helpful. An angled hydrophilic guide-wire advanced through the ureteral catheter and twisted under fluoroscopic control is usually helpful. If a straight-tipped guide-wire is used, it can be advanced through an angled Kumpe angiography catheter. A 0.025 hydrophilic guide-wire can be advanced in a similar fashion through a 4 Fr ureteral catheter and the procedure done over the 0.025 guide-wire. Similarly, a 0.018 guide-wire can be advanced through a 3 Fr ureteral catheter. This is followed by passage of a 6 Fr ureteral catheter over the 3 Fr catheter, which is then exchanged for the 0.035 guide-wire.

As a last resort, cut-to-the-light and cut-to-methylene-blue procedures have been reported, but are not advocated by this author. Briefly, nephrostomy access is obtained with a guide-wire coiled in the renal pelvis, followed by retrograde injection of methylene blue through the ureteral catheter in order to visualize the ureteral lumen. Simultaneously, the nephroscope is used to cut towards the blue lumen in the hope of creating a channel wide enough to permit guide-wire passage. In cases where the lumen is completely obliterated, a flexible ureteroscope is passed retrogradely up to the UPJ stricture and the nephroscope is used to cut a channel towards the retrograde light source. Considering the lack of outcome data, the risks involved in cutting blindly and the poor prognosis for success in view of the ischemic pathophysiology of complete ureteral fibrosis, this author prefers to abandon the procedure if guide-wire access cannot be established across the UPJ stricture. Properly consented, one can then proceed to open or laparoscopic redo pyeloplasty in this case.

A lower pole nephrostomy tube is already indwelling

This will be a common occurrence in referred cases after failed pyeloplasty. Sampaio has extensively studied the anatomy of the renal collecting system and found that lower pole access to the UPJ was possible if the infundibulum formed an angle greater than 90° with the UPJ axis. In the presence of such favorable anatomy on a nephrostogram, an attempt at lower pole nephroscopy through a minimal access sheath is reasonable. If this is not possible, a second access needs to be established, preferably via a middle calyx.

Minor bleeding that obscures endoscopy

This can occur with mucosal trauma from difficult guide-wire passage or from cold knife incision. It is more likely to be problematic with the use of very narrow endoscopes. Gentle tamponade for 10 minutes with the ureteral balloon dilator is usually effective.

Irrigant extravasation

The risk is increased by prolonged operative time, the use of high-pressure irrigation or disruption of collecting system integrity (e.g. calyceal or renal pelvic tear during dilatation of the nephrostomy tract). The access sheath should always be 4 Fr larger than the caliber of the endoscope to permit unimpeded return of low-pressure irrigation fluid. Narrower endoscopes require higher pressure irrigation for vision. Symptomatic hydrothorax or hydroperitoneum requires percutaneous aspiration/drainage and termination of the procedure with appropriate systemic support from the anesthesia team.

By how much should the percutaneous tract be dilated?

Smaller tracts are advantageous in that they take less time to create and are less likely to cause bleeding from a shearing injury of the infundibular collecting system. The 'Mini-Perc' technique uses a 13 Fr working sheath, but requires the use of endoscopes smaller than 9 Fr in order to accommodate the guide-wire and low-pressure return of irrigation fluid solution. Such small endoscopes may not be readily available. Furthermore, smaller endoscopes are more susceptible to obscured vision with minor bleeding and require higher pressure irrigation. Considering that the risk of infundibular injury is less in the dilated calyx of a hydronephrotic kidney, this author feels that a 16–18 Fr working sheath is ideal and permits the use of readily available cystoscopes.

Guide-wire access is lost

This is more likely to occur with the retrograde approach or percutaneously if a safety guide-wire is not used or if the safety wire is not immobilized to the patient. One hand must always stabilize the access sheath when removing the nephroscope. Through-and-through access with control of the guide-wire percutaneously at both the renal and urethral ends minimizes this risk, and obviates the need for a safety wire. The risk of a transected guide-wire is specific to the use of laser energy for incision, especially with the retrograde approach. Renal access can be regained under direct vision through the nephrostomy tract, though this is more successful with a mature tract. An attempt should then be made to cannulate the ureteral lumen visually with a guide-wire through the nephroscope. Likewise, retrograde cannulation of the ureteric lumen can be attempted through a ureteroscope. The risk of symptomatic irrigation fluid extravasation increases with persistence in these attempts. The procedure must be aborted and another nephrostomy tube placed if guide-wire control cannot be re-established.

Hypothermia

This will occur if irrigation fluid solution is not warmed, especially in smaller children.

The procedure takes too long

At some centers, initial nephrostomy access is created in the radiology suite on the day prior to the procedure, although this necessitates a second anesthetic. Much operative time can be wasted repositioning the patient. Performing the entire procedure with the patient in the prone position can save time, but requires an operating table that permits access to the perineum and flexible cystoscopy. Time can also be gained by substituting a 5 Fr ureteric balloon catheter from the start for the end-flushing ureteral catheter, eliminating time wasted for catheter exchanges. Development of the percutaneous tract is quicker with the dual lumen access sheath, since the safety wire can be inserted sooner. Lastly, nurses unfamiliar with the procedure should undergo a rehearsal preoperatively, particularly to verify that all catheters and guide-wires are compatible.

Inability to tolerate the internal stent postoperatively

Anti-cholinergic pharmacotherapy is indicated for bladder spasms, together with frequent, timed voiding to minimize flank pain from refluxing urine. Good endopyelotomy results have been reported with as little as 2 weeks of stenting.

COMPLICATIONS

Hemorrhage

Hemorrhage can occur from the abdominal wall tract or from the kidney and may be arterial or venous in origin. The nephrostomy tube should be clamped, but if this is not successful, it should be exchanged over the guide-wire for one of larger caliber. If bleeding persists, pressure can be applied with a Kaye tamponade or Councill balloon catheter. Close observation and serial hematocrits are necessary. If 2–4 days of tamponade are not successful, selective angiographic embolization is then required. As a last resort, partial or total nephrectomy may be necessary.

Urinoma, urinary leak

This may occur because of improper stent placement, kinking of the percutaneous stent or occlusion of stent by blood clot. Nephrostomy tube patency should be verified and the position of all tubes and stents fluoroscopically confirmed, and changed as necessary.

Pneumothorax, hydrothorax, hemothorax or urothorax

These are reported in 10 percent of upper pole accesses. Routine chest fluoroscopy is indicated at the end of the procedure when upper pole access is used. Chest tube drainage is required for symptomatic collections. Some authors will aspirate and observe asymptomatic collections if the inciting factor has been addressed.

Hyponatremia

This occurs with the inadvertent use of non-isotonic irrigation fluid solution and is compounded by extravasation. Hypertension and bradycardia are intra-operative warning signs, whereas confusion, nausea/vomiting, visual disturbances and seizure are postoperative symptoms. Furosemide or mannitol diuresis is indicated, together with isotonic intravenous supplementation. Hypertonic saline administration may cause central pontine myelinolysis.

Systemic fluid overload

Extravasation, high-pressure irrigation and prolonged surgery are all risk factors. Ventilatory support and diuresis are indicated.

Ureteral injury

Stricture, necrosis and avulsion can all occur from excessive manipulation of the ureter. Gentle passage of dilators and endoscopes is a must. The entire gamut of open corrective options may be necessary, including ureteral re-implantation with Boari flap, psoas hitch or nephropexy, trans-uretero-ureterostomy, cutaneous ureterostomy, ureteral ligation with nephrostomy until later autotransplantation or ileal interposition.

Adjacent organ injury

This can result from percutaneous access. Bleeding can occur from hepatic or splenic injury, especially in the setting of organomegaly. Hepatic injury is more likely to be controlled with conservative measures. Bowel perforation is also a possibility. Duodenal injury occurs when percutaneous access proceeds too medially. In both cases, nephroenteric fistulae are usually detected on the early postoperative nephrostogram. Colonic fistula can be conservatively managed by ensuring internal stenting of the urinary tract combined with broad-spectrum antibiotics. The nephrostomy tube is pulled back into the colon under fluoroscopy, thus creating a diverting cecostomy. If follow-up contrast studies 7–10 days later confirm healing, the cecostomy tube is removed. Open correction is indicated with intraperitoneal contamination or clinical sepsis/peritonitis. Duodenal fistula can also be managed conservatively with nasogastric suction and hyperalimentation in addition to nephrostomy and internal urinary drainage. Follow-up radiographic evaluation is deferred for 2 weeks.

Sepsis

The risk is increased with prior indwelling nephrostomy. Preoperative urine cultures and peri-operative antibiotic prophylaxis are indicated.

Recurrent UPJ obstruction

Options include open redo pyeloplasty, possibly with renal pelvic flaps, and nephropexy, ureterocalicostomy or laparoscopic redo pyeloplasty in experienced hands. Late failures of infant pyeloplasties have been repaired with repeat endopyelotomy, although outcome data are lacking. Nephrectomy can be considered with poorly functioning kidneys.

FURTHER READING

Capolicchio JP, Homsy YL, Houle AM, Brzezinski A, Stein L, Elhilali MM. Long-term results of percutaneous endopyelotomy in the treatment of children with failed open pyeloplasty. *Journal of Urology* 1997; **158**:1534–7.

Figenshau RS, Clayman RV. Endourologic options for management of ureteropelvic junction obstruction in the pediatric patient. *Urologic Clinics of North America* 1998; **25**:199–209.

Figenshau RS, Clayman RV, Colberg JW, Coplen DE, Soble JJ, Manley CB. Pediatric endopyelotomy: the Washington University experience. *Journal of Urology* 1996; **156**:2025–30.

McDougall EM, Liatsikos EN, Dinlenc CZ, Smith AD. Percutaneous approaches to the upper urinary tract. In: Walsh PC, Retik, AB, Vaughan, D, Wein A (eds), *Campbell's Urology*, 8th edn. Philadelphia: WB Saunders, 2002, 3323–40.

Nicholls G, Hrouda D, Kellett MJ, Duffy PG. Endopyelotomy in the symptomatic older child. *British Journal of Urology International* 2001; **87**:525–7.

52A

Stone management – percutaneous access

HENRY C. IRVING

INTRODUCTION

Percutaneous nephrostomy, the percutaneous insertion of a drainage catheter directly into the renal collecting system under image guidance, is a minimally invasive procedure for providing relief of obstruction which may be due to stones or other pathology. However, it is also the preliminary step in accessing the urinary tract in order to offer the opportunity for other therapeutic options, including nephroscopy for percutaneous nephrolithotomy (PCNL).

Percutaneous nephrostomy may be life-saving in the acute situation of an obstructed infected system, or when there is obstruction of a single functioning kidney. In these acute circumstances, the operator should use an approach to the kidney that offers the greatest chance of effective drainage, and the suitability of the approach for subsequent procedures is a secondary consideration. On the other hand, when percutaneous nephrostomy is the preliminary step for the provision of access for PCNL, the technique may differ in several key respects, when the prime object is to provide an access route to the collecting system which gives the surgeon the best chance of maximizing the degree of stone clearance.

Indications

- Relief of obstruction.
- Diversion of urine flow (for control of urinary fistulae and other leaks).
- Provision of access to urinary tract for elective procedures:
  - ureteric stent insertion,
  - pyelolysis (endopyelotomy),
  - percutaneous tumor therapy,
  - percutaneous nephrolithotomy.

Contraindications

- Uncontrollable bleeding diathesis.
- Inaccessible kidney:
  - intervening bowel,
  - spinal deformity,
  - malpositioned kidney, e.g. pelvic kidney.

EQUIPMENT/INSTRUMENTS

In the operating theater or interventional radiology suite.

- Image-guidance systems:
  - image intensifier (X-rays) – C-arm configuration, which may be either fixed (floor or ceiling mounted) or mobile,
  - ultrasound scanner (with a selection of transducers and needle-guide attachments).
- In theaters, suitable operating table for use with X-rays.
- In radiology suites, suitable procedures couch (when there may be irrigating fluid spillages).

All interventional uro-radiologists have their favorite selection of needles, guide-wires and catheters, which will vary according to the details of their technique. The following is a list of instruments that the author uses regularly in his practice (both for adults and children), but not all items will be used in an individual case.

- Sheathed needle (19 G).
- Guide-wires:
  - J-tipped heavy duty (0.35 or 0.38 diameter, 80–120 cm length),
  - Super-stiff (different manufacturers make different versions),
  - Terumo wire with torque control device.
- Dilators:
  - plastic, 6 Fr, 8 Fr, 10 Fr,
  - metallic, telescopic 10–30 Fr,
  - some workers (but not this author) use balloon dilatation of nephrostomy tracks, when suitable balloon catheters with back-mounted sheaths will be necessary.
- Sheaths, 18 Fr, 24 Fr, 28 Fr, 30 Fr.
- Catheters:
  - All-purpose drainage (APD) (6 Fr, 8 Fr, 12 Fr),
  - locking-loop pigtail nephrostomy catheters (6 Fr, 8 Fr, 12 Fr),
  - large-bore nephrostomy catheters, (14 Fr, 20 Fr, 24 Fr).
- Adhesive fixing discs (for retaining the drainage catheters in place).
- Urine drainage bags with connecting tubing.

The selection of dilator size will depend upon the size of catheter/sheath to be introduced, which will in turn depend upon the size of the kidney, the nature of the fluid to be drained (clear urine, pus etc.), or the size of the surgical instruments to be used (nephroscope diameter etc.). However, the underlying principle of the techniques is common – access is gained to the collecting system of the urinary tract under imaging guidance, a guide-wire is introduced, and the track is then dilated over the wire, to a diameter necessary for whatever intervention is necessary (catheter placement for drainage, or sheath insertion for the introduction of surgical instruments).

PREOPERATIVE PREPARATION

- Checking/correction of blood coagulation.
- Review of imaging studies.
- Assessment of access routes.
- Liaison with anesthetist (in older children, percutaneous nephrostomy for drainage purposes may be performed under local anesthesia with sedation).
- All percutaneous nephrostomies, whether for drainage, PCNLs or other purposes, should be performed under antibiotic cover. The antibiotics may be given at the time of anesthesia or earlier.

TECHNIQUE

Percutaneous nephrostomy for drainage

Preliminary ultrasound scanning is performed to decide upon the optimum position of the patient for the procedure, which may be performed with the patient supine, lateral, prone/oblique or prone – depending entirely on the ease of access to the target renal collecting system.

The initial step is an ultrasound-guided puncture of the collecting system with a 19 G sheathed needle. The aim should be to pass the needle assembly across renal parenchyma, through a dilated calyx, into the renal pelvis, in order to maximize the volume of collecting system along the chosen needle pathway. This will inevitably necessitate a postero-lateral oblique approach to a posterior or laterally placed calyx. For drainage purposes, it is irrelevant whether the chosen calyx is upper, lower or mid-polar – ease of access is the prime consideration and, in the vast majority of cases, a lower pole calyx will be selected. **(See Figure 52A.1)**

Once the collecting system has been punctured, the needle is removed, leaving the outer sheath in place, and backflow of urine should be seen. At this point, the technique will vary, depending upon whether it is being performed under ultrasound guidance alone or whether X-ray imaging is available.

If under ultrasound guidance alone, a J-tip guide-wire is introduced through the sheath. It will either pass down a dilated ureter or will curl up in the pelvi-calyceal system. In either case, as soon as resistance is felt, dilators are passed sequentially over the wire until the track is of sufficient diameter to permit passage of the chosen catheter. **(See Figure 52A.2)**

If X-ray screening is available, a small volume (5–10 mL) of contrast medium is injected though the sheath in order to opacify the pelvi-calyceal system. (The contrast should be sufficiently dilute, e.g. 150 mg iodine/mL, so that the guide-wires and catheters are not obscured by its density.) Guide-wires, dilators and catheters can then be introduced into the collecting system under direct X-ray screening visualization.

Once the drainage catheter is satisfactorily positioned in the collecting system, it is connected to a drainage bag and secured in place using either stitches or adhesive skin discs, according to the preference of the operator.

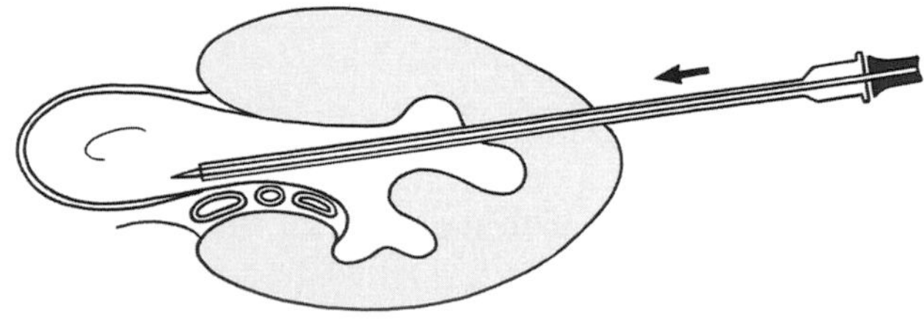

Figure 52A.1

Percutaneous nephrostomy for PCNL

This is an elective procedure and preliminary assessment of all the available imaging in consultation with the surgeon is vital in order to select the access route that will permit the best chance of achieving maximal stone clearance. As well as plain radiographs to show the size and shape of radio-opaque stones and intravenous urograms to demonstrate the anatomy of the collecting system, computerized tomography (CT) scans may often help in providing three-dimensional visualization of the stone configuration, and functional studies with isotope renograms may be needed before final decisions about intervention are made.

In contra-distinction to the performance of percutaneous nephrostomy for drainage purposes, access for PCNL necessitates careful assessment of which calyx is selected for puncture.

- If the stone is contained within a single calyx, the approach will need to be either directly into the stone-containing calyx or via a distant calyx from which the rigid nephroscope can be manipulated to reach the stone.
- If there are stones within more than one calyx, separate punctures of each stone-containing calyx may be necessary, but access via a different calyx may permit all stones to be reached from a single puncture.
- If the stone is contained within the renal pelvis, it may be possible to choose any calyx for access, although one that will permit manipulation of the nephroscope into the upper ureter may be preferable.
- If the stone occupies renal pelvis and one or more calyces, a decision is usually necessary as to how best to clear the renal pelvis and as many calyces as possible, recognizing that total clearance of a complex staghorn calculus may require more than one procedure. Occasionally, it can be predicted preoperatively that there are likely to be residual stones that may need supplementary treatment via extracorporeal shockwave lithotripsy (ESWL), and the patient/parents should be warned of this. **(See Figure 52A.3)**

In order to guide the puncture of the selected calyx under direct radiological visualization, the collecting system needs to be opacified.

Whenever possible, a ureteric catheter should be passed retrogradely at the commencement of the procedure. This will allow for:

- instillation of contrast medium into the pelvi-calyceal system,
- distension of an otherwise non-dilated collecting system,
- minimization of the chances of stone fragments passing down the ureter and causing ureteric obstruction in the postoperative period.

However, ureteric catheterisation is not always possible and other options need to be considered.

If there is an ileal conduit, opacification and distension of the upper tracts can usually be achieved by instillation of contrast medium into the conduit via a Foley (balloon) catheter, with reflux of contrast up the ureters.

Alternatively, an initial puncture of the collecting system can be performed using a fine-bore needle under ultrasound guidance and contrast injected 'antegradely'. The ideal calyx can then be selected and punctured using the larger-bore sheathed needle assembly.

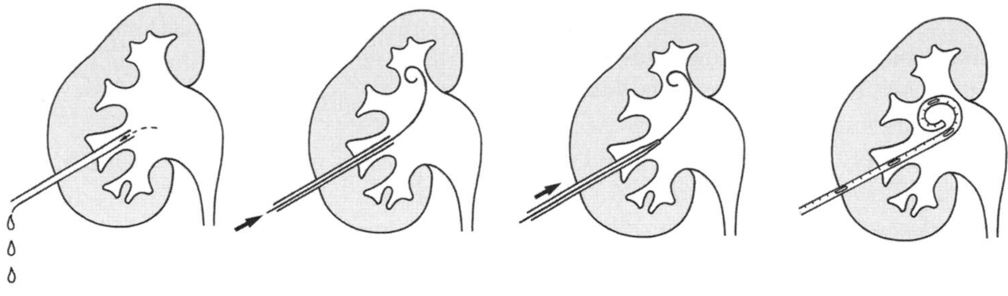

Figure 52A.2

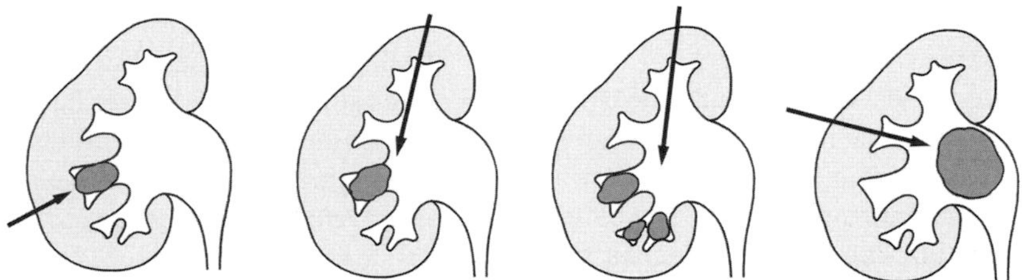

Figure 52A.3

Another option is to opacify the collecting system via an intravenous injection of contrast, but this is dependent upon sufficient renal excretory function and does not result in any significant degree of collecting system distension.

Finally, it may be necessary to perform either X-ray or ultrasound-guided puncture directly onto stone within the collecting system, and then to pass dilators and the sheath onto the surface of the stone.

In our practice, an upper pole calyceal puncture is often the preferred route of access, allowing for the clearance of maximal stone volume not only from the renal pelvis, but also from several different calyces. The approach will be a much more directly posterior route to the upper pole calyx than is necessary for a lower or mid-polar calyx, and in order to have sufficient downward (caudad) angulation to permit passage of the sheath (and subsequently the rigid nephroscope) through the collecting system, a supra-costal puncture may be necessary. Although there is then an attendant risk of traversing the pleura (see 'Complications' below), the risk of a subsequent pleural effusion or pneumothorax (treated by insertion of a pleural drain) can justifiably be offset by the improved access to complex stones.

The procedure is usually performed with the patient prone, although a lateral position may be adopted when there are particular anatomical difficulties, e.g. in some patients with marked spinal deformities or with lower limb contractures. For the usual prone position, the anesthetist will often require suitable padding or pillows to be placed under the thorax and bony pelvis in order to prevent abdominal compression that will impair ventilation – this will inevitably increase the degree of lumbar lordosis, which makes percutaneous renal access more difficult, but is a necessary measure for the overall well-being of the patient.

Following puncture of the collecting system, introduction of the guide-wire and passage of the polyethylene dilators to 10 Fr diameter, the track is then dilated further by using either metal telescopic dilators or a balloon dilatation catheter. Whilst each method has its advantages and disadvantages, this author prefers the metal telescopic dilators, which are re-usable and thus inexpensive, can be used to dilate up to any given diameter from 12 Fr to 30 Fr, and can be used to dilate a track down to the surface of a stone which is filling the collecting system. Balloon dilatation catheters are said to be less traumatic in that the expanding force is in an axial direction, but they are for once-only use and therefore more expensive, each balloon will only dilate up to a predetermined and fixed track diameter, and the catheter tip may prevent adequate dilatation of a track down to the surface of a stone.

Once the track is dilated, a sheath is introduced. Various sheaths are available, but they should have a beveled leading edge and should be constructed from firm plastic material. For pediatric practice, 18 Fr sheaths are usually adequate, but the size used is governed by the outer diameter of the nephroscope, remembering that there has to be sufficient space to allow a guide-wire alongside the scope. Once the tip of the sheath is firmly within the collecting system, the guide-wire may be dispensed with, as long as the surgeon is careful not to withdraw the sheath at any time during the ensuing stone disintegration/withdrawal procedure. Either the radiologist or a surgical assistant should remain firmly in control of the sheath in order to allow the surgeon to direct his or her full attention to the manipulation of the nephroscope and other instruments (see Chapter 52B).

At the end of the stone clearance procedure, a nephrostomy catheter (of diameter 4 Fr less than the sheath) should be introduced through the sheath, which is then withdrawn over the catheter and cut away from it. The catheter will help to minimize the risk of bleeding from the track and will allow access for a nephrostogram, for stent placement, or for re-entry to the collecting system if a second procedure is necessary.

A postoperative nephrostogram is routinely requested by some surgeons and in selected cases by others. It offers an opportunity to assess any residual stones and their position in the collecting system, and enables the detection of any stone fragments in the ureter.

Antegrade ureteric stent placement may be necessary if there has been any damage to the renal pelvis or ureter resulting in leakage of contrast into the peri-renal or peri-ureteric tissues, or if there is a risk of ureteric obstruction by residual stone fragments.

Re-entry to the collecting system may be deemed necessary if there is significant stone burden remaining after the initial procedure. A different access route may be required, but introduction of contrast or a nephroscope via the original nephrostomy track may still be helpful.

POSTOPERATIVE CARE

Whether a nephrostomy catheter has been introduced as a primary drainage procedure or following PCNL, certain principles apply.

- Dressings must be comfortable, but secure enough to prevent dislodgement of the catheter.
- Adequate analgesia must be provided and, in the case of a large-bore catheter following PCNL, a postoperative spinal or epidural anesthetic may be warranted (particularly for supra-costal punctures).
- The output from the catheter must be monitored and any possible blockage should be investigated by gentle flushing with sterile saline.
- The catheter should never be removed until it has been determined that there is no residual obstruction of the urinary tract, and an action plan for subsequent management has been agreed.

Once the catheter has been removed, urine may leak from the track for a short time, but in the absence of any residual obstruction (see above), the track will seal within a few hours.

PROBLEMS, PITFALLS AND SOLUTIONS

Percutaneous nephrostomy for drainage

The primary success rate for percutaneous nephrostomy approaches 100 percent in large published series, although there will always be an occasional case in which puncture of the collecting system and/or insertion of a drainage catheter fails. It has been shown that the success rate increases with the experience of the operator, and it is therefore worth reviewing what supplementary maneuvers may be undertaken when puncture is proving problematical.

- Ultrasound equipment.
  - There is a radiological adage 'if it can be visualized on ultrasound, it can be needled'. Ultrasound scanners vary in their image quality, and it may help to bring in an alternative machine for better visualization of the target.
  - Harmonic imaging has proven particularly useful for 'cleaning up' the image by reducing 'noise', and is now generally available on better quality equipment.
  - The use of a needle-guide attachment, rather than free-hand puncture, results in more accurate needle placement and helps reduce deviation of the needle tip away from the desired route.
- The chosen route for puncture should be re-assessed if entry into the collecting system is problematical.
  - A steeply angled (upwards) route may have been selected in order to aim at a dilated lower pole calyx, but such an approach may allow the needle tip to be deviated away from the lower pole of the kidney.
  - The shortest and most direct route for puncture should be chosen, and this is often higher and more lateral than the original route, and is also more likely to allow for direct ultrasound visualization of the passage of the needle through a calyx into the renal pelvis.
- Incomplete puncture of the collecting system. Following insertion of the sheathed needle into the collecting system, it may be possible to aspirate urine, but impossible to pass a guide-wire through the tip of the sheath. This is because the beveled tip of the needle has incompletely pierced the urothelium. The situation can be confirmed by gentle injection of contrast medium, which will both fill the pelvi-calyceal system and extravasate. The situation can be remedied by re-inserting the central needle (taking care not to puncture the side-wall of the sheath) and then advancing the assembly by a few millimeters into the system under X-ray screening guidance.
- Difficulty in passage of the guide-wire through a calyx into the pelvis is likely to be due to having punctured an anterior calyx so that the calyceal neck meets the pelvis at a steep angle. Use of an angled-tip Terumo guide-wire (rather than the conventional stiff J-tip wire) should allow this problem to be overcome.
- In pediatric practice, difficulty in the passage of dilators or the catheter over the wire is due to mobility of the kidney so that forward pressure of the dilator on either the renal capsule or urothelium pushes the entire kidney ahead of the dilator. When this happens, the operator should revert back to the smallest size dilator and recommence the dilatation procedure. The use of a central stiffener within the nephrostomy catheter is also recommended.
- Bleeding into the collecting system may result from even the most straightforward and seemingly atraumatic percutaneous nephrostomy procedure.
  - Slightly blood-tinged urine is of no concern and will clear within a few hours.
  - Heavier hematuria will also be self-limiting and is unlikely to cause any significant problem in terms of catheter blockage. As long as urine flow has been established, the naturally occurring urokinase will ensure lysis of any clots, although it may occasionally be necessary to flush the nephrostomy catheter regularly with sterile saline in order to keep it patent.
  - Patients who are in chronic renal failure may have low hemoglobin levels prior to the procedure and it may be necessary to transfuse them following a nephrostomy that has resulted in blood loss that would not be significant in other patients.
  - Very rarely, bleeding persists and selective renal arterial embolization may need to be considered (incidence of <0.001 percent in the author's experience).

Percutaneous nephrostomy for PCNL

In addition to the general problems and pitfalls described above, percutaneous nephrostomy for PCNL may pose specific difficulties in the following scenarios.

- Inability to puncture the desired calyx.
  - See previous section on 'Percutaneous nephrostomy for drainage'.
  - A specific problem for PCNL may be that the desired calyx may be so full of stone that there is no room for passage of a guide-wire into the collecting system. Several options are then available.
    - Further distension of the collecting system with saline or contrast medium in order to create space around the stone. This may not be possible and risks rupturing the collecting system.

- Choose another calyx for puncture. Total stone clearance may then not be possible, but such an approach may allow for sufficient reduction in stone bulk so that ESWL may subsequently be used for any residual stone burden.
- Puncture down onto the stone and dilate the track as far as possible so that the surgeon may then dissect onto the stone under a combination of X-ray screening and direct nephroscopic vision. This maneuver should only be attempted by experienced surgeons!

- The Amplatz sheath has been inserted, but the nephroscope does not advance into the collecting system. This occurs when the operator has failed to advance the dilators through the urothelium. One of two options is then possible.
  - The nephroscope is withdrawn and the track is re-dilated over the guide-wire, taking care to advance the dilators fully into the collecting system.
  - The surgeon may use the grasping forceps to probe ahead of the nephroscope, dissecting alongside the guide-wire under direct vision, and so enlarging the track until the nephroscope enters the collecting system. The sheath can then be advanced over the nephroscope.
- During the lithotomy procedure, the sheath becomes dislodged out of the collecting system or kidney.
  - This is not a significant problem as long as the guide-wire is in place. The dilators can be passed over the wire and the sheath re-inserted.
  - However, if the guide-wire has fallen out during the procedure (as frequently happens), the procedure will usually have to be abandoned since it is extremely difficult to re-puncture a decompressed system and any contrast instilled will simply disperse through the original puncture wound. This scenario should not be allowed to occur, and once the guide-wire has fallen out, the surgeon should have an assistant holding the sheath with the sole responsibility of preventing its dislodgement!

COMPLICATIONS

The complications of percutaneous nephrostomy are discussed here and those of PCNL in Chapter 52B.

The major complications of percutaneous nephrostomy (with the commonly quoted rates in parentheses) include the following.

- Significant hemorrhage requiring blood transfusion (up to 3.3 percent). In exceptionally rare cases, hemorrhage may need to be controlled by selective renal angiography and embolization of the bleeding vessel – a technique that should be available at all major radiological centers.
- Septicemia (up to 3 percent, despite routine antibiotic administration).
- Inadvertent puncturing of the pleura. (Up to 9 percent complication rate in supra-costal punctures for PCNL – pleural effusions, atelectasis, pneumothorax. It is therefore recommended that a chest radiograph be performed in all patients with a supra-costal puncture prior to nephrostomy catheter removal).
- Inadvertent puncturing of an intra-abdominal viscus such as the colon (0.1 percent). This risk increases when the approach is too lateral or in patients with anatomical variants, e.g. colon interposed between kidney and posterior abdominal wall. Surgical repair is usually required in intraperitoneal colonic perforation, whereas extraperitoneal colonic perforation may be treated conservatively.

Minor complications include:

- retroperitoneal urine extravasation, which may require insertion of a ureteric stent,
- significant macroscopic hematuria causing clot colic and/or catheter blockage necessitating further interventions.

FURTHER READING

Alken P. Teleskopbougierset zur permanenten Nephrostomie. *Aktuelle Urologie* 1981; **12**:216–18.

Choong S, Whitfield H, Duffy P et al. The management of paediatric urolithiasis. *British Journal of Urology International* 2000; **86** (7):857–60.

Ekelund L, Lindstedt E. Rapid dilatation of the nephrostomy track using a new type of balloon catheter. *Acta Radiologica Diagnosis* 1985; **26**:197–9.

Irving HC, Arthur RJ, Thomas DFM. Percutaneous nephrostomy in paediatrics. *Clinical Radiology* 1987; **38**:245–8.

Wah T, Weston M J, Irving HC. Percutaneous nephrostomy insertion: outcome data from a prospective multi-operator study at a UK training centre. *Clinical Radiology* 2004; **59**:255–61.

Wickham JEA, Kellet MJ. Percutaneous nephrolithotomy. *British Medical Journal* 1981; **283**:1571–2.

52B

Endo-urological management of urinary stones

AZAD NAJMALDIN, A.R. WILLIAMS AND S.N. LLOYD

INTRODUCTION

Urinary stone disease may occur in children of any age, including newborns. The incidences vary widely with geography and age. Outside the Afro-Asian stone belt, where urolithiasis is endemic, stone disease is fairly uncommon in children. There is also etiological variation. Generally, in Europe and North America, infection is the major etiological factor, although metabolic abnormalities such as hypercalciuria, cystinuria and oxaluria are important factors in multiple and recurrent stone disease. An estimated 10–80 percent of children demonstrate an underlying metabolic problem. This wide variation reflects referral patterns for different specialist units. Anatomical abnormalities such as pelvi-ureteric junction and vesico-ureteric junction obstruction or abnormalities resulting from surgery, such as an augmented bladder, are also important.

Stones may present as an incidental finding during investigations for other suspected illnesses. Infection presenting as systemic illness and hematuria are not uncommon features. Pain is often poorly localized, and typical ureteric/renal colic is relatively unusual in young children.

Since infection is a major predisposing factor, all children with stone disease should have a urine culture, metabolic screen, with serum calcium and uric acid estimation and urine collection for calcium, uric acid, oxalate and cystine estimation. The mainstays of investigations are as follows.

- Ultrasound: this is the means of diagnosis of stone disease in the majority of children. Renal anatomical details and the size, number and sites of calculi can be visualized with ultrasound. All renal and bladder calculi are visualized and the most proximal and distal ureteric calculi can also be identified.
- Plain radiography (kidney, ureter, bladder – KUB) is useful, although caution is advised when calculi are overlying bony projections or the intestine is loaded with feces or gassy. Ten percent of calculi are radiolucent and thus not visible on KUB.
- Intravenous urography (IVU) remains a useful investigation, particularly to provide an anatomical roadmap for treatment such as percutaneous nephrolithotomy (PCNL). However, IVU is becoming less popular with the improvement of ultrasound resolution, and concerns about limiting ionizing radiation in children.
- Non-contrast spiral computerized tomography (CT) scan helps in providing three-dimensional visualization of the anatomy and stone position and configuration. This is particularly so for ureteric stones. The higher radiation dose tends to preclude its use in children, although in adult practice it has become the gold standard. Magnetic resonance urography (MRU) may be used as an alternative.
- Isotope renogram: 99-technetium labeled dimercaptosuccinic acid (DMSA) provides important information with regard to renal function, which is vital in decision-making. A poorly functioning kidney with a large stone burden may be an indication for nephrectomy rather than complex intervention for clearance.
- Dynamic isotope study: mercaptoacetyltriglycine (MAG3) is useful to demonstrate reliable differential function and drainage profile in cases of suspected obstruction.

Treatment includes the eradication of infection (symptomatic or not) with appropriate antibiotics and attention to the general state of the child such as hydration and nutrition. The role of long-term prophylactic antibiotics is uncertain, and the long-term administration of analgesia must be discouraged in children. Patients with cystine stones require urinary alkalinization (pH 7–8) in order to minimize the risk of recurrence. This may be achieved by drinking large amounts of water (2 glasses per hour), which is not an easy option in children, or by using drugs such as penicillamine or alpha-mercaptopropionylglycine. However, these medications are not without significant side effects. Ideally, children with metabolic disorders should be treated under the auspices of a multidisciplinary team including a pediatric surgeon, nephrologist and metabolic medicine specialist.

Evidence of dilatation or obstruction proximal to a stone (pain, failure of drainage on radiological contrast) is an indication for early surgical intervention. Evidence of proximal dilatation and infection (positive microbiology, debris in a dilated system on ultrasound, systemic illness, pyrexia) are an indication for urgent decompression of the upper tract using percutaneous nephrostomy. This must be done as a temporary measure before further functional investigations or definitive treatment of the stone burden. In specialist units, nephrostomy in children is usually amenable to the percutaneous route (see Chapter 52A) rather than open placement but often requires a general anesthetic.

Evidence of dilatation around the stone burden (proximal and/or distal to the stone) may be an indication of an underlying condition such as pelvi-ureteric junction (PUJ) obstruction, vesico-ureteric junction (VUJ) obstruction, or raised intra-vesical pressure. Attention may be diverted first towards the cause of the stone, but both may be treated simultaneously.

Small stones may pass spontaneously (up to 3 mm in infants and small children, 5 mm in older children and adolescents). Asymptomatic small renal or bladder stones may be watched for a period of time provided they are not causing obstruction or impairment of renal function. In this situation, close observation of the general state of the child is mandatory, with particular vigilance for the signs of infection or obstruction radiologically or by ultrasound scans. Ureteric stones, on the other hand, require early surgical intervention.

Open surgical techniques have until recently been the mainstay for pediatric stone management, comprising open nephrolithotomy, pyelolithotomy, ureterolithotomy and cystolithotomy. There is still a definite role for open and/or laparoscopic surgical treatment:

- when facilities and/or experience for minimally invasive treatment are not available and referral to the regional center is not feasible;
- for stone formation secondary to PUJ/VUJ obstruction and calyceal, bladder or urethral diverticulum – both the stone and associated anatomical abnormality may be treated simultaneously through an open or laparoscopic approach;
- after failed minimally invasive therapy;
- when there is a complex large stone burden involving the upper and lower urinary tracts;
- when direct access to fragment and retrieve stones is difficult, as in post-bladder neck closure or re-implanted ureter.

Initially instrumentation proved to be the limiting factor in pediatric endo-urology, but the evolution in instrumentation of recent years has largely obviated these concerns. As with most branches of surgery, and pediatric surgical disciplines in particular, the trend towards minimally invasive treatment progresses unremittingly. Largely due to better optics and camera systems, miniaturized instruments and safer energy sources, urinary calculi that require treatment are now amenable to closed or minimal access techniques. Renal and upper ureteric stones can usually be managed satisfactorily with extracorporeal shockwave lithotripsy (ESWL). Antegrade percutaneous and retrograde endoscopic laser vaporization and/or ultrasound and lithoclast fragmentation of calculi are important advances, particularly when considering the problem of retained or distal stone burden and the subsequent indication for ureteric stenting following ESWL.

EXTRACORPOREAL SHOCKWAVE LITHOTRIPSY

Extracorporeal shockwave lithotripsy provides an excellent means of fragmentation when small fragments can be allowed to pass spontaneously and multiple treatment sessions are acceptable to clinicians, patients and carers. It is a safe technique and can produce stone clearance rates of up to 75 percent for upper urinary tract calculi. Therapeutic pressures of 10–100 MPa may be generated across a water medium by a number of sources, including piezoelectric crystals, electromagnetic eddy currents, and electrohydraulic spark.

Indications

- Single or multiple pelvi-calyceal stones.
- Staghorn calculus (as part of staged therapy with percutaneous surgery).
- Upper ureteric stones.
- Bladder stones (controversial).
- Cystine stones are notoriously resistant to fragmentation.

Contraindications

ABSOLUTE

- ESWL is not feasible for technical reasons – visualization and localization of the calculus in the focusing beam.

- The stone is associated with distal urinary tract obstruction secondary to:
  - distal stone,
  - PUJ,
  - VUJ (may include re-implanted ureters),
  - post-bladder neck closure.
- Anticoagulation.
- Sepsis.

RELATIVE

- When multiple anesthetics, if required, are thought not to be in the patient's interest.
- When facilities for stenting and minimally invasive therapy or ureteroscopic manipulation of obstructing fragments are not available.
- When the stone burden is too great.

Advantages

- Probably the least invasive method of treatment.
- Easily repeated as required.
- Applicable to all stones, especially pelvi-calyceal and upper ureteric stones.

Disadvantages

- Potential need for multiple treatment and repeat general anesthetics and post-therapy stenting or ureteroscopic manipulation.

Equipment/instruments

- Appropriate facilities and expertise to anesthetize children of all ages.
- Ultrasound and fluoroscopic screening apparatus to localize the calculi.
- Appropriate wedge, cushions and straps to maintain the position of the child on the table.
- ESWL apparatus suitable for children.

Preoperative preparation

The child must be prepared for a general anesthetic and informed consent is mandatory. Patients and carers must be informed about the nature of the procedure, success/failure rates, complications and the occasional need for post-treatment emergency instrumentation by means of stenting, ureteroscopic manipulation or even open surgery to relieve obstruction caused by dislodged stone fragments.

An up-to-date plain X-ray (KUB) and ultrasound scan should be obtained prior to treatment in case distal fragments are present causing obstruction or, indeed, the calculus remains. All children should have proven sterile urine before treatment and a prophylactic dose of broad-spectrum antibiotic is usually administered at the induction of anesthesia (gentamicin).

Technique

Extracorporeal shockwave lithotripsy is usually performed under general anesthesia. In adolescents, however, appropriate sedation may suffice (but all patients should be prepared for general anesthesia). Appropriate positioning of the patient and localization of the stone using either an ultrasound or a combination of ultrasound and fluoroscopic screening are the key to successful treatment.

The patient is positioned supine. In small children, cushion wedge and appropriate strapping are used to optimize the chance of localization. Throughout the procedure the position is maintained (usually supine or postero-lateral depending on the type of machine) such that the shockwaves are delivered to the center of the stone. A variable number of shocks (2000–3000) is administered to cause fragmentation. This may take up to 60 minutes to complete. **(See Figure 52B.1b–e)**

Postoperative care

The child may be fit soon after treatment and discharged home within hours. A patch of bruised skin at the site of delivery may be visible. The child may suffer pain, and oral analgesia may be required for 6–18 hours postoperatively. Follow-up KUB plain X-ray and/or ultrasound are arranged within 1–2 weeks of therapy. Subsequent follow-up investigations and/or management depend on the outcome of treatment. One to three sessions of lithotripsy is the norm.

Problems, pitfalls and solutions

- The ESWL table with its hatch is not suitable for very small children/infants. Minor adaptations to the lithotripter table using cushions/straps accommodate children of most sizes.
- Difficult localization of the stone is the most important aspect of the procedure, which requires an experienced operator. This is particularly so for:
  - small children,
  - small stones,
  - ureteric stones.
- An un-anesthetized older child/adolescent may prove difficult to handle. Inform the parents/carers preoperatively and prepare all children for a general anesthetic and provide attractive visual images and soothing sounds during the procedure.

(See Figure 52B.1(a))

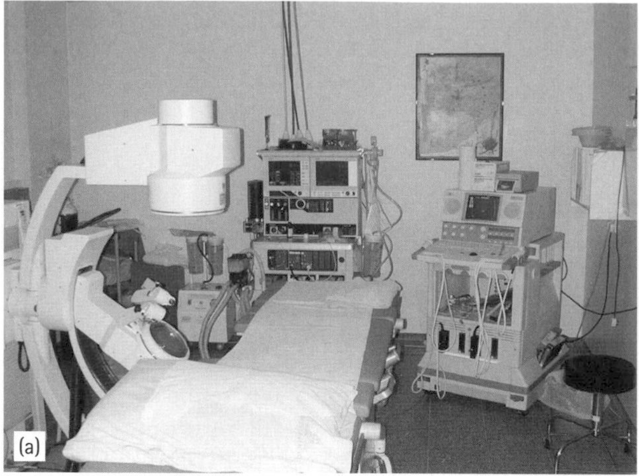

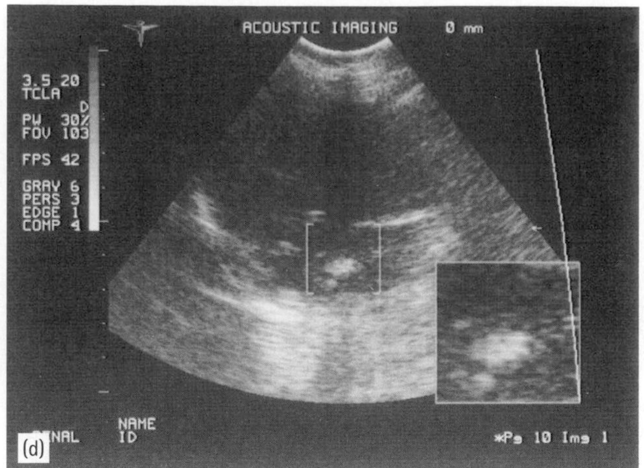

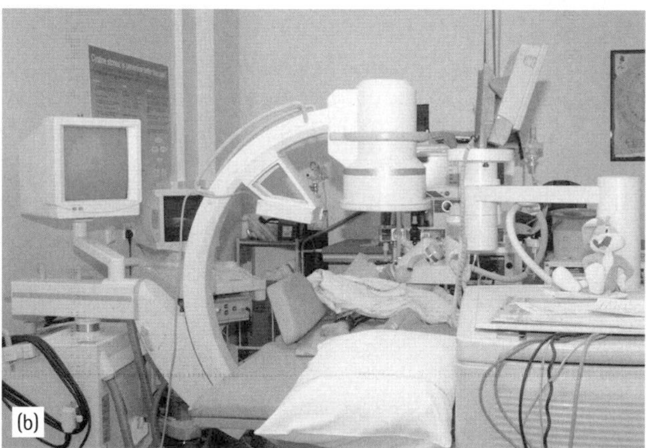

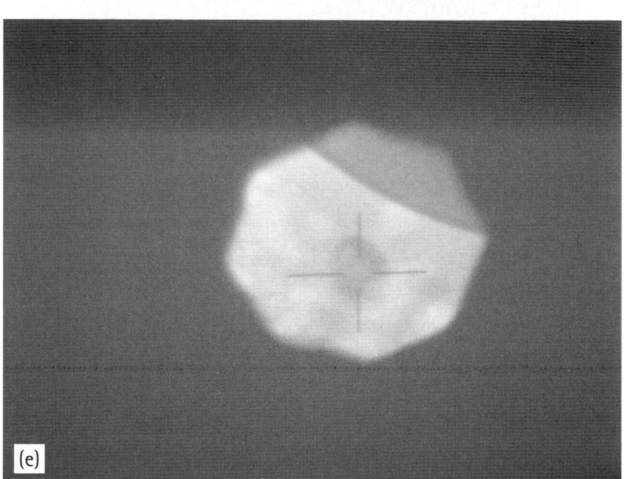

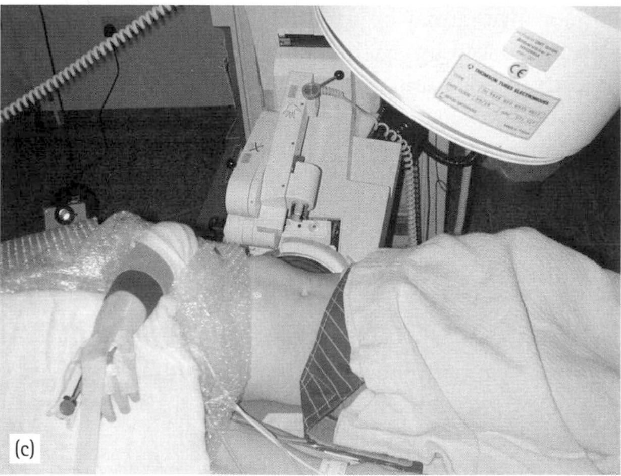

Figure 52B.1 *ESWL table; (b) supine positioning using storz lithotripter; (c) less than ideal postero-lateral positioning using an alternative machine; (d) ultrasound localization; (e) X-ray localization.*

Complications

- Transient hematuria: no active treatment is required.
- Urinary infection is rare: treat with antibiotics and ensure that there is no obstruction caused by fragments.
- Hemoptysis may rarely occur as consequence of acoustic impedance between the lung tissue and chest wall: covering the lower chest wall with a bubble-wrap dressing during the procedure can prevent this.
- Obstruction caused by fragments (the so-called Steinstrasse sign): emergency ureteroscopic manipulation to remove fragments and/or stenting to bypass obstruction and allow small fragments to pass spontaneously are usually the treatment of choice. Alternatively, insertion of a nephrostomy tube may be considered, especially if infection is suspected. **(See Figure 52B.2)**

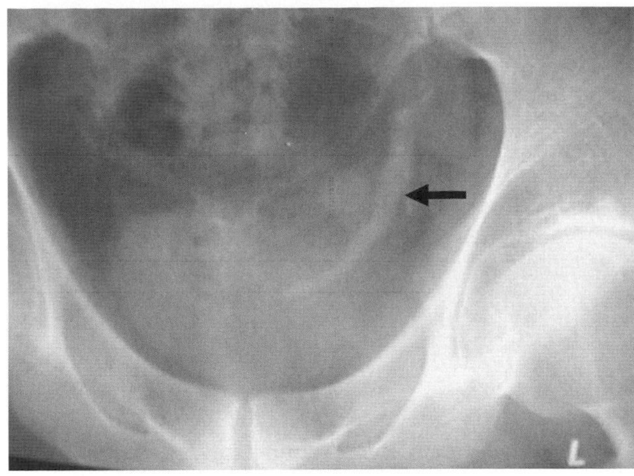

Figure 52B.2

URETEROSCOPY/URETERIC STONES

Ureteric stones may be accessed using appropriate-sized instruments in a retrograde fashion and then manipulated, fragmented and retrieved. Potentially, this technique may also allow a relatively safe retrograde approach to pelvi-calyceal stones. Flexible or rigid scopes may prove useful to pass in an antegrade fashion in the presence of percutaneous access through an upper pole renal puncture.

Indications

- Large ureteric stones. In general, stones smaller than 3 mm can reasonably be expected to pass spontaneously.
- Multiple ureteric stones.
- Symptomatic stones (pain, bleeding).
- Obstructive stones (persistent pain, signs of dilatation proximally, signs of obstruction on contrast or isotope study).
- Ureteric stones associated with infection once the infection has been treated.
- Ureteric stones associated with proximal stone burden.

Contraindications

ABSOLUTE

- Difficult access to the lower urinary tract as in post-bladder neck closure.
- Difficult access to the lower ureter as in post-Cohen's ureteric re-implantation.

In these situations, and if feasible, an antegrade approach (percutaneous through kidney approach) or even flexible endoscopy through an appropriately sited vesicostomy may be considered.

RELATIVE

- Lack of expertise and/or appropriate facilities: consider placement of a nephrostomy tube if needed due to complete obstruction and/or sepsis and referral to the nearest center for expert management.
- Significant systemic illness due to infection: consideration must be given to nephrostomy insertion as an initial measure followed by antegrade or retrograde ureteroscopy once sepsis has settled.
- Previous surgery, or known ureteric or urethral stricture.

Equipment/instruments

THE CHOICE OF URETEROSCOPE

The choice of ureteroscope will depend on local availability and the circumstances of the case. Rigid 9–12 Fr scopes with an offset eyepiece (which allows instrumentation through a straight line) allow greater functional flexibility because of the stiffness and size of the working channel, but carry an increased risk of failure to pass into the ureter of a small child and ureteric injury (perforation or stricture). The smaller 4.5–9 Fr scopes, so-called semi-rigid, with a straight eyepiece (offset working channel) are less traumatic and more appropriate to use for infants and small children, but the smaller and angled working channel restricts the range of instrumentation.

The flexible ureteroscope may occasionally prove useful, but requires an access sheath or a guide-wire for its insertion. The working channel is smaller but, with improved optics, this is becoming a very useful adjunct.

CHOICE OF ENERGY SOURCE

The choice of energy used to fragment the stone will depend on local availability and stone position.

- The laser lithotripter is finding increasing favor as it allows for stone vaporization with minimal retained fragments. Holmium laser (2150 nm wavelength) delivered in pulses is highly effective, but vaporization bubbles can sometimes obscure the view, and therefore continuous irrigation under moderate pressure is required.
- Pneumatic and electromagnetic ballistic devices achieve fast fragmentation, which is particularly good for impacted stones. The risk of mural trauma is reduced with these devices, although proximal propulsion of the fragments is a hazard. These devices are cheaper than lasers. Sizeable fragments have to be removed using appropriate stone graspers or a basket.
- Electrohydraulic lithotripters (EHLs) can also achieve good fragmentation with a high-power single spark transmitted at the tip of the probe, but carries the risk

of mural trauma if and when the tip of the probe is in contact with the urothelium.
- Ultrasound provides a safe and reasonable fragmentation alternative, although it tends to be slower and requires the use of suction to clear fragments (a suction device is a built-in component of the ultrasound probe). The limiting factor is the size of the probes, which are usually too big for the ureteroscope channels.

FRAGMENT RETRIEVAL

The method used for fragment retrieval will depend on the size of the fragments. Vaporized particles are washed away with continuous irrigation with or without hydrostatic pressure. The ultrasound probe has a built-in suction channel to clear small fragments resulting from ultrasound fragmentation. Small stones and relatively large fragments created by the lithoclast may be retrieved with either forceps or baskets. Crocodile forceps are simple to use and effective, whereas bipolar or tri-radiate forceps require a larger space (for the jaws to grasp) to function and are more effective for bulky, round stones, but they can cause trauma. Some regard these as being safer than baskets, but it is still possible to engage the ureter and cause trauma, although a stone may be released from the jaws. Baskets may be flat wire or helical in design. Flat-wire baskets can achieve reliable capture but tend to require a large lumen to function and to be traumatic, especially with moderate-sized fragments. Helical baskets are useful in smaller lumens or tortuous ureters, but achieve less reliable capture. Newer designs such as Nitinol are probably better for negotiating fragments because they tend to retain the structural memory.

ESSENTIAL

- Operating table suitable for X-ray imaging.
- Image intensifier.
- Laser/lithoclast/ultrasound energy sources and their respective probes that fit the size of ureteroscope.
- Appropriate-sized ureteroscope, preferably with an offset eyepiece and compatible camera/monitor system.
- Appropriate-sized cystoscope.
- Range of stiff, semi-flexible, slimy guide-wires of appropriate size to fit through the available cystoscope and ureteroscope.
- Appropriate-sized end-flush catheter (3–6 Fr).
- Contrast material (Urograffin).
- Appropriate-sized JJ ureteric stents.
- Urinary catheter.
- Saline giving-set and pressure pack to irrigate the ureter throughout the procedure.
- Dormia or helical wire basket.
- Atraumatic stone-grasping forceps.
- Goggles to wear if laser is employed.
- A set of open surgery instruments for emergency use in case of complications.

OPTIONAL

- Ultrasound imaging and nephrostomy kit to use for establishing proximal access/nephrostomy in case of failure or complications.

Preoperative preparation

Informed consent is mandatory, including the general risks of surgery and anesthesia, the potential need for postoperative ureteric stenting and bladder catheter, which are common. The rare possibilities of perforation and postoperative infection/sepsis and stricture formation, and the need for multiple intervention or open surgery at the time of or after ureteroscopy have to be explained. Perioperative broad-spectrum antibiotics are essential. Liaison with an interventional radiologist to help/assist in case of emergency or failure of ureterostomy is essential. A temporary nephrostomy may prove life saving when there are complications such as perforation of ureter or failed ureteroscopy in the presence of proximal obstruction/sepsis. The suitability of the operating theater for laser energy must be ensured prior to surgery.

Technique

Under general anesthesia, the patient is placed in the lithotomy position, or the Lloyd–Davis position if the child is older, as this enables easier access to the ureter. Access to and around the patient/operating table must be adequate for the use of the image intensifier, ultrasound scan, laser, lithoclast equipment etc. The normality of the urethra, bladder and ureteric openings is assessed by a preliminary cystoscopy. The site, size and number of stones and status of the ureter and proximal pelvi-calyceal system may be assessed under an image intensifier using contrast material through a suitable-sized ureteric catheter placed just within the lower end of the ureter via the cystoscope. **(See Figure 52B.3)**

Under direct vision, the ureteric orifice of the affected side is assessed and a flexible-tipped guide-wire (usually 0.25) is advanced carefully under fluoroscopic control into the renal pelvis. The cystoscope is removed and the external part of the wire is then fastened to the drape using a clip to prevent it from falling out. The wire must not be coiled, as this imparts potential energy like a coiled spring to it and the proximal end can flip out of the ureter. Passage of the guide-wire beyond an impacted stone or through a tortuous ureter may be problematic and necessitate care, time and change to a hydrophilic-coated soft wire or even ureteroscopy without a guide-wire in situ and then a wire passed subsequently once access has been established.

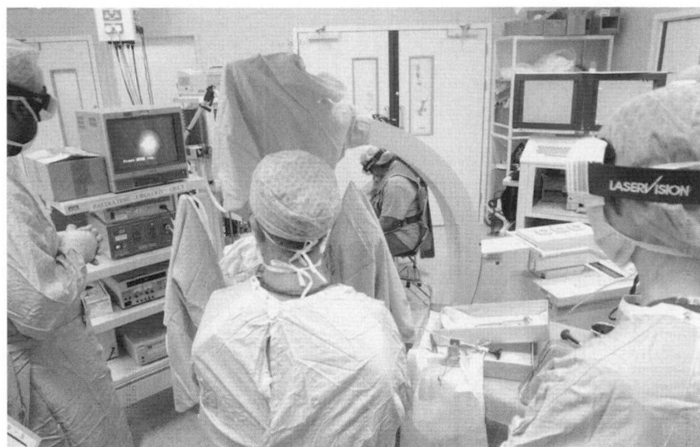

Figure 52B.3

The right hand is used to hold the ureteroscope while the left hand guides the tip of the scope into the urethra, with the light cable, wires and probes being delivered from the right of the operator. Under direct vision, the ureteroscope is then gently advanced alongside the guide-wire through the urethra and bladder into the ureteric orifice. In infants and small children, the distal ureter may have to be dilated first, with either telescopic dilators or using hydrostatic distension with saline infused under pressure. **(See Figure 52B.4)**

The attitude of the working channel to the optical channel of the ureteroscope and ureteric insertion into the bladder necessitate gentle to and fro movements or rotation of the scope by up to 180° with irrigant running under pressure (100 mmHg) to negotiate the pelvic curve of the ureter. Passage of the ureteroscope may become problematic at any stage and necessitate recourse to fluoroscopic control and retrograde ureterography to confirm the position of the scope, wire and stones in relation to the ureter and the integrity of the ureter itself. Occasionally the ureter is not large enough to accommodate the scope alongside the wire. In this case, the scope may be passed over the wire and subsequently the wire removed to free the working channel for other instrumentation, or ureteroscopy is carried out under direct vision without a guide-wire in place.

Having accessed the stone endoscopically, it may be vaporized by holmium laser or fragmented by ultrasound or lithoclast. The ureteroscope may now be passed into the left hand and the operator's right hand is free to manipulate the instruments and wires. The wire/probe is held between the thumb and index finger of the right hand and passed through a straight or gently curved working channel of the ureteroscope. The wire may be fractured by rough handling and acute angulation. The tip of the laser wire must always be kept in view and in contact with the surface of the stone, and vaporization starts peripherally, working towards the center. Care must be taken not to perforate the ureter or bore a hole in the center of the stone. **(See Figure 52B.5)**

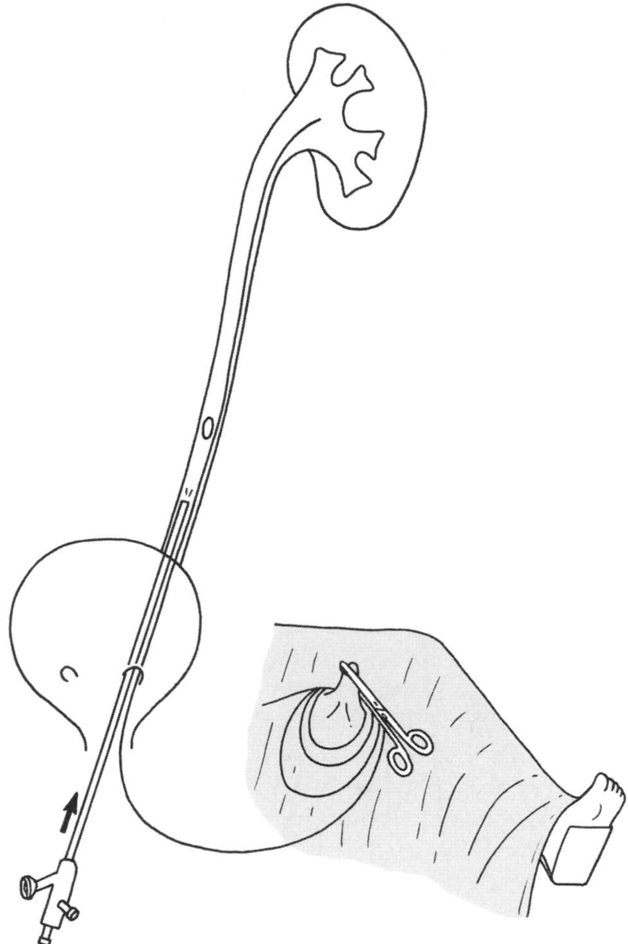

Figure 52B.4

Ultrasound is extremely safe, but slow. To maximize the energy delivered to the stone, both the ultrasound and ballistic probes are held by their handles in a straight line. The tip of the lithoclast probe is held against the center of the stone/large fragments in order to achieve maximum results and minimize the risk of mural trauma.

Very small fragments of stones will pass spontaneously. Larger fragments may have to be retrieved using graspers or a basket. The need for stenting after an apparently successful fragmentation is debatable. Stenting is necessary if:

- access is not possible – the patient can return to theater in 1–2 weeks, at which point access is always easier,
- there is an appreciable volume of stone fragments left within the ureter,
- coexisting pelvi-calyceal stones or fragments are expected to descend,
- doubt exists about the integrity of the ureter,
- there is a residual impacted stone fragment.

Stenting allows for the safe provision of drainage and facilitates the passage of small fragments. It may be left in situ for one to several weeks, depending on the circumstances

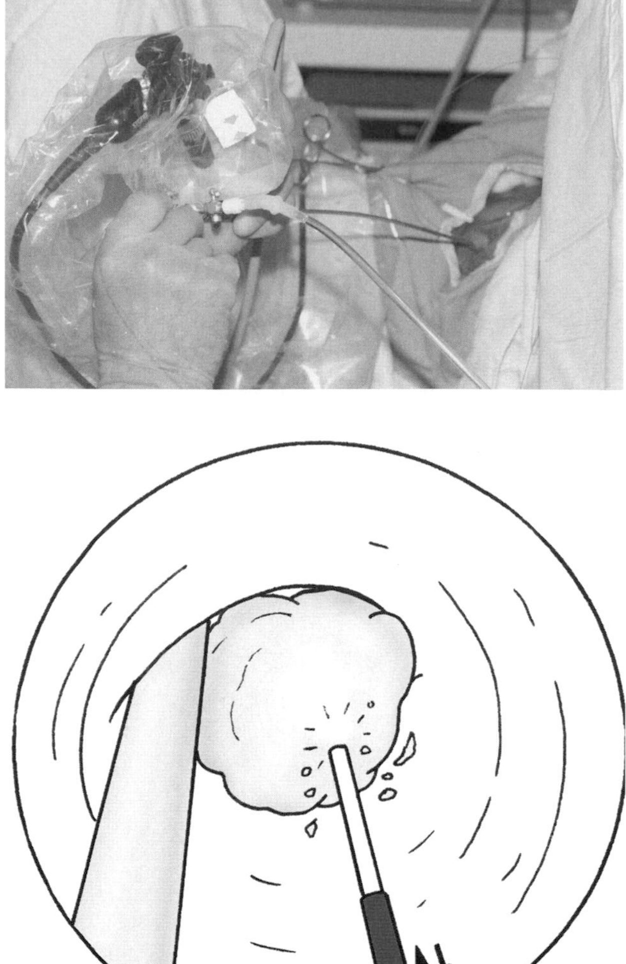

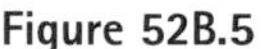

Figure 52B.5

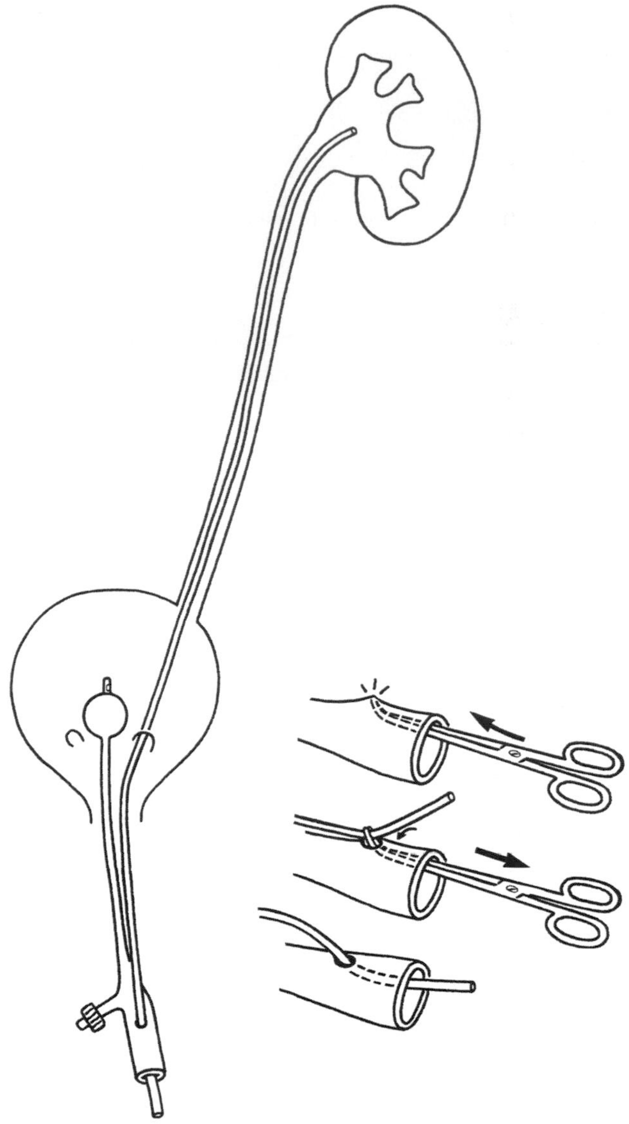

Figure 52B.6

of the case (e.g. cystine crystals deposit on stents and catheters very rapidly, and therefore stents should be left for only a short period in the treatment of cystine stones). A 24-hour maneuver to allow edema to settle and spontaneous ureteric motility to re-establish involves leaving an end-flushing ureteric catheter secured to a urethral catheter for 12–48 hours. **(See Figure 52B.6)**

Postoperative care

In uncomplicated cases (no pre-existing sepsis or perforation of ureter) a single intravenous dose of broad-spectrum antibiotics is adequate. This may be followed by prophylaxis if the child has residual stones, a stent or a coexisting anomaly such as reflux or neurogenic bladder. The child is encouraged to drink and feed within several hours and is discharged home within 24–48 hours. The parents must be informed about the possibility of postoperative pain, hematuria, infection and the passing of stone fragments.

Evidence of sepsis should be acted upon promptly with urine culture and intravenous broad-spectrum antibiotics pending definitive culture and sensitivity.

Significant pain should be investigated as ureteric obstruction from stone fragments or missed ureteric injury. Analgesia beyond the first 24 hours is not usually required. All children must have follow-up KUB plain X-ray and ultrasound scan at about 1–2 weeks postoperatively. Long-term follow-up is necessary for patients who suffer metabolic stone disease associated with anomalies of the urinary tract.

Ureteric stents are usually removed cystoscopically under general anesthesia after 6 weeks unless a second elective attempt at stone clearance is required, which would take place about 2–3 weeks after the first attempt. An alternative is to leave a thread from the distal end of the stent out of the urethra. In adults, stents are usually removed under local anesthesia using a flexible cystoscope. In cases of cystinuria, stents should be removed early (1–2 weeks) otherwise crystal deposits on the surface of the stent render its removal difficult.

Pitfalls, problems and solutions/complications

See under 'Percutaneous nephrolithotomy' below.

PERCUTANEOUS NEPHROLITHOTOMY

Percutaneous nephrolithotomy is evolving as an alternative to open surgery in children, as it is in adults. The limiting factors so far have been instrumentation and surgical expertise. PCNL is usually performed in conjunction with an interventional radiologist to establish percutaneous access (see Chapter 52A). It may be used as monotherapy or in conjunction with ESWL or ureteroscopy.

Indications

- Cases of large stone burden (a large stone or multiple stones or staghorn calculus) when stone clearance is thought to require repeated sessions of ESWL or cause distal obstruction (Steinstrasse) following ESWL.
- Unsuccessful ESWL.
- Patients who have suspected anatomical abnormalities that may render ESWL or ureteroscopic stone treatment difficult, e.g. narrow calyceal neck, calyceal diverticulum.

Contraindications

ABSOLUTE

- Lack of expertise or facilities.
- Uncorrected coagulopathy diseases.

Relative

- Very young infants or small children whose kidneys are small and mobile.
- Small, shriveled, non-dilated kidneys make percutaneous access a challenge.

Equipment/instruments

ESSENTIAL

- Operating table suitable for X-ray and image intensifier, and attachments to place the patient in the lithotomy position.
- Image intensifier.
- Appropriate energy sources, such as ultrasound scan, laser and lithoclast, and their attachments.
- Irrigation fluid (pressure-flow irrigation is avoided in PCNL because of the risk of fluid absorption).
- Appropriate nephroscope (14–16 Fr pediatric or small adult) and light source.
- Various grasping forceps that fit the working channel of the nephroscope to retrieve stones.
- Foley-type urinary catheter.
- End-flushing catheter or ureteric catheters.
- Varying types of appropriate-sized guide-wires – stiff, slippery, semi-flexible and curled tip.
- Percutaneous access kits (see Chapter 52A).
- Large tamponading nephrostomy catheter without side holes (usually an appropriately sized Foley catheter cut just proximal to its balloon) and a transfixing suture.
- Contrast material for radiography.
- A set of instruments for open surgery in case of emergency.

OPTIONAL

- Camera and screen to view endoluminal work (direct eye contact with the eyepiece of the nephroscope whilst carrying out PCNL is becoming less fashionable and bears the risk of two-way contamination). Without your assistant being able to see the operative field, it makes it very difficult to perform endo-urological intervention.
- Ultrasound apparatus with appropriate probes to scan the kidney, locate the appropriate access route, and guide the initial percutaneous insertion of the needle and guide-wire into the collecting system.

Preoperative preparation

The site, size and number of stones as well as the anatomical road map are assessed using conventional radiology imaging.

As for ESWL and ureteroscopy, informed consent is obtained, highlighting the nature and risks of the procedure including failure rates, risks of extravasation and bleeding, the possibility of retained fragments and distal stone obstruction, leaving catheter and stents, and the possibility of emergency open surgery in case of complications, or repeat PCNL for residual stone fragments, or even ESWL. Broad-spectrum intravenous antibiotics are administered at the induction of anesthesia.

Technique

General anesthesia with an endotracheal tube and full muscle relaxation are essential. The patient is placed in the modified lithotomy position and cystoscopy is performed first. An appropriate-sized soft guide-wire is placed retrogradely via the cystoscope into the renal pelvis under

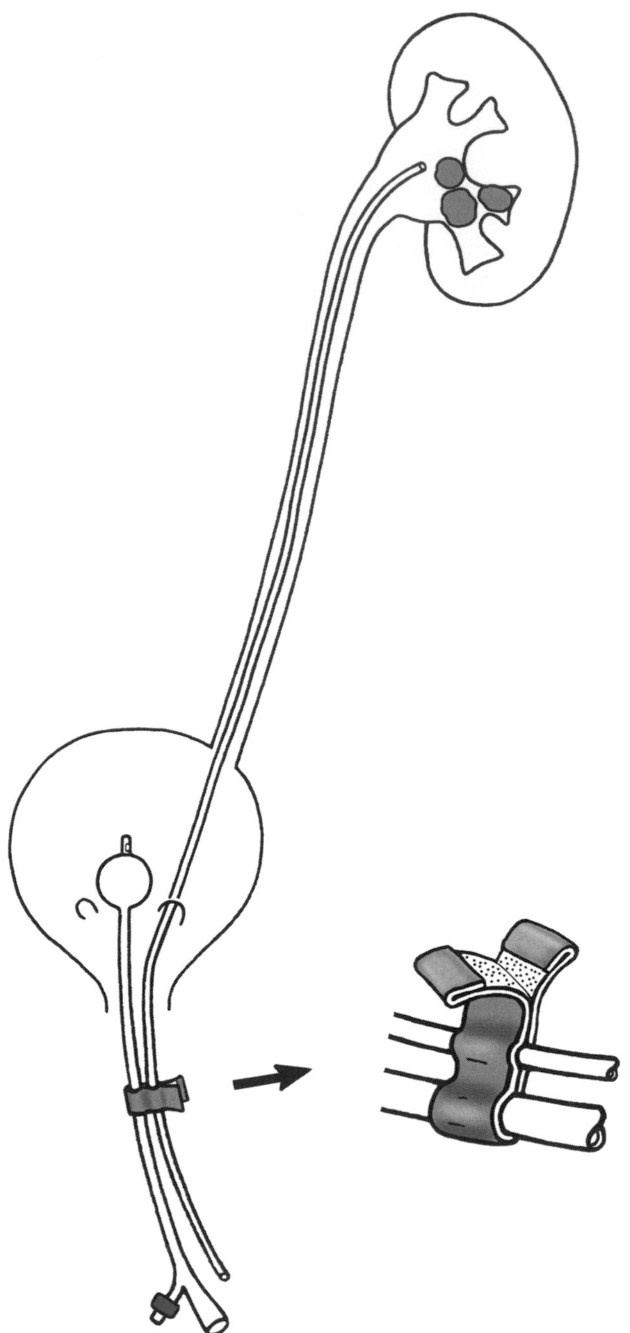

Figure 52B.7

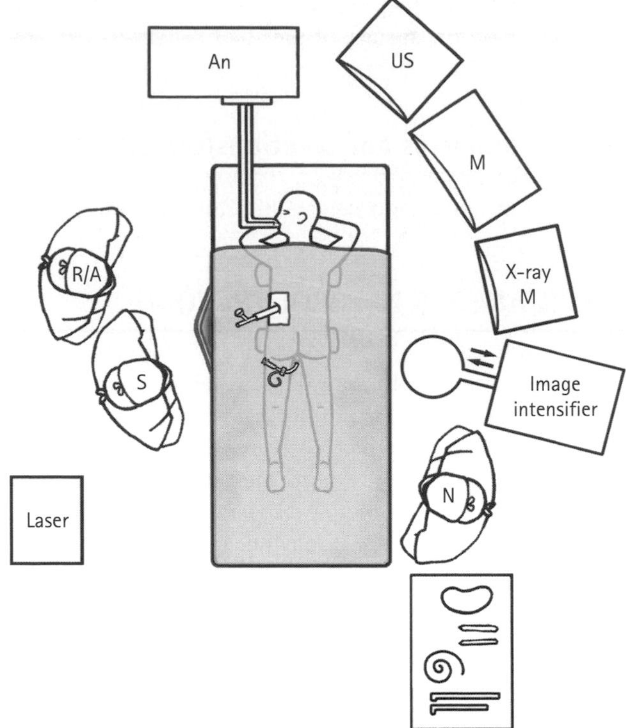

Figure 52B.8

image intensifier. Care must be taken not to expose the patient, the surgeon's hands or the theater staff to unnecessary radiation. An appropriate-sized end-flushing catheter is then passed over the guide-wire into the renal pelvis and the wire is removed. A retrograde pyelogram is performed through the catheter to confirm the optimal position of the catheter and to re-evaluate the anatomy and position of the stones. The end-flushing catheter is then secured to an indwelling Foley's urethral catheter to prevent accidental dislodgement. **(See Figure 52B.7)**

The patient is moved into the prone position and stabilized by placing pillows/cushions under the chest and pelvic regions. The patient is then covered with a purpose-made plastic drape with a side pouch to collect irrigating fluid. The previously positioned catheters (ureter and bladder) are brought to the surface in between the lower limbs posteriorly and made accessible for the radiologist/operator to inject contrast materials and/or replace a retrograde wire through the catheter during the procedure if necessary. **(See Figure 52B.8)**

The technique of percutaneous access has already been described. In brief, the accessibility of one or more previously identified calyces is confirmed (usually lower posterior for pelvic and/or upper calyx stones, middle posterior for pelvic stones upper posterior for pelvic and lower calyceal stones). Access through the upper and middle calyces allows simultaneous adequate viewing and instrumentation of the upper ureter.

Using ultrasound and/or retrograde pyelogram through the end-flushing catheter, the calyx is punctured percutaneously and its position confirmed by aspirating urine and, if necessary, injecting contrast material antegradely. Under image intensifier, an appropriate soft/J guide-wire is passed via the Teflon sheath of the needle into the renal pelvis. An appropriate-sized percutaneous track is created over the guide-wire using gradual metal or plastic dilators.

An Amplatz sheath (usually size 16–18 Fr for infants, 18–24 Fr for older children) is then passed over the dilator to maintain the track.

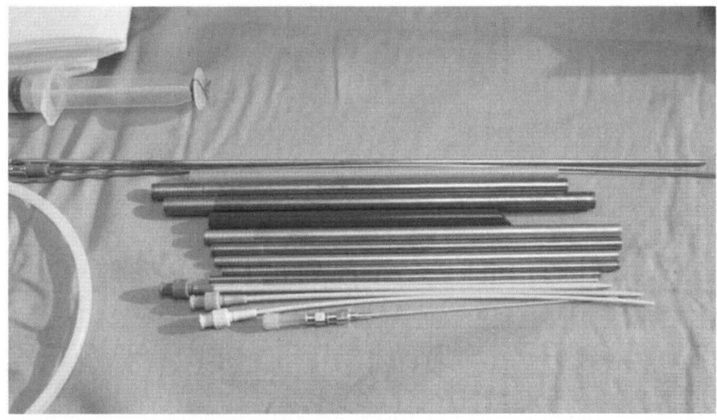

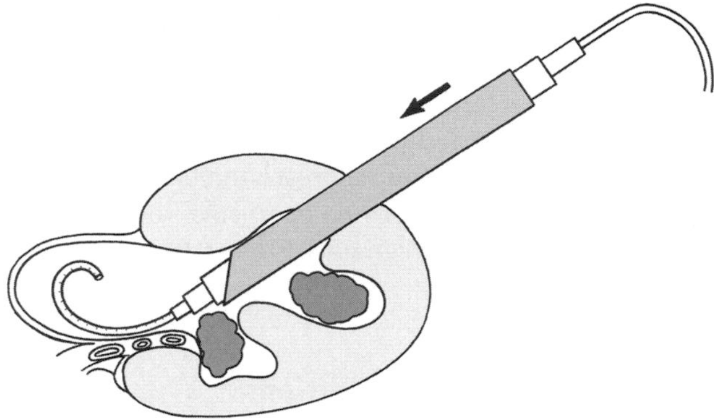

Figure 52B.9

It is absolutely crucial that the assistant keeps the Amplatz sheath and the guide-wire in position at all times. The guide-wire will be used to replace the Amplatz sheath should it become dislodged. Alternatively, a guide-wire is passed in a retrograde fashion through the end-flushing catheter and extruded through the Amplatz sheath using the nephroscope. **(See Figure 52B.9)**

The nephroscope is held in the right hand, introduced carefully through the Amplatz sheath and the stone is localized. The Amplatz sheath is rotated as necessary so that the beveled end faces the stone and/or appropriate space (pelvis or calyx). The assistant stands on the left-hand side to maintain the positions of the Amplatz sheath and the guide-wire, while the scrub nurse and the exchange of instruments and probes/wires take place on the right-hand side. The nephroscope is passed into the left hand while the right hand of the operator is freed to manipulate wires and instruments. All maneuvers take place under direct vision, preferably through the camera/monitors, and if necessary fluoroscopy and contrast materials are used. **(See Figure 52B.10)**

Fragmentation and retrieval techniques are similar to those described previously for ureteric stones, with a preference for ultrasound disintegration with associated low-pressure suction to clear fragments. Cystine stones usually require a combination of ultrasound and ballistic energy sources. Stone-grasping forceps are often used to retrieve fragments and a flexible telescope may occasionally be

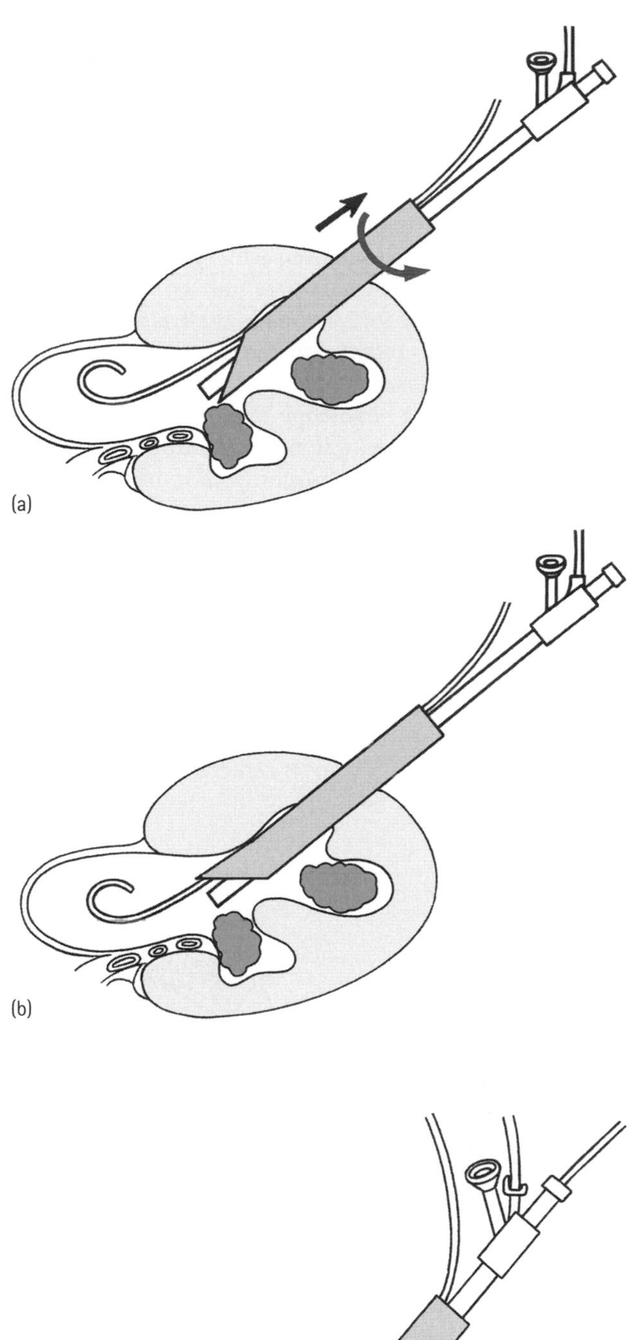

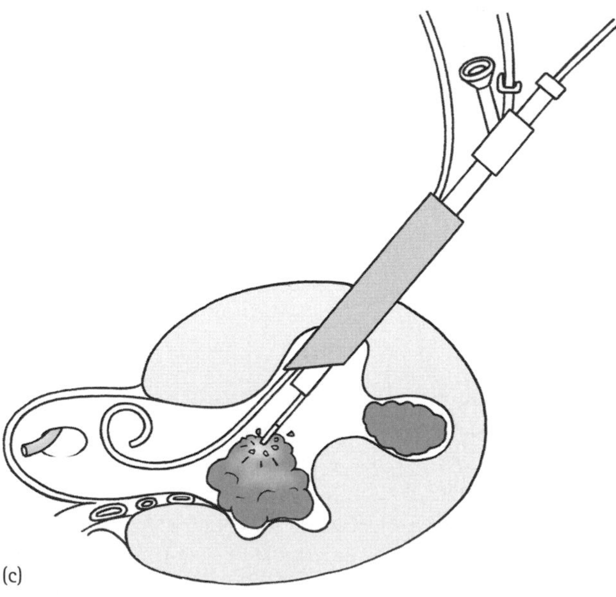

Figure 52B.10

necessary to confirm calyceal stone clearance under direct vision and to deliver laser energy to less accessible areas of the collecting system. Throughout the procedure, every effort is made to maintain the end few millimeters of the Amplatz sheath within the renal substance, otherwise hemorrhage and/or fluid extravasation and absorption may occur and jeopardize the entire procedure.

Once stone clearance has been achieved, a nephrostomy tube is inserted. A small-bore tube may be preferred, but this limits the ability to tamponade the track if bleeding occurs directly after removal of the sheath. A larger tube not only gives a better seal to the track but also maintains a track for subsequent endoscopy if a repeat procedure is required to clear retained fragments and drain the kidney. It is best to place the nephrostomy tube into the renal pelvis through the Amplatz sheath under screening, along either a safety wire or end-flushing catheter. Our preferred choice of nephrostomy tube is a rubber Foley catheter of size equal to the internal diameter of the Amplatz sheath (4 Fr less than the sheath used, i.e. 20 Fr Foley for a 24 Fr sheath), with its distal end cut distal to the balloon. To facilitate the passage of stone fragments down the ureter, the end-flushing catheter may be left in situ and re-secured to the urinary bladder catheter for 24–48 hours. **(See Figure 52B.11)**

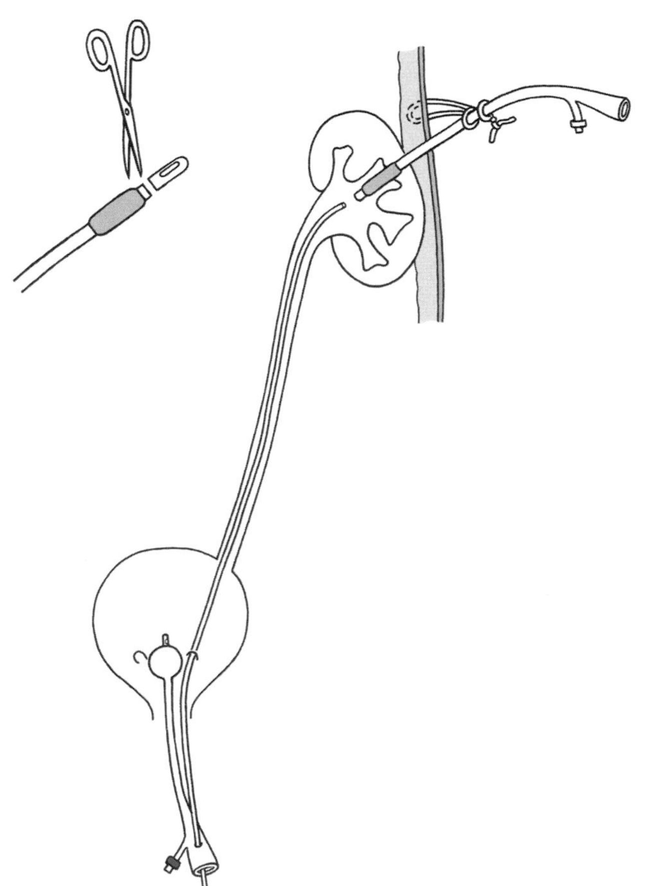

Figure 52B.11

Postoperative care

Intravenous opiate analgesia may be used within the first 8–12 hours and patients are allowed to drink and eat as soon as they are on the ward and observations appear stable. On the second postoperative day or when the drainage fluid is clear, stone clearance from the kidney and ureter is confirmed by an antegrade nephrostogram, and the catheters (nephrostomy, ureteric catheter and bladder catheter) are removed if no fragments remain. Subsequent imaging is repeated as necessary if fragments persist or if further treatment is required. If fragments remain, a second-look PCNL is recommended, as it is much easier and a clear view is obtained after the track has been established after a few days.

Obstructing ureteric stone fragments are dealt with as a matter of urgency in the fashion described previously (ureteroscopy). An antegrade approach through the nephrostomy track may be used as an alternative route to treat residual ureteric stone fragments. Here, a flexible uretroscope may prove useful.

Pitfalls, problems and solutions

COMPLEX STONE BURDEN INVOLVING BLADDER, URETER AND KIDNEY

The bladder stone has to be approached first, followed by the ureter and then the kidney stones. The bladder and ureteric stones may or may not be treated simultaneously.

POORLY FUNCTIONING KIDNEY (10 PERCENT OR LESS)

A nephrectomy or nephro-ureterectomy rather than stone clearance may be the preferred choice of treatment.

ASSOCIATED ANOMALIES

- PUJ obstruction has to be treated first or simultaneously. Combined treatment may involve an open or laparoscopic approach. An apparently successful PCNL may be followed immediately by a minimally invasive endopyelotomy (see Chapter 51).
- VUJ obstruction or ureteric stricture is to be treated first.
- Urinary reflux: re-implantation of the ureter may be considered after complete stone clearance. Subsequent passage of stones or retrograde instrumentation of the ureter can become difficult after Cohen's re-implantation of the ureter.
- Neurogenic bladder, recurrent infection and metabolic stone disease have to be kept under control.
- In bladder neck or urethral obstruction, retrograde instrumentation is difficult or impossible.

Consideration must be given to one or more of the following methods of treatment:
- laparoscopic,
- antegrade access,
- open.

DIFFICULT ACCESS

- Ureteroscopy.
  - Difficulty with positioning the guide-wire due to impacted stones, pre-existing obstruction/stricture or a tortuous ureter. Try:
    - change of wire to a softer or slippery hydrophilic wire,
    - keeping the wire below the site of obstruction,
    - inserting a ureteroscope synchronously with a wire.
  - Ureter not admitting the scope. A preliminary gentle, gradual dilatation of the lower end of the ureter may be required.
  - A small ureter not accommodating the smallest scope alongside the guide-wire. Here, the scope may be passed over the wire, or under direct vision.
- PCNL (**See Chapter 52A**).

POSITION OF AMPLATZ SHEATH

Every effort must be made to keep the sheath in an optimal position. Rotational and inward movements can be used to direct the beveled end close to the operative field/stone and must be carried out under direct vision. If vision becomes poor and renal access is lost, PCNL may have to be abandoned, but the position of the retrograde catheter is maintained in order to drain the kidney (especially if stone fragments are expected within the ureter), minimize the risk of extravasation and encourage spontaneous passage of ureteric stone fragments. This catheter will also help in further imaging done to assess the limits of extravasation and future instrumentation/treatment. These patients are kept under observation for a few days and the status of extravasation (hematoma, fluid and urine collection) is monitored by repeat ultrasound.

POOR VIEW

Ensure the telescope, camera, light source and monitors as well as the connections are compatible and functioning. In PCNL, the optimal position of the Amplatz sheath is checked. Other causes of poor view are:

- dust and fragments and vaporization bubbles resulting from the use of energy,
- bleeding from a displaced Amplatz sheath, injury from instrumentation, injury from the initial percutaneous puncture, and granulation tissue secondary to previous instrumentation or stone irritation.

A continuous adequate volume of pressurized irrigating fluid is necessary during both PCNL and ureteroscopy. Intermittent squirts of clear fluid via a 10 mL syringe attached to the side port of the scope may prove helpful.

DIFFICULT STONE CLEARANCE

Predisposing factors include:

- difficult instrumentation or access,
- poor view,
- extravasation,
- large stone burden,
- cystine stones.

For ureteric stones, a JJ stent may be left in situ and further treatment should be considered at a later date. For renal stones, a nephrostomy catheter should be placed as described previously, and a further session to clear residual stones through the established track or a new but more direct route is planned for a few days postoperatively.

ACCIDENTAL DISPLACEMENT OF STONES OR LARGE FRAGMENTS TO THE URETER (PCNL)

An antegrade or retrograde ureterolithotomy may be considered. Alternatively, the retrograde ureteric catheter is left in situ or a nephrostomy tube is placed and the patient is prepared for ureterolithotomy a few days later.

Complications

URETERAL INJURY

A relatively rare but potentially serious complication, this can occur as a result of:

- instrumentation or laser injury,
- instrumentation in the presence of impacted stones, tortuous or obstructed ureter, or inflammation.

Careful technique and manipulation under vision (ultrasound, image intensifier, camera) minimize the risk of ureteral injury. The procedure has to be abandoned and a JJ stent or percutaneous nephrostomy and antibiotic cover is necessary.

RENAL INJURY/EXTRAVASATION

This is not an uncommon occurrence during PCNL, but rarely causes significant problems. Predisposing factors include:

- difficulty with access,
- displaced Amplatz sheath,
- instrumentation or laser injury.

The procedure may be continued in the presence of a minor to moderate degree of extravasation. Adequate pelvi-calyceal drainage is maintained for a few to several days, depending on the severity of extravasation. This is achievable through the existing retrograde catheter or, better still, a JJ stent, or a nephrostomy through the access track. A separate percutaneous perinephric drain may be required and antibiotic cover is commenced.

HEMORRHAGE

Major intra-renal or extra-renal hemorrhage is a rare complication of PCNL and may occur as a result of:

- percutaneous access formation,
- displaced Amplatz sheath,
- instrumentation or laser injury.

Bleeding from the access track may be controlled by a large latex catheter through the track 'tamponade' and the lumen is occluded to encourage clot formation. Vascular embolization and occasionally open exploration may be considered, depending on the response to more conservative measures.

MAJOR SEPSIS

The risk of major sepsis is reduced significantly by the use of peri-operative antibiotics. Predisposing factors are:

- pre-existing infection,
- residual stones,
- obstruction due to impacted stones, congenital anomalies or stricture,
- stents and catheters.

An appropriate course (usually intravenous) of antibiotics is necessary. Residual stones or obstruction must be treated promptly and catheters and stents are removed as soon as possible. The role of long-term antibiotics, for residual stones, is uncertain.

BLADDER STONES

Solitary bladder stones are rare in children, with the exception of those patients having undergone bladder augmentation with intestinal segments, when mucus production, stasis and infection may predispose to stone formation. Bladder stones may occur in conjunction with anatomical abnormalities such as diverticuli and ureterocele, and the mode of the treatment is best considered in the context of the management of the associated problem.

Bladder stones are amenable to fragmentation and retrieval as described for ureteric and renal stones, with a combination of lithotripsy techniques (mechanical or laser). Transurethral retrieval may be difficult due to the small size of the urethra in children, and therefore a suprapubic percutaneous approach as for renal calculi or a laparoscopic transvesical approach should be considered. ESWL has been tried, but is often unhelpful in this situation.

Transurethral endoscopic stone treatment probably serves best those children who:

- have small stones/small fragments,
- form recurrent stones when multiple cystolithotomies are best avoided,
- will undergo other endoscopic treatment such as ureterocele incision or ureteric bladder neck injection.

If all else fails, open surgical removal through a suprapubic incision can be performed.

FURTHER READING

Al-Busaidy SS, Prem AR, Medhat M, Al-Bulushi YH. Ureteric calculi in children: preliminary experience with holmium: YAG laser lithotripsy. *BJU International* 2004; **93**: 1318–23.

Bartosh SM. Medical management of pediatric stone disease. *Urologic Clinics of North America* 2004; **31**: 575–87.

Dawaba MS, Shokeir AA, Hafez et al. Percutaneous nephrolithotomy in children: early and late anatomical and functional results. *Journal of Urology* 2004; **172**: 1078–81.

Muslumanoglu AY, Tefleki A, Savilar O et al. Extracorporeal shock wave lithotripsy as first line treatment alternative for urinary tract stones in children: a large scale retrospective analysis. *Journal of Urology* 2003; **170**: 2405–8.

Rigvi SAH, Naqvi SAA, Hussain Z et al. Management of pediatric urolithiasis in Pakistan: experience with 1440 children. *Journal of Urology* 2003; **169**: 634–7.

53

Endoscopic injection for urinary incontinence

ARNE STENBERG AND G. LÄCKGREN

INTRODUCTION

Certain congenital anatomical abnormalities, notably bladder exstrophy epispadias, spina bifida and neuropathic bladder sphincter dysfunction, lead to urinary incontinence in children as a result of inadequate function of the urethral sphincter. Urinary incontinence can have severe consequences on self-esteem and quality of life; therefore, the importance of effective treatment should not be underestimated.

The treatment of sphincter-related urinary incontinence in children generally aims to increase bladder outlet resistance, with the first priority to preserve renal function. A successful outcome is also dependent on the presence of a compliant, non-overactive bladder with an adequate capacity.

Surgical treatment of sphincter-related urinary incontinence

Currently, the treatment of sphincter-related urinary incontinence usually involves surgery, the principal procedures being:

- bladder neck plasties,
- fascial slings,
- placement of an artificial urinary sphincter.

Although these surgical procedures are well established, the outcome is unpredictable and may vary according to the patient, the technique used and the surgeon performing the procedure. Despite the inherent variability, reported response rates among patients with severe organic incontinence for all these techniques are generally 60–70 percent.

They all involve major surgery, which has a significant risk of associated morbidity and complications, including infection, urethral/rectal perforation and catheterization difficulties post-surgery. A minimally invasive treatment that can reduce the number of children undergoing open surgery is therefore worth pursuing, even if its success rate is lower than that of more invasive surgery.

Trans-urethral endoscopic injection

Trans-urethral endoscopic injection is a minimally invasive alternative to open surgery and is a similar procedure to that used in vesico-ureteric reflux (VUR). The technique, which was first investigated in the 1970s, involves endoscopic injection of a bulking agent into the submucosa of the urinary tract. Endoscopic injection may improve both passive and conscious continence through augmentation of the bladder neck and sphincter areas, respectively.

In general, the reported efficacy rates with endoscopic treatment have tended to be lower than with invasive surgery. However, the success of injection therapy is variable, depending primarily on the need for careful selection of appropriate patients, and on other factors such as the surgeon's technical expertise, the timing of treatment and the choice of bulking agent.

The surgeon's experience with the technique can affect outcome, with failure rates tending to reduce over time as the surgeon's familiarity with the procedure increases.

There is evidence to suggest that patients for whom endoscopic treatment is first-line therapy are more likely to respond successfully to treatment than those in whom, for example, bladder neck plasty is performed first. Nevertheless, several groups of patients may also benefit from endoscopic injection used as second-line treatment as a means of eliminating or reducing continuing leakage after a previous procedure.

A number of agents have been evaluated as bulking agents, with most knowledge being gained from using PTFE (Teflon), polydimethylsiloxane (silicone, Macroplastique) and bovine collagen. However, safety and efficacy concerns have prevented their widespread use in children with urinary incontinence.

A recently developed material, dextranomer/hyaluronic acid (Dx/HA) copolymer, comprises cross-linked dextranomer microspheres (80–250°μm in diameter) suspended in a 1 percent carrier gel of non-animal, stabilized sodium hyaluronate. This material is biocompatible, non-allergenic and biodegradable, ensuring an excellent safety profile. Infiltration of implanted Dx/HA copolymer with fibroblasts and in-growth of collagen stabilize the volume after injection, resulting in a bolus with long-term resilience.

The Dx/HA copolymer has been demonstrated to offer prolonged efficacy in the treatment of VUR, and there have been no safety concerns regarding its use. It is currently the only material approved by the US Food and Drug Administration for endoscopic treatment of VUR in children. The material has also been investigated for use in childhood urinary incontinence and the following methodology assumes the use of Dx/HA copolymer (different injection apparatus is required for different substances).

Indications

Children with incontinence caused purely by sphincter deficiency are most likely to respond to endoscopic injection. Satisfactory bladder function in terms of compliance and functional capacity is also required. Urethral injection may be used as primary treatment to increase bladder capacity, facilitating subsequent continence operations. Alternatively, it can be employed as secondary treatment in patients with ongoing leakage after previous surgery.

Contraindications

- Detrusor instability that is uncontrolled by pharmacotherapy.
- High-pressure bladder upon emptying.
- Presence of a urinary tract infection.
- VUR (higher grades).

EQUIPMENT/INSTRUMENTS

The following instruments are essential for performing endoscopic injection.

- Cystoscope with a minimum 4 Fr working channel. An angled viewing piece is recommended to provide a straight working channel. A 30° lens should be used.
- Flexible needle (5 Fr 23 G × 350 mm) with a Luer-Lok™ system is recommended together with a syringe pre-filled with Dx/HA copolymer.
- Video camera to record pre-procedure and post-procedure anatomy, particularly urethral coaptation following injection therapy.
- Saline infusion to ensure an adequate flow of fluid past the end of the cystoscope, maintaining good visibility by preventing folding of the urethral mucosa.

There is no requirement for an injection gun when using Dx/HA copolymer, as, unlike other injectable agents, it can be injected with finger pressure only.

PREOPERATIVE PREPARATION

Prior to the procedure, patients should undergo a full morphological and functional evaluation of the upper and lower urinary tract. A urodynamic study is needed to show a low-pressure bladder and sphincter deficiency, thus confirming the patient's eligibility for endoscopic injection therapy. A pad test and questionnaire are also used, to establish the extent and frequency of leakage, allowing the outcome of treatment to be measured objectively.

In males with incontinence caused by epispadia or bladder exstrophy, it is important that the primary operation to close the bladder and reconstruct the bladder neck is performed so that a good distance remains between the verumontanum and the bladder neck. This is to enable optimal positioning of the urethral injection.

TECHNIQUE

General anesthesia is administered intravenously supported by mask inhalation. Patients should be placed in the lithotomy position for the procedure. The surgeon sits in front of the patient and is responsible for manipulating the cystoscope and flexible needle. The assistant, who should be situated to the right of the surgeon, is responsible for injecting the Dx/HA copolymer from the syringe, thereby allowing the surgeon to maintain the position of the cystoscope and needle. Injections are usually performed transurethrally, as this provides the easiest means of observing the progress of the procedure. The flexible needle should be primed by flushing with saline and then filled with

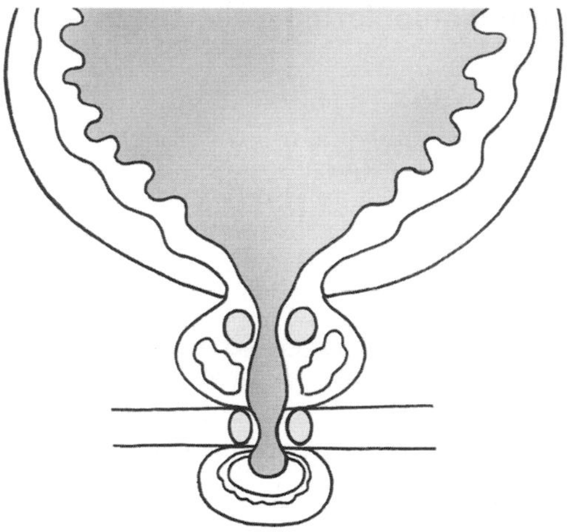

Figure 53.1

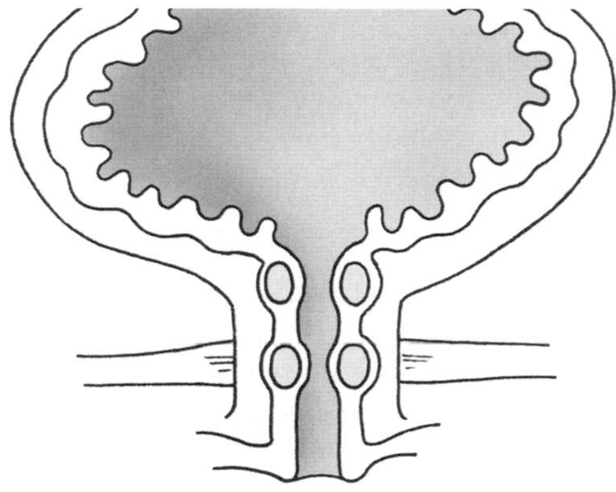

Figure 53.2

Dx/HA copolymer from the syringe. The surgeon introduces the cystoscope (with the needle retracted inside the instrument channel) into the urethra and assesses the patient's anatomy as the cystoscope is advanced towards the bladder. Once the tip of the cystoscope is inside the bladder, the needle is advanced and the cystoscope is withdrawn to the relevant position to enable injection of the urethra.

Injection points may need to be changed in accordance with anatomical differences between patients. Recommended injection points are different in male and female patients.

- Males: Dx/HA injected into both the proximal urethra (i.e. proximal to the verumontanum) and the sphincter area. **(See Figure 53.1)**
- Females: Dx/HA is injected into the whole length of the urethra. **(See Figure 53.2)**

The needle should be introduced tangentially into the submucosa by the surgeon, making sure that it is embedded quite deeply in the mucosa. The assistant injects Dx/HA copolymer from the syringe while the surgeon holds the

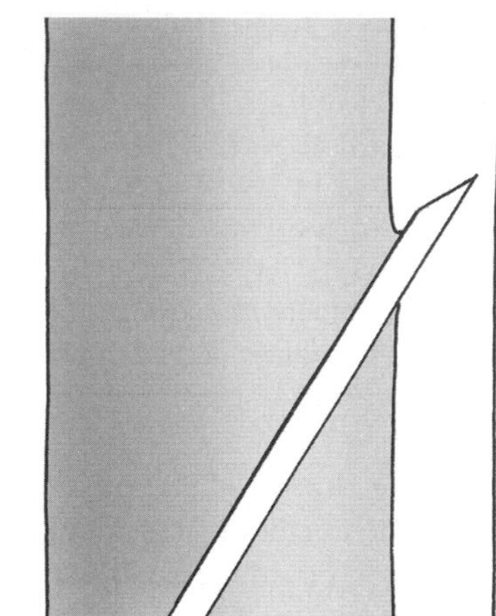

Figure 53.3

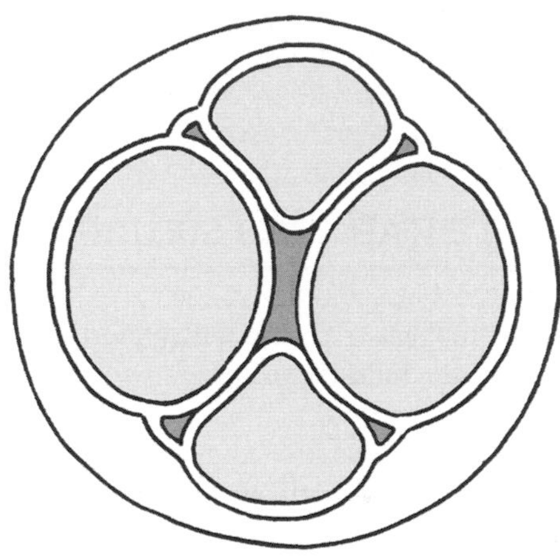

Figure 53.4

needle and cystoscope in place. Injection is continued until a prominent bolus is formed. **(See Figure 53.3)**

Injection should be continued until adequate constriction (near closure) of the urethra is achieved. To this end, four separate injections, each of approximately 1 mL of the bulking agent, are recommended, starting at the 3 and 9 o'clock positions followed by the 6 and 12 o'clock positions.

At each injection site, the needle should be kept in position for 15–30 seconds post-administration to prevent leakage of the bulking agent. **(See Figure 53.4)**

Upon completion of the injection procedure, the needle is withdrawn back into the cystoscope before it is removed from the patient's body.

It is recommended that all patients have a suprapubic catheter inserted for 3 days before being allowed to catheterize or urinate again. This is to avoid any risk of dislodging the injected substance and to allow the mucosa at the site of the injection to heal.

POSTOPERATIVE CARE

Patients may be discharged from hospital on the day of the procedure after waking from anesthesia, assuming that there are no specific problems. The suprapubic catheter is removed after 3 days.

Follow-up to evaluate the extent of any continuing incontinence is undertaken at 1, 3 and 12 months after treatment. This involves:

- recording of the number of pads used daily,
- pad tests (i.e. the weight of single pads after physical exercise during standard fluid consumption),
- questionnaires.

Urine culture and a general clinical evaluation are also recommended at 3 and 12 months. Routine annual check-ups should be performed thereafter. If post-treatment investigations reveal continued or recurrent incontinence, endoscopic injection therapy may be repeated to achieve an optimal result.

PROBLEMS, PITFALLS AND SOLUTIONS

The potential problems associated with endoscopic injection therapy include the following.

Failure to achieve a bolus upon injection of the bulking agent

If this occurs, injection should be attempted at a different site, remembering that males can be injected both at the proximal urethra and the sphincter area and that the whole length of the urethra can be injected in females.

Concerns regarding adequate closure of the urethra

It is recommended that injection is performed at the 3, 6, 9 and 12 o'clock positions until adequate constriction (near-closure) of the urethra has been achieved.

Injection depth

It is important to inject deeply into the mucosa by injecting tangentially and embedding at least the entire needle bevel. (There is evidence to show that injection into the muscle surrounding the urethra may be advantageous.)

Difficulty manipulating all of the injection apparatus

To avoid any manipulation difficulties, it is recommended that the assistant performs the injection while the surgeon concentrates on maintaining the correct position of the cystoscope and needle.

Poor visibility associated with folding of the urethra

It is important to ensure an adequate flow of fluid past the end of the cystoscope throughout the procedure to prevent this from happening.

Injection site (male exstrophy patients)

The best results are achieved when the urethra is injected proximal to the verumontanum (the feasibility of this is dependent on the primary operation). Success is less likely if injection is only possible in the sphincter region.

Anatomy (female patients)

Treatment failure is more likely if the urethra is short in length (<1 cm). This is most likely to be the case in children with previous exstrophy, bilateral single ectopic ureters, primary epispadia or a congenital short urethra.

COMPLICATIONS

An important consideration with all attempts to increase bladder outlet resistance is the potential effect on bladder volume, not least due to the requirement for good bladder volume to preserve renal function. An increase in bladder volume is likely following endoscopic injection therapy, which would be beneficial for subsequent bladder neck reconstruction. Conversely, however, there is a risk of bladder contraction and renewed incontinence, which would be exacerbated by performing a repeat endoscopic injection. In such cases, continence can only be restored by first restoring bladder capacity through augmentation techniques.

Bladder instability and urge symptoms can occur for either short or long periods of time after endoscopic injection, and these are best treated with pharmacotherapy.

Primary endoscopic treatment with Dx/HA copolymer is unlikely to jeopardize subsequent surgical procedures. In contrast, with PTFE and silicone there is a risk of sclerosis or fibrosis of tissue at the bladder neck, which may increase the difficulty of bladder neck plasty.

FURTHER READING

Caione P, Capozza N. Endoscopic treatment of urinary incontinence in pediatric patients: two-year experience of dextranomer co-polymer. *Journal of Urology* 2002; **168**:1868–71.

Dodat H, Takvorian P, Sabatier E et al. Treatment of vesicoureteral reflux in children by endoscopic injection of Teflon. Review of 3½ years' experience. *Pediatric Surgery International* 1991; **6**:273–5.

Guys JM, Fakhro A, Louis-Borrione C et al. The effect of endoscopic treatment of urinary incontinence: long-term evaluation of the results. *Journal of Urology* 2001; **165**:2389–91.

Lottman HB, Margaryan M, Bernuy M et al. The effect of endoscopic injections of dextranomer-based implants on continence and bladder capacity: a prospective study in 31 patients. *Journal of Urology* 2002; **168**:1863–7.

Mitchell M, Woodhouse C, Bloom D et al. Surgical treatment of urinary incontinence in children. In: Wein AJ (ed.), *Incontinence*, 2nd edn. Plymouth, UK: Plymbridge Distributors Ltd, 2002.

54

Extraperitoneal laparoscopy – basic technique

WALID A. FARHAT AND ANTOINE KHOURY

INTRODUCTION

Laparoscopy has become increasingly popular in pediatric urology, reducing the invasiveness of treatment and shortening the period of convalescence. Many practicing pediatric urologists and surgeons have little previous laparoscopic experience and are trying to adopt not only an additional surgical procedure, but also the completely new surgical concept of retroperitoneoscopy.

Advantages

The advantages of the retroperitoneal approach include the following.

- The technique mimics the open urological surgical procedure through the retroperitoneal approach.
- It involves a direct approach to the genitourinary organs, and therefore does not require dissection or retraction of the colon or spleen to expose the kidneys and adrenals.
- Previous transperitoneal surgery does not preclude retroperitoneoscopy.
- Postoperative hernias at the trocar sites are uncommon.
- It facilitates visualization of the posterior surface of the kidney, allowing rapid access to the renal hilum.
- The peritoneal cavity is not violated, enabling a faster postoperative recovery.

Disadvantages

- Restrictive working space may initially limit the surgeon's ability to manipulate the instruments easily. For instance, in reconstructive surgery (e.g. pyeloplasty), suturing and knot tying may be difficult. In ablative surgery (e.g. nephrectomy), the degree of technical difficulty increases if the kidney is large.
- Anatomical disorientation may initially plague the inexperienced laparoscopist.
- It involves a steep learning curve and the need for a large number of cases to master the technique.

Indications

- Total nephrectomy for a poorly functioning or non-functioning kidney.
- Partial nephrectomy for a duplicated renal system with non-function of one renal moiety.
- Distal ureterectomy for a duplication anomaly.
- Pyeloplasty for pelvi-ureteric junction obstruction.
- Pyelolithotomy and ureterolithotomy: extracorporeal lithotripsy and endo-urologic procedures have almost eliminated the need for open surgery to remove urinary stones. In some patients who have unusual anatomy, e.g. an ectopic pelvic kidney, those interventions may not be optimal and a laparoscopic approach (mainly transperitoneally rather than extraperitoneally) may be considered.
- Adrenalectomy for a cortical adenoma associated with congenital adrenal hyperplasia.

Contraindications

RELATIVE

- Previous retroperitoneal renal surgery, renal biopsy or pyeloplasty.

- Previous infectious or inflammatory retroperitoneal process (e.g. xanthogranulomatous pyelonephritis).

ABSOLUTE

- Cardiopulmonary morbidity.
- Uncorrected coagulopathy.
- Uncontrolled sepsis.
- Malignant tumors: although laparoscopy may play a role in the staging of malignant pediatric abdominal tumors such as Wilms' tumor or neuroblastoma, its role in the management of these tumors has yet to be defined. Morcellation of specimens for extraction has raised concerns about accurate pathologic staging, such that large tumors require an incision to retrieve them. In addition, the fragile consistency of the tumor may cause it to rupture during surgery.

Anatomic considerations

An understanding of the retroperitoneal anatomy is mandatory before embarking on retroperitoneoscopic surgery. The boundaries of the retroperitoneal space are as follows.

- Posteriorly and laterally: the paraspinal, psoas and quadratus lumborum muscles, which are anatomically fixed structures.
- Anteriorly: the mobile posterior parietal peritoneum and its contents.
- Superiorly: the diaphragm.
- Inferiorly: contiguous with the extraperitoneal portions of the pelvis.

The retroperitoneum contains the great vessels, kidneys, adrenals and ureters, in addition to the peri-renal adipose and areolar tissues. Since there is no actual preformed cavity in the retroperitoneal area, insufflation into the potential space is required, and can only be accomplished adequately after the adipose areolar tissue in the retroperitoneum is disrupted by insufflation; in this way the retroperitoneal space is created. (**See Figure 54.1**)

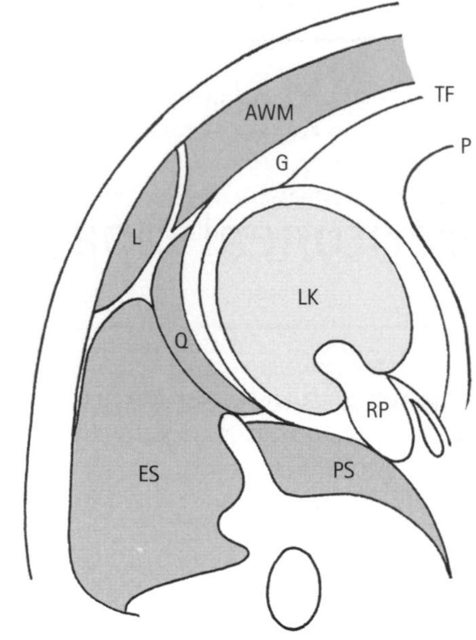

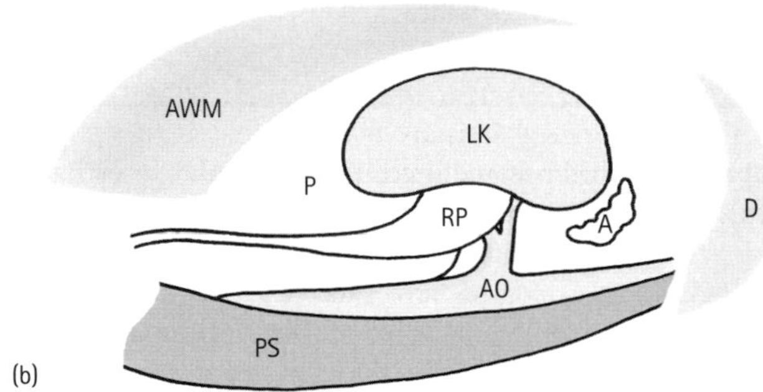

Figure 54.1 *(a) Transverse section; (b) posterior aspect of the left renal bed.*

EQUIPMENT/INSTRUMENTS

Essential

- No. 15 and No. 11 blade on a No. 3 Bard Parker handle.
- Two S-shaped Sim's retractors.
- Narrow and wide L-shape retractors.
- Three trocars: one 10 mm or 5 mm for the camera, and two 5 mm or 3 mm working ports.
- 10 mm or 5 mm 0° and 30° telescopes.
- 5 mm or 3 mm curved insulated Mayo scissors with a monopolar point.
- 5 mm or 3 mm bipolar diathermy with a smooth coagulation insert.
- Two 5 mm or 3 mm curved, fine, atraumatic, insulated grasping forceps.
- 5 mm Endoclip® applicators.

The operating room should have the capacity to support the laparoscopic procedure fully as well as accommodate conversion to an open procedure should that be required. The following additional instruments are needed for open retroperitoneal surgery.

- Abdominal wall retractors.
- Tissue scissors.
- Needle drivers.
- Suturing scissors.
- Vascular clamps.
- Vascular forceps.
- Tissue clamps.
- Tissue forceps.
- Suture materials for vascular and bowel repair.

PREOPERATIVE PREPARATION

Bowel preparation for retroperitoneoscopic renal surgery may be recommended in adults, but this has not been routinely employed in children.

Following general anesthesia, a urethral catheter is placed if intra-operative urine output monitoring is required (e.g. renal insufficiency) or retrograde filling of the bladder is indicated (e.g. after pyeloplasty) to confirm the position of a JJ stent.

Although a retroperitoneoscopic approach may be accomplished with the patient in the prone position, the flank position is preferred because it doubles the dimensions of the antero-posterior potential retroperitoneal space and displaces the peritoneum anteriorly, decreasing the chance of inadvertently opening it. The child is positioned in the full 90°-flank position as close to the surgeon as possible. To increase the retroperitoneal space further, the table is flexed and the kidney rest elevated. Pressure points are meticulously padded and an axillary roll is placed to prevent complications such as a brachial plexus palsy. The child should be taped to the table using 5 cm adhesive tape placed across the shoulder and the hips for security.

The surgeon and assistant stand on the same side and only one monitor is required. Having both surgeon and assistant in the same line of vision facilitates eye–hand coordination, particularly that of the assistant surgeon. **(See Figure 54.2)**

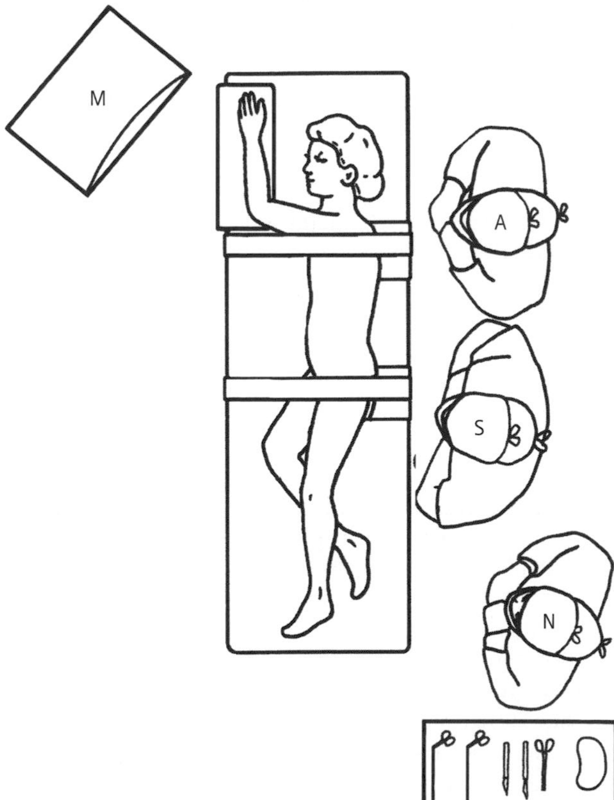

Figure 54.2

The induction and maintenance of anesthesia may be with either inhalation or intravenous agents, and intra-operative monitoring should include routine electrocardiogram, non-invasive blood pressure, O_2 saturation, temperature and inspired oxygen concentration. Although end-tidal CO_2 may not accurately reflect arterial CO_2 tension, its use is helpful to plan appropriate ventilation strategies, but in infants and children with respiratory pathology, capillary or arterial blood gas analysis might be indicated to measure CO_2 tension accurately. Maintenance volumes of fluid are usually sufficient unless there is unanticipated bleeding. Finally, it is preferable to insert the intravenous line in the arm on the same side of the surgery so that the anesthetist can then place it in a convenient position for easy access.

TECHNIQUE

Access to the retroperitoneum should be achieved by open (Hasson) or closed (Veress) techniques. The open technique is recommended for children because they have a relatively small retroperitoneum which is in close proximity to the abdominal wall and the major vessels (which are primarily retroperitoneal). In addition, since there is no actual pre-existing retroperitoneal space, placement of a Veress needle may not be accurate: inadvertent positioning deep in the retroperitoneum may cause injury to the great vessels or pneumoperitoneum, thereby complicating the procedure from the beginning. For these reasons, the most commonly employed technique is the open technique, which provides visual guidance to the correct retroperitoneal space.

In the mid-axillary line, a 1–1.5 cm long incision is made 1–2 cm below the tip of the 12th rib. The muscle fibers are split and the lumbo-dorsal fascia is incised to enter the retroperitoneum. Creation of the retroperitoneal space is an essential first step in retroperitoneoscopic surgery and there are several methods for developing it using a blunt instrument or a balloon dissector. Although commercial balloon dissectors are readily available, a cheap balloon can be made from the middle finger of a surgeon's glove tied around a catheter. The balloon is inserted anterior to the psoas muscle and outside Gerota's fascia, and approximately 400–500 mL of air are used to insufflate the balloon to create the space.

We routinely use instrument dissection to create the retroperitoneal space. The 5–10 mm trocar is inserted and the laparoscope (0°) is inserted to confirm correct placement. Prior to CO_2 insufflation, a 0 polyglactin (UR6 needle) purse-string suture is placed around the trocar in the fascia. This avoids the risk of:

- gas leakage,
- subcutaneous emphysema,
- slippage of the port.

(See Figure 54.3)

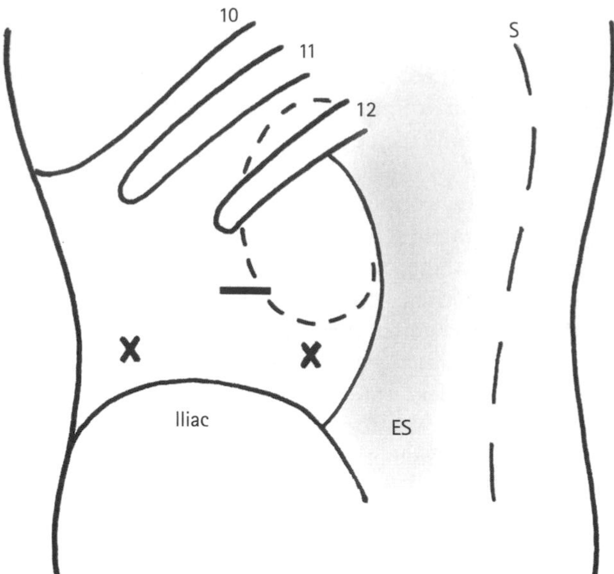

Figure 54.3

Once the depth of the trocar is well delineated, the suture is tied to the side of the port and used as a Lap-lift to enlarge the retroperitoneal space. Carbon dioxide insufflation is started at a pressure of 12 mmHg for children over the age of 2 years and 8 mmHg for children aged less than 2 years.

Blunt dissection under vision creates the retroperitoneal space: identification of the psoas muscle posteriorly is crucial. Anteriorly, the edge of the peritoneum is identified and swept medially to expose the underside of the transversalis fascia. To avoid tearing the peritoneum during placement of the secondary working trocars in the extraperitoneal space, the laparoscope should be steered lateral to medial close to the abdominal wall to uncover the internal surface of the transversalis muscle. Having created the working space, two 3–5 mm secondary trocars are inserted. The posterior secondary port is first inserted at the lateral border of the paraspinal muscles. Through this trocar, the peritoneum is further mobilized medially using a grasper to create the pelvic extraperitoneal space. The anterior secondary trocar is inserted at the anterior axillary line 2 cm superior to the iliac crest. The two secondary parts should be inserted as far apart as possible to decrease the risk of them criss-crossing in the retroperitoneum, which would limit their use in an efficient fashion. We recently modified the site of the secondary trocar insertion to be as follows: posterior trocar closer to the costovertebral angle providing direct access to renal pelvis and renal hilum.

Trocar insertion technique: a 30° laparoscope may be used to place the secondary trocars. A small skin stab is made using a No. 11 blade. A sharp-tipped obturator allows the trocars to be advanced through the muscles and fascia. Once in the retroperitoneal space, blunt-tipped obturators are exchanged for the sharp ones and the trocars are advanced further. The blunt tip prevents injury to the peritoneum and the major vessels. In addition, while inserting the trocar, it should be directed towards the area of dissection to avoid:

- constant tension on the skin during surgery,
- greater chance of gas leakage at the trocar site.

Although the sites of the telescope and other trocars are similar for all retroperitoneal renal and adrenal laparoscopic procedures, the sequence of operative strategy and the need for accessory trocars depend on the surgical procedure. Where more than three ports are required, laparoscopic guidance and bimanual palpation are recommended for accurate placement of these trocars. For instance, during retroperitoneoscopic pyeloplasty, an additional port may be required to maintain traction on the uretero-pelvic junction for better exposure; in this case, a fourth trocar (3 mm or 5 mm) is placed along the anterior axillary line at the tip of the 11th rib. Adequate dissection of the peritoneal reflection medially where the trocar is to be inserted is mandatory to avoid inadvertent peritoneotomy.

The psoas muscle and posterior aspect of the kidney are identified first and are useful landmarks for orientation in any retroperitoneoscopic renal procedure. This approach allows rapid visualization of the 'vertically' oriented main artery and vein on the screen. To facilitate exposure of the renal pedicle further, dissection of the anterior surface of the kidney is performed last. This will help keep the kidney attached to the peritoneum and provide spontaneous retraction on the renal pedicle during nephrectomy or a partial nephrectomy. In addition, it will suspend the kidney anteriorly, helping to expose the uretero-pelvic junction during pyeloplasty. The psoas muscle is a guide to the renal pedicle, which lies opposite to it; the great vessels are medial. In addition, pulsations of the renal artery and of the aorta or vena cava and ureteric contraction may help locate the renal hilum. On the right side, initial identification of the inferior vena cava on the medial aspect of the psoas muscle facilitates identification of the gonadal, renal and suprarenal veins, which are all located in the same plane. On the left side, aortic pulsation helps guide the surgeon to the renal artery. **(See Figure 54.4)**

PROBLEMS, PITFALLS AND SOLUTIONS

Malfunction of the equipment

Well-trained laparoscopy nurses should be capable of quickly recognizing equipment malfunction and responding promptly to correct. The success of the laparoscopic procedure not only depends on the surgeon's skill, but also on the proper working of all equipment. Consequently, these cases are better booked for a time when skilled staff are available so as to avoid unnecessary problems and delays. A dedicated minimal invasive suite equipped with

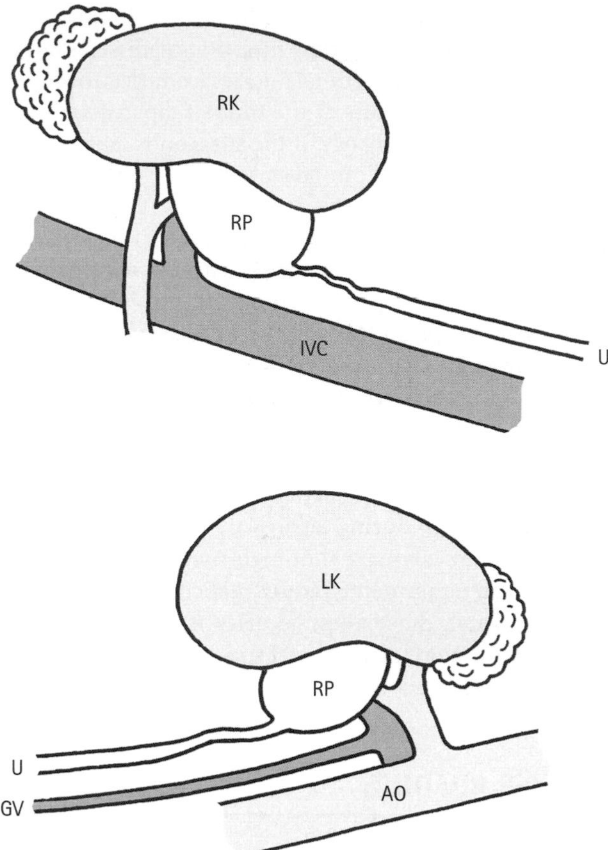

Figure 54.4 *Posterior aspects of right (RK) and left (LK) kidneys. AO: aorta, GV: gonadal vein, IVC: inferior vena cava, RP: right pelvis, U: ureter.*

trained personnel is of the utmost importance to initiate endoscopic surgery.

Inadequate visualization

Initial warming of the laparoscope in warm saline/povidone–iodine solution or using commercial defogging fluid may avoid fogging of the lens. Inadequate vision is most commonly due to gas leak around the primary trocar. This usually leads to complete collapse of the retroperitoneal space, and an extra purse-string suture around the trocar may help to decrease the leak. Another possible reason for inadequate vision is a minor peritoneal tear, which may lead to intraperitoneal insufflation that ultimately limits the retroperitoneal space. In such a case, it is best either to convert to a transperitoneal laparoscopic approach or attempt to vent the peritoneum using the technique described below.

Bleeding

Where there is peri-nephric inflammation or the patient has undergone previous retroperitoneal surgery, dissection may be difficult, and may lead to bleeding. Conversion to open surgery may be required.

Bleeding may occur during blunt dissection of the retroperitoneal space: if this occurs, the posterior secondary trocars should be placed and the bleeding vessels controlled with monopolar or the bipolar diathermy.

Subcutaneous emphysema

This problem may occur due to leakage of CO_2 around the ports. Signs include readily palpable crepitus over the flank and abdomen. Treatment involves:

- placement of a purse-string suture around the leaking port,
- changing the trocar to a larger size,
- reduction of the insufflation pressure.

Problems with insertion of the trocars

Insertion of the primary trocar in the correct space is critical. Inserting the trocar too far medially may result in peritoneal entry or colonic injury, whereas entering posteriorly in the quadratus or psoas muscles may cause bleeding. It is always advisable to create the retroperitoneal space outside Gerota's fascia, and dissect the peritoneum medially. Then a secondary 5 mm trocar can be inserted to open Gerota's fascia under vision. This facilitates the creation of the retroperitoneal space by dissecting the peritoneal reflection medially for insertion of the third trocar.

Intraperitoneal carbon dioxide insufflation

If this occurs prior to the insertion of the two 5 mm accessory trocars, consider conversion to a transperitoneal laparoscopic approach or an open procedure. If it occurs while inserting the secondary trocars (mainly the medial one, superior to the iliac spine), consider the insertion of a Veress needle or an iv cannula in the umbilicus intraperitoneally to deflate the peritoneum and change the site of the secondary trocar insertion. Since there is intraperitoneal CO_2 insufflation, the risk of injury to the bowel with the Veress needle or angiocath is minimal. If this does not improve the view, convert to either an open or transperitoneal laparoscopic approach.

COMPLICATIONS

Laparoscopic surgery always carries the risk of inadvertent injuries that may occur during the learning-curve process, and increasing experience is likely to result in a decrease in the complication rate. Although the mechanisms of injury vary, most occur during blind-access maneuvers with the first or secondary trocars. As the route of access to the retroperitoneum in open techniques is through a very small incision, this also carries a risk of damage to vascular and bowel structures, which represent the most serious injuries at this step of the surgery. For instance, at the time of the primary trocar insertion, the peritoneum may be mistaken for Gerota's fascia and opened – an additional forward vector of force while inserting the telescope is all that is necessary to injure bowel or vessels. If there is any doubt distinguishing Gerota's fascia and the peritoneum, it is recommended that further access to the retroperitoneum be obtained under vision. Finally, the instruments as well as the trocars may cause unintended injury, and the management of these injuries depends on their nature and severity.

Since the great vessels are retroperitoneal, they may be injured during laparoscopic access or dissection. In children, the distance between the abdominal wall and the retroperitoneal vessels may be as little as 5 cm. During dissection on the left side, the aorta and iliac arteries are vulnerable; on the right, injury to the inferior vena cava and/or iliac arteries may occur. For these reasons, it is advisable to tailor the length of the trocars to the patient's age and body habitus. Moreover, it is mandatory to check that the electrocautery instruments are inspected to ensure adequate insulation and decrease the risk of injury.

Features of vascular injury include bloody return from the trocar and rapid deterioration of the hemodynamic status of the patient. Once extensive vascular injury is suspected, the trocar should be left in place and an open exploration should be performed. However, if minor vascular injury is encountered during dissection (such as laceration of the gonadal vessels or adrenal vessels), hemostasis should be maintained with traction anteriorly on the kidney; which stretches these vessels and allows the bleeding to cease. The patient's vital signs should be continually observed and maintained.

The other catastrophic injury caused during retroperitoneal procedures is injury to the bowel. Although the bowel is out of sight during these procedures, bowel injuries can still occur during either trocar insertion or dissection as a result of lacerations or thermal injuries from electrocautery.

If bowel injury occurs at the time of laparoscopy, it is best dealt with immediately. If the surgeon is laparoscopically skilled, the bowel can be closed using a laparoscopic approach; otherwise, an open approach is recommended. A major contaminating injury to the small or large bowel is best handled by open repair with or without proximal fecal diversion.

The liver or spleen may also be injured during laparoscopic retroperitoneal surgery. If the injuries are superficial, bleeding can be controlled laparoscopically with gel foam or with an argon beam coagulator. If these measures fail, open exploration is recommended.

Injuries to vascular structures and bowel are an ever-present possibility during laparoscopic surgery. They are best avoided by having a thorough understanding of the anatomy and equipment, and by meticulous attention to operative detail. Since these injuries may go unnoticed, inspection of the retroperitoneal space upon entrance and prior to exiting is advised.

FURTHER READING

Radmayr C, Neumann H, Bartsch G, Elsner R, Janetschek G. Laparoscopic partial adrenalectomy for bilateral pheochromocytomas in a boy with von Hippel–Lindau disease. *European Urology* 2000; **38**(3):344–8.

Schier F, Mutter D, Bennek J, Brock D, Hoepffner W. Laparoscopic bilateral adrenalectomy in a child. *European Journal of Pediatric Surgery* 1999; **9**(6):420–1.

Waldhausen JH, Tapper D, Sawin RS. Minimally invasive surgery and clinical decision-making for paediatric malignancy. *Surgical Endoscopy* 2000; **14**(3):250–3.

55

Management of impalpable testes

ISRAEL FRANCO

INTRODUCTION

Surgical intervention for the intra-abdominal testes is considered essential for the preservation of testicular function and monitoring for testicular cancer later in adulthood. In the 1990s, laparoscopy became an established technique in the management of intra-abdominal testes. Once the testis is localized on diagnostic laparoscopy, an open definitive surgical procedure(s) may be considered. Alternatively, orchidopexy or orchidectomy can be carried out laparoscopically in one or two stages. The choice of procedure is dependent on:

- the condition and level of the undescended testes,
- the age and circumstances of the patient,
- whether a unilateral or bilateral procedure is required,
- the surgeon's preference and/or expertise.

Indications

- Intra-abdominal testes.
- Peeping testes (testes that move freely in and out of the internal ring).
- Inguinal testes with short cord in older patients.

Contraindications

There are no absolute contraindications to laparoscopic orchidopexy. However, relative contraindications may include the following.

- The presence of intraperitoneal adhesions.
- An inexperienced surgeon.

EQUIPMENT/INSTRUMENTS

Essential

Four cannulae are usually necessary. The sizes of the cannulae are dependent on the sizes of the available instruments. A 5 mm cannula is usually necessary to channel the testis down into the scrotum, and may be required for the telescope and clip applicator, but 3–3.5 mm cannulae are used for the dissecting instruments.

- 3–5 mm 0° or 30° angled telescope.
- 3–5 mm curved double jaw action insulated scissors.
- Two pairs of 3.5–5 mm atraumatic insulated grasping forceps without ratchet (one curved, the other flat) and additional 3.5–5 mm Alice forceps (or toothed forceps).
- 5 mm clip applicator with appropriate-sized clips.

Optional

- 3.5–5 mm probe or Endo-peanut.
- 3.5–5 mm needle holder.

PREOPERATIVE PREPARATION

In laparoscopic orchidopexy, the preoperative preparation is similar to that required for routine conventional surgery. Follicle-stimulating hormone (FSH), luteinizing hormone (LH) and testosterone levels are measured in cases of bilateral impalpable testes associated with micropenis and/or manifestations of hypogonadism. In these cases, laparoscopy is usually indicated unless the FSH and LH levels are extremely high. In cases of pseudohermaphrodism, complete work-up should be carried out prior to surgery. Radiological imaging, including ultrasound and computerized tomography (CT) scans, are often unreliable, with the false-positive and false-negative rates being higher than 20 percent. The role of contrast-augmented magnetic resonance image (MRI) scanning is under investigation.

Prior to surgery, informed consent must be obtained. The success rates for various procedures (depending on whether the testicular vessels are preserved or transected) and the rare possibility of intestinal and vascular injury are discussed below.

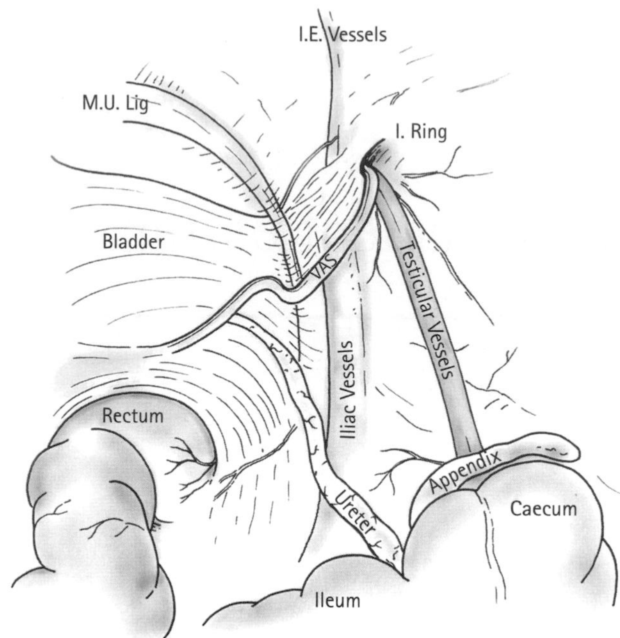

Figure 55.1 *Normal anatomy of the right iliac fossa.*

TECHNIQUE

General anesthesia with full muscle relaxation is essential (avoid nitrous oxide, as in all pediatric laparoscopy). A caudal anesthetic/analgesic provides good intra-operative and postoperative analgesia. The monitor is positioned at the foot of the operating table to facilitate viewing for both the surgeon and assistant. The patient is placed supine with the feet at the end of the operating table. A urinary catheter (8 Fr feeding tube) is usually necessary for the entire duration of the procedure.

The primary (first) cannula is placed in the infra-umbilical region using open-technique laparoscopy. A pneumoperitoneum is created at a pressure of 12 mmHg. The head-down (Trendelenburg) position may improve access. If the view of the pelvic structures is obscured by dilated loops of bowel or adhesions, the placement of additional (working) cannulae is considered for manipulation of the bowel and adhesiolysis.

The iliac fossae are inspected and the appearance of the region of the internal ring and the presence or absence of testicular vessels and vas deferens allow the surgeon to determine whether or not any additional maneuvers are required. In unilateral cases, a comparison between the normal and abnormal sides often proves helpful. **(See Figure 55.1)**

- A patent processus vaginalis is nearly always associated with an intra-canalicular testis, with the vessels and vas deferens clearly seen as they enter the ring.
- The absence of testicular vessels and vas deferens at the internal ring usually means either an absent testis or the presence of the testis somewhere in the abdominal cavity. In cases of testicular agenesis associated with absent vas deferens, the possibility of ipsilateral renal agenesis and a heterozygous carrier of cystic fibrosis should be born in mind.
- The presence of the vas deferens at the internal ring usually indicates that there is a viable or atrophic testis either in the inguinal canal or intra-abdominally.
- Atrophic or small (attenuated) vessels entering the internal ring generally indicate a probable case of in utero-torsion (absent testis). In this situation the vas-associated vessels are usually enlarged.
- The vas deferens entering the ring without testicular vessels often implies a case of looping vas deferens with the testis sitting on the medial site of the iliac vessels.

The sigmoid colon and occasionally the cecum may obscure the left and right intra-abdominal testes respectively. In cases of high abdominal testes and absent vas deferens, orchidopexy with or without (Fowler–Stephens procedure) preservation of testicular vessels is not possible, but an orchidectomy or microvascular transfer orchidopexy may be considered.

Once the testis is localized, the following options are considered.

- Open-technique surgery.
- Laparoscopic surgery:
  - orchidopexy with preservation of the vessels provided there is sufficient length to both the vas and vessels;
  - single-stage or two-stage Fowler–Stephens procedure if the testicular vessels are thought to be short;
  - orchidectomy if the testis appeared clearly abnormal and in unilateral cases of high testis associated with absent vas deferens, especially when expertise from microvascular transfer is not available.

The working cannulae are placed in the mid-clavicular lines at the umbilical level.

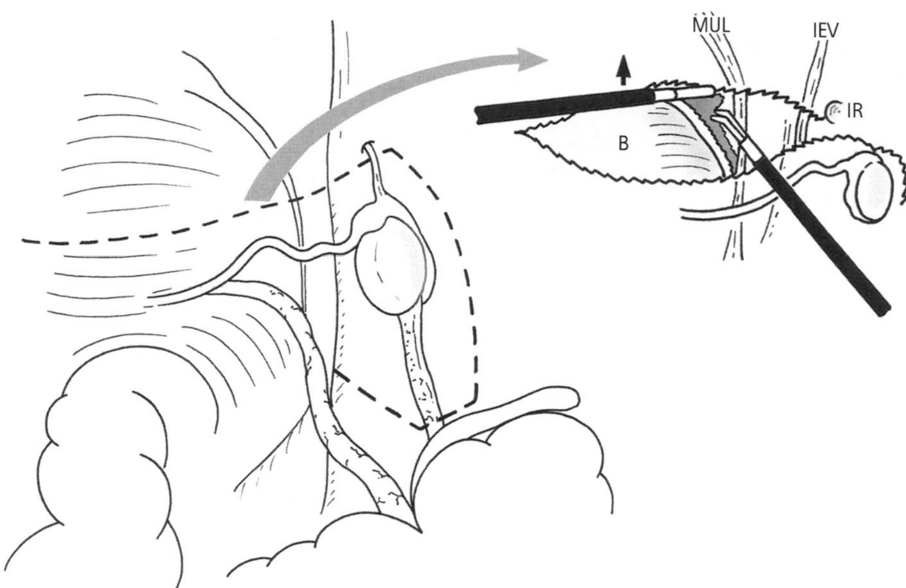

Figure 55.2

Orchidopexy

The gubernaculum is pulled out of the inguinal canal and divided using diathermy or scissors. Care must be taken not to damage the epididymis or vas deferens. The peritoneum is then incised along the lateral pelvic wall 1 cm lateral to the testicular vessel and taken as high as possible (level of the colon or beyond if necessary). The dissection of the peritoneum is then taken medially over the median umbilical ligament and across the bladder (two-thirds in unilateral cases and completely across in bilateral cases). Minimum effect and lower power electrocoagulation is used in order to avoid injury to the vessels and vas/epididymis. Once the two limbs of the dissection have been completed, attention is taken back to the upper limit of lateral dissection. The peritoneum over the testicular vessels is incised and the incision is continued towards the route of mesentery. This incision is critical to allow adequate mobilization. Care must be taken not to damage the testicular vessels, ureter and iliac vessels.

A space is then created between the bladder and the medial umbilical ligament and the pubic bone is exposed using a blunt dissector or an Endo-peanut. Extreme care is exercised not to dissect laterally to avoid damaging the femoral vein. **(See Figure 55.2)**

Once the internal dissection has been completed, a probe dissector or Endo-peanut is placed through the ipsilateral working cannula and pushed against the anterior abdominal wall over the superior edge of the pubic bone towards the external inguinal ring. The index finger is then used to invaginate the scrotum and push it towards the external inguinal ring, where the probe dissector from above is easily palpated. The probe dissector/Endo-peanut is now pushed medially through the external inguinal ring and a prominent pop is usually felt/heard. A fair amount of force is usually required. To prevent inadvertent injury to the femoral and epigastric vessels, it is important to keep the direction of force from lateral (ipsilateral cannula) to medial (external ring above the pubic tubercle).

Once through the anterior abdominal wall, the probe dissector/Endo-peanut is pushed down into the scrotum and through a pre-prepared dartos pouch/skin incision. Then a 5 mm cannula is placed over the dissector and pushed into the abdominal cavity. Once the cannula is in position, grasping forceps (Ellis) are passed cephalad and the testis (preferably remnant of the gubernaculum) is grasped carefully and pulled through to the surface of the scrotum. Care is taken not to damage the epididymis or testis. **(See Figure 55.3)**

If the cord appears tight, the abdomen is deflated, the tension on the testis is re-checked and further internal dissection is considered as necessary. Once a satisfactory position has been achieved, the testis is fixed in the scrotum and the wound is closed in the usual fashion.

A single-stage Fowler–Stephens orchidopexy may be considered for testes that would not reach a satisfactory scrotal position.

Finally, the operative field is thoroughly inspected, the cannulae are removed and the wounds are closed.

Two-stage Fowler–Stephens orchidopexy

In children who have high intra-abdominal testes and normal vas deferens, a two-stage Fowler–Stephens orchidopexy is the laparoscopic procedure of choice. However, its success is dependent on a carefully preserved, fragile collateral testicular blood supply. Therefore, it is important not to disturb the testis, vas and collateral circulation if a Fowler–Stephens orchidopexy is thought to be required and during stage one

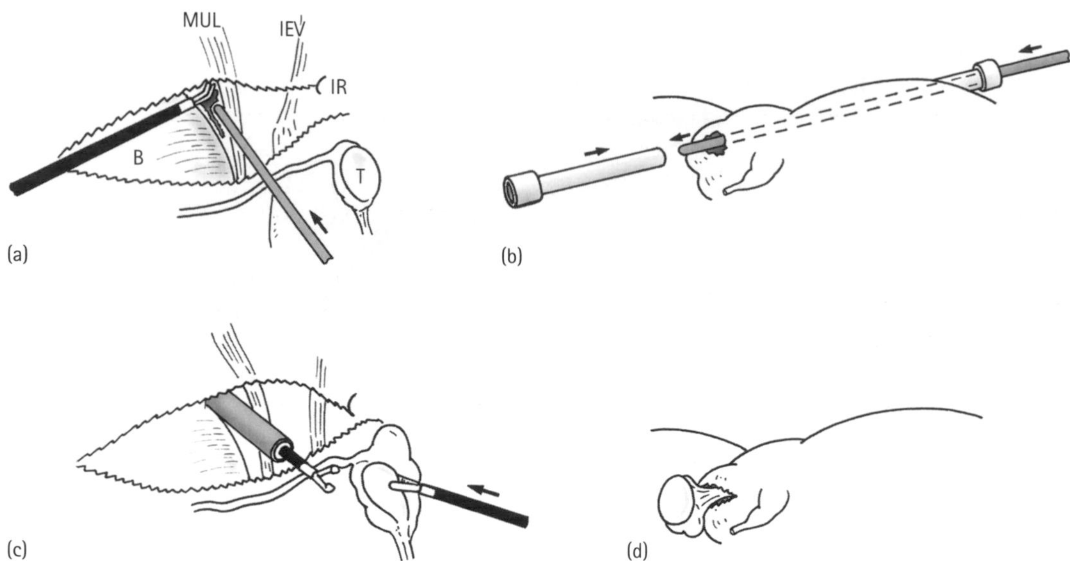

Figure 55.3

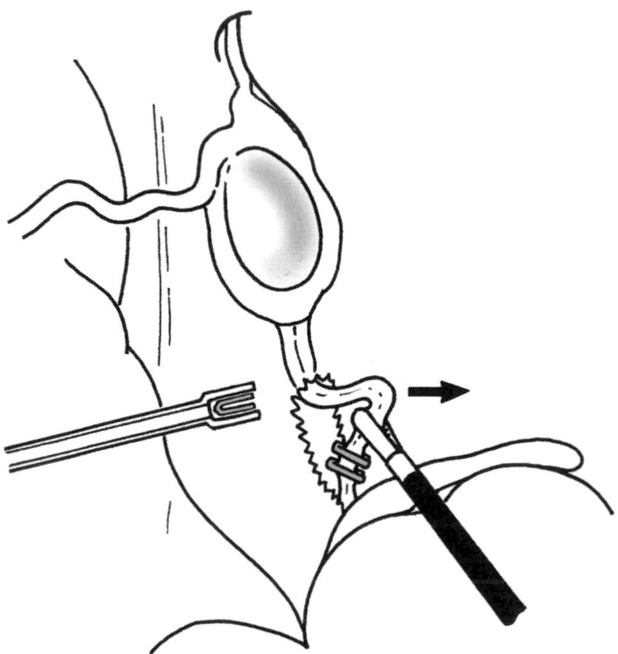

Figure 55.4

of the procedure. Access into the abdomen is obtained as for orchidopexy. The testicular vessels are grasped gently as high as possible using atraumatic forceps and divided in between Ligaclips. Alternatively, suture ligatures or bipolar diathermy may be used to secure the vessels. **(See Figure 55.4)**

Six to nine months later, the patient is re-admitted to hospital for the second stage of the procedure. Human chorionic gonadotrophin may be used in an attempt to increase the vascularity of the testis. The technique of the second stage of the Fowler–Stephens procedure is similar to that of laparoscopic orchidopexy, with the difference being already divided testicular vessels.

PROBLEMS, PITFALLS AND SOLUTIONS

Poor view

In small children, access and visibility may be improved by:

- placement of the cannulae above the umbilical level,
- use of a 5 mm instead of a 3 mm telescope,
- steep Trendelenburg position, which allows small and large bowels to move cephalad under gravity,
- decompression of the rectum/colon using a manual evacuation and/or rectal tube.

Bleeding gubernaculum

This is usually minor and may easily be avoided by pulling the gubernaculum out of the inguinal canal before it is divided using diathermy.

Dissection through the peritoneum

A gentle and appropriate technique cannot be overemphasized. Effort must be made to incise the peritoneum 1 cm clear of the epididymis, testis, vas and vessels. The seminal vesicles should never be seen. Patients who have suffered recent bladder infections tend to have peri-vesicle adhesions, which make dissection in the area more difficult than usual.

Extraction of testes

Several testicular pull-through techniques have been described. A large enough neo-inguinal ring has to be created from inside (by the technique described in this chapter) or outside using a pair of conventional artery forceps or a 5 mm laparoscopic cannula. Sometimes the testis is too large to pass through a 5 mm cannula, in which case a larger neo-ring (using a 8–10 mm cannula or gradual dilator device) is created in order to complete the procedure without damaging the testicle.

Inability to place the testis within the scrotum (short cord/vas)

- Ensure adequate mobilization without jeopardizing the blood supply/collateral circulation.
- Divide the peritoneum over the testicular vessels.
- Use the shortest route through the abdominal wall.
- Leave the testis where it reaches and re-do orchidopexy is performed 6 months later after a course of human chorionic gonadotrophin is given.
- Consider a single-stage Fowler–Stephens procedure.

Absent vas deferens

This is an anomaly usually associated with a high testis. Consider microvascular transfer orchidopexy or orchidectomy.

Prune-belly patients

In these patients, the bladder is large and densely adherent to the surrounding peritoneum. Place the camera (first/primary) cannula above the umbilicus and take care during mobilization of the bladder from the pubic bone.

COMPLICATIONS

Injury to the testis, epididymis, vas and vessels during mobilization

Careful handling and dissection and minimal use of diathermy minimize these risks.

Injury to the epigastric vessels

This may be controlled using either intracorporeal or extracorporeal ligation.

Avulsion of testicular vessels

Avulsed vessels may be ligated and the procedure continued as a single-stage Fowler–Stephens procedure.

Bleeding within the inguinal canal

This is a relatively minor problem that can be controlled with diathermy or Surgiseal.

Obstruction or injury to the ureter

The ureter may be tented up and drawn into the neo-ring if the peritoneum is not adequately mobilized. This may cause significant obstruction to the ureter. Direct injury may be avoided by keeping the proximal dissection line above and lateral to the ureter and iliac vessels.

Injury to the femoral vein

This is a potentially serious complication that may occur during the process of making the neo-ring. Keep the direction of instruments/thrust from lateral to medial using a blunt probe, Endo-peanut dissector or blunt dissecting grasper to create the neo-ring.

Injury to the bladder

Inadvertent injury to the bladder is avoided by:

- keeping the bladder empty throughout the procedure,
- careful handling of the bladder wall.

Significant perforation may be closed using intracorporeal suturing and the bladder is drained for several days.

Scrotal swelling

- Infection.
- Hematoma.
- Emphysema.

These usually resolve spontaneously, although antibiotics may be required.

Testicular atrophy

This occurs if the surgery has devascularized the testis during orchidopexy.

FURTHER READING

Baker L, Docimo S, Surer I et al. A multi-institutional analysis of laparoscopic orchidopexy. *British Journal of Urology International* 2001; **87**:484–9.

Chang B, Palmer L, Franco I. Laparoscopic orchidopexy: A review of a large clinical series. *British Journal of Urology International* 2001; **87**:490–3.

Franco I. Use of HCG stimulation for the evaluation and treatment of the impalpable testis. Hormonal evaluation and treatment in cryptorchidism. In *Dialogues in Pediatric Urology* 2001; **24**(8):37.

Franco I. Evaluation and management of impalpable testis. In: Belman AB, King LR, Kramer SA (eds), *Clinical Paediatric Urology*, 4th edn. London: Martin Dunitz Ltd, 2001.

Lindgren B, Darby E, Faiella L et al. Laparoscopic orchidopexy: Procedure of choice for the non-palpable testis? *Journal of Urology* 1998; **159**:2132–5.

Lindgren BW, Franco I, Blick S et al. Laparoscopic Fowler–Stephens orchidopexy for the high abdominal testis. *Journal of Urology* 1999; **162**:990–4.

56

Varicocele

PETER NYIRÁDY AND MILÓS MERKSZ

INTRODUCTION

Varicocele, one of the most common causes of male infertility, is due to stagnant blood in the veins of the scrotum, slowed circulation and subsequent decreased oxygenation of the testis, and possibly to the increased temperature of the testis so produced. It is relatively rare under the age of 10 years, but becomes more common between the ages of 10 and 18. Although good data on semen analysis in children and adolescents do not exist, adolescent-onset varicoceles appear to adversely affect testicular growth and function. Surgical correction may prevent infertility in prepubertal boys.

Sanchez De Badajoz et al. reported the first laparoscopic varix ligation in 1988. From the early 1990s, laparoscopic surgery has become increasingly popular in the treatment of symptomatic varicoceles in children and adolescents.

Indications

- Large (Dubin and Amelar grade III) varicocele.
- Significant (>1.5 mL) difference in testicular volume as noted on clinic examination or serial ultrasound examination.
- A standard deviation decrease of 2 in testicular size when compared with normal testicular growth curves.
- Scrotal pain or discomfort – so-called 'symptomatic varicocele'.
- Bilateral varicocele (rare).

Laparoscopic varix ligation provides an effective treatment option for varicocele, and is the approach of choice in bilateral cases and for recurrence after a failed (embolization, inguinal or sub-inguinal) operation. The technique is safe and reliable and involves a brief, minimally invasive operation with little postoperative pain and short convalescence. The anatomical structures, e.g. testicular vessels and vas deferens, are easy to see and inadvertent injury to the vas deferens can be avoided.

Contraindications

ABSOLUTE

- Hemodynamically unstable patients.
- Manifest uncorrected coagulopathy.
- Abdominal sepsis.
- Retro-abdominal or intra-abdominal compression of the venous drainage of the spermatic veins, e.g. from a retroperitoneal tumor.

RELATIVE

- Previous lower abdominal surgery and/or major scarring.
- Patients with another congenital anomaly that produces infertility.
- Any malignant disease.

RELATIVE FOR RETROPERITONEAL APPROACH

- Presence of intense peri-anal fibrosis secondary to xanthogranulomatous pyelonephritis.
- Genitourinary tuberculosis.
- Recent open surgery of the retroperitoneum.

EQUIPMENT/INSTRUMENTS

Essential

- Three 3.5–10 mm cannulae (usually one 5–10 mm and two 3.5–5 mm cannulae).
- 5 mm or 10 mm 30° angled telescope.
- 3.5–5 mm curved, insulated scissors, with diathermy point.
- 3.5–5 mm atraumatic curved and insulated forceps, without ratchet.
- 5–10 mm clip applicator.

Optional

- Unipolar and/or bipolar diathermy.
- 5 mm ultrasound dissector.
- Endoscopic ultrasound probe or Doppler probe for detection of the testicular artery.
- Special retractors for gasless operation.
- Operative laparoscope (for trocar or two-trocar technique).

PREOPERATIVE PREPARATION

Prior to laparoscopic varicocele ligation, all patients are fully informed about the available treatment options. Children and their parents (as appropriate) are told about the advantages, disadvantages, risks and complications of the operation. Preoperative abdominal ultrasound should be performed where the varicocele is on the right side, or for a left-sided varicocele that does not collapse and empty when the child is placed in the supine position, as this may be indicative of a retroperitoneal mass compressing the testicular veins.

Children are fasted for 6 hours before surgery and receive pre-medication of 0.3–0.5 mg/kg oral midazolam 60 minutes prior to the induction of anesthesia. Standard monitoring devices are attached in the operating theater.

TECHNIQUE

Transperitoneal

The procedure is performed under general anesthesia with complete muscle relaxation. Urinary catheterization is not required, but the child should be encouraged to empty the bladder before surgery. No preoperative preparation or antibiotics are required.

The patient is positioned supine. All bony prominences are padded and the extremities placed in a neutral position to minimize any postoperative neuromuscular consequences. The abdomen and genitalia are prepared and included in the operative field (access to the scrotum may be necessary). The surgeon stands on the right side of the patient. The assistant, who is responsible for controlling the camera, and the scrub nurse stand on the left side of the patient.

A small skin incision is made inferior to the umbilicus. A Veress needle is inserted to create a pneumoperitoneum and an automatic insufflator maintains an intraperitoneal pressure to a maximum of 12 mmHg. The primary trocar is introduced through the incision and the 30° laparoscope is inserted.

First the abdominal cavity is inspected in order to exclude any inadvertent intra-abdominal injury secondary to the needle and trocar insertion. Two working trocars are inserted under laparoscopic guidance, one on the right and one on the left side, midway between the umbilicus and anterior superior iliac spine. The patient may be rotated slightly (elevate ipsilateral side and slight Trendelenburg) to improve visualization. Bowel obscuring the internal ring can be swept aside using atraumatic forceps. The spermatic (testicular) vessels and vas deferens are easily identified as they enter the internal ring. **(See Figure 56.1)**

The peritoneum overlying the vessels is incised transversely from medial to lateral, 2–3 cm above the internal ring. Care is taken to avoid damage to the testicular vessels.

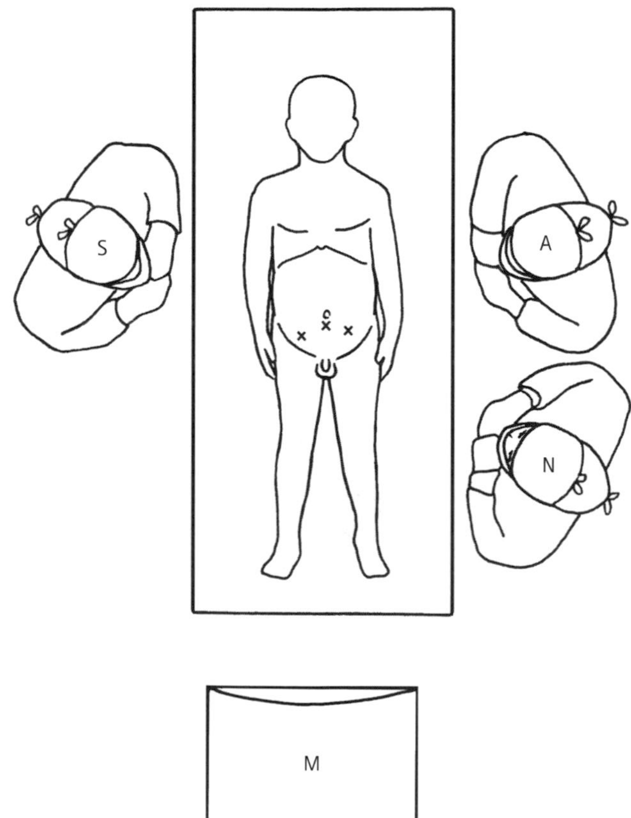

Figure 56.1

The testicular veins (usually one to three) are freed from the adjacent artery, lymphatic vessels and other tissues, and one or two clips are applied to the veins individually. The artery can be difficult to identify, and bleeding from minute vessels around the main veins can be a nuisance. All visible collateral veins are then secured using diathermy and ultrasound coagulation. **(See Figure 56.2)**

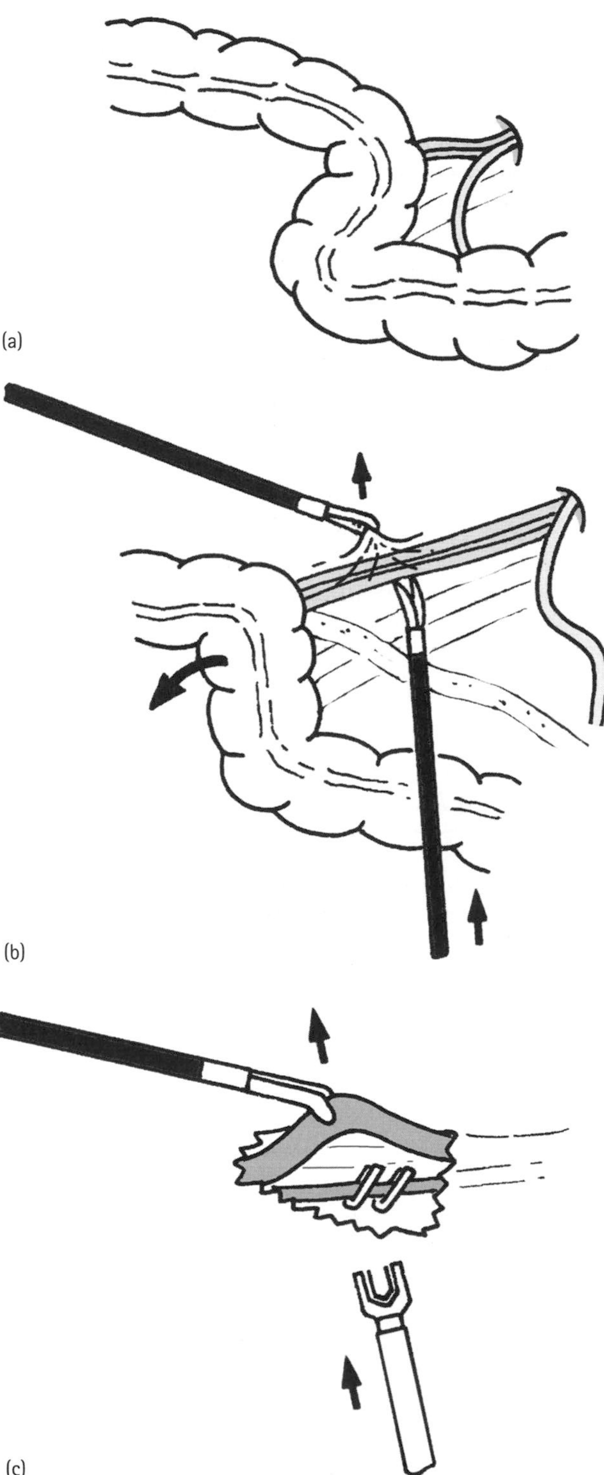

Figure 56.2

Many surgeons deliberately clip all the vessels (artery and veins) as in the first stage of a Fowler – Stephens operation (Palomo technique).

The intra-abdominal pressure is lowered to 5–6 mmHg, and hemostasis and visceral integrity are ensured. The working cannulae are removed under vision and cannula sites longer than 4 mm are closed using absorbable sutures.

Retroperiteoneal

Dilated testicular veins can be ligated easily through the retroperitoneal approach, although creating an adequate retroperitoneal space may be time-consuming. Moreover, the space is more limited for manipulation than in the transperitoneal approach. The advantage of this technique is that the intraperitoneal cavity is not opened and therefore morbidity related to its opening is avoided.

The patient is secured in the standard flank position and the space between the lowermost rib and the iliac crest is maximized by use of a kidney bridge or sand bags and cushion. **(See Figure 56.3)**

The first trocar is inserted through an initial 1.5–2 cm horizontal skin incision in the lumbar (Petit's) triangle between the 12th rib and the iliac crest. The triangle is bounded by the lateral edges of the latissimus dorsi and external oblique muscles and the iliac crest. A tunnel into the retroperitoneal space is created by blunt dissection using blunt conventional forceps. This tunnel is then dilated to allow the index finger to be introduced, pushing the peritoneum forwards and creating a small retroperitoneal space. A purpose-made trocar-mounted balloon is inserted into the retroperitoneal space and inflated with approximately 500–800 mL air. Alternatively, the finger of a surgical glove and a catheter may be used (see Chapters 54, 58 and 62B). Once the retroperitoneal space has been created, the balloon is removed and a normal cannula introduced as the first port. This cannula is fixed in position using a mattress/purse-string suture to prevent air leak. Carbon dioxide pneumo-retroperitoneum is established at 8–12 mmHg. A 30° laparoscope is inserted and two secondary ports are placed anteriorly in the anterior axillary line, taking care to avoid

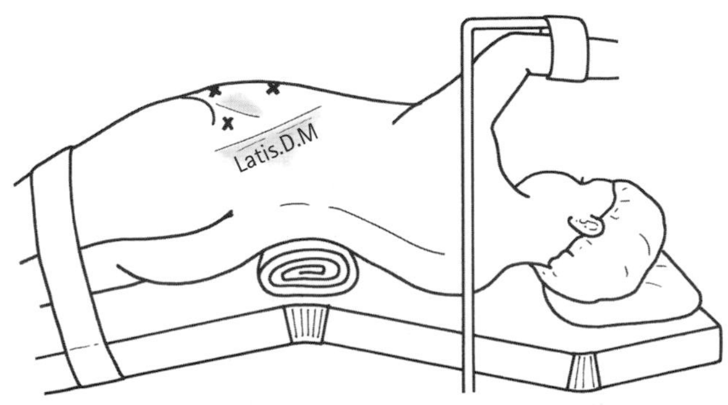

Figure 56.3

peritoneal, pleural, visceral or vascular injuries. The testicular veins are identified, dissected and secured as for the transperitoneal approach.

POSTOPERATIVE CARE

Usually oral analgesia provides sufficient pain relief, which may be necessary during the first 24 hours postoperatively. The patient is normally fit for discharge on the day of surgery.

The outcome and late complications of surgery can be determined by physical examination at 6 months postoperatively.

PROBLEMS, PITFALLS AND SOLUTIONS

Insertion of the first cannula

In difficult cases, consider open-technique laparoscopy (see Chapter 29).

Inadequate/poor view

- Dilated loops of small and/or large intestine. These are usually due to excessive intestinal insufflation at the induction of anesthesia or the use of nitrous oxide. A steep Trendelenburg position and a lateral tilt may prove helpful. An additional cannula for a retractor may be necessary.
- Intestinal adhesions and previous scarring may require adhesiolysis.
- Minor bleeding from minute vessels around the main testicular vessels can obscure laparoscopic viewing. Meticulous technique and occasionally suction and irrigation prevent and solve the problem respectively.

Identifying the artery

The artery can be difficult to see. A color Doppler endoscopic probe (artery = red, vein = blue) may help towards identifying the artery. Some surgeons routinely ligate the artery. The natural history of the latter maneuver is uncertain.

COMPLICATIONS

- Major bleeding from torn testicular vessels is very rare. The importance of careful technique cannot be overemphasized. In difficult cases, consider ligation of the entire vascular bundle (artery and vein).
- Testicular atrophy may occur with ligation of the testicular artery and vein. The incidence rate is uncertain. Some believe it is a theoretical risk, while others quote less than 1 percent.
- Phlebitis – settles spontaneously.
- A hydrocele can develop secondary to lymphatic occlusion.
- Persistent or significant recurrence of the varicocele: secondary intervention is required.
- There is a risk of injury to the vas deferens or vas-associated vessels if the collaterals around the vas deferens are disconnected.
- There is a (exceedingly rare) risk of injury to the iliac vessels, ureter and intestine.

FURTHER READING

Humphery G, Najmaldin A. Laparoscopy in the management of paediatric varicocele. *Journal of Pediatric Surgery* 1997; 32:1470–720.

57

Insertion of peritoneal dialysis catheter

AZAD NAJMALDIN

INTRODUCTION

Peritoneal dialysis is an established and effective method of treating children with renal failure and necessitates placement of a long-term, purpose-made catheter with or without omentumectomy.

Indications

- End-stage renal failure.
- When hemodialysis is not possible or contraindicated, e.g. lack of vascular access.
- When continuous ambulatory dialysis is preferred over hemodialysis, e.g. children, cost.

The conventional technique of placement of long-term peritoneal dialysis catheters requires open laparotomy. This method has the disadvantages of open surgery and the potential problems of catheter displacement, leakage and infection. The minimally invasive technique of the percutaneous insertion of catheters has a high incidence of complications, namely visceral injury, infection, catheter displacement and one-way obstruction by omentum.

Laparoscopy allows for:

- accurate and reliable positioning of a long-term catheter,
- omentumectomy if thought necessary,
- a reduced incidence of the complications of open surgery and a percutaneous procedure,
- the salvaging of existing catheters,
- assessment of the peritoneal cavity (adhesions, pre-existing infection) and intestine (colon and small bowel in hemolytic uremic syndrome).

The limitations of the laparoscopic techniques are essentially related to the experience of the surgeon, whether the patient is fit for general anesthesia and surgery, and tolerance to the creation of a low-flow, low-pressure pneumoperitoneum.

EQUIPMENT/INSTRUMENTS

Insertion of catheter alone and laparoscopic-assisted insertion of catheter and omentumectomy

- Appropriate catheter with Seldinger needle/guide-wire dilator and peel-away sheath. A 16 Fr sheath is required for a standard-size catheter.
- Minor open surgery set of instruments.
- 3.5–5 mm cannula.
- 3.5–5 mm, preferably 30/45° telescope.

Insertion of catheter and omentumectomy

ESSENTIAL

In addition to the above-mentioned instruments:

- two additional 3.5–5 mm working cannulae,
- 3.5–5 mm atraumatic grasping forceps,
- 3.5–5 mm diathermy hook or bipolar forceps,
- 3.5–5 mm curved dissecting scissors with diathermy point.

OPTIONAL

- An extra set of 3.5–5 mm atraumatic grasping forceps.
- Ultrasound shears for omentumectomy (or LigaSure™ or plasma kinetic coagulation device).
- 5 mm clip applicator and appropriate clips (or suture materials).

PREOPERATIVE PREPARATION

As for other methods of insertion of catheters, the appropriate selection of patients, preoperative measurement of electrolytes and acid–base balance, and liaison with nephrologists and the dialysis team are important preoperative measures. A thorough preoperative history, examination and abdominal ultrasound scan help towards the localization of intraperitoneal scarring. The nature and site of the catheter, the possibility of conversion to open surgery and the complications of surgery are discussed below.

TECHNIQUE

An ideally positioned catheter has the following characteristics.

- Its curled end sits in a dependent part of the abdominal cavity such as the pelvis.
- Its course through the extraperitoneal space and rectus sheath is long and oblique, 2 cm to the left of the midline.
- Its cuff sits just outside the rectus sheath *under the subcutaneous fat*. The level of the cuff depends on the size of the patient and of the catheter.
- Its outer section runs through a long and curved tunnel under the subcutaneous fat.
- Its exit through the skin is a tight fit and situated at or above the umbilical level near the anterior axillary line.

The oblique course within the rectus muscle and preperitoneal space has two important advantages:

- it minimizes the risk of dialysate leakage,
- it maintains the position and direction of the catheter in the lower abdomen and pelvis.

A long and curved subcutaneous tunnel minimizes the risks of:

- catheter displacement,
- migration of micro-organisms along the catheter and peritonitis.

Factors that affect the final position of catheter include:

- pre-existing abdominal scarring,
- the position of pre-existing stomas such as gastrostomy, vesicostomy and colostomy,

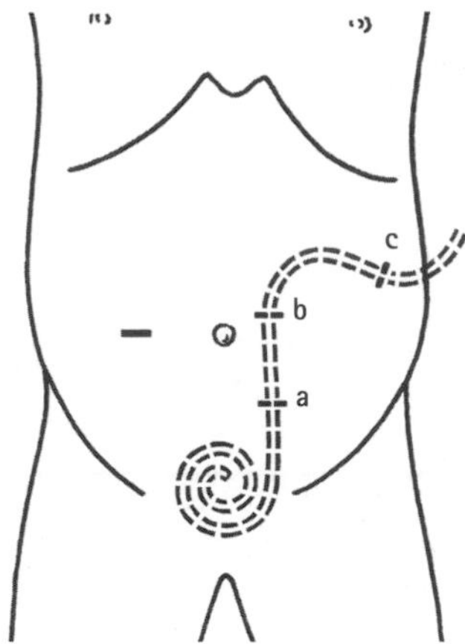

Figure 57.1

- the potential need for future surgery, e.g. renal transplantation, insertion of gastrostomy for feeding purposes etc.

The patient is positioned supine and the surgeon stands on the right side with the assistant opposite. Before starting the procedure, the length of catheter is checked against the size of the patient, and its position within the abdominal wall, including the sites of entry at both the peritoneum (a) and the anterior rectus sheath (b) as well as the exit site (c), are marked using a marker pen. To minimize the risks of dialysate leakage in an accurately positioned catheter, the distance between the pelvic peritoneum and reference point (a) must be a few to several centimeters longer than the fenestrated segment of the catheter, and the distance between (a) and (b) must be shorter than the distance between the fenestrated segment and the cuff of the catheter. **(See Figure 57.1)**

Laparoscopic insertion of catheter

A pneumoperitoneum is created (8–10 mmHg) through the primary cannula placed a few/several centimeters to the right of the umbilicus using an open technique. Alternatively, the exit site of the catheter (c) or a small midline incision a few/several centimeters above the umbilicus is used for the primary cannula. Depending on the size of the patient, a 1–2 cm transverse skin incision is made to the left of the umbilicus (b), the anterior rectus sheath is exposed, and a small pocket to fit the size of the cuff is created between the rectus sheath and subcutaneous fat. Care is taken to stay directly on the surface of the sheath and not to burrow through fat. A small cut to fit the size of the catheter is made through the anterior rectus sheath. Through this fascial incision, a needle is passed obliquely through the rectus muscle and extraperitoneally and then through the peritoneum (a) under direct vision, such that the needle is aimed down towards the pelvis 1–2 cm to the left of the midline. A suitable guide-wire, dilator and peel-away sheath

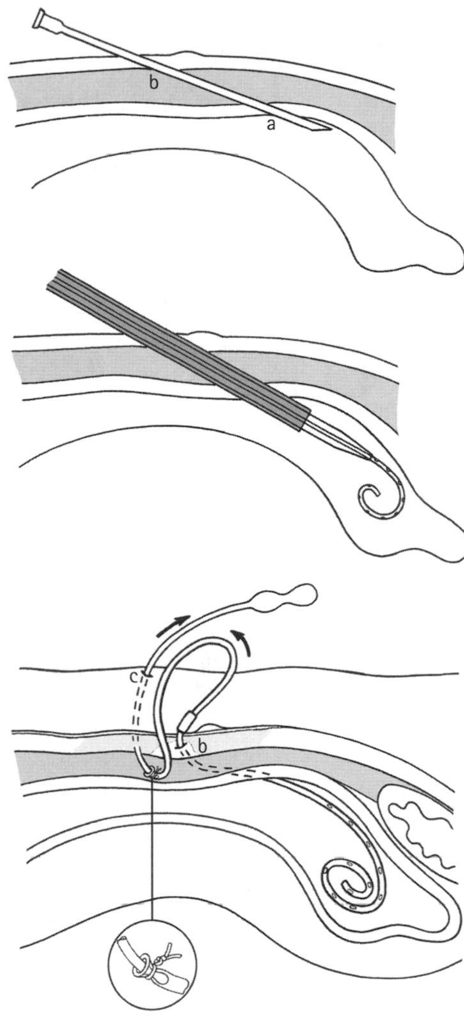

Figure 57.2

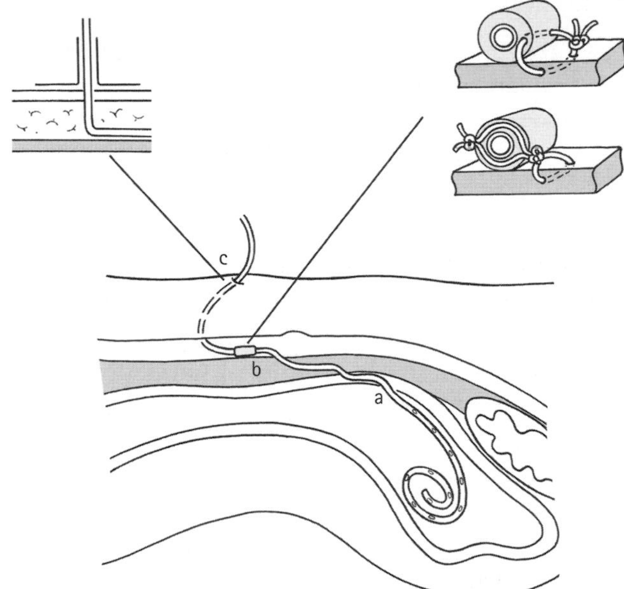

Figure 57.3

are passed under direct vision (Seldinger technique). The dialysis catheter is then passed through the sheath and the curled end positioned in the coronal plane facing the right pelvic wall. The splitable peel-away is removed, and the catheter is tunneled subcutaneously to its exit site (c) using an appropriate tunneler or a pair of conventional grasping forceps. Care is taken not to enlarge the exit incision beyond the diameter of the catheter or burrow into the subcutaneous fat or abdominal wall muscles. **(See Figure 57.2)**

To minimize the risk of catheter displacement, the cuff is fixed using an absorbable suture – 04/05 polydioxanone surgical (PDS) suture – and care is taken not to puncture the catheter. Local anesthetic agents may be infiltrated into the wound without injuring the catheter, the pneumoperitoneum is evacuated, the primary cannula is removed and the site is closed in layers meticulously (watertight). The skin incisions are closed in the usual fashion and the outer part of the catheter is fixed using a sandwich sticky dressing. The catheter may be connected to dialysate or locked with heparinized saline for later use. **(See Figure 57.3)**

PROBLEMS, PITFALLS AND SOLUTIONS

Loss of a pneumoperitoneum

This may happen through the needle, peel-away sheath or catheter. Keep a finger on the needle/peel-away sheath while preparing the catheter, and clamp the outer end of the catheter throughout the procedure using an atraumatic soft plastic clamp.

Disparity between the sizes of the catheter and patient

Use a non-touch technique and measure the suitability of the catheter to the given patient and mark the reference points (a, b and c) described earlier, which may vary depending on the size of the patient. Compared with older patients, infants require high insertion points.

Difficulty creating long/oblique tunnel

Under direct vision (through the skin incision), place the needle through the anterior rectus sheath (small nick), advance along the inner surface of the anterior sheath for a few centimeters, then dip gradually through the muscle 1–2 cm parallel to the midline towards the center of the pelvis. Through the laparoscope, the peritoneum is now seen tenting (not breached) inwards in front of the needle. Withdraw the needle by 1–2 cm, then advance extraperitoneally for a few centimeters before cutting through the peritoneum. **(See Figure 57.4)**

Difficulty passing the peel-away sheath

The delicate nature of the peel-away sheath allows indentation of the material at points of resistance such as the rectus sheath and peritoneum. Use continuous progressive pressure with gentle rotational movements.

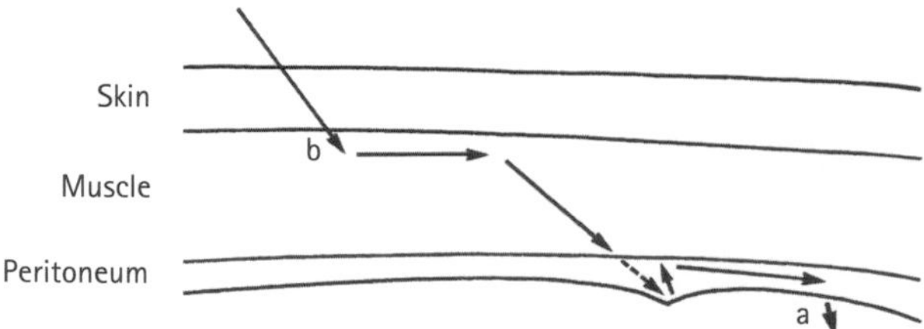

Figure 57.4

Tendency to burrow through fat during subcutaneous tunneling

Blunt instruments should be used to create a small space directly on the surface of the rectus sheath at both skin incisions and to tunnel between the two sites under the fat.

Insertion of catheter and omentumectomy

Three cannulae are placed on the right side of the abdomen, with the middle one being used for insufflation and the telescope, as previously described. Total omentumectomy is not necessary (the part that reaches the fenestrated curled end of the catheter is usually removed). Although monopolar and bipolar diathermy and scissors with or without Ligaclips or sutures are often used to divide the omentum, an ultrasound shear is by far the best tool for an effective, safe, fast and easy omentumectomy. The right edge of the omentum is grasped using an atraumatic grasper through the upper cannula and divided, usually a few to several centimeters away from the transverse colon (depending on the size of the patient), using an ultrasound shear through the lower (5 mm) cannula. Care is taken not to get too close to the colon. The omentum is then placed in a visible corner, usually the surface of the liver, for extraction at the end of the procedure. **(See Figure 57.5)**

Insertion of the catheter is now performed in a manner identical to that described earlier in this chapter. Once the catheter is secured, one of the cannula sites, usually the primary (the telescope is moved to one of the working cannulae), is enlarged slightly and the omentum is extracted. A retrieval bag is usually not necessarily and, to prevent dialysate leakage, all the cannula sites are closed, preferably in layers (watertight).

PROBLEMS, PITFALLS AND SOLUTIONS

In addition to those described above for insertion of the catheter, the following may occur.

Omentumectomy using diathermy

Fatty omentum in obese and older children can be difficult to divide using coagulation diathermy. A combination of monopolar and bipolar diathermy or diathermy with suture ligatures or clips may be tried. Alternatively, the deeper thin layer of omentum close to the transverse colon is divided first. Here, care must be taken not to cause diathermy injury to the colon.

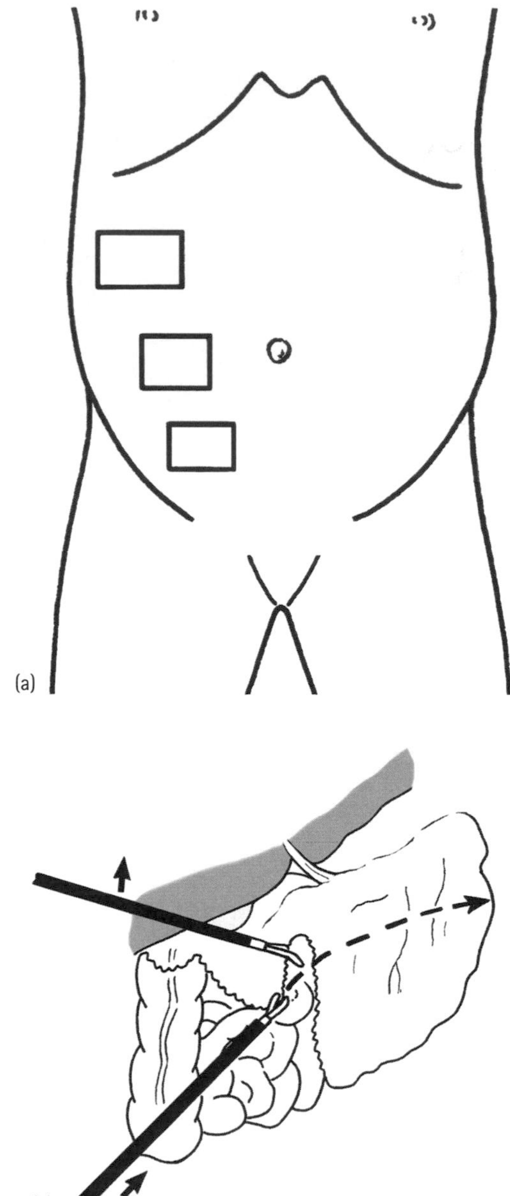

Figure 57.5

Minor bleeding from large omental vessels may be controlled using bipolar diathermy, suture ligature or clips.

Laparoscopic-assisted insertion of catheter and omentumectomy

This technique combines the speed and simplicity of extracorporeal omentumectomy with the accuracy and minimally invasive nature of laparoscopy for insertion of the catheter.

A single 2–4 cm long (depending on the thickness of the abdominal wall) supra-umbilical vertical or transverse incision is usually sufficient to complete the entire procedure. Sometimes an upper umbilical crease incision provides

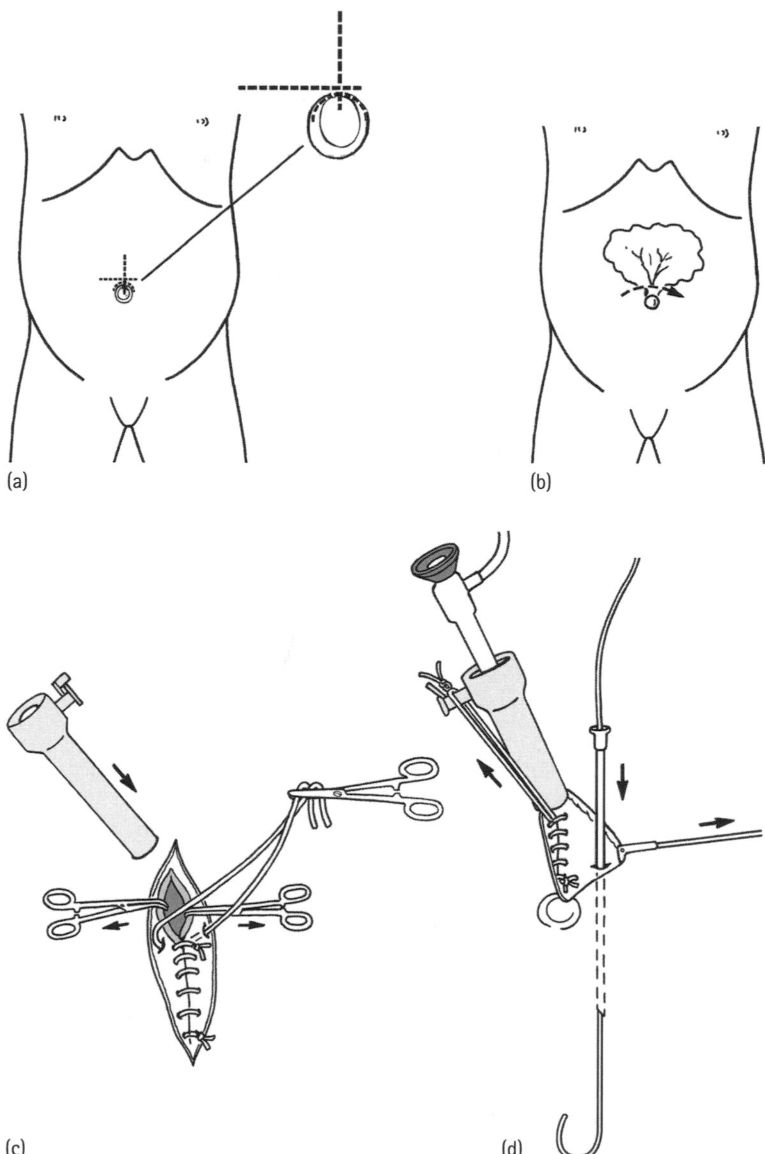

Figure 57.6

adequate exposure. Alternatively, two small skin incisions are utilized, one (2 cm) above the umbilicus for omentumectomy and the telescope cannula, and the other (1 cm) to the left of the umbilicus for insertion of the catheter.

Initial omentumectomy is performed extracorporeally after delivering the omentum through the supra-umbilical incision using conventional instruments, suture ligature and bipolar diathermy. This incision is then closed partially (from left to right in transverse incision, below cephalad in vertical incision) using continuous strong absorbable sutures before it is used for the primary cannula. The cannula is secured in position using either a purse-string or simple suture as described previously (basic technique, open method laparoscopy). **(See Figure 57.6)**

A pneumoperitoneum is created and a laparoscope is placed. The left lateral edge of the skin incision is retracted to the left, the rectus sheath is exposed and a small pocket is created subcutaneously for the catheter cuff. The insertion of the catheter is now performed in a manner identical to that described earlier in this chapter. Once the catheter is secured, the cannula is removed and the remaining deep part of the wound is closed meticulously (watertight). The skin is closed and the catheter is fixed and prepared in the usual fashion.

PROBLEMS, PITFALLS AND SOLUTIONS

The following may occur in addition to those described earlier in this chapter.

Difficulty with external omentumectomy

Total omentumectomy is not necessary. Therefore, avoid delivering the colon out through the small incision, which can become edematous and difficult to replace.

Difficult placement of the catheter

During the laparoscopy phase of the procedure, there is a tendency to pull the wound to the right, which makes retraction of the skin edge on the left difficult for insertion of the needle/guide-wire and catheter. Consider enlarging the skin incision or use a separate small incision for the catheter as described previously.

Difficult view

- Placing the laparoscope to the right of the falciform ligament and above the line of catheter insertion may cause difficulty with viewing and insertion of the catheter. A vertical (rather than transverse) supra-umbilical incision and an angled telescope may prove helpful.
- Placing the laparoscope close to the site of catheter insertion may cause difficulty with viewing. This problem is less likely with the transverse incision.

POSTOPERATIVE CARE

Adequate postoperative analgesia is usually provided by local infiltration of the wounds with anesthetic agents. Intravenous morphine infusion is rarely required and limited to the first 6–12 hours postoperatively. The line is usable immediately and care of the catheter and dialysis are as for conventional techniques.

COMPLICATIONS

Leakage of dialysate

The healing process and scar formation are slow in children who suffer chronic renal failure. In difficult cases and if possible, consider using small-volume dialysate in the first few postoperative days. The incidence is extremely low if:

- the operative details are followed carefully,
- the number and size of the skin and fascial incisions are kept to a minimum,
- the Seldinger technique and appropriate peel-away sheath are used,
- a long tunnel is created within the rectus sheath and extraperitoneally,
- a long and preferably curved subcutaneous tunnel is created,
- all muscle and fascial incisions are closed meticulously in layers (watertight),
- catheter movement is minimized (see below),
- catheter perforation during suturing and injection of local anesthetic agents is avoided.

Catheter blockage

In unscarred abdomen, the incidence of catheter blockage following laparoscopic and laparoscopic-assisted omentumectomy and insertion of the catheter is almost none. Without omentumectomy, however, the incidence rates increase (non-specific complications).

Infection/peritonitis

The incidence of technique-related catheter infection and peritonitis is low provided:

- a meticulous non-touch technique is followed,
- a long tunnel is created,
- dialysate leakage and catheter movement are prevented,
- the exit site is a tight fit around the catheter and appropriate wound care is applied.

Catheter displacement

The following minimize the risk of catheter displacement:

- Seldinger technique for insertion,
- an appropriate tunneler is used to create the subcutaneous passage,
- a long, curved tunnel is created within the abdominal wall,
- leakage and infection are avoided,
- the exit site is small and the catheter is fixed to the abdominal wall using an adhesive dressing,
- the cuff is fixed on to the surface of the rectus sheath using PDS sutures.

58

Nephrectomy and nephro-ureterectomy: transperitoneal and retroperitoneal

CRAIG A. PETERS

INTRODUCTION

Nephrectomy is usually indicated in conditions with nearly complete absence of renal function with no ureteral pathology, while nephro-ureterectomy in the pediatric patient is usually necessary for conditions leading to non-function of the renal unit and associated with complete ureteral dysfunction. In almost all situations, nephrectomy or nephro-ureterectomy is performed to prevent infection due to urinary stasis or to limit the risk of hypertension resulting from renal damage due to the associated condition. Whereas malignancies are a clear indication for nephrectomy, it is rare to need a nephro-ureterectomy, and the latter procedure has not been conducted laparoscopically in any relevant numbers to date. Pre-transplantation nephrectomy or nephro-ureterectomy is indicated for a variety of reasons, including infection, hypertension and large patient size. The most frequent indications for nephrectomy and nephro-ureterectomy are vesico-ureteral reflux with non-function of the renal unit, and obstruction of the nephro-ureteral unit. The latter is usually due to severe uretero-pelvic junction obstruction or primary mega-ureter, but may also be due to an obstructing ectopic ureter or ureterocele. Other possible causes include severe, unreconstructable ureteral strictures and poor renal function, or any cause of renal functional loss associated with ureteral obstruction distal to the mid-ureter. **(See Table 58.1)**

Selection criteria and the pathophysiology of these various conditions are detailed elsewhere, but in general there is little benefit to reconstructing a renal unit with less than 10 percent of total function on a differential renal scan. There are no data to indicate the 'correct' cut-off, below which nephrectomy should be performed, but it should be recognized that in most cases associated with a congenital condition, function less than 10–15 percent will seldom increase despite successful surgery. The actual threshold used varies widely and is largely a matter of individual preference. The complete absence of function on a renal scan is a good indication that it is reasonable to remove the affected unit. If it is more practical simply to achieve urinary drainage or absence of reflux, removal is not considered essential. The long-term risks of leaving a poorly functioning renal unit remain incompletely defined and for this reason some practitioners elect to remove the

Table 58.1 *Indications for nephrectomy and nephro-ureterectomy*

Nephro-ureterectomy	Nephrectomy
Vesico-ureteral reflux	Uretero-pelvic junction obstruction
Uretero-vesical junction obstruction	Multicystic dysplasia
Ectopic ureter (single system)	Pre-transplantation nephrectomy
Reflux and obstruction associated with posterior urethral valves, neurogenic bladder	

affected renal unit. Alternatively, some base the decision on whether the affected unit has sufficient function for the patient to be able to avoid dialysis if the contralateral unit were lost. This may be excessively stringent, in that it is generally felt that 30 percent function is required to avoid dialysis, but most surgeons would probably preserve a kidney with much less function. Perhaps optimistically, our practice has been to use a relative functional contribution of 10 percent of total uptake as the cut-off for renal salvage versus removal. It must be recognized that this is an arbitrary distinction that is not based on any outcome data.

Contraindications

There are no absolute contraindications to laparoscopic nephrectomy that do not also apply to the conventional procedure, such as profound sepsis, coagulopathy or a severely compromising medical condition. Many of these can be stabilized with temporary tube drainage or medical interventions that would permit later definitive surgical correction.

RELATIVE

- Multiple prior renal surgeries.
- Uncontrolled infection or undrained abscess.
- Uncontrolled coagulopathy.

The choice of performing the nephrectomy or nephro-ureterectomy using transperitoneal versus retroperitoneal approaches has also evolved in recent years. Our approach is to perform nephrectomy or nephro-ureterectomy retroperitoneally unless there are specific reasons to perform it transperitoneally. If a contralateral open surgical ureteral re-implantation is planned, this permits open removal of the distal ureteral stump and retroperitoneal nephro-ureterectomy.

Indications for transperitoneal technique

- Need for total ureterectomy (e.g. reflux, ectopic ureter with reflux).
- Concomitant intraperitoneal procedure (e.g. orchidopexy).
- Massive hydronephrosis.
- Prior retroperitoneal surgery (relative).

EQUIPMENT/INSTRUMENTS

- 5 mm port (for clip applicator) with reducer for 3.5 mm instruments.
- Two 3.5 mm ports.

We use 3.5 mm instruments as a reasonable compromise to minimize the size of the working ports and the efficiency of larger instruments. This size is adequate for small children up to about the age of 10 years. For older children, we tend to use all 5 mm instruments. If one uses a 3.5 mm endoscope, it may be placed into any of the ports during the procedure. If a larger scope is used, it is confined to one port, or all ports must be the larger ones.

Essential

- 3.5 mm endoscope (permits flexible positioning of endoscope during surgery).
- Scissors, 3.5 mm with cautery.
- Delicate curved grasping and dissecting instrument.
- Large grasping instrument for retraction.
- Clip applicator (5 mm). (NB Two kept in room at all times.)
- Irrigating aspirating device.
- Locking toothed grasper for specimen removal.

Optional

- Harmonic Scalpel® (5 mm) for partial nephrectomy.
- Hook cautery.

PREOPERATIVE PREPARATION

In most cases the decision to perform a nephrectomy or nephro-ureterectomy is made on the basis of a thorough evaluation; however, occasionally it is clear that renal removal is necessary, yet the functional status of the urinary tract has not been defined. The particular issues that should be addressed include the status of the contralateral kidney, the presence or absence of reflux, and the location of the affected, poorly functioning kidney. These are usually evident as long as a functional test such as an intravenous pyelogram (IVP) or dimethyl succinic acid (DMSA) scan has been performed, as well as a cystogram and, when appropriate, an ultrasound to document the presence and location of the kidney. On occasion, the kidney is so small as to make imaging difficult and some corroborative evidence that it is present should be sought. With this information, subsequent surgical decisions can be made with confidence.

Preoperative preparation also includes the following.

- Low-residue diet for 24 hours.
- Rectal suppository to unload the colon.
- Blood group and save.
- Counseling regarding the potential need for conversion to open surgery.

RETROPERITONEAL NEPHRO-URETERECTOMY

Positioning

For retroperitoneal renal access, two basic approaches are used – lateral and prone. Each has its advantages and disadvantages. The prone approach is favored by this author for all nephrectomies, but is less useful for nephro-ureterectomy when the entire ureter must be removed. Leaving a small stump is usual with the prone approach, but in general this is not of any consequence, unless there is an impairment of ureteral drainage, as in refluxing ectopic ureters. In such a case, the lateral retroperitoneal approach or a transperitoneal technique would be recommended as it permits complete ureteral resection.

The prone approach is performed in the true prone position and the first port is at the costo-vertebral angle. Secondary ports are placed above the iliac crest lateral to the sacrospinalis muscle and at the posterior axillary line. The approach permits direct access to the renal hilum without the need to retract the kidney, and has less chance of causing peritoneal injury. About two-thirds of the ureter may be removed easily from this access. **(See Figure 58.1)**

The lateral retroperitoneal approach provides more complete access to the distal ureter, if needed. It is limited by the need to retract the kidney for hilar exposure, as the kidney tends to fall down on the hilum as the dissection is undertaken. Therefore special consideration must be given to reducing exposure problems. This approach requires careful mobilization of the peritoneum from the abdominal wall and is more often associated with perforation of the peritoneum. **(See Figure 58.2)**

Whichever position is used, care is taken to provide adequate padding and support. If the operating table is to be moved during the procedure, this movement should be tested before the patient is draped to make sure that new pressure points are not produced. A bladder catheter is placed in all cases.

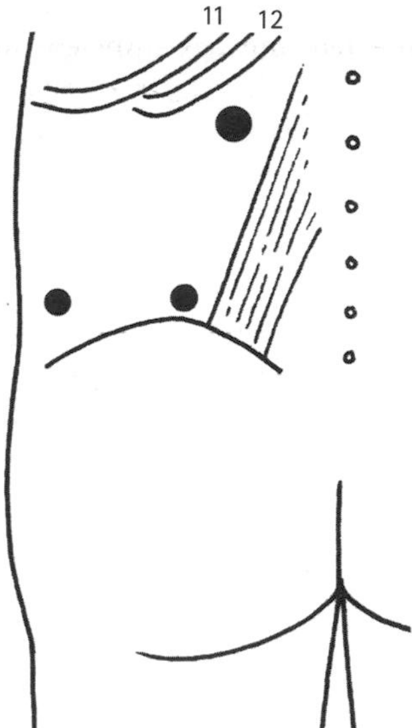

Figure 58.1

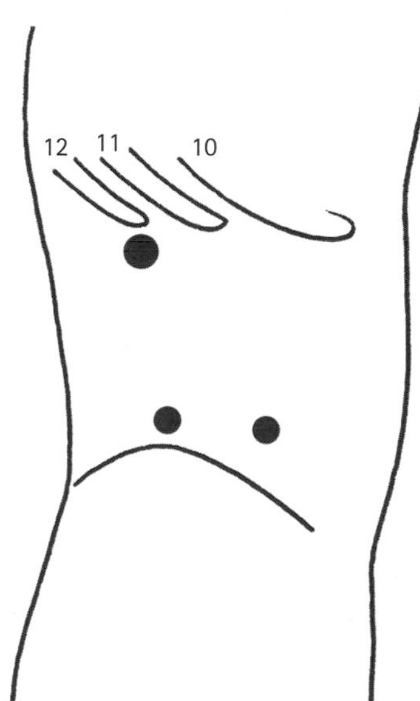

Figure 58.2

Prone retroperitoneal approach

- Simple nephrectomy.
- Partial nephrectomy with subtotal ureterectomy.

Lateral retroperitoneal approach

- Need for near-total ureterectomy (e.g. reflux with large ureter).
- Unusual renal anatomy or position.
- Obese patient.

Attention must be paid to avoiding placing the ports too close together, which will restrict movement, particularly if ports with larger heads are in use. Placing the port too far from the retroperitoneal working area runs the risk of injury to the peritoneum. Secondary ports are placed under direct vision.

Establishing the operative space in the retroperitoneum

Establishment of the working space may be the most critical step of the procedure as it provides the exposure and orientation for the nephrectomy. The initial incision is at the costo-vertebral angle, about 1 cm in length. Blunt dissection through the muscle layers, with sequential spreading at right angles, will expose Gerota's fascia. Entry through

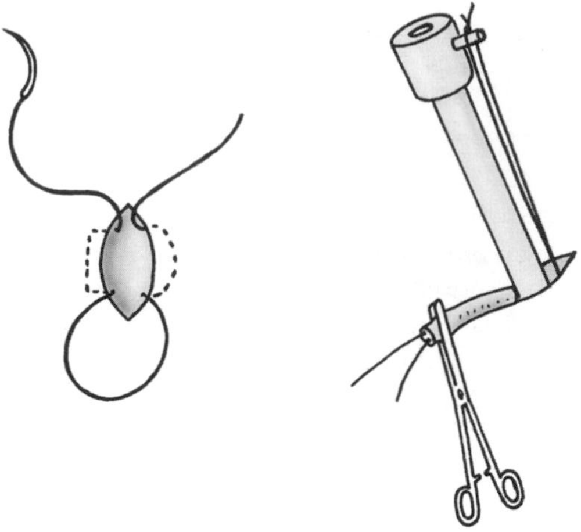

Figure 58.3

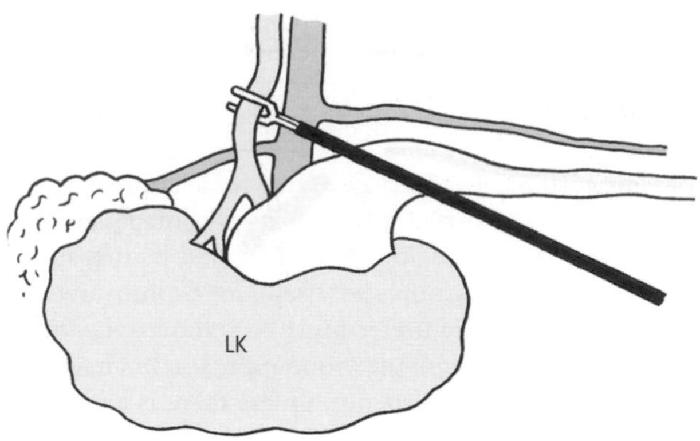

Figure 58.4 *Posterior aspect of the left kidney.*

this is indicated by a protrusion of brownish peri-renal fat. The dissecting balloon (made of the finger of a surgical glove tied over a 10 Fr catheter with two 2-0 silk sutures and lubricated) is inserted into Gerota's space and inflated with warm saline – 90 mL for infants, 150 mL for children and up to 200 mL for adolescents. The balloon is left inflated for 5 minutes, then deflated and removed, with immediate replacement by the first cannula and the endoscope.

The position in the retroperitoneum is confirmed and the kidney is identified, if possible. Blunt development of the edges of the space may be done with the endoscope, with care being taken to avoid tearing the peritoneum. The peritoneum may be identified as a white-grey demarcation line on the abdominal wall. The second port may be placed in the medial position to facilitate development of the working space further. When the position of the port and identification of the retroperitoneal working space are assured, the initial cannula is fixed in position with the pre-placed fascial suture.

The medial port is placed at the edge of the paraspinus muscles and just above the iliac crest. It may not be directly visible, but the path may be anticipated and watched. The lateral port is placed just below the tip of the 12th rib and above the iliac crest. This port has the greatest risk of entry into the peritoneum. Pre-placed fascial sutures are used in all ports to facilitate closure. **(See Figure 58.3)**

Renal exposure/control of the hilum

Renal exposure is begun with blunt dissection of the posterior surface of the kidney, with early identification of the lower pole of the kidney, if possible. When using the lateral retroperitoneal approach to the kidney, the anterior attachments are left to maintain the kidney in position. From the lower pole, the hilum is identified by superior dissection and searching for the renal artery.

From the posterior approach, the artery is seen before the vein, and is taken first. It is best to mobilize the artery medially to permit isolation of the main renal artery rather than any branches. There is a tendency to isolate the posterior branches as they are seen first, but ligation of these will leave the anterior branches to be controlled separately. To control the artery, blunt dissection of about 1 cm is needed, recognizing that the vein is just below it, and care must be taken to avoid injury. A 5 mm clip applicator is used and passed through the superior port while the camera is placed into one of the working ports. Two clips are placed on the proximal side of the artery. With ligation of the artery, the vein is usually seen just superiorly and can be isolated and controlled in a similar fashion. **(See Figure 58.4)**

Care is taken to avoid injury to the adrenal vein on the left. On the right, the vein is short, but can usually be readily isolated and controlled. It is important to recognize that what appears to be renal vein may be the cava on the right side. The exposure provided with a retroperitoneal approach is such that the cava may appear to have a transverse orientation, especially if the camera has been rotated slightly, and is of small caliber as a result of the insufflation pressure. A double-check scheme is advised for all vessel ligations. It is also important to be aware that not all vessels may have been controlled with the initial hilar dissection and, with further mobilization, these smaller vessels should be searched for.

Occasionally, it is difficult to expose the hilum, due either to fibrosis or to the angle of exposure. In these cases, the ureter is identified adjacent to the lower pole of the kidney and mobilized. It is transected at this point and used as a handle to mobilize the kidney and thereby expose the hilum. Gentle traction will provide assistance in the continued dissection of the kidney. **(See Figure 58.5)**

Mobilizing the kidney

Once the hilum has been controlled, the rest of the kidney is then mobilized from inferior to superior and usually from lateral to medial. Most of this is done bluntly, but

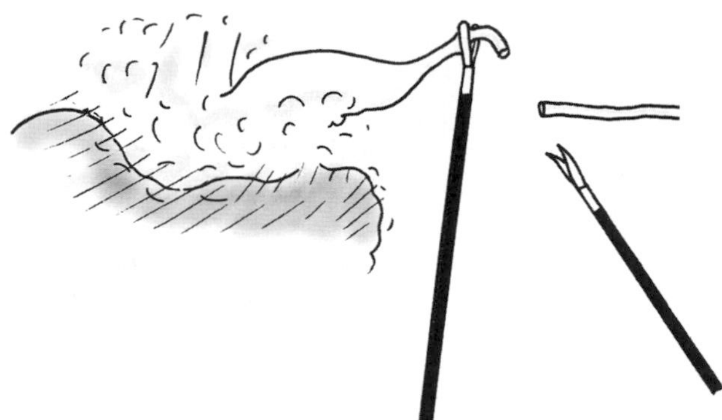

Figure 58.5 *Posterior aspect of the left kidney; retroperitoneal approach.*

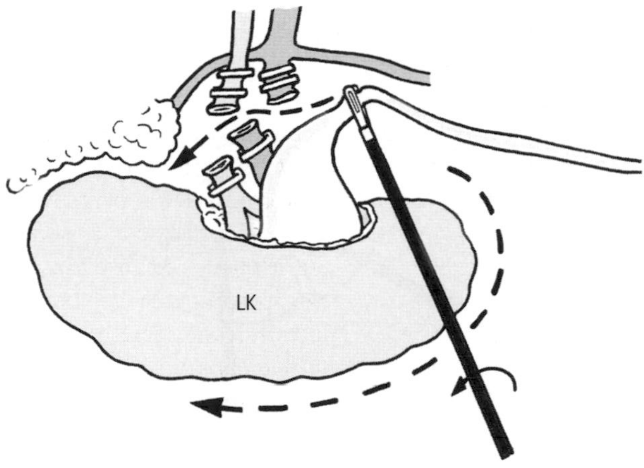

Figure 58.6

there are small vessels to be controlled superiorly. The occasional hilar vessel that was not initially controlled should be watched for. The ureter is used for traction, as it is often difficult to grasp and hold the kidney itself. Large cysts are left intact to facilitate blunt dissection; however, a decompressed cyst allows better direct traction on the wall during dissection. (**See Figure 58.6**)

Mobilization of the upper pole comes last and is not usually difficult, but it is important to be aware of the location of the adrenal gland and its vessels. Dissection should be close to the renal capsule without violating it, if possible, as this will induce bleeding.

Ureteral dissection (for nephro-ureterectomy)

When the ureter needs to be removed, as in the case of a refluxing ureter, the distal stump is grasped and mobilized with sharp and blunt dissection as far as possible. All mobilization is kept close to the ureter, and the spermatic (or ovarian) vessels are looked for. It is best to pass the ureter under these vessels to facilitate mobilization. Further dissection is done as far as reasonably possible, which is usually just to the iliac vessels. The ureter is divided with cautery and left open if obstructed, but suture ligated if it is refluxing. Clips do not stay on well, and a suture should be used.

Specimen removal

Once the ureter has been transected, it is removed directly through the port containing the grasping instrument. The kidney is then removed through the largest port, usually 5 mm, using a heavy, locking, grasping instrument with teeth. The kidney should be grasped at a pole extracorporeally with a heavy Allis or Kelly clamp and the entire instrument and port brought out. In some cases the decompressed kidney is easily removed, but sometimes it must be pulled forcefully. Twisting will often help. In very large kidneys, the port site may need to be enlarged to permit removal. We have occasionally used scissor morcellation for larger organs.

TRANSPERITONEAL NEPHRECTOMY AND NEPHRO-URETERECTOMY

Positioning

Patients are placed on an elevating wedge on the operating table to raise the ipsilateral flank. The table is then laterally tilted to drop this side of it to permit intraperitoneal access in a supine position. Once ports are placed, the table is tilted in the opposite direction to put the patient in nearly a full flank position. This still allows for rapid re-positioning into the supine position to permit urgent laparotomy. The entire abdomen is prepared and draped. A bladder catheter is placed. If a ureterectomy is to be performed, a rectal tube is placed to decompress the pelvic rectum.

Port placement

For transperitoneal nephrectomy, the initial port is in the umbilicus and is placed by the open technique using a preplaced fascial suture in a box-stitch manner. Secondary ports are placed under direct vision and secured as for the retroperitoneal approach. In small children it is best to limit the amount of cannula within the abdomen, as it may limit the working area. The upper port is placed just lateral to the midline ipsilaterally and the lower port in the mid-clavicular line ipsilaterally. For nephro-ureterectomy, it is helpful to put the upper port more laterally, and the lower abdominal port should be slightly higher.

Renal exposure and control of the hilum

In the full flank position to allow the bowel to move medially, the kidney is exposed by medial reflection of the

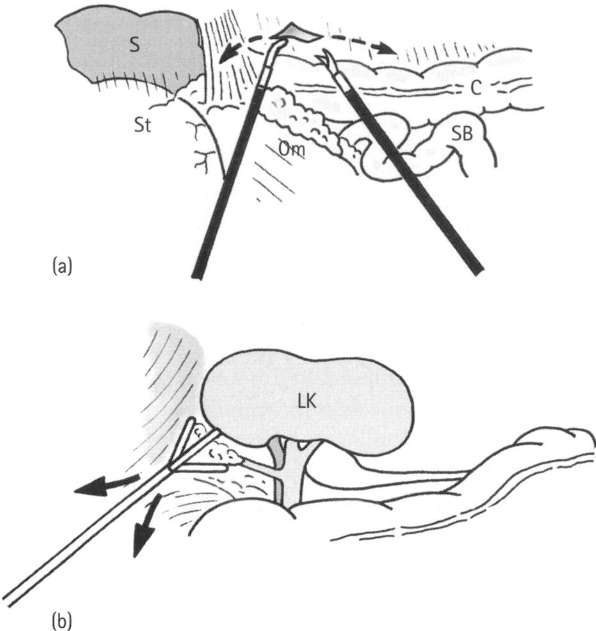

Figure 58.7 *Transperitoneal approach; left kidney.*

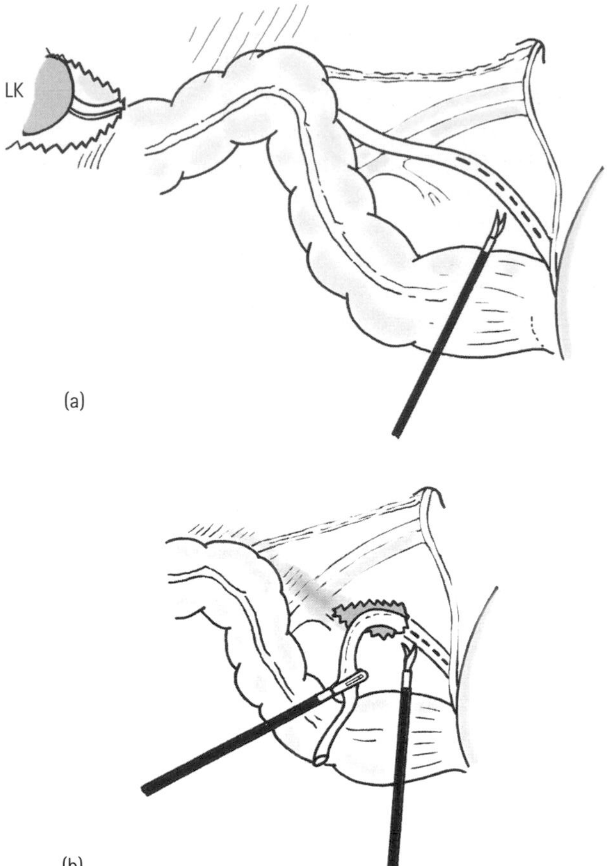

Figure 58.8

lateral edge of the colon and peritoneum. This is best carried out from the flexure of the spleen or liver to the level of the iliac vessels. A fourth port may be needed for a fan retractor to facilitate mobilizing the liver away from the kidney. The hilum is exposed first and the vessels controlled, just as in the retroperitoneal exposure. The ureter can be used for mobilization as well. (**See Figure 58.7**)

Following control of the hilum, the remainder of the kidney is mobilized, again leaving the superior and posterior aspects until last. During these dissections, it may be helpful to use the ureter for mobilization. Blunt dissection can be made more efficient using a crossing dissection, whereby the outer handles of the instruments are spread apart and the inside tips are spread in opposite directions. This enables a generous amount of movement, without the hands bumping against each other.

Ureteral dissection (for nephro-ureterectomy)

The ureter is transected below the lower pole and the ureter is dissected inferiorly with sharp and blunt dissection and cautery. Just above the level of the iliac vessels, the gonadal vessels cross over the ureter from lateral to medial, and it is necessary to pass the ureter under the vessels or sweep them laterally. Under traction, the ureter is freed of surrounding tissues to a point that will be below the vessels when the ureter is released. It is then passed under the vessels and the peritoneum inferior to the vessels is incised and the ureter brought below. It is then re-grasped for continued dissection into the deep pelvis. The iliac vessels must be protected, as well as the obturator nerve in the deep pelvis. In boys the vas deferens will be seen laterally and coursing medially over the ureter just lateral to the bladder. In the pelvis, the ureter is mobilized by incising the peritoneum over the ureter down to the level of the vas deferens and bluntly freeing the ureter of surrounding tissue. There is usually a significant vessel, feeding the distal ureter from the lateral pelvic sidewall. It should not be confused with the superior vesical artery and vein. During the dissection, the ureter is re-grasped progressively closer to the area of dissection to maximize traction and control. The ureter is taken as close to the bladder as possible. If it is a refluxing ureter, it should be suture ligated; if obstructed, it can be left open and the edges fulgurated. (**See Figure 58.8**)

Specimen removal

The kidney and ureter are removed through the umbilical port, as this can permit the widest expansion with the smallest scar, as long as any extension of the port incision is made in a circular fashion. No effort is made to suture the colon; it is simply laid back into its normal position.

Closure

Closure should be set up to be as efficient as possible. The camera port is replaced and the fascial suture tightened to permit re-insufflation. The cannulae are removed after a brief inspection of the operative field following specimen removal to ensure that there is no bleeding unmasked by the pressure release. Any irrigation can be carried out at this time. Pre-placed fascial stitches are tied securely and insufflating CO_2 is evacuated through the camera port prior to removal. Port sites are infiltrated with local anesthetic (usually bupivacaine 0.25 percent). The skin is closed with a monofilament absorbable suture and dressings are applied. A bladder catheter is left only if there is a concern regarding the bladder closure.

POSTOPERATIVE CARE

There are no special considerations postoperatively. Patients are encouraged to take fluids and begin a diet if they feel comfortable. They may ambulate on the same day and some even return home later in the day. In general, most will stay overnight and are discharged home on limited activity for 5 days with low-level analgesics. Follow-up is dependent upon the conditions for which they underwent the surgery and associated conditions. If there are no other issues, patients having had a simple nephrectomy will usually return only for a wound check 4–8 weeks postoperatively.

PROBLEMS, PITFALLS AND SOLUTIONS

Access

- In retroperitoneal techniques, perforation of the peritoneum is not uncommon and may create a pneumoperitoneum that obscures development of the retroperitoneal operative space. This can be managed by venting the peritoneum with an angiocatheter or opening it widely from the retroperitoneal position. This still provides the positioning advantages of the retroperitoneal approach, although it becomes a transperitoneal procedure. We have not seen adverse events with this maneuver.
- Dilated or cystic kidneys may be decompressed using a percutaneous needle aspiration.
- Major adhesions from previous surgery or infection may be managed with adhesiolysis. Consider conversion to an open technique.

Renal mobilization

- Mobilizing the kidney is not usually associated with high risk of injury. The position of the adrenal vessels should be borne in mind, and where the duodenum is on the right side. On the left, the tail of the pancreas may be fairly close to the medial upper pole.
- On occasion, the dissecting balloon can be placed deep to the kidney and, with inflation, the kidney is pushed up against the posterior body wall. It will be difficult to see and if it does not come into view readily, this possibility should be entertained. Withdrawal of the endoscope to visualize the posterior body wall usually reveals the kidney.
- In lateral retroperitoneal approaches, the kidney may fall medially over the hilum, making dissection difficult. For this reason the anterior and lateral attachments should not be taken down before the hilum is controlled. If the kidney falls, it may be necessary to retract with one instrument while dissecting with the other, or to place a fourth port for retraction.

COMPLICATIONS

Access

- Bowel injury.
  - Prevention: open technique.
  - Management: identify the location; if small perforation and no soilage, over-sew and irrigate.
- Abdominal wall vessel injury.
  - Prevention: perform port placement under direct vision; watch for inferior epigastric vessels.
  - Management: will usually stop while the port is in place; deep fascial stitch if persistent.

Vascular control

- Arterial injury.
  - Prevention: dissection near origin of artery to avoid branches.
  - Management: localize the source of bleeding; traction will often reduce bleeding. Clear field to permit specific ligation or cautery; avoid blind cauterization. If unable to control after 15 minutes, consider conversion to open technique.
- Venous injury.
  - Prevention: careful dissection to venous attachment to cava or over aorta; check for branches and lumbar vessels.
  - Management: may not be evident at first due to pneumoperitoneum/pneumoretroperitoneum. If concerned, reduce pressure; apply local pressure to control bleeding. Clip if possible; suture if necessary.
- Mis-identification of vessels – vena cava may appear as a large renal vein.

- Prevention: maintain camera orientation; periodically review orientation by examining wide field with kidney.
- Management: always check the origin and orientation of any large vessel to be ligated prior to slip/suture placement.

Ureteral mobilization

Complications associated with ureteral mobilization are those due to injury to the many structures adjacent to the ureter in the deep pelvis, particularly the iliac vessels, the vas deferens in boys and the uterine vessels in girls. The gonadal vessels can usually be preserved, but may cause substantial bleeding if injured. Caution should be exercised in the deep pelvis to avoid bowel injury if the rectum is not well decompressed.

FURTHER READING

Borer JG, Peters CA. Pediatric retroperitoneoscopic nephrectomy. *Journal of Endourology* 2000; **14**(5):413–16; discussion 417.

Borzi PA. A comparison of the lateral and posterior retroperitoneoscopic approach for complete and partial nephroureterectomy in children. *British Journal of Urology International* 2001; **87**(6):517–20.

El-Ghoneimi A, Valla JS, Steyaert H, Aigrain Y. Laparoscopic renal surgery via a retroperitoneal approach in children. *Journal of Urology* 1998; **160**(3 Pt 2):1138–41.

Kobashi KC, Chamberlin DA, Rajpoot D, Shanberg AM. Retroperitoneal laparoscopic nephrectomy in children. *Journal of Urology* 1998; **160**(3 Pt 2):1142–4.

59

Partial nephrectomy

PETER A. BORZI

INTRODUCTION

Minimal access partial nephrectomy is a procedure commonly performed in children for pathology related to duplex kidney and, on rare occasions, for polar pathology in a singleton system. It can be performed using a transperitoneal as well as an extraperitoneal/retroperitoneoscopic lateral or posterior approach. It is performed as an isolated excision or involving a partial or complete ureterectomy and, on occasions, involving also ureterocelectomy with lower moiety ureteric re-implantation.

Indications

COMPLICATED POLAR DUPLEX KIDNEYS

- Non-function, e.g. obstructed upper moiety, refluxing lower moiety.
- Polar infection, e.g. xanthogranulomatous pyelonephritis (XPN).

SINGLE KIDNEY

- Expanding polar renal cyst.
- Polar infection, e.g. XPN.

Contraindications

RELATIVE

- Previous retroperitoneal surgery or previous intraperitioneal surgery.
- Expected intraperitoneal adhesions.
- Expected complicating XPN.
- Suspected renal malignancy.

ABSOLUTE

- Previous renal trauma.
- Known malignancy.

The traditional open approach to partial nephrectomy has the established advantage of a wide field of exposure, but at the cost, at times, of a large incision with a slow convalescence. Minimal access partial nephrectomy, on the other hand, can allow accurate vascular definition through a small incision with excellent postoperative cosmesis. Unfortunately it often involves advanced laparoscopic techniques and is therefore not an operation for a novice in the field of laparoscopy.

Partial nephrectomy can be performed via a transperitoneal or retroperitoneoscopic approach. There is no doubt that the retroperitoneal approach does allow more rapid vascular access without the need for visceral retraction. The working space is small, with disorientation a common problem early in the learning experience. The extent of ureterectomy is limited by age and approach (lateral versus posterior). Complete ureterectomy is more likely with the posterior approach, especially in children over the age of 5 years.

Transperitoneal laparoscopic partial nephrectomy, on the other hand, allows a larger working space with much easier orientation, as intraperitoneal organs and other familiar landmarks are easily recognizable. It does, however, involve visceral retraction, with the potential risk of organ and peritoneal injuries and higher adhesion formation. Complete ureterectomy and access to the bladder base for reconstruction are easily achievable. A retroperitoneoscopic technique can be used, depending on the patient's position, via either a posterior/lumboscopic or the more traditional lateral approach. With the child placed prone, much more rapid vascular access can be achieved, without the need for constant renal retraction. The lateral approach gives a larger working space and the ability to achieve a more complete ureterectomy. It does, nonetheless, involve constant renal retraction, with vascular pedicle exposure at times compromised by the propensity of the kidney to fall onto the pedicle. Peritoneal tears are a greater risk, but are a minor clinical concern. (**See Figure 59.1**)

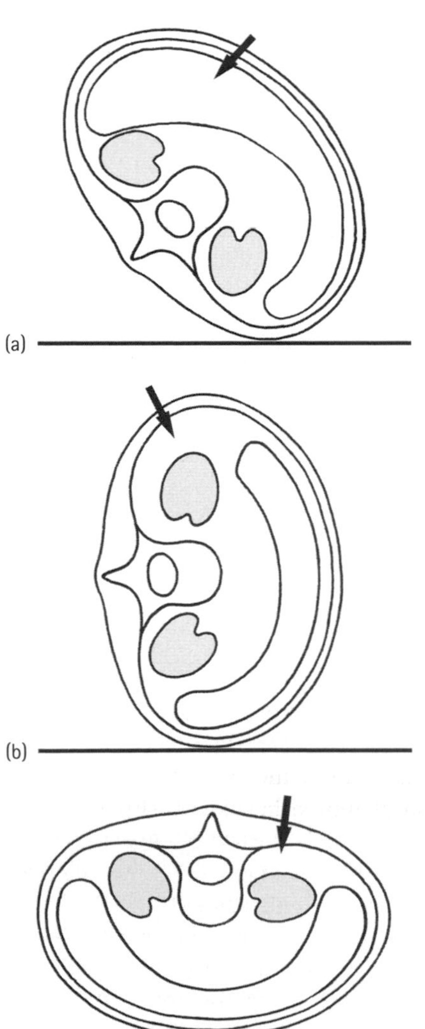

Figure 59.1 *(a) Semilateral position for transperitoneal approach; (b) lateral position for posterior retroperitoneal approach; (c) prone position for posterior retroperitoneal approach.*

EQUIPMENT/INSTRUMENTS

Essential

- 5 mm Hasson-type cannula or 5 mm port with gas tap.
- Two 5 mm ports (one with gas tap preferred).
- 5–12 mm port (retrieval bag/linear stapler).
- 30° 5 m scope.
- Scissors – diathermy insulated, double jaw action, curved.
- Hook diathermy 3.5–5 mm and bipolar.
- Suction irrigation (not necessarily on table).
- 5 mm clip applicator.
- Two sets of atraumatic grasping forceps (one ratchet, one no ratchet): curved, dolphin nose.
- Toothed grasper with ratchet.

Optional

- 5 mm atraumatic retractor.
- Advanced hemostatic shears.
- Ultrasonic dissection 5 mm bipolar sealant.
- LigaSure™ or equivalent 5 mm.
- Endoloops® (monofilament or chromic).
- Tourniquet below the level of the incision.
- 10 mm medium/large stable endoscopic clips for large vessels.

In general, 5 mm or 3.5 mm port cannulae are most commonly used. They are required with a larger 10 mm or 12 mm port for the anticipated retrieval site of the excised segment. The ports need to be well secured to the abdominal wall to prevent not only inward but also outward movement, with a tight seal around the entry wound to prevent excessive gas leakage and consequent loss of the working space, particularly with retroperitoneoscopic-surgery. The length and size of instruments are dictated by the size and age of the child. In general, young children and infants require the shorter (20 cm or 26 cm) 5 mm or 3.5 mm instruments, which are ergonomically better than the longer 5 mm version as used in adolescents and adults.

PREOPERATIVE PREPARATION

It is important to ensure that the results of renal lateralizing studies are present in the operating theater before the general anesthetic is commenced. In most instances, this would include not only a two-dimensional imaging study such as an ultrasound but also a functional study, e.g. dimethyl succinic acid (DMSA), mercaptoacetylglycine (MAG3). The presence or absence of vesico-ureteric reflux to the involved segment affects planning for postoperative bladder drainage, possible placement of a drain near the ureteric stump, as well as securing the end of the ureteric stump at the time of excision. In experienced hands, a blood sample for group and save is generally unnecessary.

PREFERRED APPROACH

Posterior retroperitoneoscopic

- Simple nephrectomy.
- Isolated upper or lower pole heminephrectomy.
- Complete ureterectomy in a patient less than 5 years old.

Lateral retroperitoneoscopic

- Complete ureterectomy in a patient more than 5 years old.
- Large hydronephrosis.

Transperitoneal retroperitoneoscopic approach

- Ectopic or concealed pelvic kidney.
- Horseshoe kidney.
- Ureterocelectomy and extravesical lower moiety re-implant.

The above recommendations are based on the strengths and weaknesses of each approach. For the novice or infrequent laparoscopist, the transperitoneal approach offers the safest environment in which to survive the learning curve before embarking on a more specialized or selective approach.

TECHNIQUE

Position

Due to the unusual positioning necessary for laparoscopic partial nephrectomy, a general anesthetic with muscle relaxation and endotracheal intubation is mandatory. Insertion of a urinary catheter is almost obligatory as overnight drainage to monitor urine output after any renal surgery as well as to reduce intravesical pressure, especially in the presence of vesico-ureteric reflux in the divided ureter. Pre-emptive local anesthetic should be administered to all potential port sites at the time of insertion, with direct injection to the peritoneum or sub-peritoneal plane creating a cylinder of local anesthetic to the skin.

Laparoscopic partial nephrectomy relies heavily on positioning to achieve maximum advantage with dissection. The posterior retroperitoneal approach involves the patient being positioned prone with pelvic and chest support, leaving the abdomen dependent and non-compressed. Strapping to the table at the mid-thorax and over the buttocks is essential, with padding to the knees as well as to the extensor aspect of the ankles. The arms are flexed superiorly. The table is then laterally rotated 30°, with the ipsilateral or affected side downwards and slight head up-tilt. The surgeon and assistant nurse stand on the affected side, with the monitor on the opposite side towards the head of the patient. In the lateral retroperitoneal approach, the patient is positioned laterally with a lumbar support and/or a kidney break in the table, which opens the lumbar space. Again, strapping at the pelvic and thoracic levels is essential if the table is to be maneuvered with a slight head up-tilt. The surgeon and assistant stand ventrally, with the monitor opposite and slightly cephalad dorsally. The transperitoneal approach can be performed in the supine or semi-lateral position with lumbar support. Particularly with the transperitoneal approach, this positioning allows gravity to play a greater role in the passive retraction of the overlying viscera. The child has a head up-tilt with a 30–40° rotation, with the ipsilateral or affected side up. This allows gravity displacement of the colon or small bowel away from the operative field. The surgeon and assistant stand ventrally, with the monitor cephalad and dorsally. (**See Figure 59.2**)

Cannula placement

In general, three ports are required for both transperitoneal and retroperitoneal minimal access surgery. Often a fourth port or direct insertion of an instrument through the abdominal wall near the costal margin allows static visceral retraction, e.g. right lobe of liver, spleen. The retroperitoneoscopic technique can create instrument clutter and it is important to allow adequate space between cannulae, particularly in infants. Inserting the cannulae at 90° if extensive inferior dissection is needed avoids the torque effect between the cannula and the abdominal wall.

Correct cannula placement is essential for good visualization and ergonomic comfort when performing a technically challenging procedure such as partial nephrectomy. The primary visualization port is placed for the creation of the retroperitoneal space. This is below the 12th rib, just lateral to the lateral edge of the erectus spinae, in the posterior retroperitoneal approach; below the tip of the twelfth rib in the mid-axillary line in the lateral retroperitoneal approach; and peri-umbilical in transperitoneal exposure. Subsequent cannula placement is either side of the visualization port in the line of vision towards the target renal moiety. Transperitoneal dissection is best done with ports placed superiorly in the mid-clavicular line and inferiorly in the anterior axillary line. In small infants, both accessory cannulae are often placed more ventrally in the mid-clavicular line above and below the umbilicus. A fourth retracting port is often necessary to deflect the liver or the lower pole of the spleen. It is best placed just below the costal margin in the

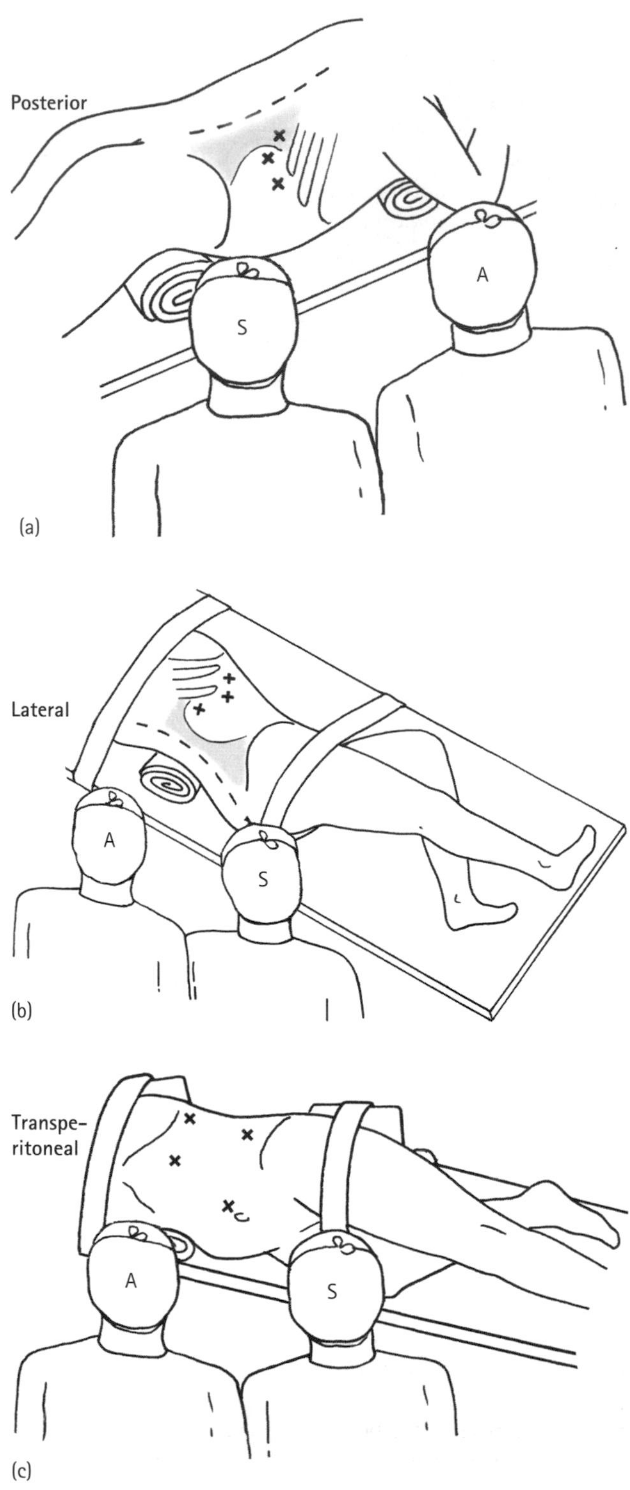

Figure 59.2

mid-axillary line. The instrument can raise the liver and be attached to the adjacent lateral abdominal wall or diaphragm as a free-standing instrument. As already mentioned, the retroperitoneum is a more restricted working space and exact port placement is crucial to a comfortable procedure. In the lateral position, one cannula is placed dorsally in the costo-vertebral angle and a second port is placed ventrally just below the tip of the eleventh rib, posterior to the peritoneal reflection. Finally, in the posterior retroperitoneal approach, cannulae are inserted more superiorly in the costo-vertebral angle and just lateral to the tip of the twelfth rib within the confines of the retroperitoneal space.

Creating the space

The space is created using an open technique cannulation, with CO_2 insufflation at a flow rate of 2–10 L/min and pressure of 10–13 mmHg, depending on the age of the child. The retroperitoneoscopic approach involves selected incision and blunt dissection through the layers of the lateral or posterior abdominal wall. Keeping the size of the entry site to a minimum restricts gas leakage and cannula slippage. A definite pop and give is experienced on entering the extraperitoneal plane. 'L' retractors allow visualization of the bulging extraperitoneal fat and can allow the option of open incision of Gerota's fascia when a larger incision is utilized. With this plane defined, there are two techniques that can be adopted to create the space. Inserting the cannula with scope dissection under vision with CO_2 insufflation is the preferred approach in the obese. Otherwise, inserting an expandable balloon or glove finger and syringe and expanding it with either air or fluid is acceptable. Care must be taken not to burst and fragment the balloon, which is difficult, if not impossible, to retrieve piecemeal. The more lateral the approach, the greater the risk of the lateral peritoneal reflection tearing and creating a pneumoperitoneum. The retroperitoneoscopic space is maintained with a flow of 5–10 L/min, with the pressure between 10 and 13 mmHg.

Defining and incising Gerota's fascia at the time of the initial port site dissection for creating the retroperitoneal space is an essential step in the lateral retroperitoneal approach. Using this maneuver and ensuring the dissection is guided dorsally, entry into the peri-renal space will leave the kidney attached and suspended on its peritoneal attachments anteriorly. Some of the difficulties encountered when the dependent kidney tends to fall onto its pedicle are avoided by utilizing passive retraction by renal suspension. On the other hand, the posterior approach and patient positioning allow the kidney to fall away with gravity. Therefore early incision of Gerota's fascia may aid orientation but is not as crucial a maneuver in the posterior approach.

Mobilization and excision

Following cannula placement and insertion of instruments, a quick orientation is helpful, especially in unfamiliar spaces such as the extraperitoneal plane in both the lateral and posterior positions. More visual cues are available in the transperitoneal approach. With the retroperitoneoscopic approach, early identification of the line of the psoas muscle and visualization of the ureters inferiorly with

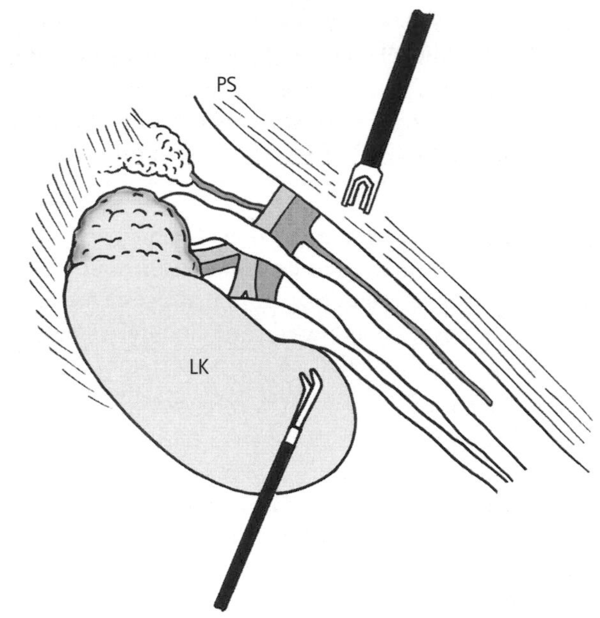

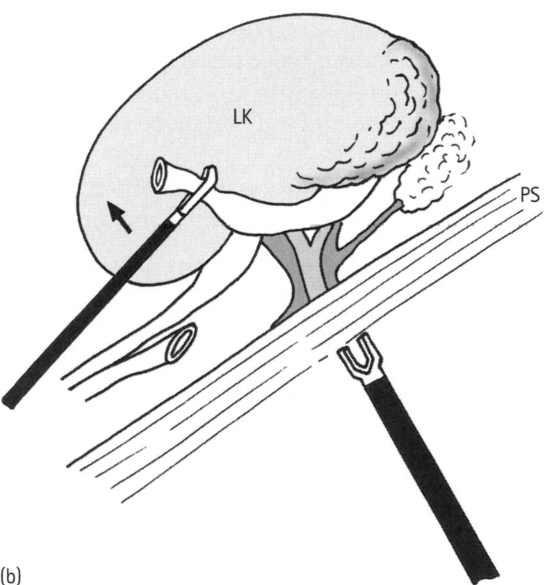

Figure 59.3 *Retroperitoneal approach. (a) Posterior; (b) lateral.*

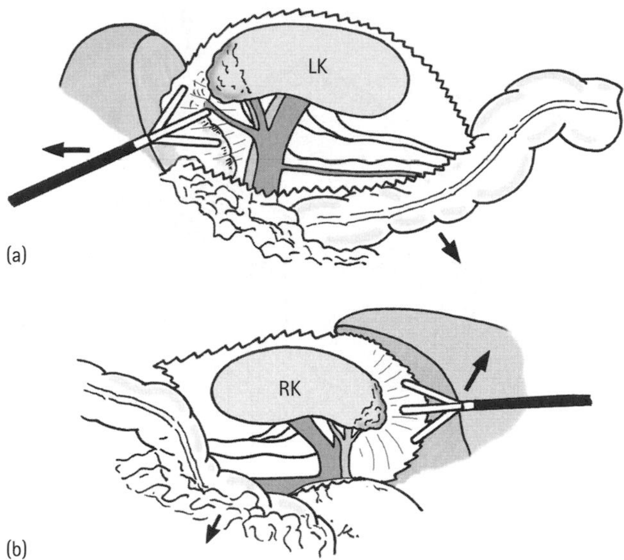

Figure 59.4 *Transperitoneal approach.*

an intact Gerota's fascia set the scene for a confident dissection and mobilization. Otherwise, after incision of Gerota's fascia and lower renal pole exposure, early identification of the duplex ureters and subsequent dissection towards the kidney is the rule. **(See Figure 59.3)**

In the transperitoneal approach, mobilization of the hepatic or splenic flexures laterally with extension superiorly to the left into the spleno-renal ligament allows visualization of Gerota's fascia. Extended release of the ligaments medially above the line of the right and left transverse colon completes adequate inferior exposure and identification of the ureters. The adjacent solid organs may need retraction. With gravity and judicious release of the spleno-renal ligament, the spleen tends to fall away. The right lobe of the liver can be elevated with a fan retractor or traumatic grasper attached to the adjacent abdominal wall. Rarely, the tail of the pancreas and duodenum need to be freed to widen exposure to the vascular pedicle. After confident early identification of the affected ureter and moiety, the ureter to be excised can be divided and used for traction and identification of the inferior or superior limit of the line of intended excision. **(See Figure 59.4)**

The wide variability of the vascular anatomy in the presence of a duplex as well as a single kidney must be considered as dissection to the hilum of the affected pole continues. Be aware that accessory or aberrant vessels are more likely in the presence of a renal anomaly. Traction on the proximal divided ureter helps to define the larger renal branch to the healthy, unaffected moiety as well as the smaller, often diminutive arterial and larger venous supply to the excised segment. The vessels are commonly paired passing anteriorly to the renal pelvis and, less commonly, posteriorly. The main renal artery is rarely visualized, with the main renal vein defined often by the insertion of the gonadal vein on the left or the proximity to the inferior vena cava on the right. The polar vessels can be divided by several methods. Although bipolar diathermy has been described with no major incident, it is suggested that an ultrasonic coagulation device or a 5 mm clip is more appropriate and secure.

After this maneuver, the line of vascular demarcation is evident, although it is often less clear with lower pole heminephrectomy due to the often superficial encroachment of healthy upper pole over the contracted lower pole moiety. The moiety can then be excised by estimating the limit of the most superior or inferior calix. Due to the inability to compress the remaining moiety during excision and thus reduce bleeding from the raw surface, two techniques have been applied with good results. One involves incising the renal

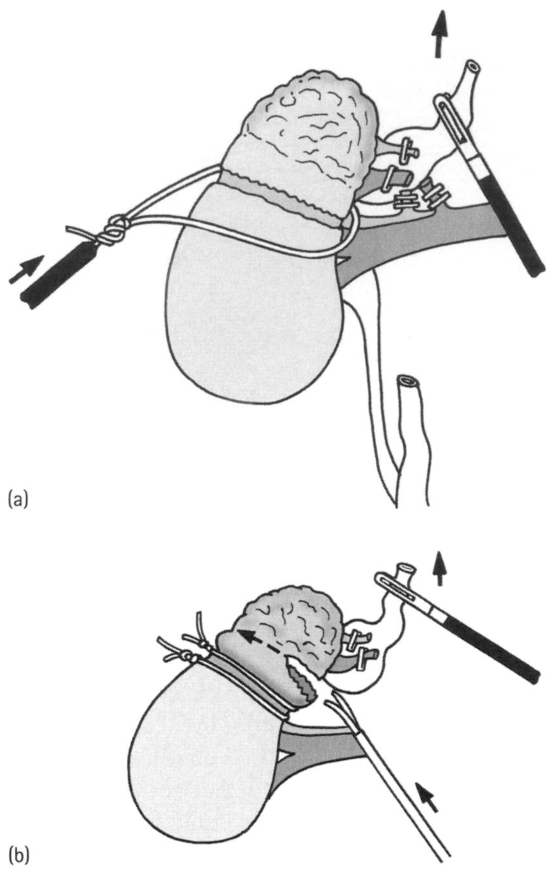

Figure 59.5

capsule over the healthy moiety 1–2 cm proximal to the line of excision and applying preferably two Endoloops® as a tourniquet. Excision can then proceed with confidence using sharp scissor dissection. Alternatively, progressive dissection and coagulation can be done with ultrasonic shears or bipolar diathermy (the former is quicker and more complete). As the excised moiety becomes free, suction irrigation is applied to check hemostasis. The integrity of the remaining moiety is then confirmed. **(See Figure 59.5)**

Complete ureterectomy is indicated in the presence of on-going or previous documented vesico-ureteric reflux or when there is a need for concomitant ureterocelectomy and lower moiety ureteric re-implantation. It is clear that a lateral retroperitoneal approach or a transperitoneal approach allows complete dissection to the detrusor hiatus. The distal ureteric stump needs to be closed with an Endoloop® clip or extracorporeal tie. An overnight extraperitoneal suction drain should be placed if there is an open-ended ureteric stump or suspected urine leakage postoperatively (e.g. de-roofed polar renal cyst).

The excised moiety and ureter can be easily retrieved by gentle stretching on the port site and splitting the abdominal wall muscles to accommodate removal. A retrieval bag may be used, but as it is a non-malignant process, fragmentation in situ can also be considered. The cannulae are removed and CO_2 evacuated. Cannula sites greater than 5 mm are closed with absorbable sutures and residual local anesthetic is infiltrated.

POSTOPERATIVE CARE

A full diet can be resumed after 4 hours, if tolerated. Intravenous morphine can be given for the first 12 hours, with the introduction of regular oral analgesia for the subsequent 24 hours as required. The urethral catheter and drainage are removed after 24 hours, or sooner if clinically indicated. The expected hospital stay is usually 24–48 hours.

PROBLEMS, PITFALLS AND SOLUTIONS

Establishing retropneumoperitoneum

- Identification of the bulging extra-renal fat ensures the correct plane for insertion of a balloon dissector or cannula for scope dissection. With insufflation of the balloon, no subcutaneous bulge should be noticeable. If it is, the dissection is likely to be intramuscular and deflation should occur and re-insertion be carried out again.
- In obese children, finding the correct plane for insertion of the balloon can be difficult, and therefore scope dissection may be preferable.
- If the glove-finger balloon ruptures during insufflation, always assume that a fragment remains in the space, which needs to be actively searched for and retrieved.

Peritoneal tear and pneumoperitoneum (retroperitoneal technique)

- Be aware of the landmarks for the lateral peritoneal reflection when planning port sites. Initial 'blind insertion' should be done medially before the space is created, with attention to the more posteriorly directed dissection. The balloon dissection will displace the peritoneal reflection anteriorly for better placement of the anterior ports.
- Continued expanding pneumoperitoneum obliterates the retroperitoneal space. Convert the exposure to an intraperitoneal space for dissection by opening the peritoneal tear widely, allowing equilibration of pressures to both spaces.
- As long as the abdominal wall is expandable without compression from the operating table and support straps, re-positioning of the operating table and gravity should not preclude continuing with the procedure.

- Alternatively, if the tear is small, continuous decompression of the peritoneal cavity with a small cannula may reduce peritoneal tension sufficiently to allow the retroperitoneal space to re-expand.
- The pneumoperitoneum will usually deflate with decompression of the retroperitoneal space. Check the tension of the abdominal wall after returning to the supine position. If the tear is small, percutaneous release of retained CO_2 may be required.

Cannula displacement and instrument clutter

- In particular, there will be a smaller working space in infants and young children. Ensuring maximum spacing, particularly with the posterior retroperitoneal approach, avoids clutter. An angled telescope is essential.
- The abdominal wall is thin and compliant in young children. Dislodgment of cannulae, both inwards and by falling out, is not uncommon with partial nephrectomy. Radially expanding sleeves, internal and external retention devices or suture fixation to rubber tubing sleeved to the cannula can be most effective.

Orientation/disorientation

- In the extraperitoneal plane with Gerota's fascia intact initially, identification of the psoas muscle, direction of the inferior vena cava on the right and movement of the kidney and extraperitoneal fat with respiration allow confident incision of the fascia and exposure of the renal capsule. Be aware that balloon dissection may create a space laterally as well as inferiorly, with the renal mass displaced quite medially as well as superomedially from the point of initial visualization.
- Early identification of both ureters inferiorly should be done before hilar dissection. The divided proximal end of the affected ureter can greatly assist as traction, and continued dissection close to the ureter allows efficient and confident identification of the variable vascular anatomy.

Line of moiety excision

Dissection close to the surface of the ureter and its respective pelvis leads into the renal sinus. Continued dissection towards the major calyces requires caution to avoid cutting the small branches of the renal artery. The change of surface texture (between normal and abnormal poles) and color (devascularization of the abnormal pole) acts as a rough guide to the line of transection.

Poor extraperitoneal visualization from light absorption

- Minor bleeding during retroperitoneal dissection can cause extensive bloodstaining of the extraperitoneal fat and peri-renal fascia. This will greatly increase light absorption and reduce visibility.
- Careful coagulation dissection for meticulous hemostasis from the outset will prevent minor continuous ooze and reduce staining.
- With established bloodstaining and increased light absorption, intermittent irrigation and suction of the retroperitoneal tissues dilute the staining and enhance light reflection.

COMPLICATIONS

Visceral injury

Electrosurgical injury is avoided by the universal use of insulated instruments, keeping the exposed coagulating end completely within the visual field. During retraction of the liver or spleen, regular checks are required to detect any shifting or undue shearing. Endeavors to increase exposure may put these adjacent organs and major vessels at risk of damage. Poor orientation, lack of depth perception, reduced operating space or careless dissection can lead to failure to appreciate adjacent intraperitoneal structures from within the extraperitoneal plane. The duodenum and inferior vena cava on the right and the colon and tail of the pancreas on the left are particularly at risk. In the presence of chronic inflammation such as polar XPN, there is a greater risk of these visceral injuries and the incidence of open conversion is higher irrespective of the learning curve.

Entry into preserved moiety-collecting system

Separate closure of the urothelium and subsequently of the renal parenchyma and capsule is difficult to achieve. Intracorporeal mass loose, interrupted or continuous absorbable suture closure of all layers with interposed extraperitoneal fat or omentum is usually sufficient. Extra renal drain and bladder catheter drainage are required for 24 hours, or for a minimum of 48 hours.

Delayed progressive urinoma

Percutaneous placement of an extra-renal drain and insertion of an internal ureteric stent with initial bladder drainage are suggested. Continued drainage is rare. If it does occur, open exposure may be appropriate.

Major bleeding

In the presence of complicated duplex systems, the vascular anatomy is often variable. Aberrant or accessory polar vessels are encountered and can be inadvertently divided during exposure and subsequent polar dissection. It is recommended that careful blunt and coagulating dissection is restricted to close to the kidney until the excised polar vessel is completely isolated. Venous bleeding can sometimes be contained by raising the insufflation pressure until the venotomy can be identified. The decision to convert to an open approach is determined by the extent of the vascular injury and the skill and confidence of the surgeon to secure hemostasis with intracorporeal suturing or stapling as indicated.

60

Pyeloplasty

C.K. YEUNG AND N.J. MAGNSOC

INTRODUCTION

Open dismembered (Anderson–Hynes) pyeloplasty has been the standard treatment for pelvi-ureteric junction (PUJ) obstruction in children. Its success rate has been reported to be greater than 90 percent. However, with the advent of minimally invasive surgery, and constant effort to overcome the shortcomings of open pyeloplasty, alternative methods for treating PUJ obstruction have been introduced, including endopyelotomy and retrograde dilatation. However, these procedures have reported success rates 10–25 percent lower than that of open pyeloplasty, and are associated with hemorrhagic complications. In 1993, laparoscopic dismembered pyeloplasty was developed in an attempt to combine the benefits of minimally invasive surgery with the higher success rates of open pyeloplasty. The goal of laparoscopic repair is similar to that of open pyeloplasty, which is to create a dependent, tension-free, watertight anastomosis. Preliminary procedures have mainly involved the transperitoneal approach, but recently the retroperitoneal approach is gaining popularity.

Indications

The indications are similar to those for open dismembered pyeloplasty.

- Primary or secondary PUJ obstruction.
- Patients with failed retrograde or antegrade percutaneous endopyelotomies.
- PUJ obstruction with associated abnormalities such as pelvic kidney or horseshoe kidney.

Contraindications

ABSOLUTE

- Severe cardiopulmonary disease or severe coagulopathy.
- Recent (within 8 weeks) or inadequately treated pyelonephritis or pyonephrosis.

RELATIVE

Transperitoneal and retroperitoneal approach

- Previous intra-abdominal or retroperitoneal surgery.
- The presence of a small intra-renal pelvis.
- A kidney with very poor function that is probably beyond salvage by operative repair.

Retroperitoneal approach

- Morbid obesity with a high-positioned kidney.
- Young infants (<6 months) with gross hydronephrosis (with transverse pelvic diameter >50 mm).

Advantages

- Can address all potential causes of obstruction.
- Optical magnification allows greater sensitivity in recognizing a causative crossing vessel or other pathologies.
- Decreased risk of hemorrhage compared with endopyelotomy, since the incisional procedures fail to appreciate the presence of crossing vessels.
- Shorter hospital stay and patient convalescence.

- Small surgical wound and decreased postoperative pain.
- Decreased risk of incisional hernias.

Disadvantages

- A need for proficiency in laparoscopic techniques.
- Longer mean operative time.

Advantages of the retroperitoneal approach over the transperitoneal approach

- Avoids mobilization and risk of injury to intraperitoneal organs.
- Not precluded by previous intraperitoneal surgery.
- Early visualization of the kidney and control of renal vessels.
- Greater sensitivity in detecting a crossing vessel since it allows quicker and more direct access to the PUJ with minimal dissection.
- Decreased postoperative ileus and risk of adhesions.

Disadvantages of the retroperitoneal over the transperitoneal approach

- Smaller and more restricted working space.
- Overcrowding of ports and instruments, leading to unfavorable ergonomics.

EQUIPMENT/INSTRUMENTS

Essential

- 5 mm 30° or 0° laparoscope.
- Two 3–5 mm working ports.
- 3 mm atraumatic grasping forceps and scissors with fine tips.
- 3 mm diathermy hook.
- 3 mm needle holder.
- 6 Fr infant feeding tube.
- 18 G venous cannula.
- 4 Fr or 5 Fr double pigtail stent over guide-wire.

Sutures

- 6-0 polydioxanone surgical (PDS) sutures for infants.
- 5-0 PDS sutures for children/adults.
- 4-0 PDS suture with a straight needle for the hitch stitch.

PREOPERATIVE PREPARATION

Patients must have documented evidence of PUJ obstruction prior to surgery. Pelvi-ureteric obstruction may be demonstrated in several ways. Initially, the patient commonly presents with flank pain and tenderness on physical examination, and urinary tract infection on urinalysis and urine culture. As well as by ultrasonography, PUJ may also be documented by radiologic demonstration of narrowing of the PUJ with proximal dilatation on excretory urography, retrograde pyelography and antegrade pyelography, or by delayed excretion on isotope renography (^{99}technetium-labeled mercaptoacetylglycine – 99Tc-MAG3). The patient is given an enema the night before surgery.

TECHNIQUE

The patient is placed under general anesthesia with endotracheal intubation. Broad-spectrum intravenous antibiotics/second-generation cephalosporin are given as prophylaxis. A Foley catheter (appropriate for the patient's age) is inserted into the bladder. The surgeon and assistant stand on one side of the operating table in line with the camera, which is pointing away (on the left of the patient for left pyeloplasty and on the right of the patient for right pyeloplasty).

Retroperitoneal approach

The patient is placed in a semi-prone position with the left flank up (left pyeloplasty) or in a 45° right lateral decubitus position (right pyeloplasty). As a result, the approach to the PUJ will be posterior for left-sided pathology and anterior for right-sided pathology.

The patient is positioned close to the edge of the operating table. Lumbar padding and support are used to extend the trunk, while straps are placed to keep the body in place. **(See Figure 60.1)**

A 1 cm incision is made over the mid-axillary line midway between the iliac crest and tip of the twelfth rib. The retroperitoneal space is entered and developed either by the combined use of a glove balloon made from the finger of a powder-free surgical glove, insinuation of a surgical sponge and sweeping motions with the laparoscope itself, or with a balloon trocar system. Videoretroperitoneoscopy is performed using a 5 mm 0° or 30° laparoscope. Pneumoretroperitoneum is maintained at a pressure of 10–12 mmHg. Two additional 3–5 mm ports are inserted, one above and one below the camera port, under direct videoscopic guidance.

The peritoneal reflection is identified and Gerota's fascia is entered. The lower pole of the kidney and the renal pelvis are exposed. The PUJ and upper ureter are then mobilized.

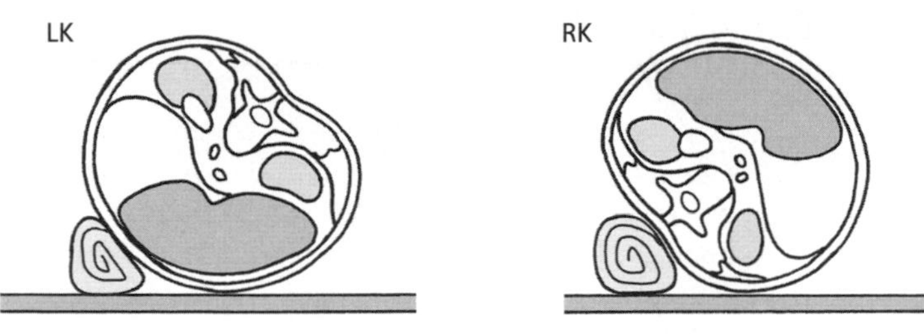

Figure 60.1

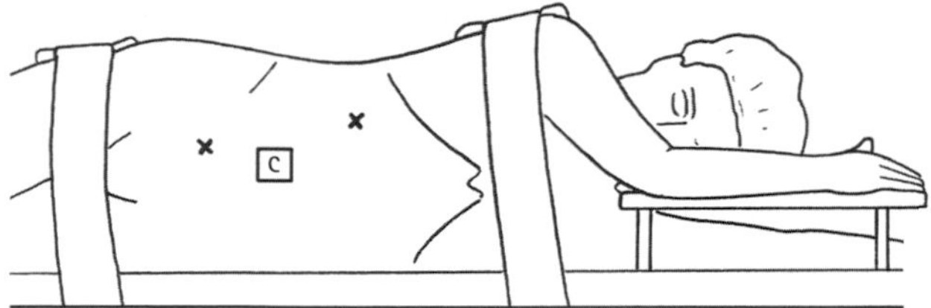

Figure 60.2

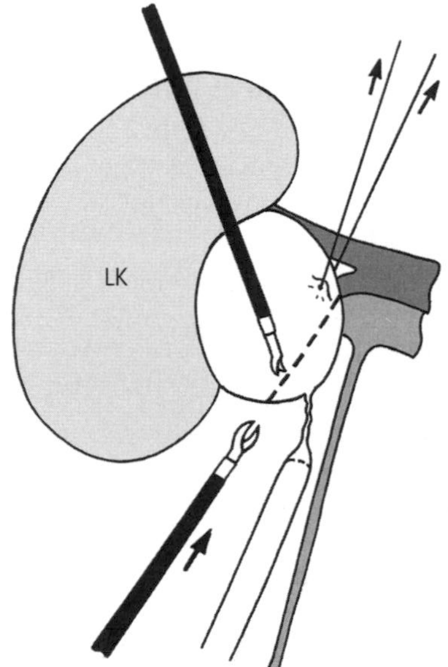

Figure 60.3

At this point, possible causes for the PUJ obstruction may be identified, such as a crossing blood vessel or a fibrotic band.

Transperitoneal approach

The patient is positioned semi-laterally close to the edge of the operating table, with the ipsilateral side elevated, and is secured by placing a sandbag or padding to support the back. The patient is stabilized by being strapped to the operating table with adhesive bandage to allow rotation, if required. The approach to the PUJ will be anterior.

A 5–7 mm Hasson trocar is introduced at the umbilicus. The incision is closed around the port using purse-string sutures to prevent gas leakage. Two additional 5 mm instrument ports are introduced under direct vision, one on the ipsilateral upper quadrant, the other port between the umbilicus and symphysis pubis. **(See Figure 60.2)**

The colon is mobilized and allowed to fall away medially from the renal bed, thus exposing Gerota's fascia, which is entered with limited mobilization. The PUJ is identified by tracing the dilated renal pelvis medially until the gonadal vessels are seen crossing the pelvis. Identification of the PUJ is facilitated by lifting the renal pelvis up towards the anterior abdominal wall. The peri-renal fat is dissected as the lower pole of the kidney and the upper ureter are identified and mobilized. Care must be taken to preserve the peri-ureteric vasculature. Any fibrotic band kinking the ureter is divided. The PUJ is identified and the incision line for pelvic reduction and pyeloplasty is planned.

Continuation for both the retroperitoneal and transperitoneal approaches

A 4-0 PDS suture over a straight needle is passed percutaneously through the abdominal wall to the upper pole of the renal pelvis, and passed back through the abdominal wall at the same entry point. This stitch serves to mark the upper limit of the line of the pyeloplasty during pelvi-ureteric anastomosis. More importantly, it also serves as a hitch stitch to stabilize and present the pelvis to facilitate intracorporeal suturing during the anastomosis. It is important to leave a long external length of suture to allow for intra-operative adjustment of the tension. **(See Figure 60.3)**

The renal pelvis is dismembered above the area of the pathology. If a concomitant intra-renal calculus is present, intervention at this point is ideal using a flexible scope. If crossing vessels are present, the ureter and renal pelvis are transposed to the opposite side of them.

The redundant renal pelvis is excised adequately and the proximal ureter is spatulated laterally. **(See Figure 60.4)**

A short segment of a 6 Fr feeding tube is inserted through a working port and into the open end of the spatulated proximal ureter to separate the anterior and posterior walls. The stent allows accurate placement of the first corner suture over the apex of the spatulated upper ureter.

Anastomosis of the most dependent part of the reduced pelvis and the ureter is performed using continuous 6-0 PDS sutures for infants and younger children and 5-0 PDS sutures for older children on a 3/8 round-body needle. Suturing is started at the wall of the reduced renal pelvis

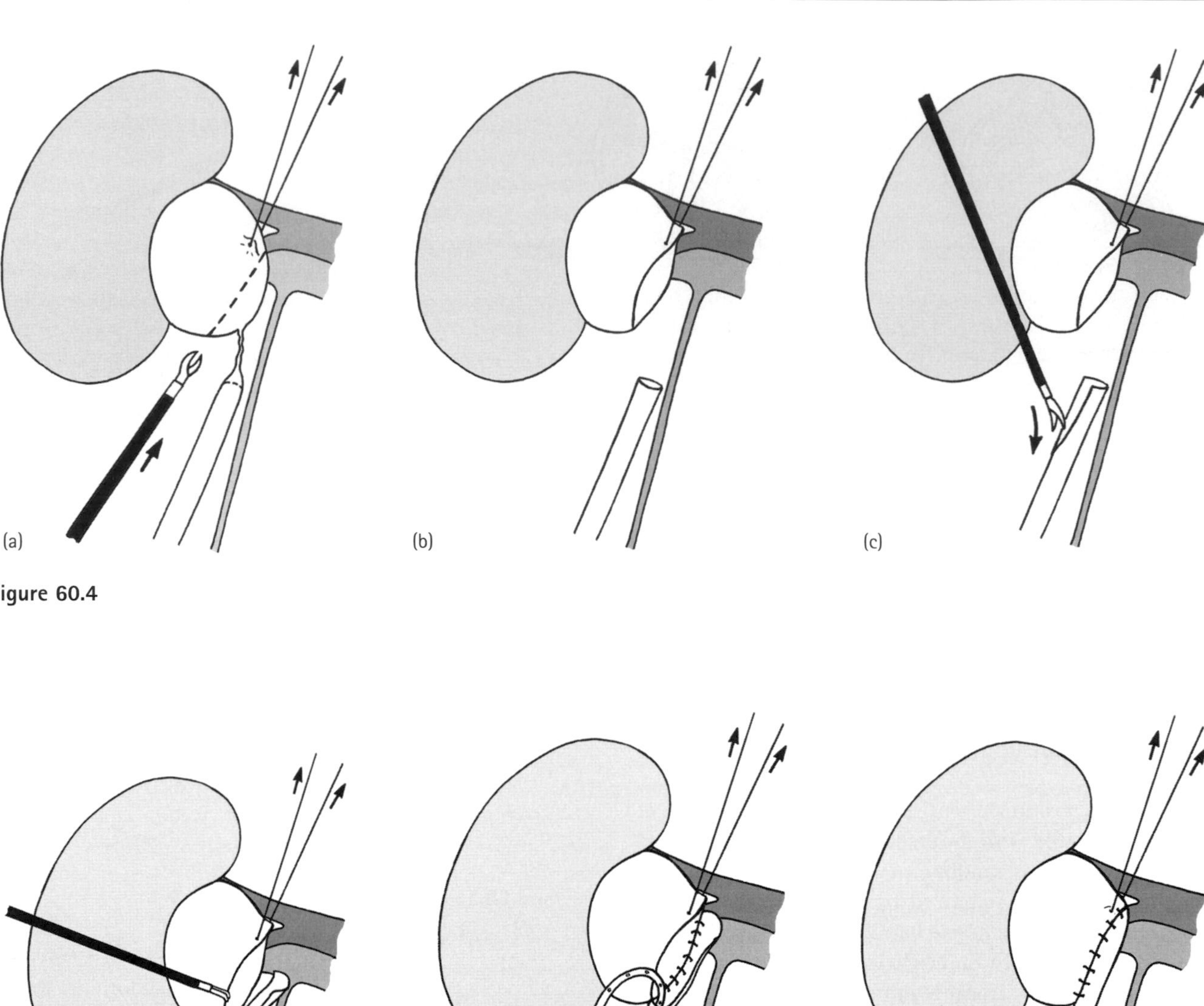

Figure 60.4

Figure 60.5

that is away from the surgeon. So, if the approach to the PUJ is anterior, the posterior wall is sutured initially; if the approach is posterior, the anterior wall is sutured initially. Care must be taken to ensure that there are no mucosal flaps. **(See Figure 60.5)**

After completion of the first side, a trans-anastomotic double pigtail stent is inserted. Insertion of the stent is facilitated by first passing a 18 G venous cannula through the abdominal wall. A flexible guide-wire is then inserted through the cannula and manipulated into the upper ureter and advanced to the bladder. The venous cannula is withdrawn and a 4 Fr or 5 Fr double pigtail catheter is passed over the guide-wire into the bladder, with the proximal end of the pigtail stent positioned in the renal pelvis. Entry of the stent into the bladder may be sensed by a sudden yield as it passes through the vesico-ureteric junction. Backflow of urine from the bladder may also be noted from the stent upon withdrawal of the guide-wire. The location of the pigtail stent may be confirmed radiologically. The anterior layer of the pelvi-ureteric anastomosis is completed with continuous fine PDS sutures and tied intracorporeally at the upper corner with the suture from the posterior anastomotic sutures.

Additional running or interrupted sutures may be placed in the area of the pelvis which was not opposed by the initial suturing. The hitch stitch is released and the PUJ and upper ureter are inspected to ensure a good tension-free anastomosis and that no kinking has occurred.

The retroperitoneal cavity is desufflated and hemostasis is ascertained. Insertion of a drain is usually not necessary. The ports are then removed. For 5 mm ports, the port sites are repaired by interrupted absorbable sutures. There is no need to repair the port site if 2–3 mm mini-ports are used. For the transperitoneal laparoscopic approach, the previously inserted purse-string suture over the umbilical port is tightened, thereby closing the defect.

POSTOPERATIVE CARE

The patient is started on a normal diet as tolerated on day one postoperatively and progressed accordingly. Postoperative analgesia is given until discharge. The Foley catheter is removed after 2 days. Antibiotic prophylaxis is resumed, and discontinued only when the double pigtail stent is removed, which is around 3–4 weeks after surgery. The patient is followed up with ultrasonography and MAG3 diuretic renal renography 3 months after removal of the stent.

PROBLEMS, PITFALLS AND SOLUTIONS

- The main technical problem for laparoscopic dismembered pyeloplasty occurs when a retroperitoneoscopic approach has been adopted for very young infants with a huge hydronephrotic renal pelvis, due to a combination of restriction of operative space, difficulty in orientation of the huge pelvis and manipulation of instruments. A transperitoneal approach is recommended for young infants less than 6 months of age with a grossly hydronephrotic pelvis (transverse renal pelvic diameter >50 mm).
- Poor visualization in the retroperitoneal space due to peritoneal perforation and hence difficulty in maintaining pneumoretroperitoneum. This can be solved by repairing the perforation or inserting a Veress needle in the peritoneal cavity if the perforation is small, or by liberally enlarging the perforation to convert the retroperitoneal and intraperitoneal spaces into a single cavity.

COMPLICATIONS

These may either be intra-operative or postoperative.

- Urine leak/urinoma.
  - The importance of a good watertight anastomosis cannot be over-emphasized.
  - Improper placement or kinking of the pigtail stent: ensure adequate placement of the stent intra-operatively.
- Urinary ascites: this occurs more commonly with the transperitoneal approach.
- Transient ileus: this occurs more commonly with the transperitoneal approach.
- Bowel serosal injury: this occurs more commonly with the transperitoneal approach.
- Abdominal wall hematoma: this may occur inadvertently during incision of the skin when inserting a port. Adequate hemostasis of the layers of the abdominal wall must be confirmed when the ports are removed.
- Pyelonephritis: this can usually be treated medically; however, an obstructive etiology must be excluded.
- Re-stenosis of repair: this may also be found in open pyeloplasty.
- Acute obstruction after stent removal.
- Urinary calculi formation.

FURTHER READING

Eden CG, Cahill D, Allen JD. Laparoscopic dismembered pyeloplasty: 50 consecutive cases. *British Journal of Urology International* 2001; **88**(6):526–31.

Janetschek G, Peschel R, Frauscher F, Franscher F. Laparoscopic pyeloplasty. *Urologic Clinics of North America* 2000; **27**(4):695–704.

Jarrett TW, Chan DY, Charambura TC, Fugita O, Kavoussi LR. Laparoscopic pyeloplasty: the first 100 cases. *Journal of Urology* 2002; **167**(3):1253–6.

Tan HL. Laparoscopic Anderson–Hynes dismembered pyeloplasty in children. *Journal of Urology* 1999; **162**(3 Pt 2):1045–7; discussion 1048.

Yeung CK, Tam YH, Sihoe JD, Lee KH, Liu KW. Retroperitoneoscopic dismembered pyeloplasty for pelvi-ureteric junction obstruction in infants and children. *British Journal of Urology International* 2001; **87**(6):509–13.

61

Re-implantation of the ureter

AZAD NAJMALDIN

INTRODUCTION

Open surgical re-implantation of the ureter, both transvesical and extravesical, has been successfully undertaken for many decades. However, these operations have the morbidity of open surgery, with failure rates up to 19 percent and re-operation rates up to 9 percent (recurrent or persistent vesico-ureteric reflux or distal ureteric obstruction).

In experienced hands, the sub-ureteric injection of bulky agents for the treatment of vesico-ureteric reflux has a failure rate of 11–16 percent after one to four injections.

Although different minimally invasive techniques for re-implantation of the ureter have been described (extravesical, transvesical and cystoscopic-assisted transvesical), this chapter describes a technique of endoscopic transvesical Cohen's re-implantation of the ureter.

Indications

- Primary vesico-ureteric reflux.
- Secondary vesico-ureteric reflux.
- Vesico-ureteric junction obstruction.
- Ectopic ureter.
- In association with other procedures.

EQUIPMENT/INSTRUMENTS

Essential

Depending on the age and size of the patient, 3.5–5 mm instruments are used. In general, 3.5 mm working instruments are easier to use than larger instruments.

- One 5 mm primary and two 3.5 mm secondary cannulae.
- 5 mm 30–45° scope allows a better view.
- Two sets of atraumatic grasping forceps.
- Scissors.
- Suction irrigation.
- Monopolar diathermy hook.
- Appropriate-sized Foley catheter (6–10 Fr) to distend and drain the bladder preoperatively and postoperatively – or, alternatively, a simple straight tube.
- Stents of appropriate sizes to use per-operatively and postoperatively. Usually, size 4–8 Fr, depending on the size of the ureter and the nature of the procedure; simple plastic tubes such as nasogastric tubes work well.
- Absorbable but strong suture materials of appropriate sizes, preferably on atraumatic tapering needles.
  - 2-0 Vicryl® for purse-string and/or hitching bladder suture around the primary cannula.
  - 3-0/4-0 Vicryl® or polydioxanone surgical (PDS) to transfix the ureter around the stent and repair the bladder defect per-operatively.
  - 5-0/6-0 Vicryl® or PDS for the anastomosis and repair of the bladder mucosa per-operatively. The needles may have to be straightened out so that they can be passed through the cannulae or percutaneously into the bladder. Alternatively, use size 8 or 10 mm needles, which may be passed through 3.5 mm cannulae.

Optional

- Extra cannulae and/or working instruments or telescopes.

- Self-retaining (balloon inside, flange outside) purpose-made cannulae that minimize the risk of cannula displacement and extravasation of fluid or gas.
- Appropriate sizes of needle and peel-away sheath for insertion of suprapubic tubes and catheters.

PREOPERATIVE PREPARATION

The preoperative preparation is the same as for the open technique. Before planning surgery, complete assessment of the urinary system is essential in order to identify and/or exclude the following.

- Primary causes for reflux or obstruction that may require attention first and/or continuous postoperative management, e.g. neurogenic bladder and obstructed urethra.
- Associated anomalies that may require assessment and treatment at the same time as re-implantation, e.g. ureterocele, contralateral ureteric abnormality, bladder diverticulum, urolithiasis.
- Prognostic factors such as other system abnormalities, renal scarring and bladder malfunction.

The specific investigations may include ultrasound scan with or without plain X-rays, micturating cystourethrogram, dynamic isotope renogram, dimethyl succinic acid (DMSA) renogram, urodynamics, cystoscopy and occasionally intravenous urogram. Urinary infection must be excluded and/or treated appropriately prior to surgery.

TECHNIQUE

Under general anesthesia with complete muscle relaxation, the patient is positioned supine. The abdomen, genitals and perineum are prepared thoroughly and the patient is draped in such a fashion that the genitals and the external urinary meatus remain sterile, accessible and protected throughout the procedure. A bladder catheter and ureteric stent are placed per-urethrally. In the supine position, catheterization of the female urethra is less easy than that of the male. One may therefore place these catheters/tubes either per-urethrally prior to preparing and draping the patient (in which case the tubes need to be fixed with tape and their ends cleaned and included in the outside operating field for access) or suprapubically using a peel-away needle or sheath. The balloon of the catheter is inflated sufficiently to prevent it and the tubes from falling out. **(See Figure 61.1)**

The right-handed surgeon stands on the left side of the patient for re-implantation of the right ureter and bilateral surgery, and on the right side of the patient for left re-implantation of the ureter. The assistant and nurse may stand on either side of the table. The bladder is distended to its maximum capacity using a large bladder syringe and normal saline through the urethral catheter. Often the bladder can be distended to or just below the umbilicus. A small (usually 2 cm) vertical or transverse incision is made at the upper limit of the bladder. The dissection is deepened and the upper part of the anterior wall of the bladder is exposed extraperitoneally. (In lean patients a large bladder is easily accessible through the usual sub-umbilical cannula crease incision.) A purse-string suture is placed in the bladder wall using strong suture material (deep and relatively wide mucosa-sparing bites). The primary cannula is placed through the purse-string into the bladder and secured with a double throw of suture, thereby preventing a fluid leak. The suture is then secured around the gas port of the cannula to prevent the cannula from falling out and allowing 1–2 cm of the cannula to remain inside the bladder. Alternatively, two simple but strong hitching sutures are used instead of the purse-string. The telescope is now placed inside the bladder and two working cannulae are introduced under direct vision, one on each side, strictly at the outer edges of the bladder. The working cannulae are fixed, allowing 2–3 cm of their length to remain inside the bladder. A cuff of pre-adjusted rubber tube on the cannula may be used to prevent it falling into the bladder. Care must be taken not to allow fluid to escape through or around the primary and working cannulae before they are appropriately positioned and fixed firmly.

Once the cannulae are in position, normal saline is aspirated through the catheter or a suction tube through one of the working cannulae and the bladder is re-distended using CO_2 at a pressure of 8–12 mmHg. **(See Figure 61.2)**

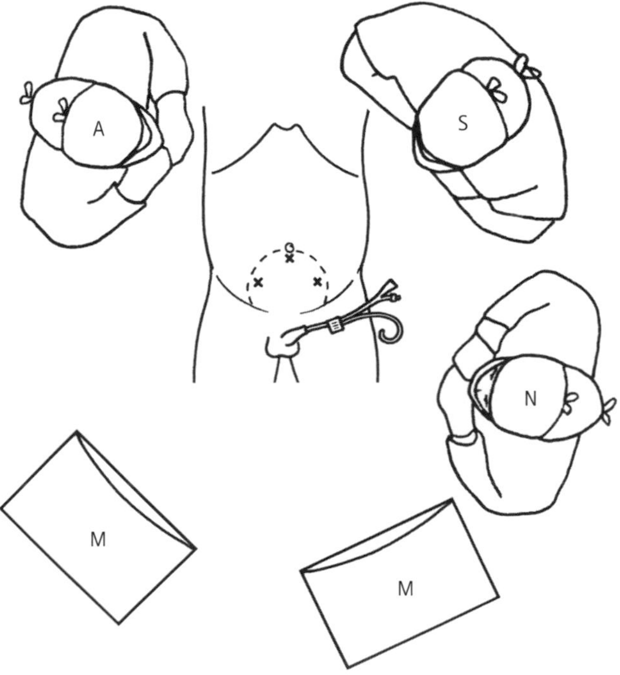

Figure 61.1

Mobilization of the ureter, repair of the bladder and tunneling, anastomosis and stenting of the ureter are performed in a manner identical to that used for open technique Cohen re-implantation of the ureter.

The pre-positioned stent is pushed as high as possible into the ureter and transfixed using a figure-of-eight suture. The transfixed stent is held in the left hand while a circumferential incision is made around the ureteric orifices using a monopolar diathermy hook (or needle) through the right working cannula. The incision is deepened and an adequate length of distal ureter is mobilized carefully using sharp and/or blunt dissection with a monopolar diathermy hook, scissors or fine atraumatic grasping forceps. Care is taken not to damage or de-vascularize the ureter, cause bleeding by cutting large peri-ureteric vessels or cut the transfixation suture. Aggressive and excessive direct manipulation of the ureter should be avoided. A set of accessory atraumatic grasping forceps inserted through an additional cannula may facilitate safer and higher mobilization of the ureter. **(See Figure 61.3)**

The site of re-implantation is marked and a submucosal tunnel is made using a combination of sharp and blunt dissection with scissors and atraumatic grasping forceps respectively. If necessary, the bladder wall at the site of mobilization of the ureter is repaired using interrupted, inverted, absorbable sutures. **(See Figure 61.4)**

The ureteric stent is either removed or cut 1 or 2 cm distal to the transfixation suture and the ureter is passed through the tunnel. If necessary, the distal end of the ureter is re-fashioned and the anastomosis is carried out using interrupted fine absorbable sutures. The bladder mucosa at the site of mobilization is repaired using continuous absorbable sutures. **(See Figure 61.5)**

The ureter is stented and the bladder catheterized using either the pre-existing catheters and stents or appropriate-sized fresh materials through:

- the urethra,
- the working or even primary cannula,
- separate suprapubic peel-away sheaths.

The working cannulae are removed under vision (no repair is required for the 3.5 mm cannulae) and the site of the primary cannula is formally closed using the pre-positioned purse-string and/or hitching sutures or additional

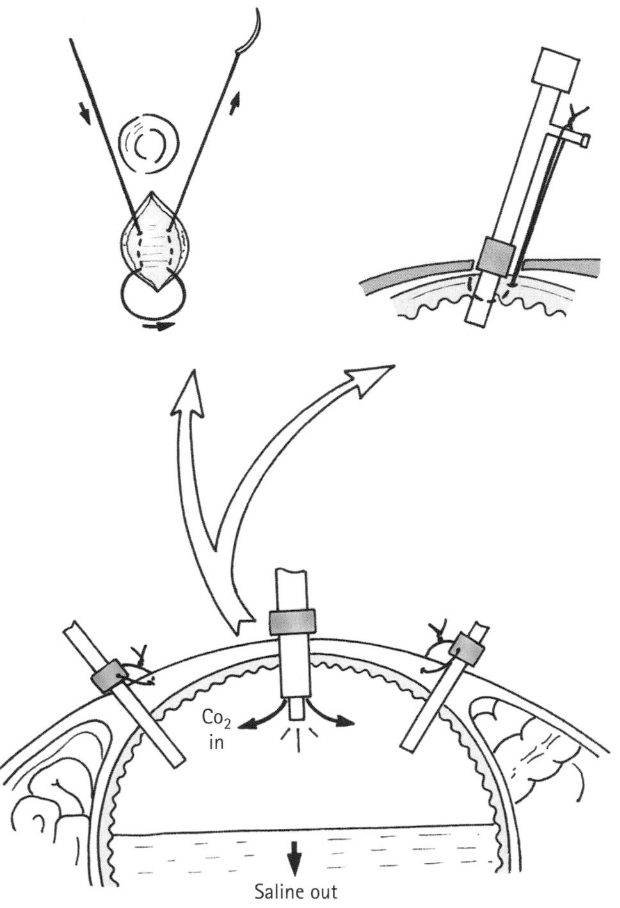

Figure 61.2

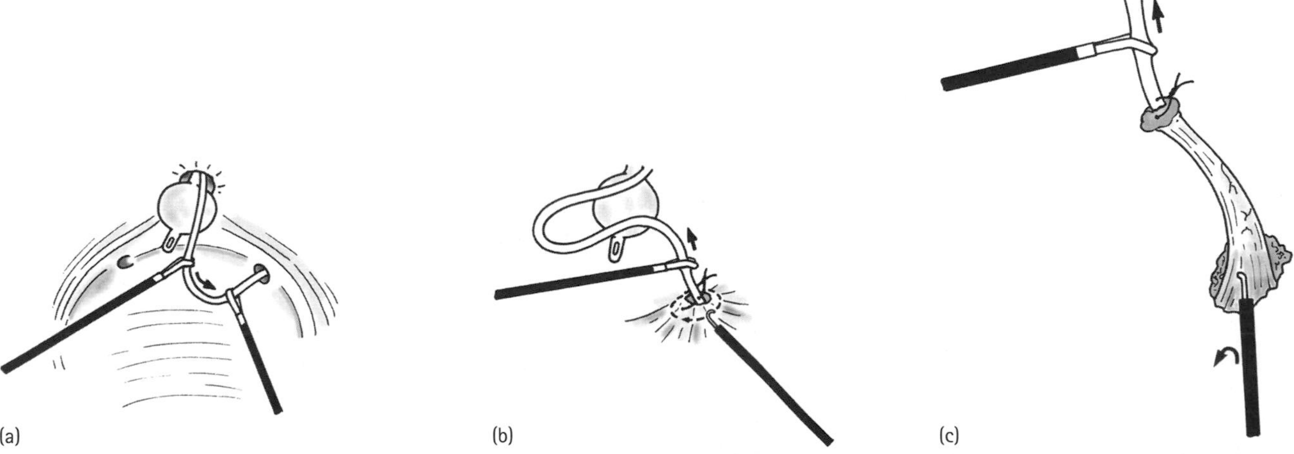

Figure 61.3

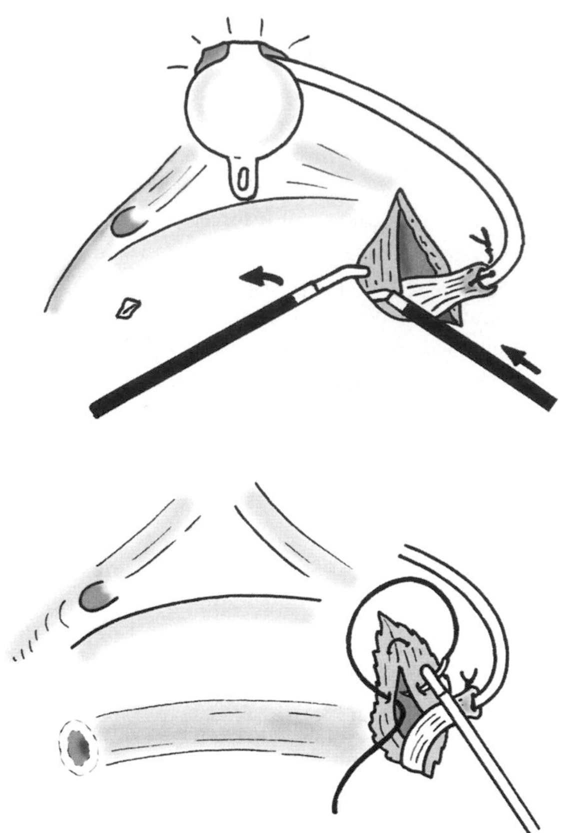

Figure 61.4

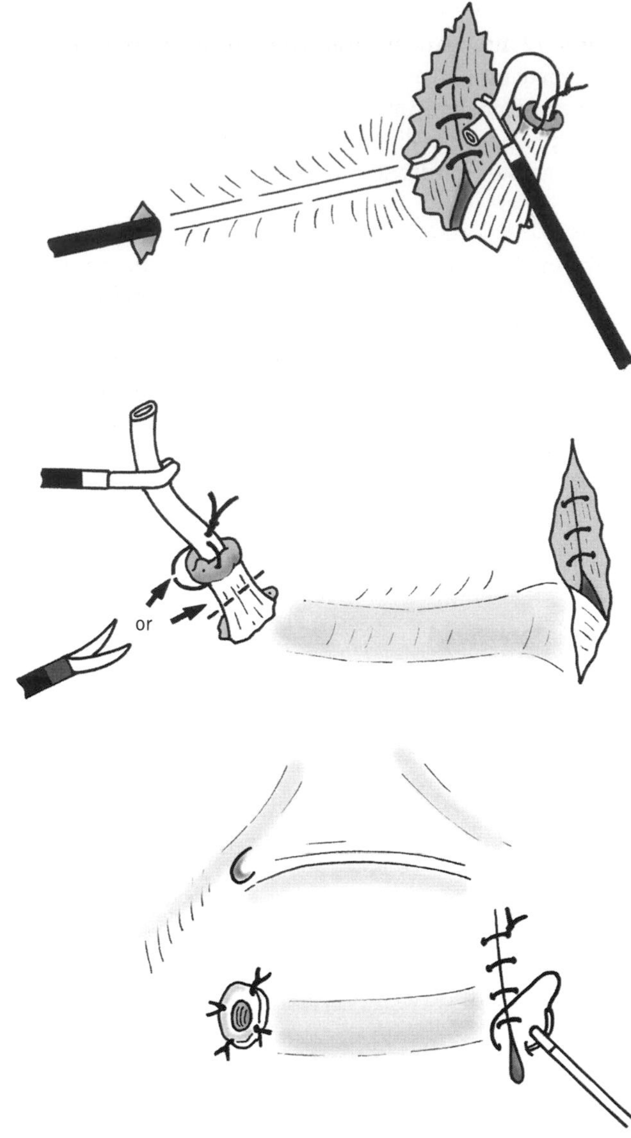

Figure 61.5

sutures. The wounds are infiltrated with appropriate local anesthetic agents and the catheters/stents are connected to an appropriate urine bag. **(See Figure 61.6)**

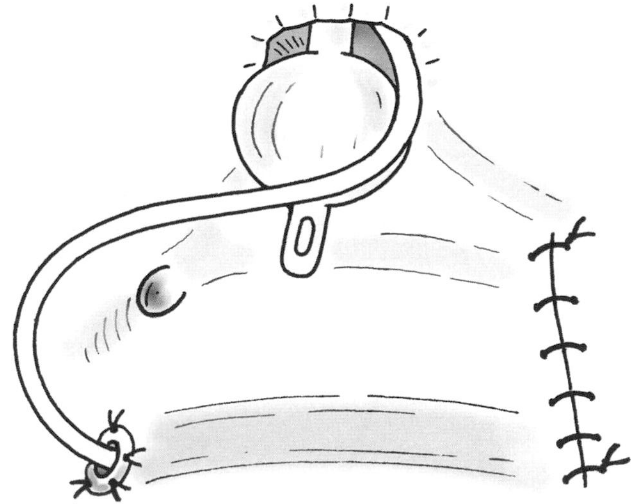

Figure 61.6

POSTOPERATIVE CARE

Oral analgesia with or without antispasmodic agents usually provides adequate postoperative pain relief. Intravenous morphine and/or epidural or caudal analgesia may be required for the first 12 hours postoperatively. The patient is usually ready to leave the hospital 12–24 hours after surgery and is re-admitted as a day patient for removal of the stent and catheter with or without sedation at 5–6 days postoperatively.

PROBLEMS, PITFALLS AND SOLUTIONS

Access

- In the majority of patients who may benefit from laparoscopic re-implantation of the ureter, the bladder is a highly compliant structure. To create a working space safely, first distend the bladder with normal saline to its maximum capacity, then insert and fix both the primary and working cannulae, and finally drain and insufflate the bladder with CO_2 to a pressure of 8–12 mmHg (start insufflation from above while draining the bladder from below).

- Intermittent bladder spasm is more common with direct gas insufflation than it is when saline is used prior to the CO_2 insufflation technique. Antispasmodic agents may be tried.
- Every effort should be made to stay extraperitoneally during insertion of the primary and working cannulae.
  - Distend the bladder to its maximum capacity before insertion of the cannulae.
  - Place the cannulae just inside the palpable margins of the bladder (dome for the primary, lateral for the first and second working cannulae, and suprapubic for additional cannulae).
  - Maintain maximum bladder distension and prevent saline leak by:
    - a single attempt at cannula insertion (avoid multiple stabs),
    - locking the gas port/valves of the cannulae,
    - fixing the cannulae in position immediately.
- In open technique vesicostomy, an over-distended bladder may cause extravasation of saline at the site of the purse-string/hitching sutures and/or primary cannula. The suture bites must be wide and deep; make an effort to stay outside the mucosa, and quickly push the cannula through the purse-string or in between the two hitching sutures and tie the sutures snugly around the cannula.
- Peripherally sited cannulae allow better working space but less direct view/access compared with centrally positioned cannulae, which have the opposite effect (less working space and more direct view).
- Cannulae displacement and extravasation of saline/gas are preventable by:
  - appropriate technique, as described above,
  - using small rather than large cannulae and fixing them in position immediately using either sutures and a rubber cuff, as described above, or self-retaining devices, e.g. balloon and phlange inside and outside respectively.

Mobilization of the ureter

- The balloon of the urethral catheter may obstruct viewing and suturing. Deflate the balloon partially or completely as necessary. Alternatively, use a non-balloon straight plastic tube.
- Per-urethral stenting of the ureter may prove difficult, especially in boys. Use suprapubic access through a needle and peel-away sheath.
- Longer than usual mobilization of the ureter (as in dilated or obstructed ureter) within the confined space of the bladder may prove difficult. An additional cannula and instruments may facilitate wider dissection. **(See Figure 61.7)**

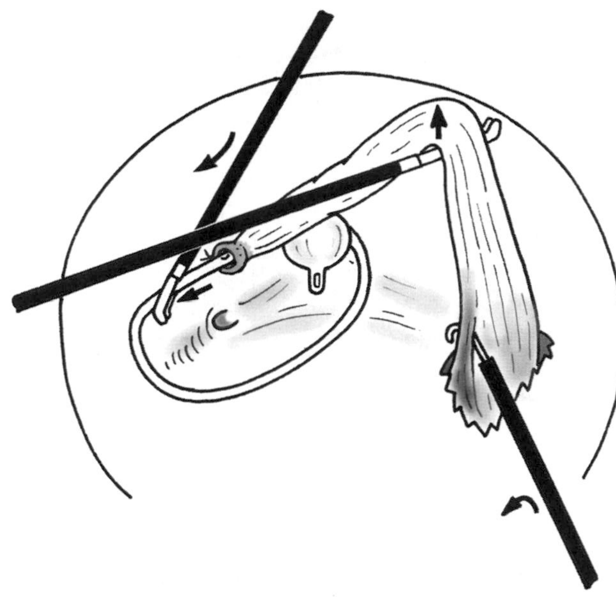

Figure 61.7

Tunneling for the ureter

When tunneling becomes difficult, incise the bladder mucosa, undermine the edges and re-suture once the ureter is fixed in position.

Postoperative drainage

- Per-urethral catheter and ureteric stenting may be difficult, undesirable or inconvenient for the patient.
- The catheter or ureteric stent, or both, may be positioned suprapubically using a needle and peel-away sheath.
- Alternatively, one or more cannula sites are used for the bladder catheter and/or ureteric stents. Here, a straight tube is passed through the cannula under telescopic vision before the actual cannula is removed. Alternatively, a guide-wire is used through the cannula under vision before it is replaced by a drainage/stent tube.

COMPLICATIONS

- Complications of anesthesia, surgery and laparoscopy in general.
- Complications of re-implantation of the ureter in general:
  - injury to the ureter, vas deferens, vagina and rectum,
  - extravasation and herniation (diverticulum) at the site of re-implantation,
  - infection,
  - persistent and/or recurrent reflux or obstruction.

- Extravasation and peri-vesical collection at the site of cannula entry. Use small rather than large cannulae, stay extraperitoneally during cannula insertion, avoid cannula dislodgement, formally close larger cannula sites (open technique cannula insertion and probably any cannula site 5 mm and over) and drain the bladder postoperatively for a few days.

FURTHER READING

Chertin B, DeCaluwe D, Puri P. Endoscopic treatment of primary grade IV and V vesicoureteral reflux in children with subureteral injection of polytetrafluoroethylene. *Journal of Urology* 2003; **169**:1847–9.

Elder JS, Peters CA, Arant BS Jr, Ewalt DH, Hawtrey CE, Hurwitz Rs et al. Pediatric vesicouretral reflux guidelines: panel summary report on the management of primary vesicoureteral reflux in children. *Journal of Urology* 1997; **157**:1846–51.

Elder JS. Guidelines for consideration for surgical repair of vesicoureteral reflux. *Current Opinions in Urology* 2000; **10**:579.

Mouriquand PDE. Surgical treatment of vesicoureteric reflux. In: L Spitz and AG Coran (eds) *Rob and Smith Operative Surgery (Pediatric Surgery)*, 5th eds, pp. 643–53. London: Chapman and Hall, 1995.

62A

Transperitoneal adrenalectomy

AZAD NAJMALDIN AND SATISH K. AGGARWAL

INTRODUCTION

Laparoscopic adrenalectomy has already become a gold standard for selected adult patients. In pediatrics, experience is slowly growing. The advantages related to minimal access are best exemplified by laparoscopic adrenalectomy because the open approach carries the morbidity of a large incision and difficult exposure. This is particularly so in bilateral adrenalectomy. The technique allows for excellent exposure and is suitable for a wide range of conditions, including tumors.

Both, retroperitoneal and transperitoneal approaches have been used for adrenalectomy. This chapter describes the more commonly used transperitoneal approach.

Indications

UNILATERAL ADRENALECTOMY

- Benign functional tumors of the adrenal (up to a few centimeters):
  - cortical adenoma (Cushing's),
  - aldosteronoma,
  - pheochromocytoma.
- Adrenal hyperplasia.
- Adrenal cyst.
- Small neuroblastoma detected on screening.

BILATERAL ADRENALECTOMY

- Adrenal hyperplasia due to failed treatment of pituitary Cushing's disease.
- Ectopic adrenocorticotrophic hormone (ACTH) production that has not responded to medical treatment.
- Bilateral adrenal hyperplasia.
- Bilateral benign tumors and cysts.

Contraindications

ABSOLUTE

- Large, clinically detected neuroblastoma.
- Adrenocortical carcinoma.
- Existing contraindication to laparoscopic surgery.

RELATIVE

- Large, benign, non-cystic adenomas.

EQUIPMENT/INSTRUMENTS

Essential

- Four 3.5–12 mm cannulae.
- 5–10 mm, preferably 30–45°, telescope.
- Two sets of 3.5–5 mm atraumatic curved insulated grasping forceps without ratchet.
- 3.5–5 mm curved double jaw action insulated scissors with diathermy point.
- 3.5–5 mm hook monopolar diathermy.
- 5 mm clip applicator with appropriate clips.
- 3.5–5 mm retractor.

- 3.5–5 mm suction irrigation probe.
- Non-permeable retrieval bag.

Optional

- Additional cannulae and grasping forceps.
- Ultrasound shear, LigaSure™ or plasma kinetic instrument as an alternative to electrocoagulation and clips for controlling small and major vessels.
- Suture to ligate major vessels.

PREOPERATIVE PREPARATION

Preoperative preparation is essentially the same as for open adrenalectomy. Diagnostic evaluation is conducted in consultation with the endocrinologist and/or oncologist. This includes blood and urine hormonal assays and appropriate imaging – ultrasound scan, computerized tomography (CT) or magnetic resonance imaging (MRI) – to assess the nature and size of the lesion and whether there is local invasion or distant metastasis. Patients with Cushing's disease and functional adenomas should receive stress doses of intravenous hydrocortisone. Blood counts, serum electrolytes and blood pressure are monitored and corrected.

An appropriate quantity of blood is cross-matched. Consent is obtained from the patient and parents for both laparoscopic and open surgery in case conversion to an open technique becomes necessary.

TECHNIQUE

The operation is performed under general anesthesia with muscle relaxation. A nasogastric tube may improve exposure, particularly for left adrenalectomy. The patient is positioned in a semi-lateral position (approximately 45°) and appropriately padded and strapped to the table. A lumbar support (break in the table or a soft towel under the dependent loin/lower chest) opens up the flank. The access may be improved further by tilting the table laterally and raising the head end. The surgeon and camera operator stand in front of the patient. A second assistant and the scrub nurse stand opposite. A supine position with lateral tilts and additional cannulae for the second retractor may allow bilateral adrenalectomy. Alternatively, a change of position will be necessary.

A 5–12 mm primary cannula is inserted in the respective hypochondriac region using an open technique. A pneumoperitoneum is created with a flow rate of 0.5–1.0 L/min and pressure of 8–12 mmHg. Following an exploratory laparoscopy, the site, size and number of working cannulae

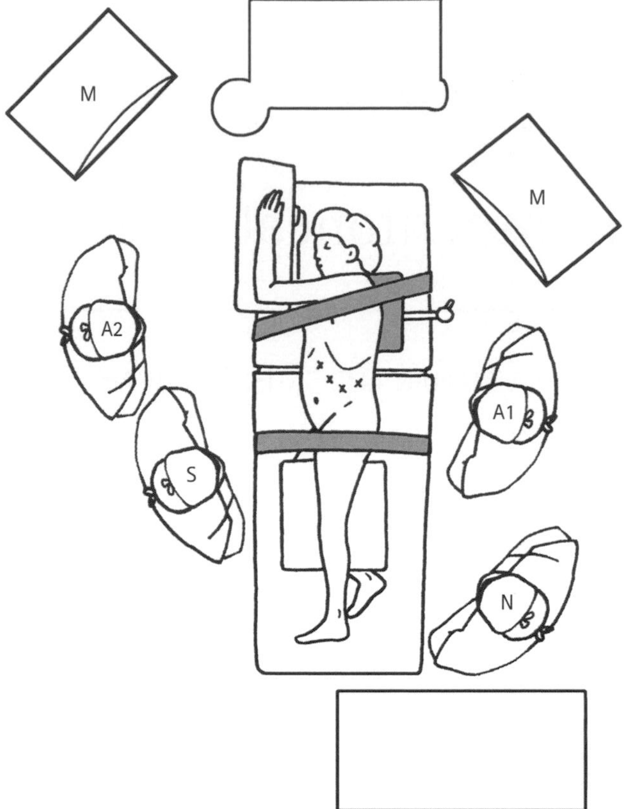

Figure 62A.1

are decided. Three secondary 'working' cannulae are generally necessary, one in the epigastric region and the other two below and lateral to the primary cannula. The retractor may be placed through the epigastric cannula and the other instruments, particularly the telescope, are moved from one cannula to another to improve viewing/access. A fourth working cannula for an additional retractor/instrument may prove helpful. **(See Figure 62A.1)**

Familiarity with normal anatomy and its variations is the key to a safe and successful operation. Adrenals are retroperitoneal organs, embedded in Gerota's fascia and surrounded by retroperitoneal fat. They are highly vascular, with multiple arteries from the aorta, inferior phrenic and renal arteries. Each gland has a single central vein. The right adrenal vein is short and courses medially to drain directly into the inferior vena cava. The left vein is long and runs inferiorly to drain into the left renal vein. Accessory veins may be present on both sides. The right adrenal is pyramidal in shape and sits over the upper pole of the right kidney in direct contact with the diaphragm posteriorly. The anterior surface is crossed by the right triangular ligament of the liver above and the duodenum below. The inferior vena cava forms the immediate medial relation and a portion of the gland lies beneath it. The left gland is flattened and is in intimate contact with the medial surface of the upper pole of the left kidney. Anteriorly, the gland is covered

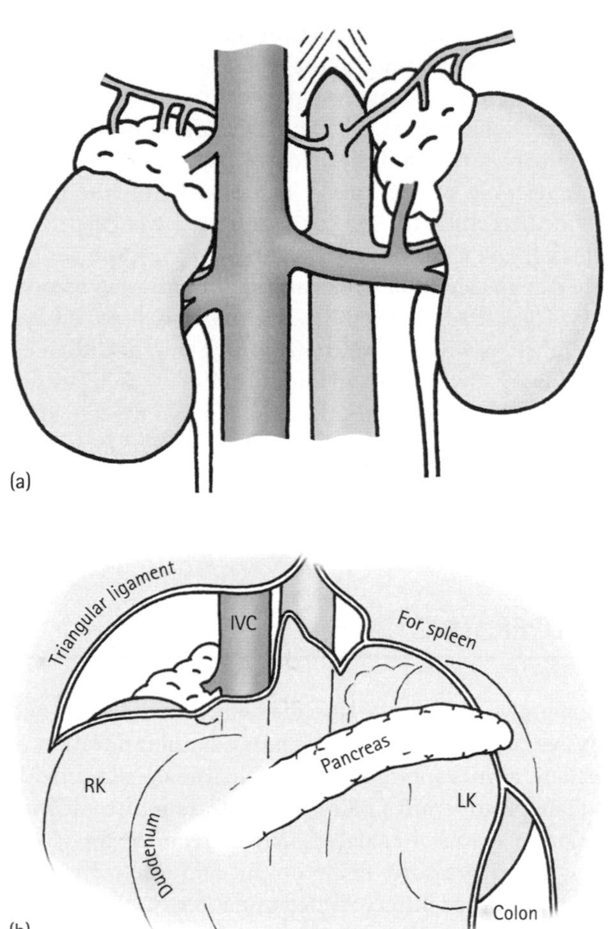

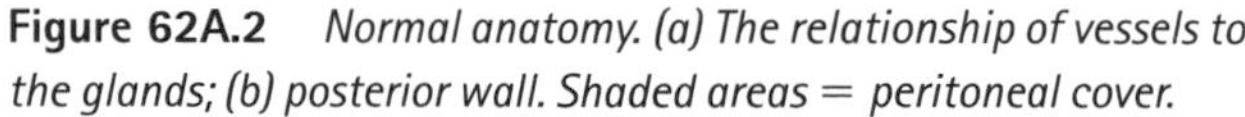

Figure 62A.2 *Normal anatomy. (a) The relationship of vessels to the glands; (b) posterior wall. Shaded areas = peritoneal cover.*

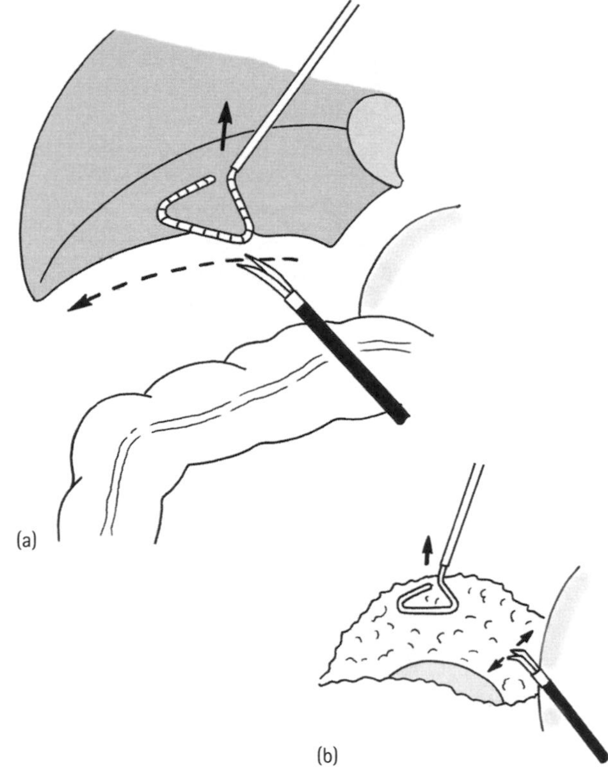

Figure 62A.3

by the omental bursa and spleen above and pancreas below. The left renal vein is close inferiorly and the gland rests on the left crus of the diaphragm posteriorly. **(See Figure 62A.2)**

Right adrenalectomy

The right lobe of liver is retracted cephalad using a retractor through the epigastric cannula. The posterior peritoneum overlying the upper pole of the kidney is incised transversely using scissors and/or diathermy, and the underlying Gerota's fascia is opened. The retractor is then re-positioned within Gerota's fascia and the anterior surface of the gland is exposed. The adrenal gland is easily identifiable by its distinct rich-yellow color and position over the kidney. **(See Figure 62A.3)**

The key step in right adrenalectomy is exploration and secure ligation of the main adrenal vein. Careful dissection is started on the medial border of the gland using a combination of blunt and sharp dissection (atraumatic curved grasper/scissors). The plane between the inferior vena cava and the adrenal is entered and the right adrenal vein is carefully exposed. Excessive retraction and the use of diathermy are avoided. The vein is then clipped – doubly on the vena cava side and singly on the gland side – and divided. Alternatively, the vein is secured using suture ligature, LigaSure™ or plasma kinetic coagulation. An accessory vein, which drains the gland superiorly into the inferior vena cava or the hepatic vein, is found in 20 percent of cases. **(See Figure 62A.4)**

The dissection is continued inferiorly, then superiorly and finally postero-laterally. Connective tissue and small adrenal arteries are secured and divided using monopolar or bipolar diathermy or ultrasound shear. In general, the dissection is kept close to the capsule, and glands containing functional tumors are handled as little as possible. Once the gland has been mobilized, the operative field is checked, hemostasis is ensured and an appropriate-sized non-permeable bag is inserted through the large cannula. The free gland is then placed into the bag and retrieved through the cannula (small glands). The retractors, instruments and cannulae are removed under vision. For large glands, the site of the cannula is extended and both the bag and the cannula are removed in one move. In this situation, the other instruments and working cannulae may be removed under vision first, since the pneumoperitoneum disappears following retrieval of the specimen. Wounds greater than 4 cm are closed in layers. Local anesthetic agents are infiltrated into the wounds. **(See Figure 62A.5)**

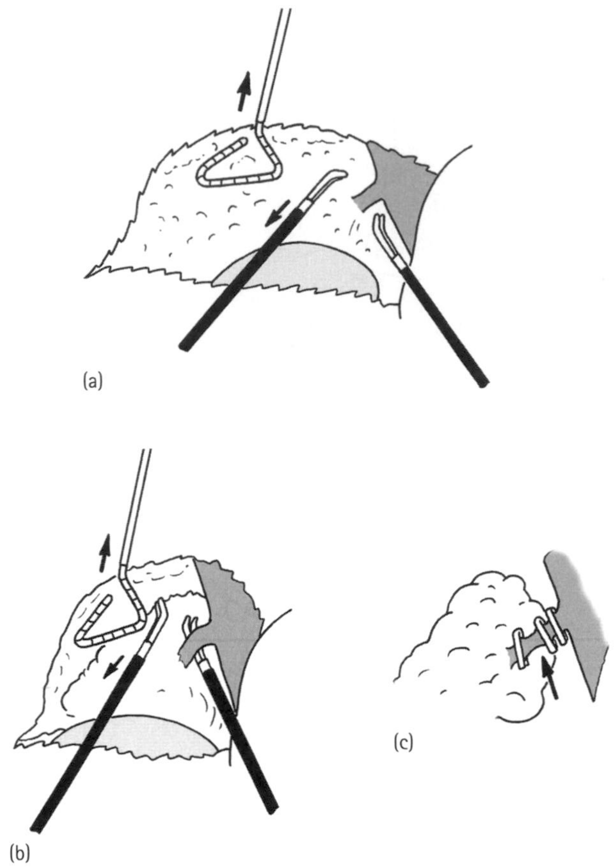

Figure 62A.4

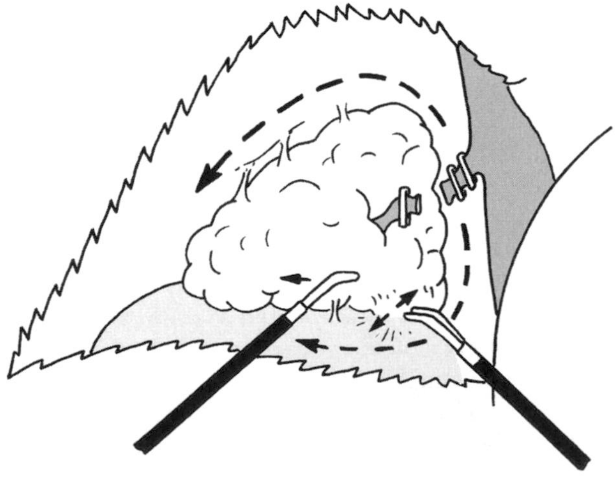

Figure 62A.5

Left adrenalectomy

The first step is complete division of the spleno-renal ligament. This allows the spleen to fall medially under gravity. Sometimes this incision is extended lateral to the splenic flexure. A retractor is then placed through the epigastric cannula and the spleen, its pedicle and the tail of the pancreas are retracted downwards and medially. The left adrenal gland is identified at the medial aspect of the upper pole of the kidney. Using low-power coagulation hook or fine forceps diathermy, the connective tissue between the tail of the pancreas and the splenic hilum on one side and the upper pole of the kidney and adrenal on the other is divided carefully to expose the inferio-medial aspect of the gland. The positions of the retractor, telescope and/or diathermy instruments are changed or readjusted as necessary. The left adrenal vein is visualized and dissected free to its junction with the left renal vein. The vein is divided between two proximal and one distal clips or ligatures. Aberrant phrenic vein may descend and join the left adrenal vein before it drains into the renal vein. This may have to be secured using diathermy coagulation. The remaining part of the procedure is continued as for right adrenalectomy. **(See Figure 62A.6)**

POSTOPERATIVE CARE

Postoperative care can be provided on a general ward, and intensive care is usually not necessary. Local infiltration of anesthetic agents and oral non-steroidal analgesics provide adequate postoperative pain relief. Intravenous morphine infusion or epidural analgesia may be required for 12–24 hours. Blood pressure, urine output and electrolytes are closely monitored and corrected as necessary. Appropriate hormonal replacement is ensured and the patient is watched for acute adrenal crises. Oral feeding is started on the first postoperative day and the patient may be discharged from hospital within a few days, depending on the background condition. Long-term follow-up and hormone replacement therapy, especially after bilateral adrenalectomy, are planned in consultation with the pediatric endocrinologist and/or oncologist.

PROBLEMS, PITFALLS AND SOLUTIONS

Large gland

Access to and around a large gland may prove difficult. Consider the following.

- Further lateral and head tilts to assist gravity.
- Additional cannula for a second retractor or telescope, or an additional working instrument.
- Wider mobilization of the surrounding structures.
- Move the telescope and/or other instruments from one cannula to another.
- Change of position in bilateral adrenalectomy (right semi-lateral for right gland, and vice versa).
- A benign cystic gland may be aspirated prior to mobilization.
- Open surgery.

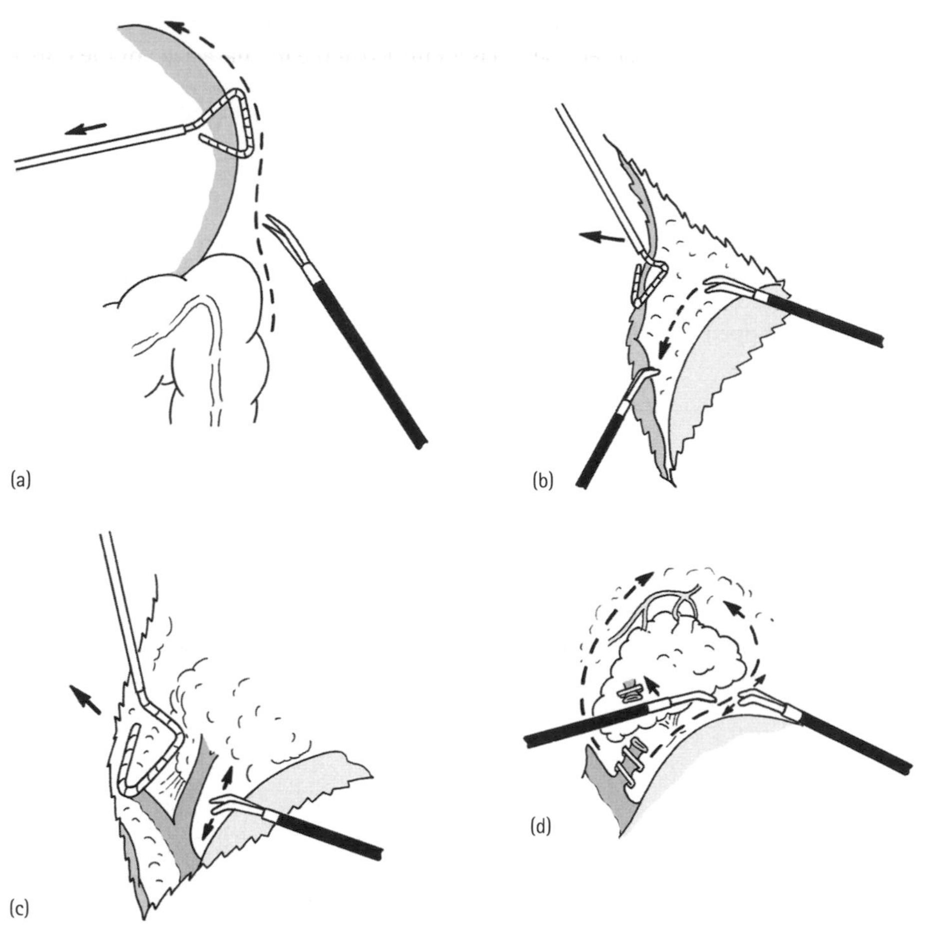

Figure 62A.6

Adhesions around the gland

This may result from previous hemorrhage, surgery or malignant transformation. Careful dissection and low-power diathermy minimize the risk of injury to the surrounding structures. Consider conversion to an open procedure.

Gland extending around major vessels (inferior vena cava, renal, aorta)

Meticulous technique and the need for additional working instruments cannot be over-emphasized.

Short adrenal vein or difficult exposure

Retract the gland away from the inferior vena cava on the right and the renal vein on the left. Effort must be made to divide the vein leaving a reasonable stump attached to the inferior vena cava or renal vein, respectively. The newly devised coagulation instruments (LigaSure™, plasma kinetic) may prove immensely helpful. Alternatively, clip or ligate first and then divide the vein on the surface of the gland, followed by a further coagulation of the bleeding point on the surface of the gland, if necessary. Application of a pre-tied ligature (Endoloop®) to the vein stump adds further security. **(See Figure 62A.7)**

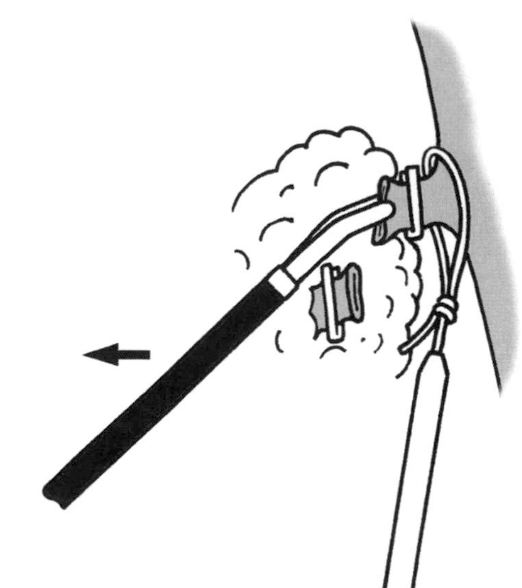

Figure 62A.7

COMPLICATIONS

- Acute hypertensive crises: preoperative and postoperative preparation minimizes the risk.
- Acute adrenal insufficiency in total/subtotal adrenalectomy: continuous adequate supply of steroid peri-operatively is mandatory.
- Bleeding: a rare but potentially serious complication. It often results from difficult dissection at and around the main adrenal vein. Consider conversion to an open procedure expeditiously, especially if the source is inferior vena cava or renal vein.
- Injury to surrounding structures.

FURTHER READING

Najmaldin AS, Aggarwal SK. Laparoscopy in tumors. In Zacharious Z (ed.), *Laparoscopy in Infants and Children – Hospitalisation Laparoscopic Paediatric Surgery*. Heidelburg: Springer-Verlag (CD ROM), 2004.

62B

Extraperitoneal adrenalectomy

ALLAN M. SHANBERG AND GARRETT S. MATSUNAGA

INTRODUCTION

Adrenal pathology is uncommon in children and therefore few large series of laparoscopic adrenalectomies in children have been reported. However, with increasing familiarity with laparoscopic techniques and the development of smaller instruments, laparoscopic adrenalectomy in the pediatric population is rapidly replacing the open technique as the gold standard.

Indications

- Pheochromocytoma: rare, usually associated with MEN-2b and Von Hipple–Lindau disease.
- Aldosteronoma: rare – 15 reported cases to date.
- Primary pigmented nodular adrenocortical disease: a rare cause of Cushing's syndrome, usually occurring as part of the Carney complex. Treatment involves bilateral adrenalectomy.
- Benign adenoma causing Cushing's syndrome.

Contraindications

- Carcinoma or suspected carcinoma: in these situations, the need for more extensive exploration and the risk of tumor spillage preclude the use of laparoscopy.
- Neuroblastoma: although this is the most common pediatric adrenal tumor, the majority of adrenal tumors are large and advanced at the time of surgery. However, localized stage I/II neuroblastoma is not considered to be a contraindication to laparoscopic adrenalectomy.

Both the intraperitoneal and retroperitoneal laparoscopic approaches to the adrenal gland share the benefits of decreased postoperative pain and morbidity, reduced hospital stay and cosmetic advantage compared to open adrenalectomy. In our experience, avoiding the peritoneal cavity by utilizing a retroperitoneal approach has several additional advantages over the transperitoneal approach. Postoperative shoulder-tip pain and other symptoms of diaphragmatic and peritoneal irritation from carbon dioxide insufflation are virtually eliminated. Intra-abdominal adhesions from previous abdominal surgery are avoided and new adhesions are not created. Analgesic requirements after surgery are decreased with the retroperitoneal approach. Most transperitoneal adrenalectomy techniques describe mobilization of the colon to expose the adrenal gland. In our experience with both techniques, eliminating this step reduces the risk of bowel injury or perforation, shortens operative time and decreases the incidence of postoperative ileus. Lastly, the scant amount of peri-renal fat in children improves visualization and eases dissection, making them ideal candidates for a retroperitoneal approach.

The combination of the above benefits translates into a shorter hospital stay and convalescence for the retroperitoneal approach. In addition to medical cost savings, children return to their daily activities faster or may commence postoperative chemotherapeutic regimens sooner.

The difficulties of creating an adequate retroperitoneal space can be reduced using either commercially available or 'home-made' retroperitoneal dissecting balloons. In fact, much of the initial dissection is completed once the balloon is inflated in the retroperitoneum. Commercially available dissecting balloons should be used with caution in the pediatric population, as they seem to tear the peritoneum easily.

The location of the right adrenal vein high under the inferior vena cava limits the visualization and dissection of the right adrenal vasculature. For this reason, right-sided laparoscopic adrenalectomy is somewhat easier using a transperitoneal approach, although we have had success with the retroperitoneal technique. Occasionally, conversion from an extraperitoneal to a transperitoneal approach is necessary.

EQUIPMENT/INSTRUMENTS

Essential

- 5 mm and 10 mm 30° angled telescopic lens.
- 10 mm self-retaining Hasson trocar.
- Two 3.5 mm trocars.
- One or two 5 mm trocars.
- 3.5 mm laparoscopic cautery scissors.
- 3.5 mm laparoscopic grasping forceps.
- 5 mm laparoscopic clip applicator.
- Harmonic Scalpel® (5 mm).

Optional

- Laparoscopic sac.
- LigaSure™ bipolar electrocautery device (5 mm).
- Fan retractor (5 mm).
- Suction irrigator (5 mm).

PREOPERATIVE PREPARATION

It is important in the work-up for an adrenal tumor to determine if the patient has a pheochromocytoma. In this situation, alpha-blockade should be commenced 2 weeks prior to surgery and short-acting beta-blockade 24 hours prior to surgery. These measures combined with volume expansion and a well-informed anesthesiologist will avoid complications from an adrenergic crisis.

TECHNIQUE

After the induction of general anesthesia with endotracheal intubation and muscle relaxation, an orogastric tube and urethral catheter are placed. Nitrous oxide should be avoided by the anesthesiologist to prevent bowel distension.

Patient positioning

The patient is placed in the flank position with the kidney rest elevated and the table in full flexion. This maximizes the space between the costal margin and the iliac crest. A beanbag is used to secure the older child in this position, whereas towel rolls taped in place may suffice for a younger child. When positioning the smaller patient in the right lateral flexed position, care must be taken not to compress the vena cava, which could result in hypotension. Lastly, axillary rolls and padding between the legs and beneath the downside bony prominences should be used as appropriate. **(See Figure 62B.1)**

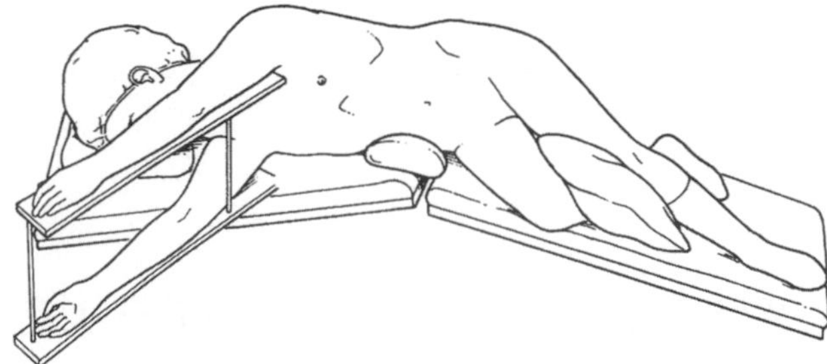

Figure 62B.1

Entering the retroperitoneum

- Right-side tumor: mid-axillary line below the costal margin.
- Left-side tumor: mid-axillary line above the iliac crest.

A 10 mm incision is made in the mid-axillary line below the costal margin or above the iliac crest for a right-sided or left-sided approach, respectively. Tonsil clamps are carefully advanced under direct vision in a muscle-spreading fashion into the retroperitoneal space. Directing the tip of the clamp posteriorly towards the quadratus lumborum muscle reduces the risk of injury to the peritoneum and its contents. Psoas muscle fat should be clearly seen. After developing the tract by spreading the clamps widely, the space between Gerota's fascia and the psoas fascia is developed further by blunt digital dissection. The incision should easily accommodate the fifth finger if the surgeon's index finger is too large. Sweeping a finger along the anterior surface of the quadratus lumborum and psoas muscles minimizes the risk of opening the peritoneum inadvertently.

Creation of the retroperitoneal working space

A 'home-made' retroperitoneal balloon dissecting catheter can be made by tying the end of the middle finger of a No. 8 rubber Triflex orthopedic glove to the end of an 18 Fr red rubber catheter. The catheter is advanced into the retroperitoneum and then filled with 50–300 mL of ice-cold saline, depending on the size of the patient. **(See Table 62B.1)**

The balloon dissector is left inflated for 5 minutes to develop the retroperitoneal space and tamponade any small

Table 62B.1 *Retroperitoneal balloon dissection guide*

Patient age (years)	Patient weight (kg)	Amount of ice-cold saline (mL)
<1	<10	50–100
1–3	10–15	100–200
4–10	20–30	200–300
10–14	30–50	300–400
>14	>50	400–500

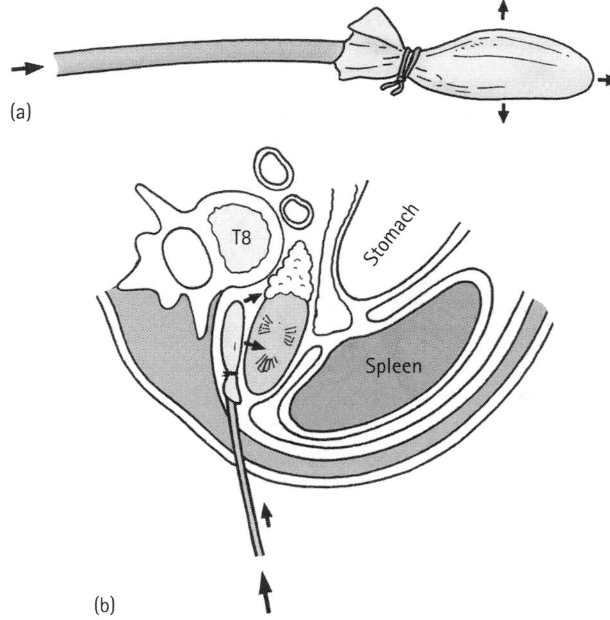

Figure 62B.2

bleeding vessels. The fingertip of the glove adapts to the contour of the retroperitoneum, which seems to result in improved dissection and less trauma. In our experience, the incidence of inadvertent peritoneal laceration using this 'home-made' dissector is considerably less than with the commercial retroperitoneal dilators used in adults. Additionally, the reduced cost of using this 'home-made' dissector makes it preferable to other commercially available models. **(See Figure 62B.2)**

Trocar placement

Once the balloon dissector has been deflated and removed, a 10 mm Hasson self-retaining balloon trocar is introduced into the retroperitoneal space through the initial incision. Sealing the tract between the inner balloon and the outer foam cuff decreases subcutaneous emphysema. Insufflation with CO_2 to a pressure of 12–14 mmHg is maintained. Two working trocars are introduced under direct vision in the anterior and posterior axillary lines approximately midway between the costal margin and iliac crest. We choose to use a 3.5 mm and a 5 mm trocar, placing the 5 mm port where

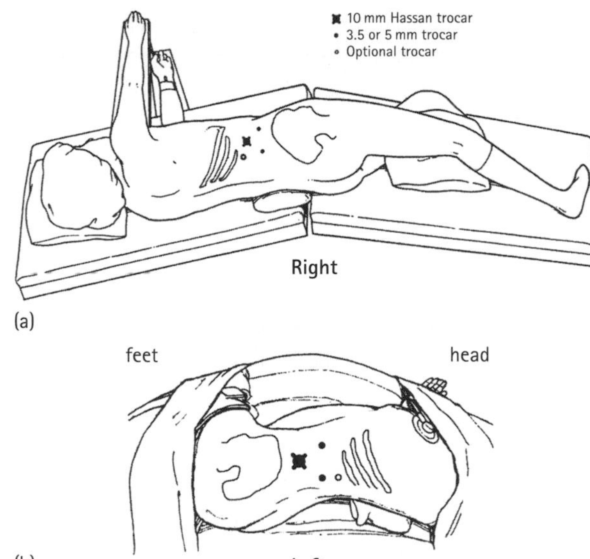

Figure 62B.3

the Harmonic Scalpel® will be used. A 5 mm camera is placed through the 10 mm Hasson trocar. An optional fourth 5 mm trocar can be placed superior to the most posterior port, through which a retractor can be inserted to retract either the spleen or the liver. **(See Figure 62B.3)**

The surgeon faces the patient's back, with the camera assistant on the opposite side of the table. As with all laparoscopic surgery, the camera and surgeon should be facing the same direction to avoid operating 'backwards'. Occasionally, with larger adolescent patients, it is more comfortable for the surgeon and camera assistant to work facing the patient's front.

Creating adequate exposure in the retroperitoneum

The peritoneum is carefully separated off Gerota's fascia with both blunt and Harmonic Scalpel® dissection. Gerota's fascia is opened widely and posteriorly. On the right side, the attachments behind and lateral to the liver are divided, while on the left, the spleno-renal ligaments are released. These critical maneuvers release the liver and spleen, respectively, allowing them to be retracted cephalad to create an adequate exposure.

Locating the adrenal gland

Using the Harmonic Scalpel® (or cautery scissors) and a grasping clamp, the quadratus lumborum and psoas muscles are exposed to use as the initial landmark. Regardless of side, Gerota's fascia must be opened to identify the kidney. Continue to dissect Gerota's fascia superiorly off the upper pole of the kidney until the adrenal gland is identified.

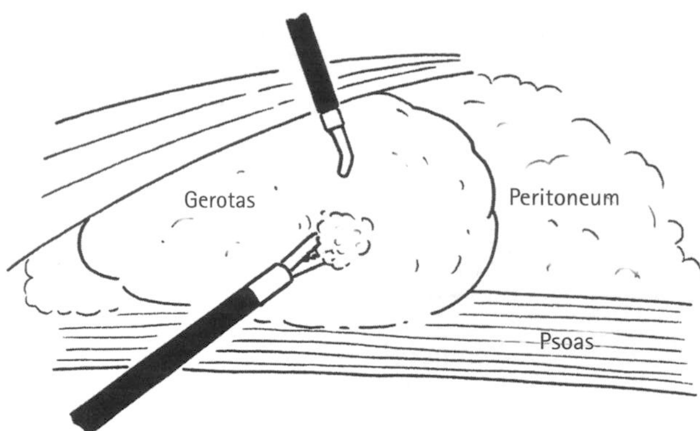

Figure 62B.4 *Retroperitoneal approach. Posterior aspect of the right kidney and gland.*

Care should be taken to avoid the tail of the pancreas on the left. (**See Figure 62B.4**)

Excision of adrenal gland

If a pheochromocytoma is suspected, early identification and ligation of the adrenal vein should be performed with minimal manipulation of the adrenal gland.

For a right-side tumor, the vena cava is identified medial and superior to the kidney. Dissection is carried up the vena cava utilizing a small, 5 mm, fan retractor to lift the liver and peritoneum and facilitate exposure. The right adrenal vein is very short and must be dissected very carefully where it inserts into the inferior vena cava. The adrenal vein should be triple clipped proximally and double clipped distally. It is extremely important that this step is completed first, as avulsion of the adrenal vein can easily occur during dissection and traction of the right adrenal gland. Once the vein is controlled, the remainder of the gland is dissected free, securing hemostasis of the phrenic and aortic adrenal vessels with the Harmonic Scalpel®. The arterial supply to the adrenal gland comprises three small vessels arising from the aorta, renal artery and phrenic arteries. These should be cauterized with the Harmonic Scalpel® if small or clipped if larger.

On the left side, the left adrenal vein drains into the left renal vein. If needed, a fan retractor can be used to retract the spleen cephalad. (**See Figure 62B.5**)

Removal of the adrenal gland

The adrenal gland is placed into an entrapment sac inserted through the 10 mm port. A 5 mm camera is introduced into one of the working ports and the 10 mm Hasson trocar is removed. The adrenal gland is then grasped with heavy forceps or removed in the entrapment bag under direct visualization through the 10 mm skin incision. The Hasson trocar is replaced and the pneumoretroperitoneum re-established to ensure or gain hemostasis. The working ports are all removed under direct vision and the skin sites closed with subcuticular sutures. The 10 mm site is closed in two layers: the fascia with 3-0 Vicryl® suture and the skin with subcuticular suture.

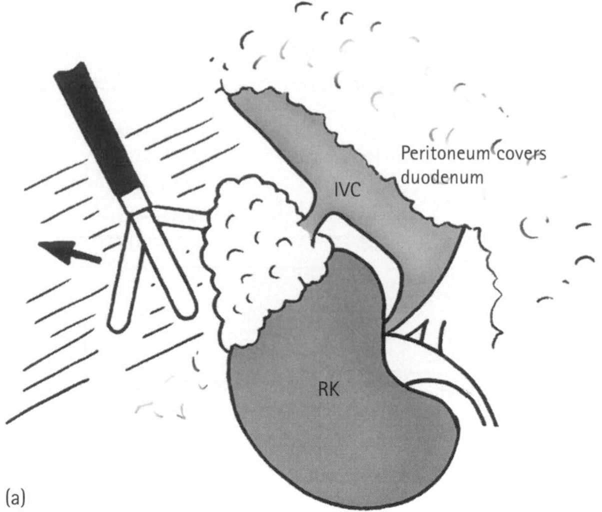

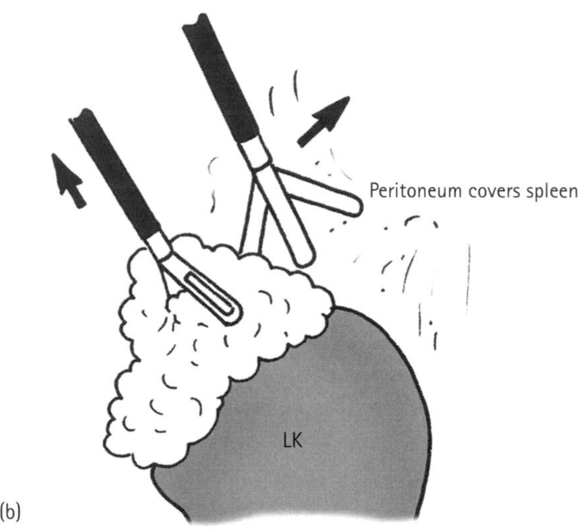

Figure 62B.5 *Posterior aspect of the glands. (a) Right; (b) left.*

POSTOPERATIVE CARE

The trocar sites are infiltrated with 0.5 percent bupivacaine, and a single dose of ketorolac (0.5 mg/kg) is administered prior to awakening the patient. The orogastric tube and urethral catheter are removed prior to extubation. Children can be discharged home later the same day, or early the next morning if surgery starts late in the day. Patients who have had a bilateral adrenalectomy or for whom open conversion has been necessary are admitted for observation overnight. Children rarely require more than acetaminophen or ibuprofen for analgesia.

Parents are instructed to keep children at home with limited activity for 2–3 days. After this, they can resume full activity and school. Sports participation may be resumed 2 weeks postoperatively.

PROBLEMS, PITFALLS AND SOLUTIONS

Inadequate visualization

- Ensure the patient is properly positioned in full flexion with kidney rest elevated. This opens up the space between the costal margin and iliac crest.
- Use finger dissection along the quadratus, and then balloon dissection, and avoid entering the peritoneum.
- Using a 5 mm camera rather than a 10 mm camera through the 10 mm Hasson trocar decreases 'cluttering' of the retroperitoneal space with instruments.
- Use retractors to displace the liver or spleen via the fourth optional port.

Loss of pneumoretroperitoneum

- Check to ensure there is no leak between the trocar and skin.
- Use a reducer if placing a 5 mm instrument/camera through the 10 mm port.
- Ensure vents on trocars are closed.
- Look for a peritoneal tear.

Peritoneal laceration

A small peritoneal tear will function as a one-way valve, expanding the peritoneum at the expense of the retroperitoneal space. In this circumstance the peritoneal opening should be widened to prevent ball-valve expansion of the pneumoperitoneum. A further trocar can be placed to introduce a retractor to hold the peritoneal contents away from the field of dissection.

Locating the adrenal gland

Regardless of side, the easiest and most reliable way to locate the adrenal gland is to locate the superior pole of the ipsilateral kidney first. Carefully dissecting Gerota's fascia while advancing along the superior pole of the kidney will lead one to the adrenal gland.

Pheochromocytoma

The best way to avoid the complications of hormonal surges during intra-operative adrenal manipulation is to perform a thorough preoperative evaluation. Knowing if the adrenal tumor is hormonally active allows for optimal preoperative preparation (i.e. alpha or beta blockade), anticipation of complications of anesthesia, and proper surgical technique (i.e. early renal vein ligation).

COMPLICATIONS

Bowel injury (especially in smaller children)

Although we have never seen an injury to bowel, there are several theoretical areas where this may occur. Electrocautery along the peritoneum should be used with caution, as spread of current to bowel on the opposite side could injure bowel serosa, resulting in delayed bowel perforation. For this reason, we prefer to use the Harmonic Scalpel® for dissection. Injury to bowel from trocar placement should not occur with open placement of the Hasson trocar and placement of the remaining trocars under direct vision.

If a bowel injury is suspected, another trocar can be placed intraperitoneally to explore the bowel and repair it laparoscopically if indicated. Open exploration and repair remains an option.

Hemorrhage

Bleeding is often encountered during dissecting around the adrenal gland. With the use of the Harmonic Scalpel®, small tributaries to the adrenal are sealed, decreasing bleeding. Other techniques to control bleeding include:

- argon beam coagulator – it is important to open vents while using this device to prevent complications such as pneumothorax,
- oxidized regenerated cellulose (Surgicell®) – this can be welded to tissue with the argon beam coagulator,
- gelatin-based matrix and thrombin solution (Floseal®),
- 5 mm LigaSure™ is excellent to control the adrenal vein.

Open conversion

Conversion to an open procedure should not be considered a failure on the part of the surgeon. Rather, it demonstrates wise judgment when it is consistent with the best interests of the patient.

FURTHER READING

Castillo LN. Laparoscopic adrenal surgery in children. *Journal of Urology* 2002; **168** (1):221–4.

Shanberg AM. Laparoscopic retroperitoneal renal and adrenal surgery in children. *British Journal of Urology* 2001; **87**(6):521–4.

63

Intersex

JOHN M. HUTSON AND CHRIS KIMBER

INTRODUCTION

Laparoscopy has limited use in intersex patients, many of whom are diagnosed without direct visualization of the internal genitals. Congenital adrenal hyperplasia, for example, rarely needs laparoscopy, as the internal genitalia are normal (as confirmed on ultrasonography) and reconstruction of the external genitalia is done via the perineum. There are, however, a number of clear situations in which laparoscopy is indicated.

Indications

- Diagnosis of intra-abdominal anatomy when this is in doubt.
- Biopsy or excision of dysplastic gonads containing Y chromosomes.
- Excision of internal genital ducts as a single procedure or as part of an abdomino-perineal reconstruction.

Diagnosis of internal genital anatomy

This is required in patients in whom chromosomal analysis shows the presence of a Y chromosome, as seen in a range of (mostly rare) conditions. This is because normal or dysplasic gonads containing the Y chromosome have a variable degree of testicular differentiation and a propensity to undergo progressive dysplasia, possibly related to the intra-abdominal temperature (37 °C). **(See Table 63.1)**

Table 63.1 *Y chromosome-containing conditions*

Condition	Karyotype	Pelvic anatomy
CAIS/PAIS	46XY	Testes in pelvis/inguinal hernia, absent vas deferens and uterus
Mixed gonadal dysgenesis	45X0/46XY	One testis (dysplastic) and vas, one streak and uterine tube
Ullrich–Turner	45X0/46XY	Turner phenotype but streak gonads contain some Y cells
True hermaphrodite	XX/XY	Testis + ovary
	XX	Testis + ovotestis
	Intragonadal mosaicism	Ovotestis + ovotestis
	Intragonadal mosaicism	Ovary + ovotestis
Pure gonadal dysgenesis	46XY	Streak gonads and female internal ducts
Persistent Mullerian duct syndrome	46XY	Testes plus both male and female ducts

CAIS, complete androgen insensitivity syndrome; PAIS, partial androgen insensitivity syndrome.

Androgen insensitivity syndrome

Androgen insensitivity is caused by an X-linked mutation in the androgen receptor, making the target tissues more or less insensitive to circulating androgens. It is the most common cause of male pseudohermaphroditism in which genetic males (46XY) with testes do not have a normal male phenotype. In the complete form of androgen insensitivity syndrome (CAIS), the androgen receptor is non-functional and the external genitals are unambiguously female, and the vagina is short and blind ending. Both Mullerian and Wolffian ducts are absent. Secondary sex characteristics are normal female apart from the absence of pubic and axillary hair, as testosterone is converted in peripheral tissues into 17-beta-estradiol.

Patients with CAIS may present early in childhood as females with inguinal hernia or, more commonly, as adolescents with primary amenorrhea.

A small percentage of AIS patients have a less severe mutation of the androgen receptor, leading to partial insensitivity (PAIS), and external ambiguity because of partial virilization. The Mullerian ducts are absent (Mullerian inhibitory substance is functioning normally), but the Wolffian ducts are partly preserved (the epididymis and proximal vas deferens).

Laparoscopy is not always needed for the diagnosis of CAIS to be made, as the testis is usually found within the inguinal hernia, and absence of the vas deferens confirms the diagnosis. In patients having laparoscopic herniotomy, the presence of testes and the absence of a uterus will indicate the anomaly. If the diagnosis has been made preoperatively (chromosome or testosterone analysis, pelvic ultrasound or rectal examination fails to identify a cervix), gonadectomy can be performed at the time of herniotomy. Alternatively, where a testis is found unexpectedly in a hernial sac, it is better to biopsy the gonads to confirm the diagnosis and replace it in the abdomen. Laparoscopy can be undertaken at a later date to perform bilateral gonadectomy and confirm the internal genital anatomy. **(See Figure 63.1)**

In PAIS, laparoscopy may aid diagnosis, although the gonads are usually located in labioscrotal folds, and the status of the internal anatomy can be confirmed by ultrasound or magnetic resonance imaging (MRI).

Mixed gonadal dysgenesis

In mixed gonadal dysgenesis the karyotype is commonly 45XO/46XX, but other patterns have been described. The mosaicism is usually expressed to a different extent in each urogenital ridge, leading to gonadal and genital duct asymmetry. In the commonest variant, one gonad is testicular (with an accompanying vas deferens) and the other is an undifferentiated streak gonad (with adjacent Mullerian duct structures).

Laparoscopy is useful in mixed gonadal dysgenesis to confirm the internal anatomy, as well as to remove one or other genital structures, depending on the gender of rearing.

True hermaphroditism

The external genitalia are often asymmetrical and a number of chromosomal arrangements occur, although the commonest is 46XX.

Laparoscopy will reveal the retained ovary or ovotestis, allowing a management plan to be formed. One of the common varieties shows an intra-abdominal left ovary and female genital tract (round ligament, hemi-uterus and tube and ovarian vessels). On the other side, the vas deferens and gonadal vessels may disappear through the internal inguinal ring. Gonadal excision or other procedure (e.g. orchidopexy) will depend on the gender chosen for rearing. **(See Figure 63.2)**

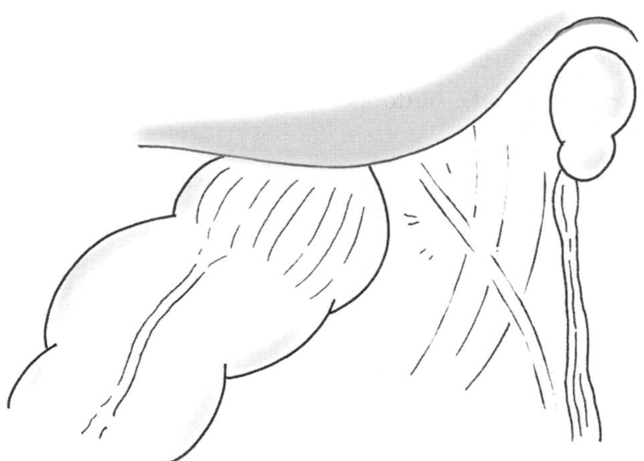

Figure 63.1

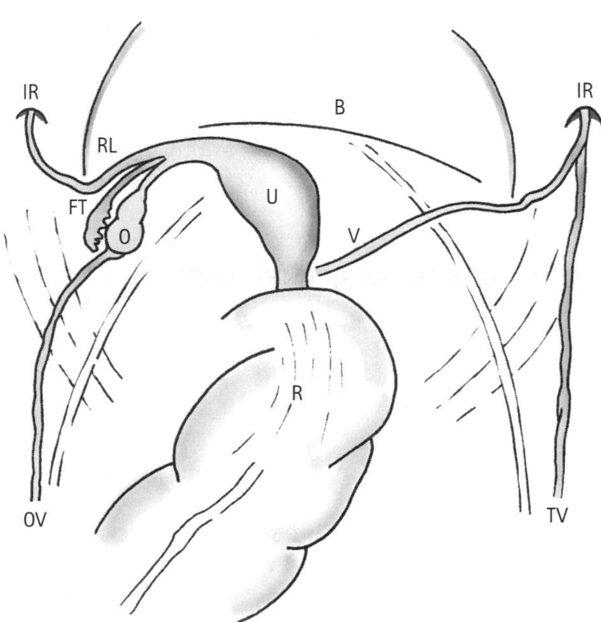

Figure 63.2

Pure gonadal dysgenesis

These children usually present in adolescence with failure of pubertal development, as the appearance at birth is unambiguously female. Gonadectomy is required for the prevention of malignancy, and puberty is induced by hormone treatment. The internal genitalia are feminine because of an absence of testosterone and Mullerian inhibition substance, so pregnancy is possible by in-vitro fertilization of a donor egg from a female relative.

Persistent Mullerian duct syndrome

This rare form of genital anomaly presents with normal male external genitalia with either impalpable testes or a hernia ipsilateral to an impalpable testis (hernia uteri inguinalis). Endoscopy provides an excellent way of documenting the location of the gonads as well as of identifying and/or removing the retained Mullerian ducts (hypoplastic uterus and Fallopian tubes).

Biopsy/excision of gonads

Gonadal biopsy should be performed in any situation in which the diagnosis remains uncertain despite all other investigations. Where the gonad is heterogeneous, the possibility of true hermaphroditism or secondary tumor (gonadoblastoma or malignant seminoma) should be considered, and multiple biopsies with frozen section may be needed. In true hermaphroditism, the gonad may contain adjacent ovarian and testicular tissue forming an ovotestis: the ovarian tissue may be at one or both poles with testicular tissue between. To avoid missing the diagnosis, a longitudinal wedge biopsy should be taken.

Excision of gonads is required where there is gonadal tissue discordant with the gender of rearing, intra-abdominal gonadal tissue containing a Y chromosome. Undifferentiated streak gonads are excised easily, as their blood supply is very meager and can be diathermied. More substantial gonads or gonadal tumors need formal ligation of the gonadal vessels.

Excision of internal genital ducts

Laparoscopic excision of the genital ducts is required for children with female internal ducts who are being raised as males (e.g. with intersex conditions such as mixed gonadal dysgenesis and true hermaphroditism with unilateral Mullerian duct retention, and persisting Mullerian duct syndrome with bilateral duct retention). Also, there are some males with androgenic dysfunction in whom there is a remnant of the urogenital sinus (primitive vagina).

In children being raised as females, laparoscopic removal of Wolffian duct remnants may be required, as in some true hermaphrodites.

EQUIPMENT/INSTRUMENTS

Essential

- Three 3.5–12 mm cannulae, with appropriate reducers as required.
- 3.5 mm or 10 mm 30° angled telescope.
- 3.5–5 mm curved, insulated scissors with diathermy connection.
- Two pairs of 3.5–5 mm atraumatic grasping forceps, one with a ratchet.
- Fine 3.5–5 mm hook monopolar and bipolar diathermy.
- 3.5–5 mm suction/irrigation device.
- 5 mm clip applicator or Endoloop® sutures.
- 3.5 mm or 5 mm needle holder.

Optional

- 3-0 or 4-0 atraumatic suture for transabdominal retraction of the bladder.

PREOPERATIVE PREPARATION

Adequate preoperative imaging and molecular diagnosis are the main preoperative steps. Ultrasonography will determine the presence of a uterus or hemi-uterus in most cases, although MRI is useful if in doubt. More important is the determination of the presence or absence of the urogenital sinus (remnant of the lower vagina): retrograde urogenital sinugram and/or urethroscopy are the best investigations. Where any uncertainty persists, urethroscopy at the start of the operation will resolve the issue. However, recognition and interpretation of normal anatomy and its variations require surgical and radiological expertise.

TECHNIQUE

Under general anesthesia, the patient is positioned supine. A pad under the buttocks is often helpful to elevate the pelvis. In babies, a cross-table position is advantageous, with the lower legs dangling over the edge. A crossbar over the head protects the anesthetic apparatus and access to the airway by the anesthetist, but allows the surgeon to stand at the patient's head. The relative positions of the anesthetist and nurse depend on the handedness of the surgeon. The patient should be prepared with antiseptic to include the entire abdomen and genitalia, as well as the upper thighs. The passage of a urinary catheter ensures the bladder is completely empty. **(See Figure 63.3)**

A supra-umbilical incision and Hasson technique (open technique laparoscopy) allow insertion of the telescope

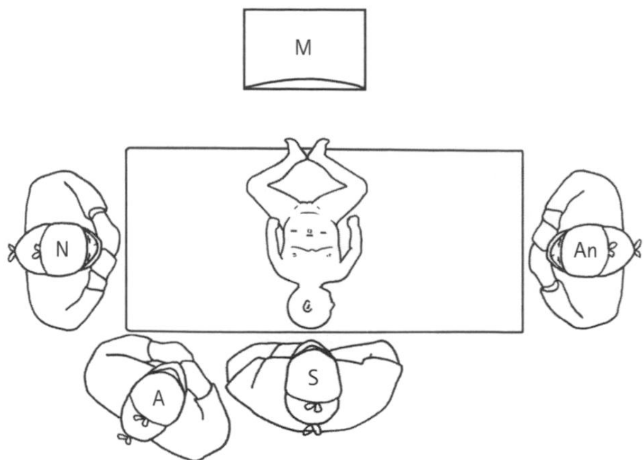

Figure 63.3

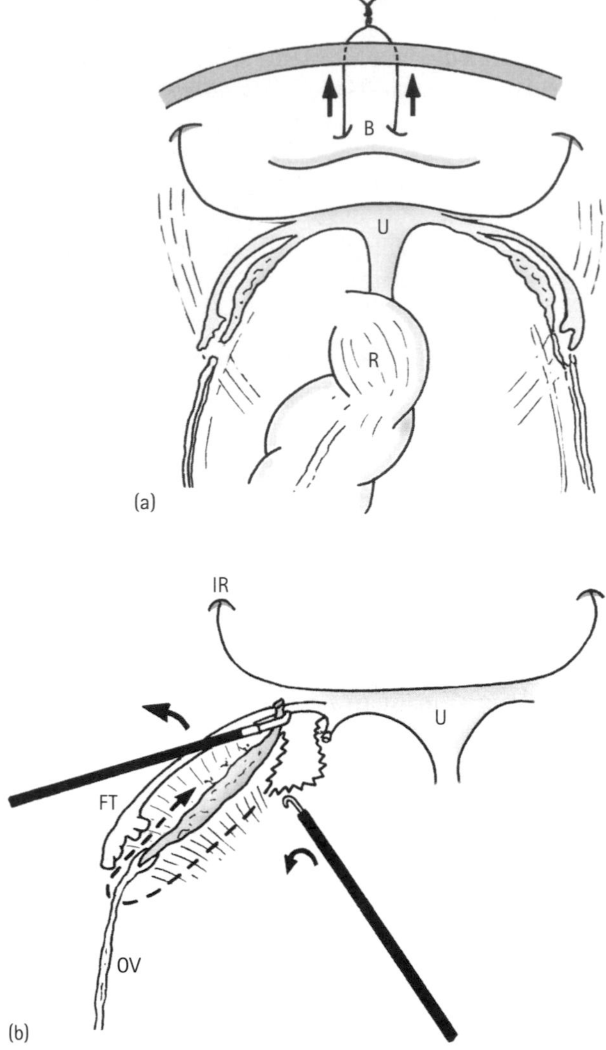

Figure 63.4

(primary) port and creation of a pneumoperitoneum. Two working ports are established, one each side of the umbilicus. In babies they are better placed higher in the epigastrium, although in older patients this is not necessary.

The table should be tilted to place the baby in the Trendelenburg (head-down) position to facilitate exploration of the pelvic viscera. If the bladder is obscuring the pelvic organs, it can be lifted out of the way by a transabdominal suture passed through the lower abdomen that picks up its wall.

Inspection of the internal genitalia will reveal whether a streak gonad or ovotestis is present, and the status of the genital ducts.

If a uterus is present, it is picked up with the grasping forceps at its fundus to reveal the relative positions of the streak gonad and primitive Fallopian tube.

A streak gonad usually runs close to the Fallopian tube, with its medial and lateral ends almost inseparable from the uterus and fimbriated end of the tube, respectively. The gonad can be grasped with the other instrument; a ratchet allows the position to be maintained. Excision of a streak gonad can be performed with diathermy hook, scissors and diathermy, or bipolar diathermy. Clips or sutures are often not needed for the gonadal vessels, as these are usually hypoplastic. If the vessels are more substantial, a clip or Endoloop® can be used. One must take care not to damage the uterus and its vessels medially, the Fallopian tube anteriorly, and the fimbriated end and ureter laterally.

When the streak gonads are removed in girls with Ullrich–Turner syndrome (which contain a Y chromosome), the Fallopian tube can be preserved to allow the maximum flexibility for subsequent assisted reproduction. **(See Figure 63.4)**

If an ovotestis is identified with adequate distinction between the ovarian and testicular tissue (one pole of the gonad has a spherical testicular appearance, while the other pole appears ovarian), a hemi-gonadectomy is possible. A right ovotestis with a left ovary is a relatively common circumstance in patients with true hermaphroditism. Excision of the testicular half of the gonad is straightforward. **(See Figure 63.5)**

The gonad is likely partially to descend through the internal inguinal ring when testicular tissue is present. Traction on the vessels and internal ducts delivers the gonad back into the peritoneal cavity. Partial or total unilateral gonadectomy is carried out using fine-hook diathermy, depending on the degree of delineation. Complete gonadectomy is a safer course of action where there is doubt about the testicular nature of the gonad.

In persistent Mullerian duct syndrome, both testes may be intra-abdominal, or one (or both) testes may be prolapsed through the internal inguinal ring; if so, the testes should be pulled back into the abdomen, which is easy, as they are not attached by the gubernaculum. The infantile uterus and tubes are in a floppy broad ligament, which also encloses the vas deferens. The latter ducts run across the ligament to the lower end of the infantile uterus and then merge

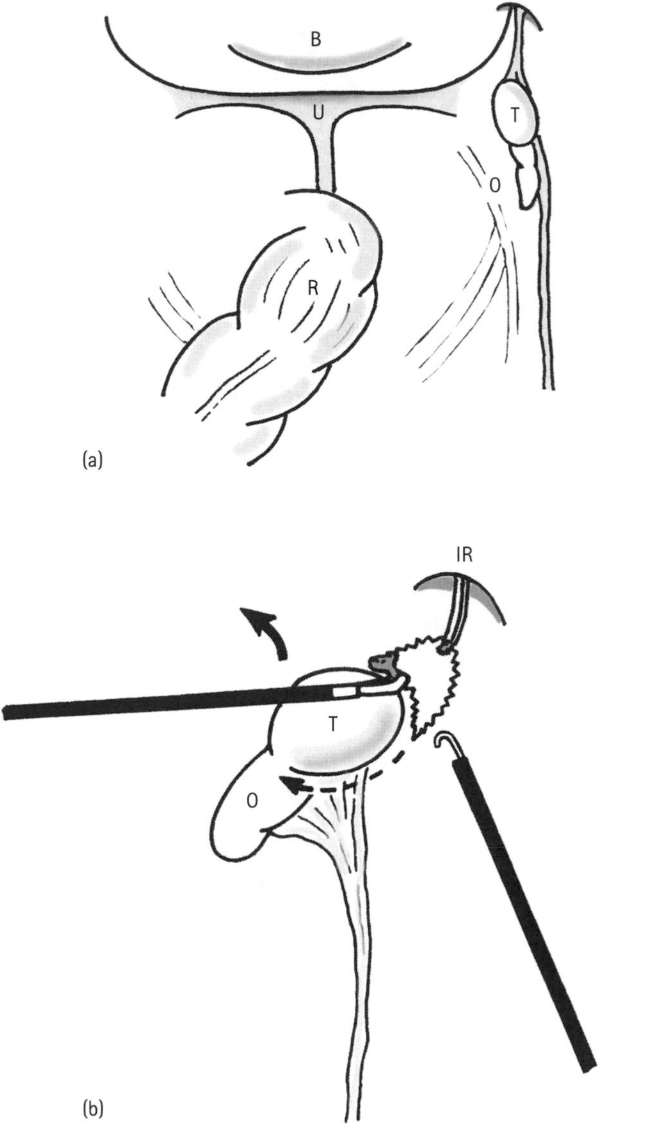

Figure 63.5

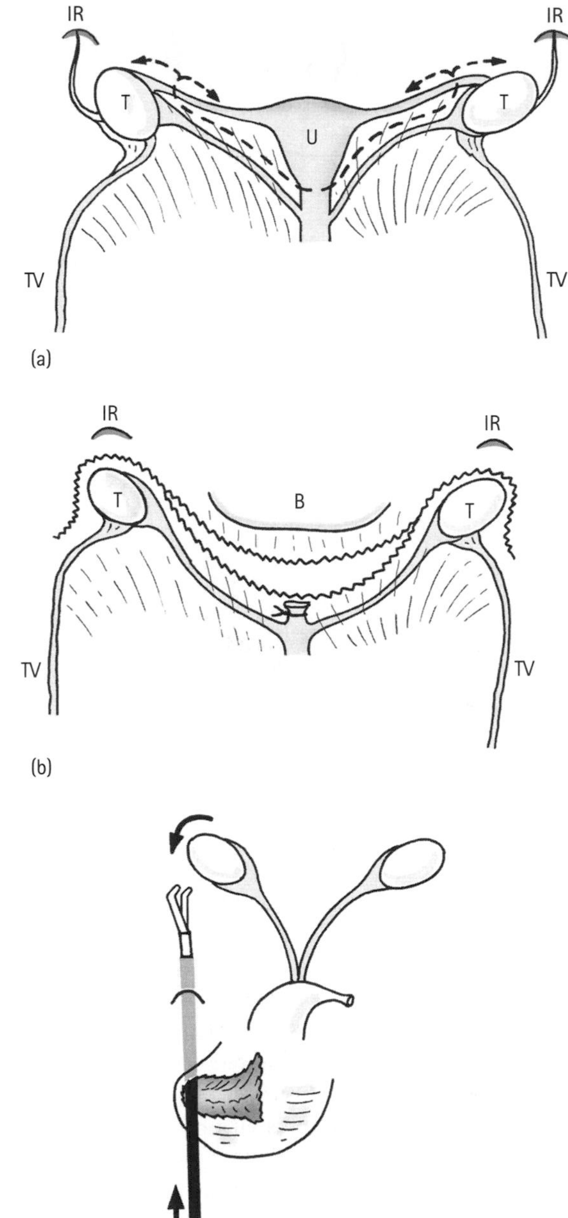

Figure 63.6

into the wall. Excision of the female genital tract, therefore, should only include the Fallopian tubes and upper uterus, and the cervix and hypoplastic vagina should be left in situ.

Traction on the Fallopian tubes allows diathermy hook dissection through the broad ligament, sticking close to the Mullerian duct structures. The lower part of the uterine body is amputated just above the site of fusion with the vasa deferentia. An Endoloop® or single transfixion suture can be applied to seal the uterine cavity. Orchidopexy can now be carried out (as described elsewhere), with the testes brought down through the same or separate canals, depending on mobility. Usually the length of the vas deferens is adequate to reach the scrotum, although sometimes the proximity of the two testes to each other prevents orchidopexy independently on each side. Where the testes are close together, the scrotum can be opened in the midline to create a pocket on each side. Grasping forceps are passed up to and through the inguinal canal, entering the abdomen on either side of the inferior epigastric vessels, and both testes are pulled down to the scrotum, once the track has been dilated. The testes are then positioned on either side of the scrotal septum. **(See Figure 63.6)**

In some boys with gonadal dysgenesis, there is a residual remnant of the lower vagina (derived from the persisting urogenital sinus). The vas deferens usually drains into the vault of the cavity, creating a conical or V-shaped structure. The peritoneum is opened transversely behind the bladder

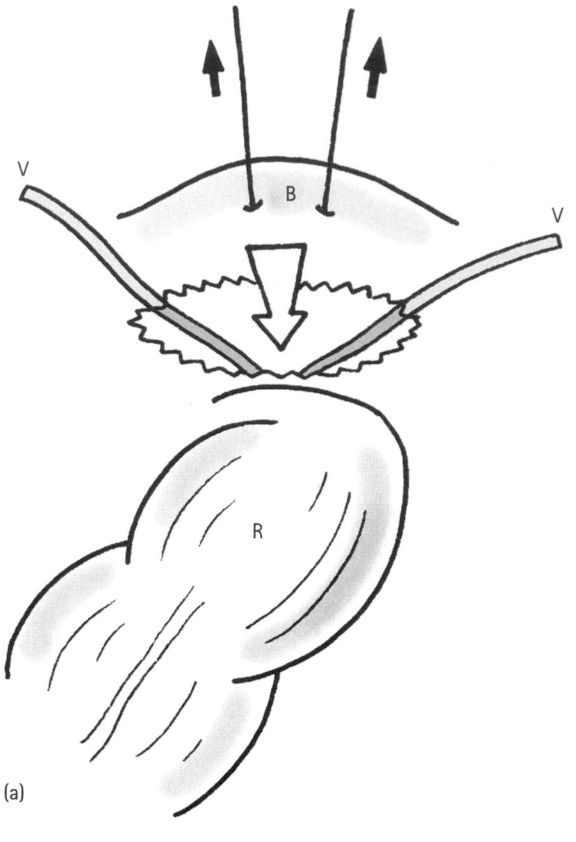

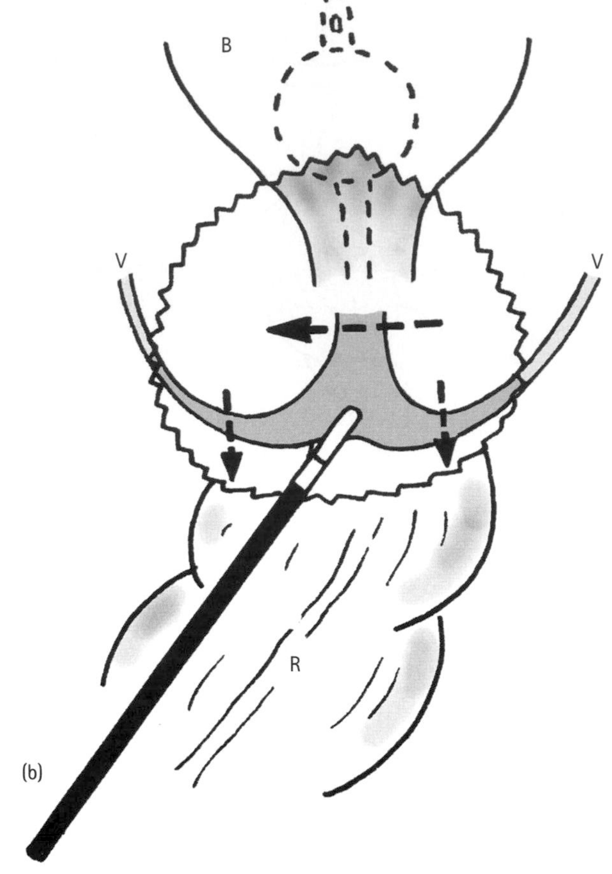

Figure 63.7

using the diathermy hook or fine scissors, and the vasa deferentia are dissected off the back of the bladder to expose the vaginal remnant. This is dissected down to its connection with the posterior urethra, which is identified by the presence of a catheter or metal sound. Excision of the vagina requires transection of the vas deferens, which can be done at any convenient level, and then an Endoloop® or single suture ligation is used to close the lower vagina at its entry point into the posterior urethra. The vasa are divided with diathermy or scissors. If the epididymis has developed, the ipsilateral dilated vas deferens is excised at the internal inguinal ring, and its distal end is clipped or closed with an Endoloop® or suture ligature. **(See Figure 63.7)**

POSTOPERATIVE CARE

Local anesthetic in the port sites, plus some oral or narcotic analgesia for the first 12–24 hours postoperatively, is usually adequate. Diet and fluids can be resumed immediately. A urinary catheter should be left in situ for a short while (12–24 hours) if dissection has included extraperitoneal exposure of the bladder neck and posterior urethra. Discharge home should be possible after catheter removal the next day.

PROBLEMS, PITFALLS AND SOLUTIONS

The most common problem is likely to be confusion about the anatomy, because of the possibility of variable male and female structures. This can be avoided by careful preoperative planning. Biopsy and photography and termination of the operation will allow the diagnosis to be made correctly.

Difficult access or poor view

- Ensure Trendelenburg position and that the bladder is empty.
- Use a transabdominal traction suture on the bladder if it is flopping down and obscuring the retrovesical structures. Alternatively, insert an extra port to enable the assistant to hold the back wall of the bladder up.

Bleeding

This is rarely a major problem, as the gonadal and uterine vessels are often small because of the poor development of the structures. If bleeding occurs, proximal occlusion of the gonadal vessels with grasping forceps will usually control it, until clips, suture or diathermy have been applied.

Dissection behind bladder neck/urethra

'Tenting up' the urethra by traction on the vaginal remnant may risk damage to the sphincter or create a fistula. The use of a stiff urethral catheter or a metal sound in the urethra will ensure this is not included in the dissection or excision margin.

COMPLICATIONS

- Inadequate gonadal excision, leaving potentially malignant streak gonadal tissue, or residual gonadal tissue from the opposite sex. Careful review of the biopsy/excised material together with postoperative hormonal assessment (if needed) should determine whether repeat excision is required.
- Incorrect excision of gonadal/ductal tissues. This can be avoided by delaying surgery until the surgeon is absolutely sure of the diagnosis and the state of the anatomy. Biopsy, photography/video recording, and termination of the procedure until further advice is sought provide a reliable means of avoiding this disaster.
- Incomplete excision of vaginal remnant may lead to recurrent or persisting urosepsis, breakdown of vaginal closure and retrovesical abscess. This can be avoided by very careful positioning of the Endoloop® (or clips) at the urethra–vagina junction.
- Persisting epididymitis following retrograde spread of organisms may require a course of postoperative antibiotics. If epididymitis has occurred preoperatively, the ipsilateral vas deferens is usually dilated and/or inflamed, and this should be excised at the internal ring and the distal end closed with a clip or Endoloop®.
- Posterior urethral fistula or sphincter damage can be avoided by keeping dissection close to the wall of the vaginal remnant, and keeping a metal sound in the urethra. The assistant can manipulate the sound while the surgeon observes the posterior urethra, to ensure that the dissection finishes at the correct point.
- Potential injury to adjacent pelvic structures, particularly iliac vessels and ureter, can be avoided by careful instrumentation and dissection.

FURTHER READING

Heloury Y, Plattner V. Laparoscopy and intersex. In: Bax NMA, Georgeson KE, Najmalden A, Valla JS (eds), *Endoscopic Surgery in Children*. Berlin: Springer-Verlag, 1999, 427–30.

64

Ovarian cysts and tumors

ANTOINE DE BACKER

INTRODUCTION

Ovarian masses are uncommon in children. These lesions, whether cystic, solid or mixed, span a spectrum of pathology from functional (non-neoplastic) ovarian cysts to ovarian torsion, and from benign lesions to highly aggressive malignant neoplasms. About 45 percent of ovarian masses are functional benign cysts such as follicle cysts and corpus luteum cysts. Another 40 percent are benign neoplasms, most commonly benign cystic teratomata (dermoid cysts). The remaining 15 percent are malignant neoplasms. **(See Table 64.1)**

Ovarian masses may occur at any age, in infants as well as in adolescents. They may be unilateral or bilateral, cystic unilocular or multilocular, or solid. They come to surgical attention in a variety of ways. Some are detected incidentally during ultrasound examination prenatally or postnatally, whereas others present insidiously as painless abdominal swellings. Most patients suffer from (acute or chronic) abdominal pain. Acute symptoms may be caused by torsion, bleeding or rupture of large cysts. Constipation, nausea and vomiting, as well as fatigue, are also reported. More rarely, there may be symptoms of precocious puberty or of virilization, and a pelvic mass is often palpated.

Table 64.1 *Clinical classification of ovarian masses*

Non-neoplastic lesions (±45%)	Neoplastic lesions (40% benign, 15% malignant)
Luteinoma of pregnancy Hyperthecosis Simple cyst Corpus luteum cyst Endometriosis Inflammatory lesions Parovarian cysts Polycstic ovaries (Stein-Leventhal syndrome) Inclusion cysts	*A. Epithelial tumors* 1. Serous 2. Mucinous 3. Endometrioid 4. Clear cell 5. Brenner 6. Mixed 7. Undifferentiated *B. Sex cord-stromal tumors* 1. Granulosa-stroma a. Granulosa b. Theca-fibroma 2. Androblastoma 3. Gynandroblastoma *C. Lipoid cell tumors* *D. Germ cell tumors* 1. Dysgerminoma 2. Endodermal sinus tumor (yolk sac tumor) 3. Embryonal cancer 4. Polyembryoma 5. Choriocarcinoma 6. Teratoma (mature/immature grade I-II-III) 7. Mixed forms *E. Gonadoblastoma* *F. Soft tissue tumors* *G. Unclassified tumors* *H. Metastatic tumors*

Indications

Not every ovarian cyst has to be explored surgically; smaller cysts or larger cysts in neonates often resolve in the first months after birth and do not need surgery.

Asymptomatic smaller cysts (<5 cm) in postmenarchal girls without sonographic findings suggestive of malignancy can also be followed by imaging without surgical intervention.

As already mentioned, ovarian masses are very rare in the pediatric population. There is little consensus as to the indications for treatment and the ideal approach to their management. For simple, presumably functional, cysts in neonates and postpubertal girls, most surgeons adopt a conservative attitude, consisting of follow-up by imaging with neither surgical interference nor puncture for evaluation. Some surgeons advocate single or repeated ultrasound-guided punctures instead of cystectomy.

The generally accepted operative indications include the following.

- Antenatally diagnosed 'simple' ovarian cysts of more than 5 cm in diameter that fail to resolve in the first months after birth.
- Uncomplicated large (>5 cm, completely anechoic) 'simple' cysts in older children.
- Radiologically 'simple' cysts in prepubertal girls.
- Complicated cysts on ultrasound (fluid-debris level, septation, clots), either symptomatic or asymptomatic.
- Suspicion of torsion, rupture or hemorrhage.
- Suspicion of tumor.

Experience with adult patients has shown that the ovary is accessible and suitable for laparoscopic surgery. Even large ovarian cysts and cystic tumors may be safely dealt with via a minimally invasive approach. Excellent results have been reported for the aforementioned indications. *The only controversial indication for laparoscopy is ovarian malignancy*, for which the role of laparoscopic surgery is yet to be determined, in part because of the rarity of ovarian malignancy in children. The danger of the laparoscopic treatment of malignant ovarian tumors is rupture of the tumor causing tumor spillage during its removal. That aside, all other steps of the procedure (inspection of the entire abdomen, aspiration and analysis of ascites, biopsy of suspect distant lesions and oncologically safe adnexectomy) can be performed as adequately as (if not better than) with laparotomy. The risk of tumor spillage is probably higher with the larger tumors; therefore, it may be reasonable to use an entirely laparoscopic approach for the smaller tumors (for instance <6–7 cm), and to remove larger tumors by laparotomy.

In recent years, great emphasis has been placed on the preservation of fertility. There is substantial evidence that laparoscopy is associated with fewer adhesions than conventional open surgery. In ovarian surgery, the prevention of adhesions is of the utmost importance; this goal seems to be best achieved with laparoscopic surgery. Other benefits of a laparoscopic approach, such as quick recovery from surgery and nearly invisible scars, are applicable also to ovarian laparoscopic surgery.

Contraindications

ABSOLUTE

The only absolute contraindication to a laparoscopic procedure is the presence of a medical condition unrelated to the ovarian pathology that prohibits general anesthesia or laparoscopy itself.

RELATIVE

High radiological and clinical suspicion of malignancy preoperatively. Some authors continue to recommend a conventional laparotomy in such instances. However, diagnostic laparoscopy can be carried out first without compromising the child's condition. Conversion to laparotomy can take place subsequently if judged necessary (as in cases where the tumor is very large).

EQUIPMENT/INSTRUMENTS

Ovarian cysts may develop in newborns as well as in adolescents and young adult girls. The diameter and length of cannulae and other instruments must be adapted to the size of the patient.

Essential

- 5 mm or 10 mm cannula with stopcock, blunt-tipped trocar, length 55 mm.
- Two (preferably threaded) 5 mm cannulae without stopcock, shielded obturator, length 55 mm.
- 5 mm or 10 mm 30° angled telescope.
- Bipolar cauterization forceps, curved, with fine tip.
- 5 mm curved, preferably insulated, mini-scissors with diathermy point.
- 5 mm fine, atraumatic, preferably curved, grasping dissecting forceps.
- Fine 5 mm hook monopolar diathermy.
- 5 mm suction irrigation device.
- 5 mm clip applicator.
- Small retrieval bag.
- Two 5 mm needle holders.
- Pre-tied suture loops or 4-0 sutures on a ski-shaped needle.

Optional

- For babies, short 3 mm instruments.
- Ultracision Harmonic Scalpel®.

PREOPERATIVE PREPARATION

On clinical grounds, it is nearly impossible to differentiate between masses that need surgical treatment and others that do not, or between benign and malignant lesions. The age of the patient may give a clue as to the likely nature of a cystic ovarian tumor: most cysts found during the neonatal period are functional and develop because of stimulation by maternal hormones. Functional cysts are also found in postmenarchal girls. In prepubertal girls, on the other hand, cysts are unlikely to be functional because the ovaries are still inactive. In this age group, therefore, every ovarian mass has to be considered malignant until proven otherwise.

The presence of endocrinopathy, whether isosexual (precocious puberty) or heterosexual (virilization), does not assist in distinguishing benign from malignant lesions because endocrinopathies are seen in both. In postmenarchal girls, a pregnancy test should be performed to rule out (ectopic) pregnancy, although the test may produce a false-positive result in the case of a human chorionic gonadotrophin (hCG)-producing germ cell tumor. Serum assays for alpha-fetoprotein (AFP), beta-hCG and (less importantly in children) CA125 will be needed. Elevated AFP levels are seen with endodermal sinus tumors (yolk sac tumors) and germ cell tumors. CA125 is more important in adult women with epithelial tumors. Plain abdominal X-ray films may demonstrate calcification, highly suggestive of a teratoma, but cannot distinguish between benign mature and immature teratoma or other malignant tumors. Ultrasonography is the imaging modality of choice for the initial assessment of pelvic pathology. The size and location of the mass, its extent, the echogenicity of its internal structures and the presence of ascites are analyzed.

Investigation with high-resolution equipment may allow the experienced pediatric radiologist to distinguish 'simple' non-neoplastic cysts from 'complicated' cysts, pure cysts from cystic tumors, and benign from malignant pathology. Color Doppler is able to demonstrate neovascularization in the cyst wall, a criterion for malignancy. Cysts >5 cm in diameter, with thick septae, the presence of intracystic papillomatous vegetations or irregular solid parts, indefinite margins and the presence of ascites are all suggestive of malignancy. In adult women, the use of transvaginal ultrasonography has improved the diagnostic accuracy: for obvious reasons, this approach has limited application in the child. Computerized tomography (CT) is superior to ultrasonography for the detection of abdominal metastatic disease. Magnetic resonance imaging (MRI) provides more soft tissue contrast than CT and is biologically safer: it may be more sensitive and specific than either CT or ultrasonography in the evaluation of an ovarian mass, and more sensitive but less specific than ultrasonography in discriminating malignant from benign conditions.

Despite all the technical advances and innovations, however, diagnostic accuracy by imaging will never reach 100 percent. Since ovarian masses represent a very heterogeneous group of conditions, a thorough knowledge of this pathology is needed in order to deal appropriately with every situation.

TECHNIQUE

General anesthesia with endotracheal intubation and muscle relaxation is essential. A Foley urinary catheter and a nasogastric tube are inserted. Antibiotic prophylaxis is not needed. Since the procedures described below may be performed on small babies as well as adolescent girls, the size of the instruments and the position of the ports have to be adapted to the age and size of the patient.

At the commencement of the procedure, a careful general laparoscopic examination of the entire abdominal cavity is carried out. Any fluid in the pouch of Douglas should be collected for cytology. The abdominal cavity, greater omentum and liver are inspected, followed by careful inspection of both adnexae. The presence of small follicular cysts is a common and normal finding in neonatal and postpubertal ovaries. These cysts usually regress spontaneously and do not need to be resected. Where there is a tumor, a search for distant metastases must be undertaken.

The goal of surgery is to remove the benign cyst preserving as much healthy ovarian tissue as possible. This will maximize the child's opportunity for subsequent normal endocrine and reproductive function.

The procedure is performed with the patient in the supine position with some degree of Trendelenburg and lateral tilt to the normal side. The surgeon and camera operator stand on the side of the patient opposite to that of the adnexa to be operated upon (left side for right adnexa and vice versa). For huge cysts for which it has been impossible to determine the exact location preoperatively, the surgeon usually stands on the left side of the patient. The first cannula with blunt-tipped trocar is inserted through a small infra-umbilical incision under direct visual control (10 mm in older girls, 5 mm in babies). A pneumoperitoneum is created using a flow rate of 1 L/min and a pressure of 8–10 mmHg (babies) to 12–14 mmHg (teenage patients).

After a preliminary thorough laparoscopic inspection, the position of the two extra ports is decided. For a right-sided lesion, a cannula can be placed in the right flank two or three fingerbreadths under the costal margin, and a second one either a bit lower in the left flank or in the left suprapubic region (on the opposite side for a left-sided lesion). However, if the cyst is lying freely in the abdominal cavity secondary to auto-amputation, only one supplementary port will be needed. Once the working ports have been introduced, the CO_2 flow rate is set to medium (4–10 L/min). **(See Figure 64.1)**

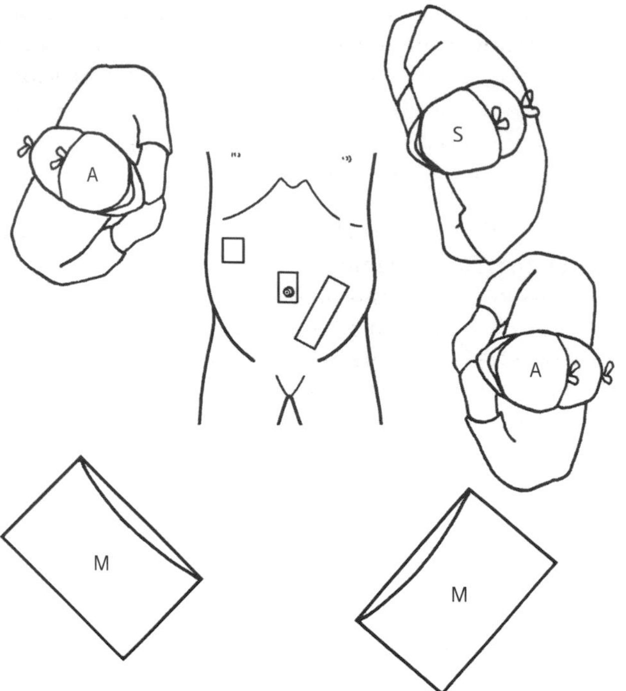

Figure 64.1

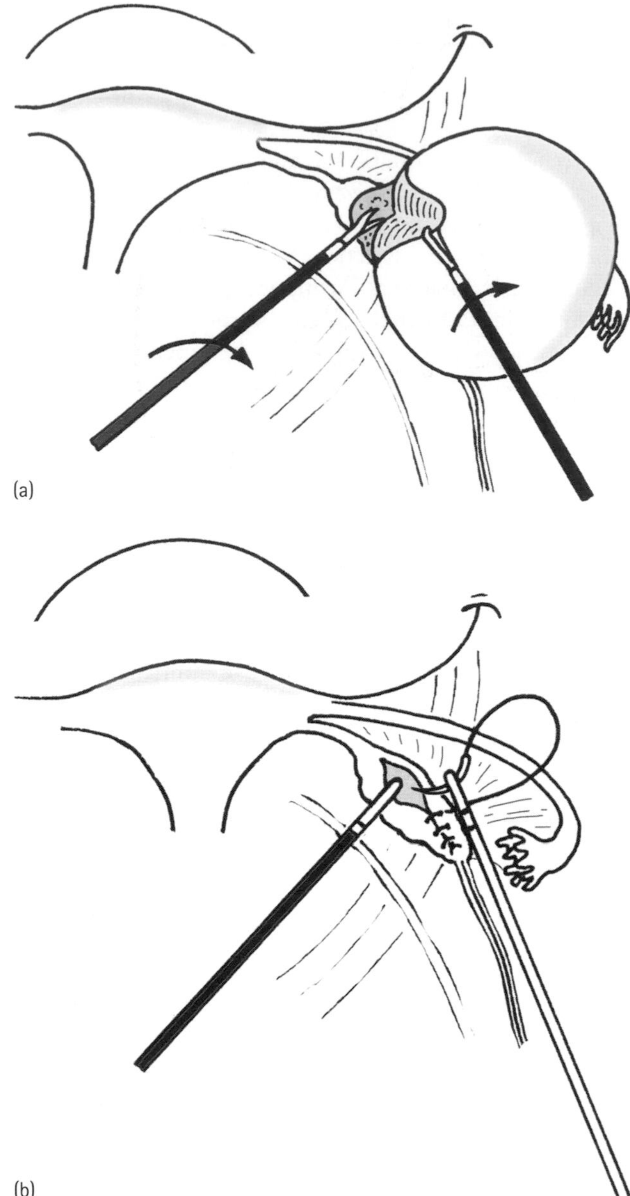

Figure 64.2

Cystectomy with preservation of ovarian tissue

If the appearance of the lesion is characteristic of a simple, non-neoplastic cyst (large unilocular cyst with a smooth surface and no evidence of malignancy), conservative surgical management with preservation of normal ovarian tissue is indicated. In these instances the ovary has become somewhat flattened and attenuated as an elongated plaque of gonadal tissue. This plaque has to be separated from the cyst and, if possible, reconstructed. In most cases, it is preferable not to empty the cyst first, so that it can be mobilized more easily and dissection is facilitated.

The cyst is grasped close to the ovarian plaque and slightly pressed into the pelvis; this maneuver creates a certain tension on the vascular pedicle. The cyst wall is incised around the thickened plaque of ovarian tissue, at the anti-mesenteric portion of the ovary, away from the blood vessels of the hilum. This can be achieved with fine bipolar cauterization followed by incision with fine scissors. Monopolar coagulation with a hook may cause thermodestruction of the remaining ovarian tissue. Thereafter, a plane of dissection can be developed between the gonadal plaque and the cyst. With careful dissection using fine bipolar coagulation and fine scissors, the cyst can be completely freed from the ovary without leakage of its contents. Alternatively, this dissection can be done with the Harmonic Scalpel® if the equipment is available.

To reconstruct the ovary (to prevent adhesions), the cyst is 'parked' somewhere outside the operating field. The ovarian plaque is closed with a running stitch of 4-0 Vicryl® using two laparoscopic needle holders. In addition, a piece of anti-adhesion barrier sheet can be draped over the reconstructed ovary to prevent the formation of adhesions. Others recommend the use of tissue glue. Laparoscopic ovarian reconstruction is quite complicated in small children and more studies are needed to evaluate the necessity of this maneuver. **(See Figure 64.2)**

The cyst may now be removed; this can be done in two ways. The first option involves puncturing and emptying the cyst and then removing it through a port. The cyst is punctured with a long needle passed percutaneously, rather than trying to introduce the suction cannula into it. The latter procedure is more likely to result in spilling of the cyst's contents – although this may not be important in the case of a follicular cyst, it should be avoided in cases of

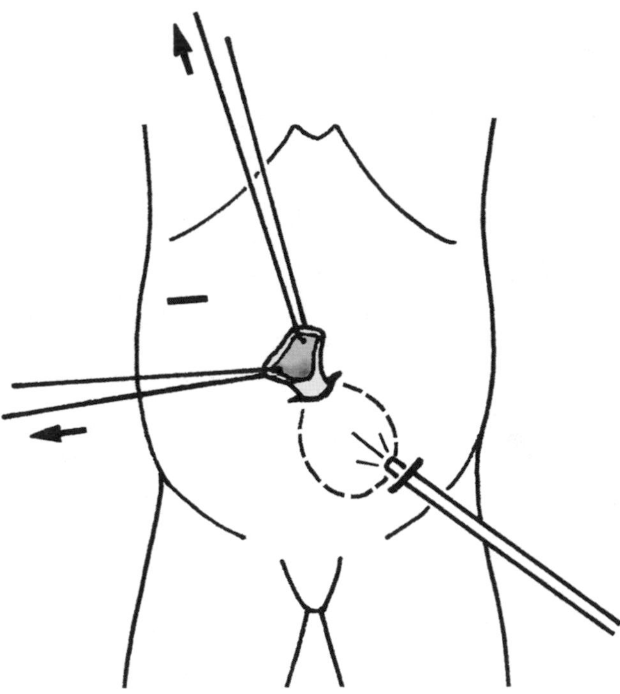

Figure 64.3

cystic teratoma or mucinous cystadenoma. A 5 mm laparoscope is introduced in the right flank port. Grasping forceps, inserted via the 10 mm umbilical cannula, are used to grasp the empty cyst, which is then removed.

A second option consists of not puncturing the cyst, and removing it in the same way as the gallbladder is removed after cholecystectomy. Grasping forceps, inserted via the 10 mm umbilical cannula, are used to grasp the cyst firmly and the umbilical port and the lesion are delivered partially. The cyst wall is grasped with two ordinary clamps or held with two sutures, and is completely emptied by puncture or with the suction cannula after incision; the collapsed cyst is then delivered. The cyst content must be submitted for cytologic analysis, and the cyst wall for histologic examination. Finally, the abdomen is rinsed with warm saline. The remaining ports are removed and the wounds closed (Vicryl® 3-0 to close the fascia, 4-0 for the subcutis). **(See Figure 64.3)**

Even where no residual ovarian tissue appears to be present macroscopically, the same technique should be applied, since microscopic studies have shown the presence of oocytes in the hilar attachment (under the ovarian albuginea close to the hilum).

Unroofing of the cyst – partial cystectomy

Instead of dissecting the intact cyst out of the ovary, which is not always an easy procedure, some advocate simple unroofing of the cyst or partial cystectomy, both of which are said to be as efficacious as complete cystectomy. Unroofing or partial cystectomy (comparable procedures except that a larger part of the cyst wall is removed in partial cystectomy) has the advantages that the procedure is easier and quicker, and that the risk of thermodestruction of the oocytes in the ovariumrest is minimal if not absent. The disadvantages are that in partial cystectomy only part of the cyst can be examined by the pathologist, and theoretically islands of suspect tissue could be left behind. Moreover, the cyst has to be emptied first, which is difficult to do without contaminating the abdominal cavity. In benign situations, this is probably of no consequence, but it is not always easy to be absolutely certain of the benign nature of the cyst before histologic analysis is carried out.

Technically, the cyst must be emptied first, either with a long needle passed percutaneously under direct vision or by opening it with scissors and aspirating the contents with the suction cannula. The technique of unroofing consists of excising the top part of the cyst wall with scissors after monopolar coagulation. In partial cystectomy, a larger part of the cyst is excised, the line of dissection remaining sufficiently far from the ovarian hilum. Ablation of the remaining inner cyst lining can be obtained using bipolar coagulation, but this again may destruct adjacent oocytes. The ovary must not be reconstructed after partial cystectomy.

Removal of an auto-amputated cyst

It is not unusual to find a cyst that is completely loose in the abdominal cavity due to auto-amputation. Such auto-amputated cysts are always benign. They may be found in the pelvis, but also are located in other parts of the abdomen (in the upper abdomen, for instance). The entire abdomen and both adnexae are inspected with a laparoscope inserted through the first umbilical cannula. If no other cysts are present, a second 5 mm port is inserted in the right iliac fossa or suprapubic region. Grasping forceps are used to bring the cyst into the pelvis, where it is punctured and emptied as described earlier. The collapsed cyst is then delivered through the suprapubic trocar.

Oophorectomy for benign tumors

The accepted surgical treatment of benign ovarian tumor is oophorectomy. More recently, ovarium-sparing tumorectomy has been recommended for benign dermoid cysts (especially in bilateral tumors). It is of paramount importance not to rupture the tumor. Rupture of dermoid cysts may lead to peritonitis and adhesion formation. Rupture of cystadenomas may lead to local recurrence.

Oophorectomy is done with bipolar diathermy and fine scissors or with a hook. It is important to mobilize the adnexa to ensure the vessels are easily exposed at a sufficient distance from the pelvic wall and to facilitate the identification of important structures such as the ureter as it courses beneath the peritoneum, and the iliac vessels. The mesosalpinx and ligamentum ovarii proprium are coagulated and incised. The ovarian vessels are ligated with an Endoloop®. The tumor is placed in a retrieval bag and removed after enlargement of the abdominal wall incision. During this procedure, one has to be extremely careful not to harm the ureter, particularly when cautery and Endoloops® are used, as it may be very close.

Whenever feasible, and if the tube is uninvolved in the tumoral process, salpingectomy should be avoided. However, situations may be encountered whereby complete adnexectomy seems the most logical operation to perform. In this situation, the Fallopian tube must be transected first close to the uterus and then removed together with the ovarian tumor. More recently, the safety of ovarium-sparing surgery has been documented for benign cystic teratomas (dermoid cysts), especially in the 10 percent of cases that are bilateral. This technique is identical to the one described for cystectomy. **(See Figure 64.4)**

Malignant tumors

There is no consensus regarding the place of laparoscopic surgery in the treatment of *malignant* ovarian tumors, but it is possible there might be a place for it in the treatment of smaller tumors. Malignancy has to be suspected when the tumor is irregular, where there is tumoral ingrowth, distant metastases or ascites. Despite refinements in imaging techniques, malignancy is not always demonstrated preoperatively. When confronted with a high suspicion of malignancy, the entire abdomen has to be inspected first, ascites sampled for cytologic analysis, and suspect lesions biopsied. Frozen-section histology may be useful in some uncertain cases. Extreme care must be taken not to rupture the tumor. The risk of spreading the cancer if an ovarian malignancy is ruptured may compromise the patient's survival. For larger tumors, conversion to laparotomy seems wise.

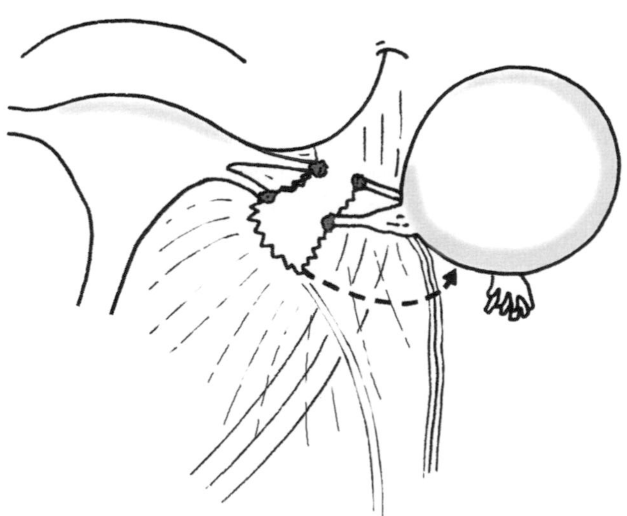

Figure 64.4

Acute torsion

If torsion of an ovarian cyst/tumor is found during laparoscopy, the first step is to untwist the adnexa with two pairs of grasping forceps, to allow assessment of the viability of the organ.

If the adnexa and the cyst are necrotic, adnexectomy is indicated, as described earlier. The necrotic mass is best placed into a retrieval bag introduced through the 10 mm umbilical port. Before doing so, the 10 mm laparoscope is removed and replaced by a 5 mm laparoscope inserted via one of the other 5 mm ports. The cyst is punctured, and the bag removed.

If the twisted adnexa and cyst regain a good blood supply after untwisting, which is often the case, cystectomy (complete or partial) with preservation of the healthy ovarian tissue is carried out as described previously.

Laparoscopy-assisted mini-laparotomy

This operation starts with a diagnostic laparoscopy, followed immediately by a 3–4 cm suprapubic mini-laparotomy through which the adnexa is exteriorized after the cyst has been aspirated, if necessary. The cyst or cystic teratoma is dissected free from the ovarian cortex, and the ovarium is reconstructed. This technique can be applied to cases of adnexal torsion, as well as to cases of benign cystic/tumoral pathology.

POSTOPERATIVE CARE

All procedures described in this chapter are usually well tolerated. The nasogastric tube and the Foley catheter are removed at the end of the operation. Postoperative analgesia is achieved with intravenous paracetamol. Intravenous opiates are not given routinely. Patients are allowed to drink after a few hours, are fed orally the day after surgery and are discharged on the second or third day.

Patients with non-neoplastic cysts are followed up for 1 year with serial ultrasonography. Patients with benign germ cell tumors are followed up for 5 years with serial ultrasonography and measurement of AFP levels. Those with malignant tumors (immature teratomas Grade III, endodermal sinus tumors [yolk sac tumors] etc.) are referred to a pediatric oncologist for adjuvant therapy.

PROBLEMS, PITFALLS AND SOLUTIONS

- Laparoscopic procedures on the ovary are not usually difficult. Moderately experienced laparoscopic surgeons should be able to carry out these operations with success, provided their knowledge of ovarian pathology is adequate, and provided they perform the interventions meticulously. The umbilical port should be inserted by the open technique: especially in large ovarian cysts, blind insertion of the first sharp-tipped trocar may injure the cyst.

One should not hesitate to insert a fourth 3mm or 5mm trocar whenever this is judged to be necessary.

- It is preferable to carry out cystectomy on an intact cyst. An un-emptied cyst helps in the mobilization of the ovarian plaque. Should the cyst be emptied first, the cyst wall and ovarian plaque become very mobile, making dissection much more difficult.
- Bleeding from the residual ovary tissue is usually minor. Careful dissection and bipolar diathermy minimize this risk.
- Castration-sparing operations must be carried out where benign disease is bilateral.
- If the procedure cannot be fully achieved laparoscopically, a mini-laparotomy is performed (suprapubic area, left or right). The deflated cyst with the ovary from which it originates is delivered through the incision, the cyst is removed and the ovary reconstructed.

COMPLICATIONS

- Monopolar diathermy is best avoided to salvage the maximum number of residual ovarian follicles.
- Care must be taken not to disseminate the contents of the cyst into the peritoneal cavity, particularly if it is a dermoid cyst or malignancy is a possibility. Dermoid material produces significant peritonitis. Copious lavage with warm saline has been shown to bring inflammation and adhesion formation close to control levels. The content of mucinous cystadenomas also must not be spilled into the peritoneum.
- The most serious complication during adnexectomy is transection, thermodestruction or inadvertent ligation of the ureter. Transection of the ureter may require conversion to open surgery and repair by suture of the ureter over a ureteric stent.
- Major bleeding is uncommon. Care must be taken to secure the ovarian/tube blood supply and not to cause inadvertent injury to the iliac vessels.

FURTHER READING

Dass DL, Hawkins E, Brandt ML et al. Surgery for ovarian masses in infants, children and adolescents: 102 consecutive patients treated in a 15-year period. *Journal of Pediatric Surgery* 2001; 36:693–9.

Lazar EL, Stolar CJH. Evaluation and management of pediatric solid ovarian tumors. *Seminars in Pediatric Surgery* 1998; 7:29–34.

Shalev E, Bustan M, Romano S et al. Laparoscopic resection of ovarian benign cystic teratomas: experience with 84 cases. *Human Reproduction* 1998; 13:1810–12.

Silva PD, Ripple J. Outpatient minilaparotomy ovarian cystectomy for benign teratomas in teenagers. *Journal of Pediatric Surgery* 1996; 31:1383–6.

Steyaert H, Meynol F, Valla JS. Torsion of the adnexa in children: the value of laparoscopy. *Pediatric Surgery International* 1998; 13:384–7.

65

Ovarian transposition

AZAD NAJMALDIN AND SATISH K. AGGARWAL

INTRODUCTION

Ovarian failure is a serious side effect of pelvic irradiation for cancer in young girls and premenopausal women. An ovary lying directly in the field of radiation is likely to be damaged irreversibly at a relatively low dose of radiation. Ovarian transposition away from the field of radiation has been shown to preserve ovarian function in 70–80 percent of cases in adults, and there are reports of subsequent successful pregnancy. The procedure is now being increasingly performed laparoscopically and has the following advantages.

There are essentially two types of ovarian transposition: *median transposition* behind the uterus and *lateral transposition* outside the true pelvis. The choice is determined by the field and mode of radiation. Median transposition is used for inverted Y-field of radiation in Hodgkin's disease, which is rare and associated with high scatter radiation. Lateral transposition just outside the true pelvis is suitable for brachytherapy (midline tumors such as vaginal, uterine and bladder tumors), while more lateral transfer is necessary for external radiation.

Indications

- Conditions requiring abdominal/pelvic radiation where ovaries fall in the field of radiation.

Contraindications

ABSOLUTE

- Major uncorrectable bleeding diatheses.
- Terminal cancer.

RELATIVE

- Cancers requiring high-dose chemotherapy. Oophorectomy for cryopreservation may be offered to this group and the procedure may be carried out laparoscopically.

Advantages

- It allows for assessment and biopsy of the tumor in deep peritoneal recesses.
- Radiotherapy can commence almost immediately after the procedure, unlike open surgery, after which one has to wait for the wounds to heal.
- It allows for concomitant visualization of pelvic anatomy and safe insertion of radium rods for brachytherapy.

EQUIPMENT/INSTRUMENTS

Essential

- Three 3.5–5 mm cannulae.
- 5 mm straight or 30° telescope.
- 3.5–5 mm curved insulated scissors with diathermy point.
- Two sets of 3.5–5 mm atraumatic grasping forceps without ratchet.
- Fine 3.5–5 mm hook, or needle monopolar and bipolar diathermy.
- 5 mm clip applicator with appropriate titanium clips – metal clips interfere with magnetic resonance imaging (MRI).

- 3.5–5 mm needle holders.
- Needle and suture: polypropylene 5-0–3-0, depending on the size of the patient. Some surgeons and oncologists may prefer absorbable suture, i.e. polydioxanone surgical (PDS) suture, which may allow spontaneous re-positioning of the ovary.

Optional

- Additional cannulae.
- LigaSure™, plasma kinetic or ultrasound shear – as an alternative to clips and ligatures to control major vessels.

PREOPERATIVE PREPARATION

Full cancer work-up is undertaken in consultation with the oncologist and radiotherapist. The radiation field is clearly marked and dosage and mode of radiation are worked out.

The rare possibility of conversion to an open technique and the success rate of the technique are formally discussed with the patient and care providers. Further, the possibility of future pregnancy and the need for re-positioning of the ovary are also discussed.

TECHNIQUE

General anesthesia with muscle relaxation is necessary. The patient is positioned supine; however, lateral and head-down tilts may improve access during the operation. The bladder is emptied by expression and a urinary catheter is rarely necessary. The monitors are placed at the foot of the table and the surgeon stands on the right side of the patient for the left ovary and vice versa. The primary cannula (5 mm) is placed at or above the umbilicus, depending on the size of the patient. Once a pneumoperitoneum is created at a pressure of 8–10 mmHg, a preliminary survey of pelvic anatomy is made and the sites for secondary cannulae are decided. This may vary between unilateral and bilateral procedures. However, a straight-line formation, horizontal, oblique centered at the umbilicus, or vertical starting at the umbilicus, covers all eventualities. The remaining part of the procedure is dependent on the nature of the transposition to be executed. **(See Figures 65.1 and 65.2)**

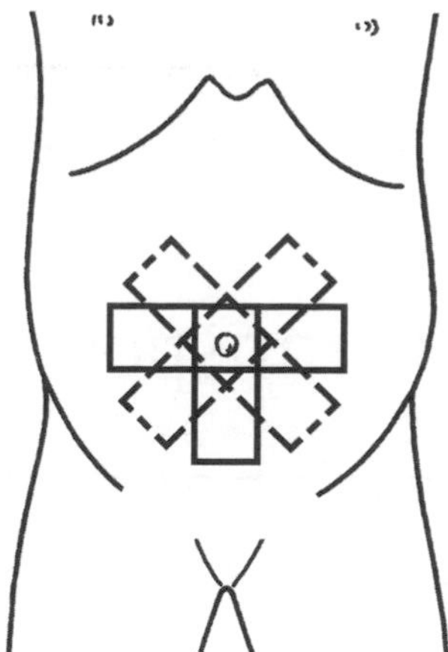

Figure 65.1 *Position of cannulae. Broken lines indicate left and right unilateral surgery. Solid lines represent horizontal and vertical line formation for bilateral surgery.*

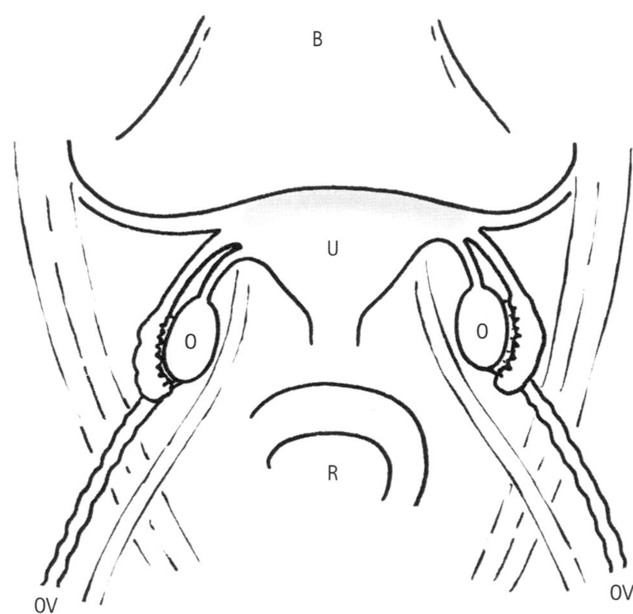

Figure 65.2 *Normal anatomy.*

Median ovarian transposition

The uterus is pushed anteriorly with a blunt instrument, and the ovaries are exposed. Alternatively, a suprapubic suture, passed percutaneously through the abdominal wall, middle of the uterus and back through the abdominal wall, allows full retraction of the uterus. The suture must be removed at the end of the procedure. The ovarian ligaments are held close to the ovaries with atraumatic graspers, and moved towards the midline behind the uterus. Both ligaments are then held in one instrument and fixed using either two clips or a single non-absorbable or absorbable suture. The tubo-ovarian relationship is preserved and care is taken not to link the tubes. **(See Figure 65.3)**

Lateral ovarian transposition

The ovary is fixed outside the true pelvis – lateral to the iliac vessels. This may be achieved by either a simple suture fixation or partial mobilization of the ovary (if the medial attachments are tight).

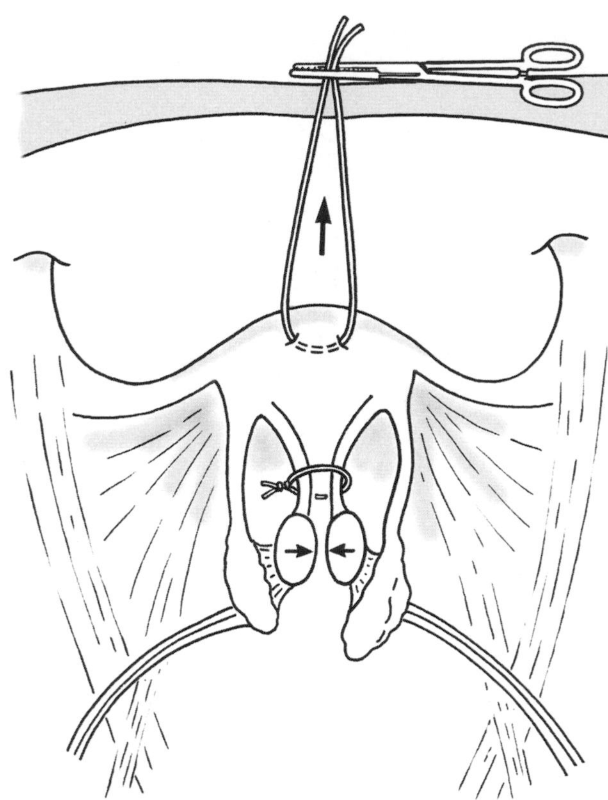

Figure 65.3

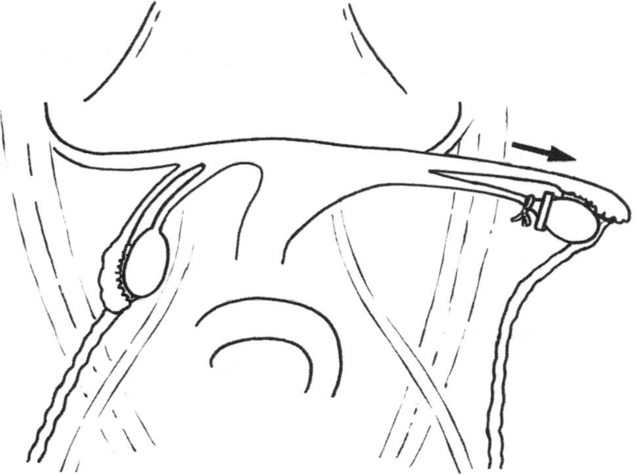

Figure 65.4

The meso-ovarium is kept taut and divided using a monopolar hook or needle diathermy or diathermy on scissors. The tubo-ovarian relations at the fimbrial end are left undisturbed. Care is taken not to damage the ureter, iliac vessels, uterus and Fallopian tube. The ovary is then taken lateral to the iliac vessels and fixed in the iliac fossa using one or two stitches through the divided end of the ovarian ligament – tunica albuginea – and the ovary is marked with a titanium clip. **(See Figure 65.5)**

Simple suture fixation

A short piece of 5-0–3-0 suture on a straightened-out ski or curved needle (depending on the size of the working cannula) is introduced through a working cannula or percutaneously. The ovarian ligament close to the ovary is held gently using atraumatic graspers. The ovary is then lifted out of the pelvis and moved across the iliac vessels to the iliac fossa. A single stitch is taken through the tunica albuginea close to the ovarian ligament and the ovary is fixed securely to the ilio-psoas muscle. The ovarian position is marked with a titanium clip through the ovarian ligament at the surface of the ovary. Care must be taken not to grasp the ureter or injure the iliac vessels. **(See Figure 65.4)**

Partial mobilization of the ovary

The uterus is retracted anterio-medially using either an atraumatic instrument through a third working cannula or a percutaneously applied suture as described earlier. The ovarian ligament is picked up midway between the uterus and the ovary and a window is created in the meso-ovarium using a fine curved atraumatic grasper. The ovarian branches of the uterine vessels and the ovarian ligament are then divided between clips or ligatures. The ovarian end of the divided ligament is carefully held in a grasper and the ovary is retracted to facilitate further dissection.

Mobilization of the ovary and pedicle

A wider radiation field (external radiation) necessitates complete lateral mobilization of the ovary with an intact ovarian pedicle.

In addition to division of the ovarian ligament and meso-ovarium as described above, the *ovary is dissociated from the fimbrial end of the Fallopian tube* using a diathermy needle. Care is taken not to cause thermal injury to the ovary. Alternatively, the tube is clipped or ligated medial to the fimbriae and divided, leaving a portion of the tube attached to the ovary. The ovary is then picked up by the attached remnant of ovarian ligament and the ovarian vessels are carefully mobilized cephalad to the desired level by dividing the peritoneum on either side using scissors. Electrocautery and ultrasound shear may cause vascular thrombosis. The ovary is then anchored to the lateral abdominal wall lateral to the cecum/right colon. Care is taken not to twist the vascular pedicle. **(See Figure 65.6)**

POSTOPERATIVE CARE

Local infiltration of anesthetic agents and oral non-steroidal analgesics provide adequate postoperative pain

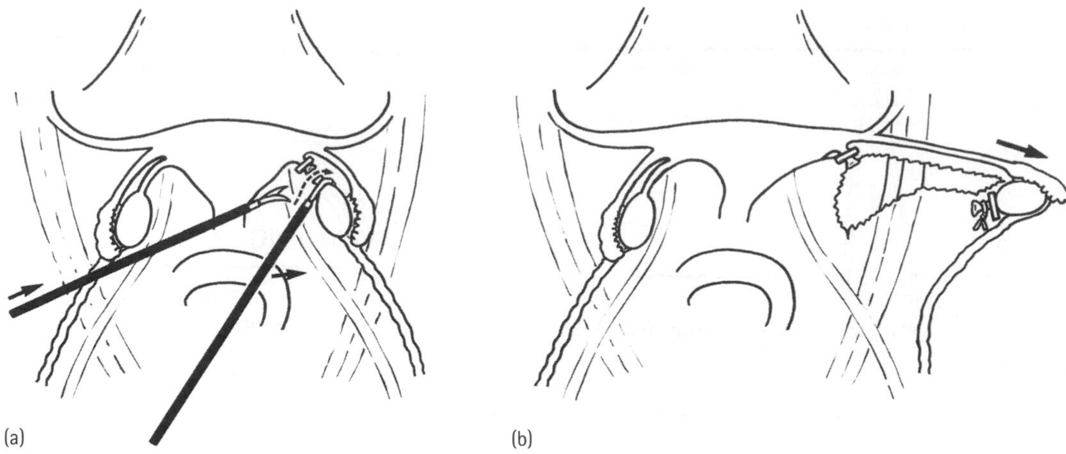

Figure 65.5

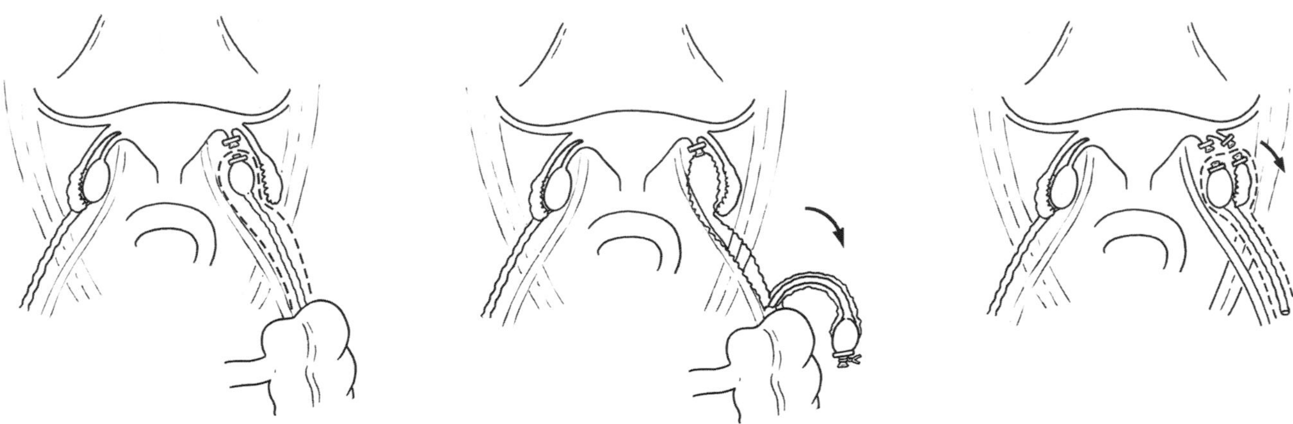

Figure 65.6

relief. The patient is allowed to feed within several hours of surgery and discharged home within 8–24 hours. Radiotherapy may commence straightaway. The position of the ovary is checked by a plain X-ray, which demonstrates the location of the marker clip.

PROBLEMS, PITFALLS AND SOLUTIONS

Difficult access and view

- Distended colon and small bowel loops may hinder the view. The head-down position and/or lateral tilt often improve exposure.
- A distended bladder may require catheterization or suprapubic aspiration.
- The uterus has a tendency to fall posteriorly, especially in older children and adolescents. A percutaneously placed suprapubic suture through the fundus/middle of the uterus allows adequate retraction. This suture must be removed at the end of the procedure.
- Consider placing an atraumatic instrument or a retractor through an additional cannula to retract the uterus or dilated loops of intestine.
- Adhesions from previous surgery may require adhesiolysis.

Handling the ovary

- The ovarian ligament and meso-ovarium can be short, particularly in small children. Care must be taken not to damage the ovary. If necessary, sacrifice the Fallopian tube.
- Handle and anchor the ovary through the ovarian end of the divided or undivided ovarian ligament whenever possible.

Metastatic ovarian cancer

- Oncological advice must be sought.
- Limit the procedure to the healthy ovary or abandon it in the case of bilateral disease.

COMPLICATIONS

Early complications are rare; however, late complications are not uncommon.

- Injury to the nearby structures, namely the uterus, Fallopian tube, ureter, iliac vessels, intestine and bladder. Appropriate technique should minimize this risk.
- Injury or early ischemia to the ovary. Handle the ovary carefully and avoid excessive use of electrocoagulation. Dissection at and around the main ovarian vessels must be carried out using scissors only. Care must be taken not to twist the ovarian pedicle during lateral transposition.
- Bleeding from the divided vessels is often not significant, and the problem is avoided by the appropriate use of clips and electrocautery.
- Inadequate anchoring is prevented by taking deep sutures through the fascia/muscle of the abdominal wall rather than just the peritoneum.
- Late effects are related to cyst formation in the ovary, infertility due to tubal adhesions or disconnection, and ovarian failure secondary to scattered radiation.

FURTHER READING

Bisharah M, Tulandi T. Laparoscopic preservation of ovarian function: an underused procedure. *American Journal of Obstetrics and Gynecology* 2003; **188**:367–70.

Morice P, Castaigne D, Haie-Meder C et al. Laparoscopic ovarian transposition for pelvic malignancies: indications and functional outcomes. *Fertility and Sterility* 1998; **70**:956–60.

Najmaldin AS, Aggarwal SK. Laparoscopy in tumors. In: Zacharious Z (ed.), *Laparoscopy in Infants and Children – Hospitalisation Laparoscopic Paediatric Surgery.* Heidelburg: Springer-Verlag, CD-ROM, 2004.

Tan HL, Scorpio RJ, Hutson JM et al. Laparoscopic ovariopexy for pediatric pelvic malignancies. *Pediatric Surgery International* 1993; **8**:379–81.

Thibaud E, Ramirez M, Brauner R et al. Preservation of ovarian function by ovarian transposition performed before pelvic irradiation during childhood. *Journal of Pediatrics* 1992; **121**:880–4.

Index